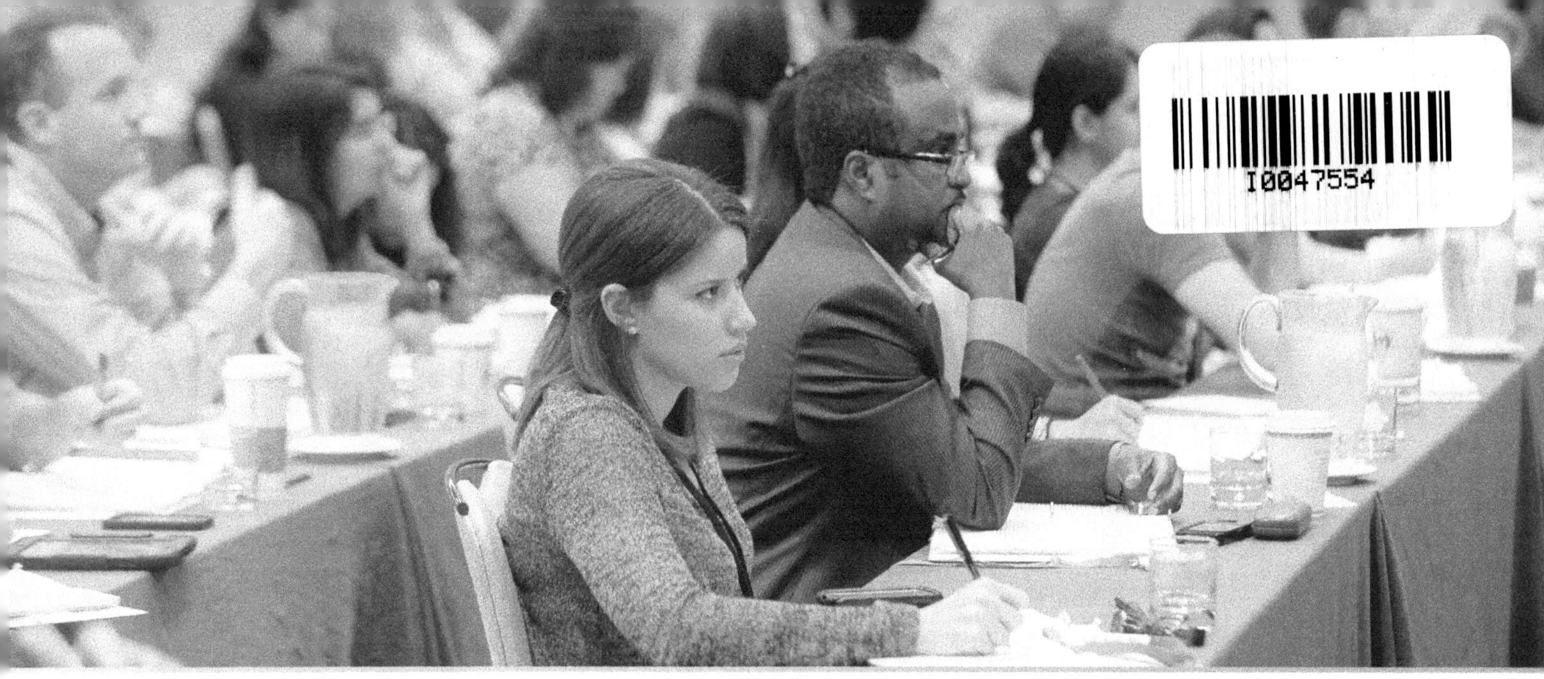

EBR CEU

ENDOCRINE BOARD REVIEW
CLINICAL ENDOCRINOLOGY UPDATE

2018 SAVE THE DATE

NEW THIS YEAR! CEU EXPANDS TO TWO CITIES—MIAMI AND ANAHEIM—MAKING IT MORE CONVENIENT FOR YOUR SCHEDULE. EBR WILL OCCUR IN MIAMI ONLY.

EBR/CEU

MIAMI, FL

ENDOCRINE BOARD REVIEW
SEPTEMBER 4-5, 2018

CLINICAL ENDOCRINOLOGY UPDATE
SEPTEMBER 6-8, 2018

CEU

ANAHEIM, CA

OCTOBER 19-21, 2018

ENDOCRINE.ORG/CEU

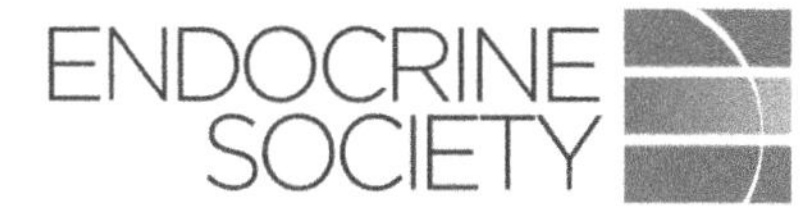

FROM THE EXPERTS IN ENDOCRINOLOGY

ENDO 2018

MEET-THE-PROFESSOR

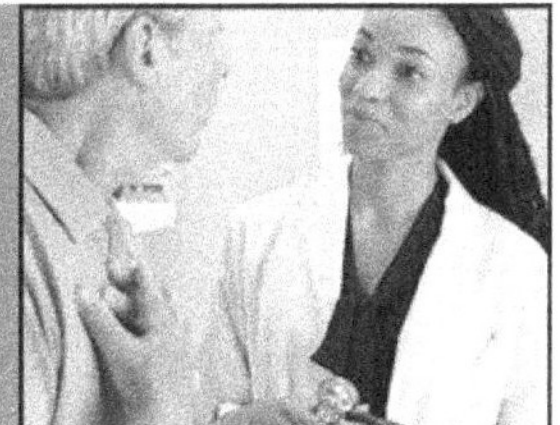

REFERENCE EDITION

ENDOCRINE

CASE MANAGEMENT

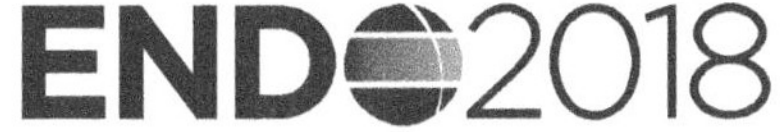

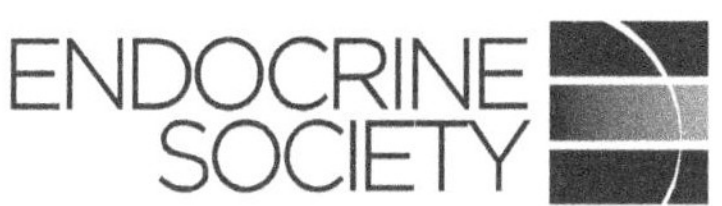

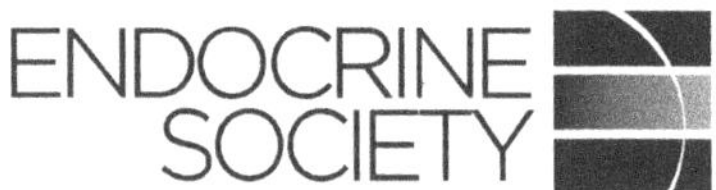

2055 L Street, NW, Suite 600
Washington, DC 20036
www.endocrine.org

Other Publications:
https://www.endocrine.org/publications

The Endocrine Society is the world's largest, oldest, and most active organization working to advance the clinical practice of endocrinology and hormone research. Founded in 1916, the Society now has more than 18,000 global members across a range of disciplines.

The Society has earned an international reputation for excellence in the quality of its peer-reviewed journals, educational resources, meetings, and programs that improve public health through the practice and science of endocrinology.

Physician-In-Practice Chair, ENDO 2018
Ann Danoff, MD

ISBN: 978-1-879225-53-4
eISBN: 978-1-879225-46-6
Library of Congress Control Number: 2019951421

On the Cover:
Large central image: © Shutterstock. Doctor attending and listening to her patient. (By Rocketclips, Inc.).
Smaller image, top left: © GlobalStock. Two doctors standing together.
Small science image, to right of smaller image: © Shutterstock. Digital illustration of DNA. (By hywards).

ENDO 2018 CONTENTS

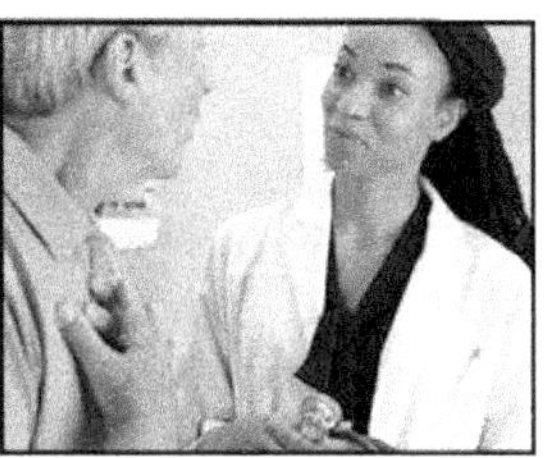

ENDO 2018 FACULTY

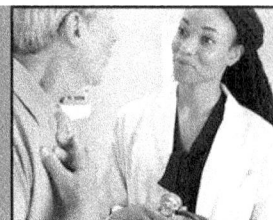

2018 MEET-THE-PROFESSOR CASE MANAGEMENT FACULTY

Robert Adler, MD
McGuire Veterans Affairs Medical Center

S Faisal Ahmed, MD, FRCPCH
Royal Hospital for Children

Bradley Anawalt, MD
University of Washington

Simon Aylwin, MA, MB, BChir, PhD, FRCP
King's College Hospital

Irina Bancos, MD
Mayo Clinic

Daniel Bichet, MD
Université de Montréal

Jeffrey Boord, MD, MPH
Parkview Health

Pierre-Marc Bouloux, BSC, MD, FRCP
Royal Free Hospital

Gregory Brent, MD
UCLA David Geffen School of Medicine

Rebecca Brown, MD
National Institutes of Health

Paul Carroll, MD
Guy's & St Thomas' NHS Foundation Trust

Frederic Castinetti, MD, PhD
La Conception Hospital

Laurie Cohen, MD
Boston Children's Hospital

Ellen Connor, MD
University of Wisconsin Hospital

Natalie Cusano, MD, MS
Lenox Hill Hospital

Ramona Dadu, MD
University of Texas MD Anderson Cancer Center

Jaime Davidson, MD
University of Texas Southwestern Medical Center

Jaydira Del Rivero, MD
National Cancer Institute/NIH

Sara DiVall, MD
University of Washington

Gerard Doherty, MD
Harvard Medical School

Henry Dufour, MD
University de la Méditerranée

Richard Dunbar, MD, MSTR
University of Pennsylvania

Richard Eastell, MD
University of Sheffield

Peter Ebeling, AO
Monash University

David Ehrmann, MD
University of Chicago

Lauren Fishbein, MD, PhD
University of Colorado School of Medicine

Peter Gaede, MD
Slaglese Hospital

Anne Goldberg, MD
Washington University School of Medicine

Steven Grinspoon, MD
Massachusetts General Hospital

Ashley Grossman, MD, FRCP
University of Oxford

Mark Gurnell, PhD, MA(Medicine), FHEA, FAcadMedicine, FRCP
University of Cambridge

Stephanie Hahner, MD
University Hospital of Wuerzburg

Gary Hammer, MD, PhD
University of Michigan

Niki Karavitaki, FRCP
University of Birmingham

Laurence Katznelson, MD
Stanford University

Susan Kirk, MD
University of Virginia

Karen Klein, MD
Children's Hospital and Health Center

Bente Langdahl, DMSc
Aarhus University Hospital

John (Jack) Leahy, MD
University of Vermont College of Medicine

Jonathan Leffert, MD
North Texas Endocrine Center

Michael Levine, MD
Children's Hospital of Philadelphia

Susan Mandel, MD, MPH
University of Pennsylvania

Kathryn Martin, MD
Massachusetts General Hospital

Barbara McGowan, MBBS, PhD
Guy's & St. Thomas's NHS Trust

John Miell, MD, DM, FRCPE, FRCP
Lewisham Healthcare

Mark Molitch, MD
Northwestern University

Lisa Neff, MD
Northwestern University

Mary Patti, MD
Joslin Diabetes Center

Anne Peters, MD
University of Southern California

Vera Popovic-Brkic, MD, PhD
University of Belgrade

Richard Quinton, MD, FRCP
Newcastle University

Jane Reusch, MD
Denver Veterans Affairs Medical Center

Scott Rivkees, MD
University of Florida

Richard Ross, MBBS, MD, FRCP
University of Sheffield

Micol Rothman, MD
University of Colorado Denver

Elizabeth Seaquist, MD
University of Minnesota

Mark Sherlock, MB, BCh, BAO, MRCPI
Tallaght Hospital

Mark Sperling, MD
Mount Sinai School of Medicine

Antoine Tabarin, MD
University de Bordeaux

Lisa Tannock, MD
University of Kentucky

Peter Trainer, MD
The Christie NHS Foundation Trust

Guillermo Umpierrez, MD, CDE, FACP, FACE
Emory University School of Medicine

Joseph Verbalis, MD
Georgetown University

W Edward Visser, MD, PhD
Erasmus Medical Center

Steven Waguespack, MD
University of Texas

John Wass, MD
Churchill Hospital

Margaret Wierman, MD
University of Colorado School of Medicine

Teresa Woodruff, PhD
Northwestern University

ENDO 2018 OVERVIEW

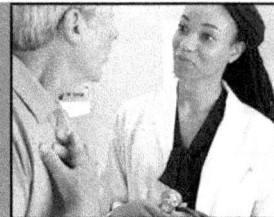

OVERVIEW

The *Meet-The-Professor Case Management* reference book is intended primarily for consultation relating to endocrinology. As a reference book, educational credits are not available. For information on educational products that include educational credit, please visit endocrine.org/store.

LEARNING OBJECTIVES

Meet-The-Professor Case Management will allow learners to assess their knowledge of all aspects of endocrinology, diabetes, and metabolism.

Upon completion of this educational activity, learners will be able to:

- Recognize clinical manifestations of endocrine and metabolic disorders and select among current options for diagnosis, management, and therapy.
- Identify risk factors for endocrine and metabolic disorders and develop strategies for prevention.
- Evaluate endocrine and metabolic manifestations of systemic disorders.
- Use existing resources pertaining to clinical guidelines and treatment recommendations for endocrine and related metabolic disorders to guide diagnosis and treatment.

TARGET AUDIENCE

Meet-The-Professor Case Management provides case-based education to clinicians interested in improving patient care.

ANNUAL MEETING STEERING COMMITTEE CLINICAL CHAIRS

John Newell-Price, MA, PhD, FRCP, ENDO 2018 Chair
University of Sheffield

Samuel Dagogo-Jack, MD, MBBS, Clinical Science Chair
University of Tennessee Health Science Center

Ann Danoff, MD, Physician-In-Practice Chair
University of Pennsylvania

ANNUAL MEETING STEERING COMMITTEE CLINICAL PEER REVIEWERS

Guillaume Assié, MD, PhD; Felix Beuschlein, MD; Lisa S. Chow, MD; Mark Cooper, BM, BCH, PhD, FRCP, FRACP; David A. D'Alessio, MD; Matthew T. Drake, MD, PhD; Maralyn Druce, MA, MBBS, FRCP, PhD, MMed, SFHEA; Robert Eckel, MD; Richard A. Feelders, MD, PhD; Larry A. Fox, MD; Megan R. Haymart, MD; Anders Juul, MD, PhD, DMSC; Lawrence S. Kirschner, MD, PhD; Peter Kopp, MD; Ana Luiza Maia, MD, PhD; Sally Radovick, MD; Stephanie B. Seminara, MD; Nalini Shah, DM; Adrian Vella, MD, FRCP; Bulent Yildiz, MD

STATEMENT OF INDEPENDENCE

The Endocrine Society has a policy of ensuring that the content and quality of this educational activity are balanced, independent, objective, and scientifically rigorous. The scientific content of this activity was developed under the supervision of the Endocrine Society's Annual Meeting Steering Committee.

DISCLOSURE POLICY

The faculty, committee members, and staff who are in position to control the content of this activity are required to disclose to the Endocrine Society and to learners any relevant financial relationship(s) of the individual or spouse/partner that have occurred within the last 12 months with any commercial interest(s) whose products or services are related to the content. Financial relationships are defined by remuneration in any amount from the commercial interest(s) in the form of grants; research support; consulting fees; salary; ownership interest (eg, stocks, stock options, or ownership interest excluding diversified mutual funds); honoraria or other payments for participation in speakers' bureaus, advisory boards, or boards of directors; or other financial benefits. The intent of this disclosure is not to prevent planners with relevant financial relationships from planning or delivering content, but rather to provide learners with information that allows them to make their own judgments of whether these financial relationships may have influenced the educational activity with regard to exposition or conclusion. The Endocrine Society has reviewed all disclosures and resolved or managed all identified conflicts of interest, as applicable.

The following faculty reported relevant financial relationship(s): The following faculty reported relevant financial relationships, as identified below:

S.F. Ahmed: is a consultant for Acerus; and receives grant support from Diurnal. **P.V. Carroll:** serves on the advisory board of Shire; receives grant support from Shire; is a research investigator for Ipsen and Novo Nordisk.; and is member of the speakers' bureau of Shire. **L.E. Cohen:** is a study site principal investigator for Versartis, Ascendis, and Opko; and received an honorarium from Scherer Clinical Communications, which received grant support from Novo Nordisk. **N.E. Cusano:** is a member of the speakers' bureau of Shire. **R. Dadu:** serves on the advisory board of Bristol-Myers Squibb. Consulting fee, Eisai. **J.A. Davidson:** serves on the advisory board of Jansen Pharmaceuticals, AstraZeneca, Intarcia, Merck & Co., Novo Nordisk, and Sanofi; is a consultant for AspireBariatrics; and is member of the speakers' bureau of AstraZeneca, Jansen Pharmaceuticals, and Novo Nordisk. **R.L. Dunbar:** serves on the advisory board of Akcea Therapeutics; received grant support from Akcea Therapeutics, AstraZeneca, Amarin, Zydus, Regeneron, and Kowa. **A.C. Goldberg:** serves on the advisory board of Esperion, Regeneron Pharmaceuticals, and Sanofi; is a consultant for OptumRX; is a research investigator for Ionis Pharmaceuticals Inc., Amgen Inc, Pfizer, Inc., Sanofi, Regeneron Pharmaceuticals, and Amarin.; and serves as editor of the

Merck Manual. **S.K. Grinspoon:** is a consultant for Theratechnologies; is a research investigator for Theratechnologies, KOWA, Gilead, and Navidea. **G.D. Hammer:** is a consultant for HRA Pharmaceuticals, Millendo Therapeutics, Orphagen, and Embara; is an owner of Millendo Therapeutics; owns stock in Millendo Therapeutics, HRA Pharmaceuticals, and Embara. **N. Karavitaki:** receives grant support from Pfizer, Inc.; and is member of the speakers' bureau of Ipsen. **L. Katznelson:** serves on the advisory board of Novartis Pharmaceuticals, Versartis, and Pfizer, Inc.; is a research investigator for Novartis Pharmaceuticals, and Versartis. **K.O. Klein:** serves on the advisory board of Abbvie; is a consultant for Abbvie; and is member of the speakers' bureau of Abbvie. **B.L. Langdahl:** serves on the advisory board of Amgen Inc, UCB Pharmaceuticals, and Eli Lilly; receives grant support from Novo Nordisk; is a research investigator for Amgen Inc and Mereo; and is a member of the speakers' bureau of Amgen Inc, Eli Lilly & Company, Teva Pharmaceutical Industries Ltd., and UCB Pharmaceuticals. **J.L. Leahy:** serves on the advisory board of Novo Nordisk, Merck & Co., Sanofi, Valeritas, Janssen Research & Development Company; and is a member of the speakers' bureau of Merck. **J.D. Leffert:** is a research investigator for Novo Nordisk, Mylan GMBH, Boehringer Ingelheim, Sanofi-Aventis, Abbvie, AstraZeneca, Bristol-Myers Squibb, and KOWA Research Institute. **K.A. Martin:** is an employee of Up To Date. **B.M. McGowan:** serves on the advisory board of Novo Nordisk; is a consultant for Novo Nordisk, Boehringer Ingelheim, and Orexigen; receives grant support from Novo Nordisk; is a research investigator for Novo Nordisk; and is member of the speakers' bureau of Novo Nordisk, Sanofi, Jansen Pharmaceuticals. **M.E. Molitch:** is a consultant for Merck, Pfizer, Inc., Novartis Pharmaceuticals, Chiasma; receives grant support from Bayer, Inc., Novartis Pharmaceuticals, Novo Nordisk, Chiasma, and Jansen Pharmaceuticals; and his spouse owns stock in Amgen Inc. **M.E. Patti:** is a consultant for Eiger; receives grant support from Jansen Pharmaceuticals, Medimmune, and Xeris Pharmaceuticals; and is a research investigator for XOMA. **A. Peters:** serves on the advisory board of Abbott Laboratories, Boehringer Ingelheim, Eli Lilly & Company, Lexicon Pharmaceuticals, Inc., Merck, Novo Nordisk, and Sanofi; is a research investigator for Mannkind Corporation; and is a member of the speakers' bureau of Eli Lilly & Company, and Dexcom. **J.E. Reusch:** receives grant support from AstraZeneca, Merck & Co.; and is member of the speakers' bureau of Sanofi-Aventis and Novo Nordisk. **R.J. Ross:** owns stock in Diurnal. **M.S. Rothman:** serves on the advisory board of Ultragenyx. **E.R. Seaquist:** is a consultant for Eli Lilly & Company, Medtronic Diabetes, Novo Nordisk, and Sanofi; serves on the advisory board of Zucara; and is consultant for 360 Marketing Services. **M.A. Sperling:** serves on the advisory board of Novo Nordisk. **A. Tabarin:** serves on the advisory board of Novartis Pharmaceuticals, HRA Pharmaceuticals, and Ipsen; is a consultant for HRA Pharmaceuticals and Novartis Pharmaceuticals; receives grant support from Novartis Pharmaceuticals, and Pfizer, Inc.; and is a research investigator for Novartis Pharmaceuticals, Ipsen; and is member of the speakers' bureau of Novartis Pharmaceuticals, Ipsen, and HRA Pharmaceuticals. **P.J. Trainer:** is a consultant for Strongbridge; serves on the advisory board of Versartis, Chiasma, Novartis Pharmaceuticals, Ipsen, ONO-Pharma, and Antisense Pharmaceuticals; and is a research investigator for Novartis Pharmaceuticals. **G.E. Umpierrez:** received grant support from Aventis Pharmaceuticals, Novo Nordisk, Merck, AstraZeneca, and Boehringer Ingelheim. **J.G. Verbalis:** serves on the advisory board of Corcept; and is a consultant for Ferring Pharmaceuticals and Otsuka. **W.F. Young:** is a consultant for Nihon Medi-Physics.

The following faculty reported no relevant financial relationships: **R. Adler; B. Anawalt; S. Aylwin; I. Bancos; J. Boord; P-M Bouloux; G. Brent; R. Brown; F. Castinetti; E. Connor; J. Del Rivero; S. DiVall; G. Doherty; H. Dufour; R. Eastell; D. Ehrmann; L. Fishbein; P. Gaede; A. Gharib; A. Grossman; M. Gurnell; S. Hahner; S. Kirk; M. Levine; S. Mandel; J. Miell; L. Neff; V. Popovic-Brkic; R. Quinton; S. Rivkees; M. Sherlock; L. Tannock; W.E. Visser; S. Waguespack; J. Wass; M. Wierman; T. Woodruff.**

The following AMSC peer reviewers reported relevant financial relationship(s): **G. Assié**: Speaker, Novartis; **F. Beuschlein:** Speaker, Ipsen, HRA Pharma; **L.S. Chow:** Grant support, Eli Lilly, Medtronics; **S. Dagogo-Jack:** Principal Investigator/Co-investigator for Clinical Trials Contracts to University of Tennessee from AstraZeneca, Novo Nordisk, Boehringer Ingelheim, Consultant, Amgen, Merck, Sanofi, AstraZeneca, Novo Nordisk, Boehringer Ingelheim, Janacare, Janssen, Perle Bioscience, Response Scientific, Inc.; Stock Owner: Dance Pharma, Janacare; **D.A. D'Alessio:** Consultant, Lilly, Merck, Janssen, Intarcia, Novo Nordisk, Grant Suport, Merck; **M. Drake:** serves on the advisory board for Amgen and Ultragenyx; **M.R. Druce:** Advisory Board, Ipsen; **R. Eckel:** Consultant, Sanofi Aventis, Regeneron Pharmaceuticals, Novo Nordisk - Scientific Advisor; **R.A. Feelders:** Grant support, Novartis, Ipsen; **Juul, Anders:** Speaker, Novo Nordisk, Pfizer, Ferring, Merck, Bayer; Clinical Trial; **J.D.C. Newell-Price:** The Pituitary Foundation (Patient support charity) Trustee; Advisory Board Member, Novartis, Ipson, HRA Pharma; Partridge, Nicola C: Consultant and Research Contract, Orthofix, Inc.; **S. Radovick:** Consultant, CVS Caremark; Support, NESGAS, PORIYA; **L.S. Kirschner:** Advisory Board, Corcept Therapeutic; **A.V. Vella:** Principal Investigator, Novo Nordisk, Obesity Society, XOMA, Member of Advisory Board, VTV Therapeutics.

The following AMSC peer reviewers reported no relevant financial relationships: **M.S. Cooper; A. Danoff; L.A. Fox; M.R. Haymart; P. Kopp; S.B. Seminara; N.S. Shah; B.O. Yildiz.**

The medical editor for this program reported no relevant financial relationships.

The Endocrine Society staff associated with the development of content for this activity reported no relevant financial relationships.

DISCLAIMERS

The information presented in this activity represents the opinion of the faculty and is not necessarily the official position of the Endocrine Society.

USE OF PROFESSIONAL JUDGMENT:

The educational content in this enduring activity relates to basic principles of diagnosis and therapy and does not substitute for individual patient assessment based on the health care provider's examination of the patient and consideration of laboratory data and other factors unique to the patient. Standards in medicine change as new data become available.

DRUGS AND DOSAGES:

When prescribing medications, the physician is advised to check the product information sheet accompanying each drug to verify conditions of use and to identify any changes in drug dosage schedule or contraindications.

POLICY ON UNLABELED/OFF-LABEL USE

The Endocrine Society has determined that disclosure of unlabeled/off-label or investigational use of commercial product(s) is informative for audiences and therefore requires this information to be disclosed to the learners at the beginning of the presentation. Uses of specific therapeutic agents, devices, and other products discussed in this educational activity may not be the same as those indicated in product labeling approved by the Food and Drug Administration (FDA). The Endocrine Society requires that any discussions of such "off-label" use be based on scientific research that conforms to generally accepted standards of experimental design, data collection, and data analysis. Before recommending or prescribing any therapeutic agent or device, learners should review the complete prescribing information, including indications, contraindications, warnings, precautions, and adverse events.

ACKNOWLEDGMENT OF COMMERCIAL SUPPORT

This activity is not supported by educational grant(s) or other funds from any commercial supporter.

PUBLICATION DATE: February 2018

ENDO 2018 TOPIC INDEX

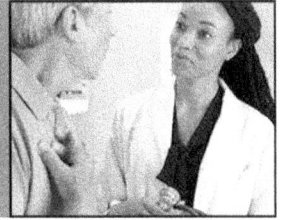

ADIPOSE TISSUE, APPETITE, AND OBESITY

ADRENAL

BONE AND MINERAL METABOLISM

CARDIOVASCULAR ENDOCRINOLOGY

DIABETES MELLITUS AND GLUCOSE METABOLISM

ENDOCRINE DISRUPTION

NEUROENDOCRINOLOGY AND PITUITARY

PEDIATRIC ENDOCRINOLOGY

REPRODUCTIVE ENDOCRINOLOGY

THYROID

MISCELLANEOUS

ENDO 2018 SPEAKER HANDOUT INDEX

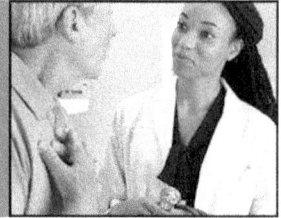

n/a = Handout not available

ADIPOSE TISSUE, APPETITE, AND OBESITY

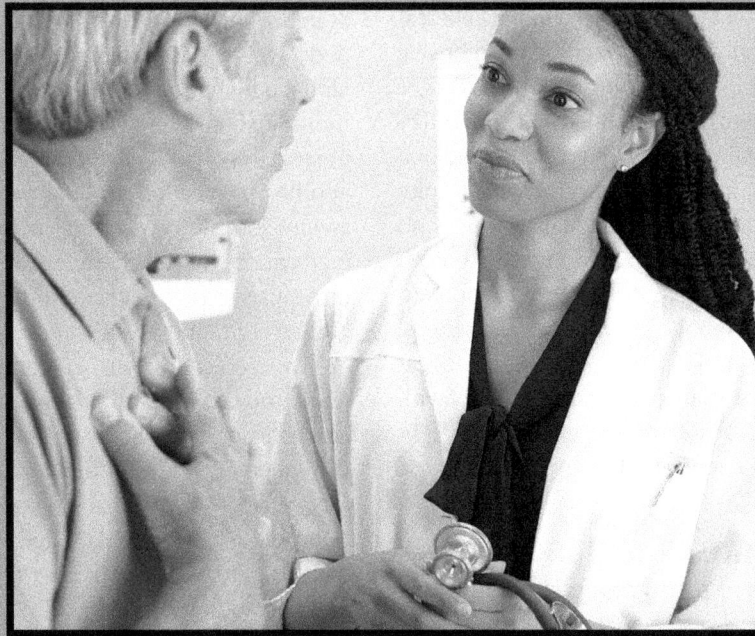

Obesity Management: Effective Use of Pharmacotherapy and Bariatric Surgery

M09
Presented, March 17–20, 2018

Lisa M. Neff, MD. Division of Endocrinology, Metabolism and Molecular Medicine, Northwestern University Feinberg School of Medicine, Chicago, Illinois 60611, E-mail: l-neff@northwestern.edu

SIGNIFICANCE OF THE CLINICAL PROBLEM

One third of American adults are obese. Obesity affects all organ systems and increases the incidence of diabetes, cardiovascular disease, cancer, fatty liver disease, and other comorbidities. Lifestyle modification is the cornerstone of obesity management; weight loss in the range of 2% to 10% can produce clinically important improvements in comorbidities, with greater weight loss producing more improvements (1). In the Look AHEAD (Action for Health in Diabetes) trial, almost one quarter of individuals engaged in an intensive lifestyle intervention were able to maintain a weight loss of 5% to 10% at 8 years, and one quarter maintained a loss of ≥10% (2). However, one quarter maintained a loss of <5%, and one quarter were unable to maintain any weight loss despite substantial support and education. Individuals who try to maintain a reduced body weight face numerous extrinsic and intrinsic challenges, including an obesogenic environment and a variety of adaptive metabolic and hormonal changes, similar to those seen in starvation, that occur with modest weight loss (3-6). Given these challenges, many patients with obesity would benefit from the use of effective tools for weight management, such as medications and bariatric surgery.

BARRIERS TO OPTIMAL PRACTICE

Barriers to the optimal care of patients with obesity include patient, physician, and medical system factors. Patient factors include frustration, embarrassment, fear of failure, fear of potential treatment risks, lack of family or community support, lack of time to devote to self-care, and lack of motivation. Physician factors include lack of time to provide counseling, fear of offending the patient, lack of knowledge about treatment options, skepticism about potential efficacy or benefits of treatment, and weight bias. Medical system factors include a lack of coverage for physician counseling about obesity, dietitian referrals, obesity medications, and bariatric surgery.

LEARNING OBJECTIVES

As a result of participating in this session, learners should be able to:

- Explain the benefits and potential risks of pharmacotherapy for obesity
- Discuss the benefits and potential risks of bariatric surgery
- Identify patients who may benefit from treatment with medications or surgery for obesity
- Recognize common barriers to the effective use of tools for weight management (medications or surgery)

STRATEGIES FOR OBESITY MANAGEMENT

According to expert guidelines, pharmacotherapy should be considered for patients who have a body mass index (BMI) ≥ 30 kg/m^2, if adequate weight loss has not been achieved with lifestyle (7-9). Pharmacotherapy also can be considered for individuals with a BMI ≥ 27 kg/m^2 when weight-related comorbidities are present.

Goals of pharmacological treatment include the loss of ≥5% of initial body weight and long-term maintenance at a reduced body weight. Treatment guidelines suggest that if an individual patient does not lose ≥5% after 3 months of treatment, therapy should be discontinued. However, patients who are unresponsive to 1 pharmacological agent may respond to another medication. Once a patient has achieved successful weight loss (≥5% of initial body weight) with the help of a medication, most patients will benefit from continued (long-term) use of that medication to help to maintain their lower body weight and avoid weight regain.

Five medications are currently approved by the US Food and Drug Administration for long-term use in obesity management: orlistat (Xenical; Genentech, South San Francisco, CA), phentermine/topiramate (Qsymia; Vivus, Campbell, CA), lorcaserin (Belviq; Eisai, Woodcliff Lake, NJ), naltrexone/bupropion (Contrave; Orexigen Therapeutics, La Jolla, CA), and liraglutide (Saxenda; Novo Nordisk, Plainsboro, NJ). In addition, other medications, such as the sympathomimetic phentermine, are approved for short-term use (3 months). However, as indicated, a long-term approach to obesity management is essential, and long-term off-label use of phentermine is common in clinical practice. Obesity medications have a variety of different mechanisms, leading to reduced hunger, increased fullness, reduced cravings or drive to eat, or a combination of these effects. An overview of medications is shown in Table 1. Recent practice guidelines and reviews offer a more detailed discussion of pharmacological therapies for obesity (8, 10).

Insurance coverage of weight loss medications varies widely but has been increasing in recent years. When coverage is available, prior authorization often is required to ensure that patients meet predetermined plan eligibility

Table 1. Medications for Obesity

Medication	Mechanism of Action	Dosage/Administration	Contraindications	Adverse Effects
Orlistat	Lipase inhibitor	120 mg three times a day with meals	Pregnancy, chronic malabsorption syndromes, cholestasis, warfarin use	Oily stools, flatus with discharge, fecal urgency, fat-soluble vitamin deficiencies
Phentermine/ topiramate	Sympathomimetic/ γ-aminobutyric acid receptor modulator	3.75/23 mg every morning for 14 d, then 7.5/46 mg every morning If weight loss inadequate (<5% at 12 wk), may increase to 11.25/69 mg every morning for 14 days then 15/92 mg every morning	Pregnancy, CAD, uncontrolled HTN, glaucoma, hyperthyroidism, anxiety disorder, seizures, MAOI use	Dry mouth, constipation, paresthesia, memory impairment, dizziness, dysgeusia, mood changes
Lorcaserin	5-HT_{2C} receptor agonist	10-mg tablet twice a day or 20-mg ER tablet once daily	Pregnancy; caution if bradycardia; CHF; valvular disease; concomitant triptan, SSRI, SNRI, or MAOI use	Headache, dizziness, dry mouth, constipation, fatigue, mood changes, memory impairment
Naltrexone/ bupropion	Opioid receptor antagonist/ norepinephrine and dopamine reuptake inhibitor	8-mg/90-mg ER tablet taken as follows: one tablet in the morning for 1 wk, then one tablet twice a day for 1 wk, then two tablets in the morning and one tablet every evening for 1 wk, then two tablets twice a day	Pregnancy, history or risk of seizures, uncontrolled HTN, glaucoma, opioid use, MAOI use, anorexia or bulimia	Nausea, constipation, headache, dizziness, insomnia, dry mouth, diarrhea, increased heart rate or BP, mood changes
Liraglutide	Glucagon-like peptide 1 analog	0.6 mg subcutaneously once daily for 1 wk, then 1.2 mg once daily for 1 wk, then 1.8 mg once daily for 1 week, then 2.4 mg once daily for 1 wk, then 3 mg once daily	Pregnancy, medullary thyroid cancer, MEN2, caution if history of pancreatitis	Nausea, vomiting, diarrhea, constipation, reflux, fatigue
Phentermine	Sympathomimetic	Multiple doses/formulations available: 8-mg tablets: one tablet three times a day before meals 15-, 30-, or 37.5-mg capsules: one capsule every morning 37.5-mg tablets: one tablet every morning or 1/2 tablet twice a day	Pregnancy, CAD, uncontrolled HTN, glaucoma, hyperthyroidism, anxiety disorder, seizures, MAOI use	Dry mouth, constipation, insomnia, irritability, increased heart rate or BP, headache

Abbreviations: BP, blood pressure; CAD, coronary artery disease; CHF, congestive heart failure; ER, extended release; HTN, hypertension; MEN2, multiple endocrine neoplasia type 2; MAOI, monamine oxidase inhibitor; SNRI, serotonin-norepinephrine reuptake inhibitor; SSRI, selective serotonin reuptake inhibitor.

criteria (*e.g.*, a diagnosis of obesity, previous ineffective trial of lifestyle modification, planned use of lifestyle modification along with medication). When insurance coverage is not available, some patients may consider paying out of pocket with the help of a savings program from the manufacturer.

Current bariatric surgical procedures include laparoscopic-adjustable gastric banding, sleeve gastrectomy (SG), Roux-en-Y gastric bypass (RYGB), and biliopancreatic diversion with duodenal switch (BPD-DS). Bariatric surgery produces large and durable weight loss, reduces morbidity and mortality, lowers medication usage, and improves health-related quality of life

(11, 12). Therefore, bariatric surgery should be considered for patients with a BMI ≥40 or ≥35 kg/m^2 when considerable weight-related comorbidities are present (13). Weight loss after bariatric surgery may vary depending on the patient and the procedure, but losses of 20% to 35% of initial body weight are typical. Expert recommendations regarding patient selection, types of procedures, and pre- and postoperative care are presented in two recent practice guidelines (13, 14).

Bariatric procedures have three main mechanisms of action. First, in all procedures, gastric capacity is restricted, leading to enhanced fullness. Second, in SG, RYGB, and BPD-DS, there is a modulation of gastrointestinal hunger and satiety hormones, including ghrelin, glucagon-like peptide 1, and peptide YY. Finally, in BPD-DS and long-limb RYGB (but not RYGB with a standard limb length), induction of macronutrient malabsorption contributes to the greater weight loss seen with these procedures. However, this also increases the risk of nutritional deficiencies. In addition to the three main mechanisms of action, other potential mechanisms, such as alterations in the gut microbiome, have been suggested and may play a role in the metabolic improvements seen after bariatric surgery.

Numerous barriers to weight management exist at the patient, physician, and health system level. Patient factors, such as frustration, embarrassment, fear of failure, fear of potential treatment risks, and lack of motivation may be overcome by using neutral, bias-free language with patients (*e.g.*, talking about weight instead of obesity), creating a collaborative relationship focused on the patient's goals, and using motivational interviewing to help guide behavior change. Physicians can also reduce the feeling of shame or failure that patients may feel by educating them about the many factors that influence weight, including the hormonal and metabolic changes that occur with weight loss, such as decreased energy expenditure, decreased leptin, and increased ghrelin. Importantly, patients who understand these factors may be more open to a discussion about pharmacotherapy or bariatric surgery as a tool to augment their efforts with lifestyle modification.

MAIN CONCLUSIONS

Pharmacotherapy and bariatric surgery are effective and safe weight management tools that should be offered to appropriate patients with obesity. Patient education and a respectful patient-physician relationship can overcome the barriers that influence patients' acceptance of these important tools.

CASES

Case 1

Ms. K. is a 38-year-old woman with concern about weight gain. She has not seen a physician for several years because of embarrassment about her weight. She reports fatigue of several years duration and is concerned about the possibility of hypothyroidism.

She has a history of weight cycling (Fig. 1) and is currently at her highest weight. Factors that have contributed to weight gain are stress eating, consuming food items left over by her young child, lack of time for meal planning, a sedentary lifestyle, and a 40-lb weight gain during pregnancy with retention of much of the gained weight. In the past, Ms. K. has had some weight loss success (5 to 15 lb per attempt) with commercial diet programs, tracking food intake, and increasing physical activity.

A typical day's intake includes one or two eggs, one or two slices of toast with butter, and black coffee 3 days a week for breakfast at 7:00 AM. She skips breakfast 4 days a week. A typical lunch is consumed at noon and consists of a southwest chicken salad or turkey sandwich and soup (from chain restaurant). Around 5:30 PM she often engages in unplanned eating of her child's dinner leftovers, such as chicken nuggets or macaroni and cheese, because she's very hungry. A typical dinner is consumed at 8 PM with her husband and might consist of a baked chicken breast, sautéed or steamed vegetables, and small potato. Around 10:00 PM, she often has two to three cookies for a snack, noting that she is not hungry but craves sweets while relaxing after a stressful day. Her physical activity includes walking the family dog twice a day for 5 minutes. In the past, she enjoyed aerobics classes and yoga, but finding time for structured exercise is difficult now that she has a child.

Ms. K. has no known medical history. Her family history includes type 2 diabetes in her mother and hypertension in her father. Review of systems is negative other than mild fatigue. Her current medications include an intrauterine device and an occasional multivitamin. Physical examination is unremarkable except for generalized obesity (height, 5 ft, 7 in; weight 220 lb; BMI, 34.5 kg/m^2) and prehypertension [blood pressure (BP), 136/86 mm Hg]. She has no thyromegaly or Cushingoid features.

Laboratory testing done after the visit reveals the presence of prediabetes and low high-density lipoprotein. Her results show a fasting glucose of 108 mg/dL; hemoglobin A_{1c}, 6.2%; low-density lipoprotein, 99 mg/dL; high-density lipoprotein, 40 mg/dL; triglycerides, 134 mg/dL; and thyrotropin,

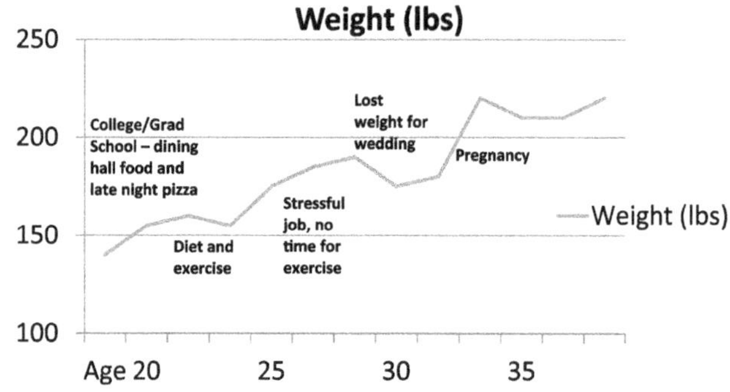

Figure 1. Ms. K.'s weight graph.

2.34 μIU/mL. Renal function, liver function, and electrolyte test results were normal.

You use motivational interviewing techniques to help Ms. K. to identify lifestyle modification goals (plan a healthy afternoon snack, begin tracking food intake, increase walking to 10 minutes twice a day). You also refer her to a dietitian for additional dietary guidance and support. She is interested in pharmacotherapy for weight management.

Question

Which medication options would you consider for this patient and why? In this young, relatively healthy woman, any of the medications approved by the Food and Drug Administration for long-term use could be considered, but specific clues in her history may suggest the following options:

- Extended-release phentermine/topiramate is an attractive option because of its dual mechanisms of action, convenient once-daily administration, and robust average weight loss of ~6% to 9%. Many patients describe having less hunger as well as a reduction in cravings and thoughts about food (likely a result of γ-aminobutyric acid receptor modulation). The appetite suppressant action would help the patient to reduce portions at lunch and dinner and avoid nibbling on her child's leftovers. With fewer cravings, she may also be able to reduce her evening sweets eating. In young women of child-bearing age, the use of topiramate can be a concern because of an increased risk of birth defects. However, this patient has an intrauterine device and has no interest in expanding her family. Although she has prehypertension, this is not a contraindication. Monitoring of BP should occur regularly because increases can occur. However, a reduction in BP with weight loss is more likely than an increase.
- Because the patient has prediabetes, liraglutide also is an excellent choice, as it would provide her with independent benefits for satiety and blood sugar control. Cost and insurance coverage can limit access for some patients.
- Naltrexone/bupropion could also be considered given the patient's history of stress eating and cravings. This choice might be less effective for this patient than extended release phentermine/topiramate because it acts on satiety rather than on hunger. However, it could be a reasonable option, particularly if the patient does not tolerate or respond to phentermine/topiramate.

Case 2

Mr. R. is a 62-year-old man with sleep apnea, hypertension, and type 2 diabetes. He reports gradual weight gain over the years, particularly after he was started on medication for diabetes and hypertension (Fig. 2). He had a successful weight loss of just >20 lb ~15 years ago through diet and exercise. He kept the weight off for a few years. He also lost 5 lb after starting liraglutide for diabetes but has regained the weight as a result of a more hectic work schedule and financial stressors. He has been working with a dietitian for several years and has a generally healthy diet but admits that he has trouble with portion control. He denies eating to the point of discomfort or feeling a loss of control over eating. His physical activity consists of walking with his wife for 30 minutes 3 to 4 days a week.

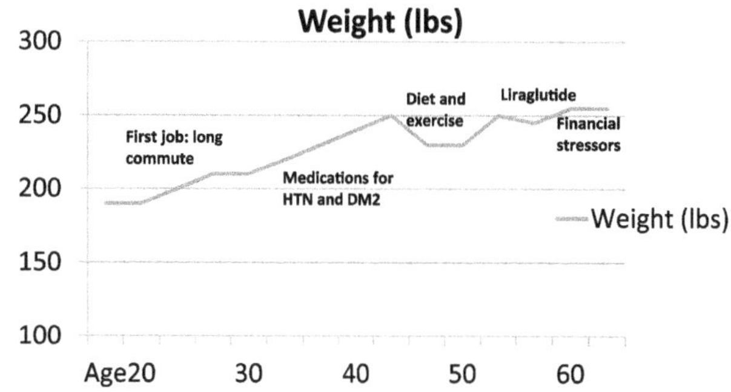

Figure 2. Mr. R.'s weight graph.

His medical history includes sleep apnea, hypertension, and type 2 diabetes. He has no surgical history. His medications include lisinopril 20 mg daily, metoprolol 100 twice a day, atorvastatin 40 mg, metformin 1000 mg twice a day, glipizide 10 mg daily, and liraglutide 1.8 mg every day. He uses continuous positive airway pressure most nights and feels rested. His review of systems is positive for heartburn 3 days a week after dinner. He takes over-the-counter antacids (calcium carbonate).

Mr. R.'s physical examination is remarkable only for obesity (weight, 255 lb; height 5 ft, 10 in; BMI, 36.6 kg/m^2), a few scattered skin tags at the neck, and mild acanthosis. His BP is 128/84 mm Hg. His laboratory test results reveal a hemoglobin A_{1c} of 7.1% and normal kidney and liver function panels. Foot examination is normal. Cholesterol panel (on statin) was ordered by his primary physician 6 months prior and was unremarkable.

Question 1

What treatment option should be recommended for this patient, and why? Given his comorbidities, bariatric surgery should be recommended. Mr. R. should be counseled that bariatric surgery is the treatment most likely to provide him with considerable and sustained weight loss as well as improvement and possibly resolution of his sleep apnea, hypertension, diabetes, and reflux. He should be counseled that studies indicate that bariatric surgery is likely to reduce his risk of cardiovascular disease and death and improve his quality of life.

RYGB is the treatment of choice for this patient. His history of reflux makes SG a less-attractive option because reflux can be exacerbated by this procedure. In contrast, reflux typically resolves after RYGB. Diabetes remission rates are also higher with RYGB than with SG.

Question 2

If the patient is not willing to consider bariatric surgery at this time, which medication options could be recommended? Several options could be considered, including lorcaserin, switching from liraglutide 1.8 mg/d to liraglutide 3.0 mg/d, bupropion/naltrexone with monitoring of BP, addition of a sodium/glucose cotransporter 2 inhibitor, or orlistat.

Given the patient's report of difficulty with portion control, lorcaserin, higher-dose liraglutide, and bupropion/naltrexone may be most helpful because they increase satiety. Sodium/glucose cotransporter 2 inhibitors do not increase satiety but could have beneficial effects on blood sugar, BP, cardiovascular risk, and weight. Orlistat similarly does not affect satiety but could be considered for a small weight benefit. Phentermine/topiramate could also be considered if other options are not viable or effective, but cardiac evaluation should be undertaken before starting phentermine given the patient's many risk factors for cardiovascular disease.

REFERENCES

1. National Heart, Lung, and Blood Institute. Managing overweight and obesity in adults: systematic evidence review from the Obesity Expert Panel, 2013. Available at: https://www.nhlbi.nih.gov/health-topics/managing-overweight-obesity-in-adults. Accessed 18 December, 2017.
2. Look AHEAD Research Group. Eight-year weight losses with an intensive lifestyle intervention: the Look AHEAD study. *Obesity (Silver Spring)*. 2014;**22**(1):5-13.
3. Goldsmith R, Joanisse DR, Gallagher D, Pavlovich K, Shamoon E, Leibel RL, Rosenbaum M. Effects of experimental weight perturbation on skeletal muscle work efficiency, fuel utilization, and biochemistry in human subjects. *Am J Physiol Regul Integr Comp Physiol*. 2010; **298**(1):R79-R88.
4. Rosenbaum M, Hirsch J, Gallagher DA, Leibel RL. Long-term persistence of adaptive thermogenesis in subjects who have maintained a reduced body weight. *Am J Clin Nutr*. 2008;**88**(4):906-912.
5. Rosenbaum M, Sy M, Pavlovich K, Leibel RL, Hirsch J. Leptin reverses weight loss-induced changes in regional neural activity responses to visual food stimuli. *J Clin Invest*. 2008;**118**(7):2583-2591.
6. Rosenbaum M, Goldsmith R, Bloomfield D, Magnano A, Weimer L, Heymsfield S, Gallagher D, Mayer L, Murphy E, Leibel RL. Low-dose leptin reverses skeletal muscle, autonomic, and neuroendocrine adaptations to maintenance of reduced weight. *J Clin Invest*. 2005; **115**(12):3579-3586.
7. National Heart, Lung, and Blood Institute. Clinical Guidelines on the Identification, Evaluation, And Treatment of Overweight and Obesity in Adults: The Evidence Report. Bethesda, MD: National Heart, Lung, and Blood Institute; 1998. NIH publication no. 98-4083.
8. Apovian CM, Aronne LJ, Bessesen DH, McDonnell ME, Murad MH, Pagotto U, Ryan DH, Still CD; Endocrine Society. Pharmacological management of obesity: an Endocrine Society clinical practice guideline. *J Clin Endocrinol Metab*. 2015;**100**(2):342-362.
9. Jensen MD, Ryan DH, Apovian CM, Ard JD, Comuzzie AG, Donato KA, Hu FB, Hubbard VS, Jakicic JM, Kushner RF, Loria CM, Millen BE, Nonas CA, Pi-Sunyer FX, Stevens J, Stevens VJ, Wadden TA, Wolfe BM, Yanovski SZ, Jordan HS, Kendall KA, Lux LJ, Mentor-Marcel R, Morgan LC, Trisolini MG, Wnek J, Anderson JL, Halperin JL, Albert NM, Bozkurt B, Brindis RG, Curtis LH, DeMets D, Hochman JS, Kovacs RJ, Ohman EM, Pressler SJ, Sellke FW, Shen WK, Smith SC Jr, Tomaselli GF; American College of Cardiology/American Heart Association Task Force on Practice Guidelines; Obesity Society. 2013 AHA/ACC/TOS guideline for the management of overweight and obesity in adults: a report of the American College of Cardiology/American Heart Association Task Force on Practice Guidelines and The Obesity Society. *Circulation*. 2014;**129**(25):S102-S138.
10. Saunders KH, Shukla AP, Igel LI, Kumar RB, Aronne LJ. Pharmacotherapy for obesity. *Endocrinol Metab Clin North Am*. 2016;**45**(3): 521-538.
11. Sjöström L. Review of the key results from the Swedish Obese Subjects (SOS) trial - a prospective controlled intervention study of bariatric surgery. *J Intern Med*. 2013;**273**(3):219-234.
12. Schauer PR, Bhatt DL, Kirwan JP, Wolski K, Aminian A, Brethauer SA, Navaneethan SD, Singh RP, Pothier CE, Nissen SE, Kashyap SR; STAMPEDE Investigators. Bariatric surgery versus intensive medical therapy for diabetes—5-year outcomes. *N Engl J Med*. 2017;**376**(7): 641-651.
13. Mechanick JI, Kushner RF, Sugerman HJ, Gonzalez-Campoy JM, Collazo-Clavell ML, Guven S, Spitz AF, Apovian CM, Livingston EH, Brolin R, Sarwer DB, Anderson WA, Dixon J. American Association of Clinical Endocrinologists, The Obesity Society, and American Society for Metabolic & Bariatric Surgery Medical guidelines for clinical practice for the perioperative nutritional, metabolic, and nonsurgical support of the bariatric surgery patient. *Endocr Pract*. 2008;**14**(Suppl 1):1-83.
14. Mechanick JI, Youdim A, Jones DB, Garvey WT, Hurley DL, McMahon MM, Heinberg LJ, Kushner R, Adams TD, Shikora S, Dixon JB, Brethauer S; American Association of Clinical Endocrinologists; Obesity Society; American Society for Metabolic & Bariatric Surgery. Clinical practice guidelines for the perioperative nutritional, metabolic, and nonsurgical support of the bariatric surgery patient—2013 update: cosponsored by American Association of Clinical Endocrinologists, The Obesity Society, and American Society for Metabolic & Bariatric Surgery. *Obesity (Silver Spring)*. 2013;**21**(Suppl 1)S1-S27.

Lipodystrophy

M17
Presented, March 17–20, 2018

Rebecca J. Brown, MHSc. Diabetes, Endocrinology, and Obesity Branch, National Institute of Diabetes and Digestive and Kidney Diseases, National Institutes of Health, Bethesda, Maryland 20892, E-mail: brownrebecca@mail.nih.gov

SIGNIFICANCE OF THE CLINICAL PROBLEM

Lipodystrophy syndromes are rare, heterogeneous disorders that have in common either generalized or regional deficiency in body fat. Deficient body fat leads to low levels of the adipocyte derived hormone leptin, causing hyperphagia and ectopic lipid deposition in the liver and muscle. This frequently leads to severe metabolic disease that is refractory to conventional medications, including insulin resistance and diabetes, hypertriglyceridemia and acute pancreatitis, nonalcoholic fatty liver disease (NAFLD), and polycystic ovarian syndrome (PCOS). Many patients have early mortality related to cirrhosis, pancreatitis, complications of diabetes, or cardiovascular disease.

Most health care providers are not familiar with lipodystrophy, and thus, many patients remain undiagnosed, especially males and those with partial lipodystrophy, which may be mistaken for obesity or Cushing's syndrome. Moreover, few practitioners are comfortable managing patients who may require high doses of insulin. Accurate diagnosis is important to provide optimal disease management, appropriate screening for medical complications of lipodystrophy, and genetic counseling if relevant.

BARRIERS TO OPTIMAL PRACTICE

- Lipodystrophy syndromes are rare, heterogeneous, and challenging to diagnose.
- Patients with lipodystrophy often have severe metabolic disease that is poorly responsive to conventional medical therapy.

LEARNING OBJECTIVES

As a result of participating in this session, learners should be able to:

- Recognize physical examination and metabolic features of generalized and partial lipodystrophy
- Perform appropriate screening for comorbidities in patients with lipodystrophy
- Develop a treatment plan for metabolic complications of lipodystrophy

STRATEGIES FOR DIAGNOSIS, THERAPY, AND MANAGEMENT

Diagnosis of Lipodystrophy

Classification (Table 1)

Lipodystrophy syndromes are broadly categorized based on their etiology (genetic or acquired) and the distribution of missing adipose tissue, which may involve the entire body (generalized lipodystrophy) or only certain adipose tissue depots, typically the limbs and buttocks (partial lipodystrophy). Progeroid and autoinflammatory disorders are complex, multisystem diseases associated with variable degrees of lipodystrophy.

Clinical Presentation

A lipodystrophy syndrome should be suspected in a patient with regional or generalized absence of adipose tissue, particularly in the presence of concomitant metabolic disease that is typically associated with excess adiposity. It is critical to distinguish the absence of fat in a patient with lipodystrophy from both the variable distribution of body fat (*e.g.*, apple or pear body types) in the general population and the healthy low body fat without metabolic disease seen in lean, athletic individuals. There is no diagnostic test for all forms of lipodystrophy, although genetic testing may be confirmatory in genetic cases. Leptin levels are low (1.1 ± 0.7 ng/mL; range, 0.25 to 5.3 ng/mL) in patients with generalized lipodystrophy (2) but are quite variable in patients with partial lipodystrophy (6.2 ± 3.4 ng/mL; range, 0.6 to > 15 ng/mL), and there is no leptin level that is diagnostic for lipodystrophy.

Patients may present to a variety of providers at many stages of life. Common presentations are listed in Table 2 and include:

- Muscular appearance or failure to thrive in infancy
- Insulin-resistant diabetes or acanthosis in a lean child, adolescent, or young adult
- Nonalcoholic fatty liver disease (increased abdominal girth, hepatomegaly, elevated transaminases) in a lean child, adolescent, or young adult
- PCOS features in lean adolescent/young adult women
- Severe hypertriglyceridemia or its complications at any age (acute pancreatitis, xanthomata)
- Metabolic disease out of proportion to adiposity in patients with partial lipodystrophy

Screening for Comorbidities of Lipodystrophy

As reported by Brown *et al.* (1), patients with lipodystrophy are at high risk for metabolic complications, including diabetes/insulin resistance, dyslipidemia (high triglycerides with low high-density lipoprotein [HDL] cholesterol), NAFLD, reproductive dysfunction (PCOS), and cardiovascular disease

Table 1. Major Subtypes of Lipodystrophy

Subtype	Inheritance Pattern	Lipodystrophy Phenotype	Genes Involved
Congenital generalized lipodystrophy	Autosomal recessive	Near total absence of body fat Generalized muscularity Metabolic complications	*AGPAT2, BSCL2, CAV1, PTRF, PCYT1A*
Progeroid syndromes	Autosomal recessive, autosomal dominant, *de novo*	Partial or generalized absence of body fat Progeroid features Variable metabolic complications	*LMNA, FBN1, CAV1, POLD1, KCNJ6, PIK3R1, ZMPSTE24, SPRTN, WRN, BANF1*
Familial partial lipodystrophy	Autosomal dominant, rarely autosomal recessive	Absence of fat in limbs Metabolic complications	*LMNA, PPARG, AKT2, PLIN1, CIDEC, LIPE, PCYT1A*
Autoinflammatory diseases	Autosomal recessive	Variable absence of fat Variable metabolic complications	*PSMB8*
Acquired generalized lipodystrophy	NA	Near total absence of body fat Metabolic complications	None
Acquired partial lipodystrophy	NA	Absent fat in upper body; increased fat in lower body Mild or no metabolic complications	None

Adapted from Brown *et al.* (1).
Abbreviation: NA, not applicable.

(cardiomyopathy, rhythm disturbance, coronary artery disease). All patients with generalized and partial lipodystrophy should undergo screening for these conditions at diagnosis. Ongoing screening should be conducted as follows, except in patients with acquired partial lipodystrophy, in whom metabolic disease is infrequent.

- Diabetes screening should be conducted annually.
- Triglycerides should be measured at least annually or if signs or symptoms of severe hypertriglyceridemia (xanthomata or pancreatitis) occur. Complete fasting lipid panel should be performed annually after age 10 years.
- NAFLD should be evaluated annually with alanine aminotransferase (ALT)/aspartate aminotransferase (AST). Liver ultrasound should be performed at diagnosis and subsequently as clinically indicated. Liver biopsy should not be performed routinely but may be clinically indicated in many patients, especially those with *BSCL2* mutations, who are at high risk for cirrhosis in childhood, and those with acquired generalized lipodystrophy, who may develop autoimmune hepatitis in addition to steatohepatitis.
- Oligomenorrhea/amenorrhea, hyperandrogenism, and subfertility are common. Evaluation for PCOS (sex steroids, gonadotropins, pelvic ultrasound) should be performed as clinically indicated. Pubertal disorders are common, and children should undergo annual pubertal staging.
- Screening for cardiovascular complications of lipodystrophy should include at least annual blood pressure monitoring and electrocardiogram and echocardiography annually (in congenital generalized lipodystrophy and progeroid disorders) or as clinically indicated (in familial partial lipodystrophy and acquired generalized lipodystrophy). Evaluation for cardiac ischemia and rhythm disorders should be considered in patients with progeroid disorders and certain *LMNA* mutations associated with cardiomyopathy.
- Proteinuric nephropathy is common in lipodystrophy, including diabetic nephropathy, focal segmental glomerosclerosis, and membranoproliferative glomerulonephritis. Urine protein excretion should be measured annually, and kidney biopsy should be performed as clinically appropriate.

Treatment of Lipodystrophy

As reported by Brown *et al.* (1), there is no cure for lipodystrophy and no way to regrow missing adipose tissue. Thus, the treatment of lipodystrophy is targeted toward its complications.

Diet and Exercise

Lifestyle modification, especially diet, is essential in all patients with lipodystrophy. Most patients should follow a diet with balanced macronutrients (50% to 60% carbohydrates, 20% to 30% fats, ~20% protein); low-fat diets are appropriate in the context of acute pancreatitis. Avoid the temptation to overfeed infants with generalized lipodystrophy in cases of failure to thrive. Because these infants lack body fat, it is normal to have a low weight for length. If normal linear growth is maintained, supplemental feeding in children should be avoided, because it may worsen metabolic disease. Caloric restriction will help control metabolic disease, but it can be

Table 2. Clinical Features That Increase the Suspicion of Lipodystrophy

Features
Essential feature
Generalized or regional absence of body fat
Physical features
Failure to thrive (infants and children)
Prominent muscles
Prominent veins (phlebomegaly)
Severe acanthosis nigricans
Eruptive xanthomata
Cushingoid appearance
Acromegaloid appearance
Progeroid (premature aging) appearance
Comorbid conditions
Diabetes mellitus with high insulin requirements
≥200 U/d or ≥2 U/kg/d
Requiring U-500 insulin
Severe hypertriglyceridemia
≥500 mg/dL with or without therapy
≥250 mg/dL despite diet and medical therapy
History of acute pancreatitis secondary to hypertriglyceridemia
Nonalcoholic steatohepatitis in a nonobese individual
Early-onset cardiomyopathy
PCOS
Other historical clues
Autosomal dominant or recessive pattern of similar physical features or metabolic complications
Substantial hyperphagia (may manifest as irritability/aggression in infants/children)
Adapted from Brown *et al.* (1).

challenging to implement in hyperphagic patients and must be balanced by energy requirements for growth in children. Most patients should be encouraged to exercise, and anecdotally, metabolic disease may be greatly ameliorated in high-performance athletes with lipodystrophy. However, patients predisposed to cardiomyopathy should have cardiology clearance before beginning an exercise program, and contact sports should be avoided in patients with lytic bone lesions (typically *AGPAT2* mutation) or severe hepatosplenomegaly.

Metreleptin

Leptin replacement with recombinant human methionyl leptin (metreleptin) is the only drug approved specifically for generalized lipodystrophy. It is approved as an adjunct to diet to treat the complications of acquired or genetic forms of generalized lipodystrophy. Metreleptin is available only under a risk evaluation and mitigation strategy program, meaning that prescribers must complete an online training module to become certified prescribers, and it may not be prescribed off label (*i.e.*, for partial lipodystrophy). The major clinical effects of metreleptin in patients with generalized lipodystrophy are as follows:

- Reduction in appetite and body weight (if excessive weight loss occurs, especially in growing children, the dose should be reduced)
- Improved glycemia (A1c reduction 2% after 1 year) and insulin resistance; many young patients with good beta cell function can discontinue insulin entirely, even when starting at high doses (many hundreds of units per day)
- Decreased triglycerides (60% reduction after 1 year)
- Decreased hepatic steatosis and biopsy measures of nonalcoholic steatohepatitis (note, however, that metreleptin is not US Food and Drug Administration approved specifically for the treatment of nonalcoholic steatohepatitis)
- Decreased proteinuria
- Improved fertility and decreased sign/symptoms of PCOS

Although metreleptin has some benefits in ameliorating metabolic complications of partial lipodystrophy, responses are of lesser magnitude and more heterogeneous than in generalized lipodystrophy. Benefits tend to be greater in patients with more severe leptin deficiency (< 4 ng/mL), more severe hypertriglyceridemia (> 500 mg/dL), and/or poorly controlled diabetes (A1c > 8%). Importantly, metreleptin may not be prescribed off label to patients with partial lipodystrophy and is only available to these patients through clinical trials and compassionate use programs in the United States.

Other Medications

Metformin is an appropriate first-line agent for diabetes. In patients with high insulin requirements (>200 U/d or >3 U/kg/d in children), concentrated insulin such as U-500 should be considered (3). Insulin glargine and degludec should be avoided because their prolonged duration of action requires subcutaneous fat. Dyslipidemia should be treated according to current guidelines for the general population. Statins are appropriate first-line therapy in most adults. Fibrates should be used for triglycerides >500 mg/dL and may be considered for triglycerides >200 mg/dL.

MAIN CONCLUSIONS

Diagnosis of lipodystrophy requires careful history taking and physical examination. Patients are at high risk for metabolic complications and may respond poorly to conventional medications, including high-dose insulin. Leptin replacement with metreleptin is an effective treatment option for patients with generalized forms of lipodystrophy.

DISCUSSION OF CASES AND ANSWERS

Case 1

A 4-month-old African American girl was noted to appear muscular at birth. Breastfeeding was discontinued after 1 month because the baby was never satisfied and always seemed hungry. Despite her excessive appetite, she had poor weight gain and was admitted for failure to thrive at 4 months of age. Physical examination reveals hepatomegaly and generalized muscular appearance with absence of subcutaneous fat. Laboratory testing reveals dyslipidemia, with nonfasting triglycerides of 832 mg/dL, glucose 103 mg/dL, insulin 45 µIU/mL, and A1c 4.9%. Serum leptin is 0.2 ng/mL.

Question

1. What is the likely diagnosis?

Answer

Congenital generalized lipodystrophy. Given the patient's African American descent, she likely has the most common genetic form, caused by recessive mutation in *AGPAT2*.

Question

2. How should she be treated?

Answer

Dietary management is appropriate first-line therapy. A pediatric dietician should be consulted given the patient's young age and specialized needs. This infant was prescribed a high-calorie (30 kcal/oz) specialized formula containing medium-chain triglycerides as the primary source of fat to manage her hypertriglyceridemia. Metreleptin was initiated as an adjunct to dietary treatment at 1 year of age at a dose of 0.06 mg/kg/d. She weighs 10 kg; thus, her dose is 0.6 mg of a 5-mg/mL solution. Her parents measure this as 12 unit markings on an insulin syringe.

Question

3. After initiating metreleptin, the patient loses 1 kg, and her weight for length decreases from the 25th centile to < third centile. What should be done?

Answer

The dose should be decreased to maintain a dose of 0.06 mg/kg/d based on her current body weight. For her current weight of 9 kg, the dose is 0.54 mg. This is measured as 11 unit markings on an insulin syringe.

Question

4. At age 3 years, the patient weighs 11 kg, maintaining her weight for length in the third centile. Fasting laboratories show triglycerides 540 mg/dL, HDL 16 mg/dL, glucose 96 mg/dL, A1c 5.4%, ALT 24, and AST 17. Her metreleptin dose is still 0.54 mg. What should be done to manage her dyslipidemia?

Answer

Her metreleptin dose should be increased based on her weight gain. For a weight of 11 kg, 0.06 mg/kg/d equals 0.66 mg, measured as 13 unit markings on an insulin syringe. The patient's diet should be reviewed, with a goal composition of 50% to 60% carbohydrates, 20% to 30% fat, and ~20% protein.

Question

5. The patient maintains good metabolic control for years, with periodic adjustments in metreleptin dose based on growth. At age 12 years, she develops polyuria and polydipsia. A1c is 9.3%. Triglycerides are 1100 mg/dL. Her metreleptin dose is still 0.06 mg/d. Why has her metabolic control deteriorated?

Answer

The most common reason for acute metabolic decompensation in a patient with generalized lipodystrophy who has previously responded to metreleptin is noncompliance with metreleptin. As in most chronic diseases, noncompliance commonly develops during adolescence. In addition, patients with lipodystrophy will experience worsening of insulin resistance during puberty and usually require higher metreleptin doses, typically ~0.12 to 0.15 mg/kg/d. Rarely, neutralizing antibodies to leptin might be a cause of nonresponsiveness to metreleptin in a patient who previously responded to treatment.

Case 2

A 17-year-old white girl with history of juvenile idiopathic arthritis was diagnosed with type 2 diabetes at age 14 years and treated with metformin. A1c at diagnosis was 7.5% but gradually climbed to >9%, and insulin was initiated. By age 17 years, she required >3.5 U/kg/d of insulin by pump (total daily dose, 196 units) with poor control and A1c 9.5%. Triglycerides at the time of diabetes diagnosis were >600 mg/dL, with HDL 27 mg/dL, and the highest documented triglyceride level was >2000 mg/dL. Current medications are: simvastatin, fish oil, insulin, metformin, glyburide, and combination oral contraceptive pill. Both parents have type 2 diabetes. Physical examination reveals a well-appearing adolescent with body mass index of 22.4 kg/m^2 (75th centile).

Question

1. What features in the patient's history should raise suspicion for lipodystrophy?

Answer

Insulin requirement of >3 U/kg/d in a lean adolescent, combined with high triglycerides and low HDL, should raise suspicion for a syndromic cause of severe insulin resistance, including lipodystrophy. Careful physical examination should be performed to evaluate fat distribution. In this patient, skinfold examination revealed normal subcutaneous fat in the trunk and arms, with diminished subcutaneous fat in the gluteal area and lower extremities, suggestive of partial lipodystrophy.

Question

2. What testing should be performed to confirm a diagnosis of lipodystrophy?

Answer

There is no single diagnostic test for lipodystrophy. The patient has a history of autoimmune disease; however, her fat distribution is more consistent with genetic forms of partial lipodystrophy (characterized by missing fat in buttocks and limbs) rather than autoimmune acquired partial lipodystrophy (characterized by missing fat in the upper body). Given the strong family history of diabetes, a genetic form of lipodystrophy was suspected. The two most common genes causing familial partial lipodystrophy are *LMNA* and *PPARg*. This patient was found to have a mutation in *PPARg*.

Question

3. What screening tests should be performed to evaluate metabolic complications of lipodystrophy?

Answer

The patient already has a diagnosis of diabetes and should undergo standard screening for complications. Fasting lipid panel should be conducted to evaluate dyslipidemia. Screening for NAFLD should include ALT, AST, and liver ultrasound. Screening for proteinuric nephropathy may include spot urine protein-to-creatinine ratio or 24-hour urine protein. Screening for PCOS should be performed as clinically appropriate based on history and physical examination. Screening for cardiovascular disease other than hypertension is not routinely indicated in a young patient with familial partial lipodystrophy.

Question

4. What treatment options exist for this patient?

Answer

Healthy diet and exercise are the mainstays of treatment for lipodystrophy. Given the patient's high insulin requirements, U-500 insulin should be considered for management of diabetes. In addition to a statin and fish oil, fibrates may be used to manage hypertriglyceridemia. The oral contraceptive should be discontinued because it may exacerbate hypertriglyceridemia; barrier contraceptives and intrauterine devices are safer choices in patients with lipodystrophy. Metreleptin is only available to patients with partial lipodystrophy in clinical trials.

REFERENCES

1. Brown RJ, Araujo-Vilar D, Cheung PT, Dunger D, Garg A, Jack M, Mungai L, Oral EA, Patni N, Rother KI, von Schnurbein J, Sorkina E, Stanley T, Vigouroux C, Wabitsch M, Williams R, Yorifuji T. The diagnosis and management of lipodystrophy syndromes: a multisociety practice guideline. *J Clin Endocrinol Metab.* 2016;**101**(12):4500–4511.
2. Diker-Cohen T, Cochran E, Gorden P, Brown RJ. Partial and generalized lipodystrophy: comparison of baseline characteristics and response to metreleptin. *J Clin Endocrinol Metab.* 2015;**100**(5):1802–1810.
3. Lane WS, Cochran EK, Jackson JA, Scism-Bacon JL, Corey IB, Hirsch IB, Skyler JS. High-dose insulin therapy: is it time for U-500 insulin? *Endocr Pract.* 2009;**15**(1):71–79.

Hypoglycemia After Bariatric Surgery

M27
Presented, March 17–20, 2018

Mary-Elizabeth Patti, MD. Joslin Diabetes Center and Harvard Medical School, Boston, Massachusetts 02115, E-mail: mary.elizabeth.patti@joslin.harvard.edu

SIGNIFICANCE OF THE PROBLEM

Hypoglycemia occurring after bariatric and other forms of upper gastrointestinal surgery is increasingly recognized as a condition commonly presenting to clinical endocrinologists (1). Although the true frequency of this condition remains uncertain, due to differences in diagnostic criteria and diverse populations under study (2), postbariatric hypoglycemia can be severe and disabling for some patients, with neuroglycopenia, seizures, falls, loss of consciousness, motor vehicle accidents, and job and income loss. Moreover, repeated episodes of hypoglycemia can result in hypoglycemia unawareness, further impairing safety and requiring the assistance of others to treat hypoglycemia.

After bariatric and other upper gastrointestinal surgery (such as fundoplication), undigested food empties out of the stomach rapidly, contributing to postprandial "spikes" in glucose. Together with robust prandial incretin secretion (*e.g.*, GLP1), high postprandial glucose levels trigger excessive insulin secretion, leading to extremely rapid drops in glucose. These rapid drops in glucose make it very difficult for patients to detect and successfully treat low blood glucose levels before neuroglycopenia develops. Additional defects contributing to hypoglycemia include reduced insulin clearance and insulin-independent glucose uptake (3). Thus, initial prevention strategies are focused on reducing postprandial glucose and insulin secretion by reducing intake of simple carbohydrates and slowing absorption with disaccharidase inhibitors.

BARRIERS TO OPTIMAL PRACTICE

- The need to differentiate whether symptoms are caused by hypoglycemia or other conditions commonly present in postbariatric patients
- The need to define the underlying cause of hypoglycemia
- Incomplete efficacy of current therapies

LEARNING OBJECTIVES

As a result of participating in this session, learners should be able to:

- Summarize the pathophysiology of postbariatric hypoglycemia
- Identify diagnostic strategies for evaluation of possible hypoglycemia in a postbariatric patient
- Identify staged management approaches for postbariatric hypoglycemia

STRATEGIES FOR DIAGNOSIS, THERAPY, AND MANAGEMENT

Diagnosis

The diagnosis of hypoglycemia is challenging in any patient, but even more so in a patient with a history of bariatric or other gastrointestinal surgery. The adrenergic and cholinergic symptoms of hypoglycemia are nonspecific and overlap considerably with those of the dumping syndrome. Thus, it is essential to first determine whether hypoglycemia is indeed present, whether it is associated with the symptoms, and whether symptoms respond to treatments that increase glucose (Whipple triad). Moreover, accurate determination of the glucose level in a venous sample at the time of symptoms is essential, as capillary glucose values determined by a glucometer can be misleading in the setting of poor blood flow (*e.g.*, cold exposure or Raynaud disease). Simultaneous assessment of β-cell peptides would be ideal if hypoglycemia is confirmed. If glucose is not low at the time of symptoms, additional considerations would include dumping syndrome, anxiety, orthostatic hypotension, or cardiovascular disease.

Once hypoglycemia is diagnosed, the next step is to determine the cause of hypoglycemia. Detailed history, exam, and laboratory testing should be focused on the potential role of systemic and hormonal disease, such as adrenal insufficiency, nutritional adequacy, ethanol intake, and medications that may induce hypoglycemia.

Additional details more specific to the possibility of postbariatric hypoglycemia would include the following: (1) type and date of bariatric surgery, (2) weight trajectory postoperative, (3) nutritional adequacy, and (4) history of diabetes or gestational diabetes preoperatively. Specific details about hypoglycemia episodes should include the severity (frequency, neuroglycopenia, and requiring assistance of others) and timing (relationship to meals, provocative foods, activity, and fasting). Detailed records of symptoms, food, and activity can be helpful to identify patterns linked to hypoglycemia. Although continuous glucose monitoring (CGM) is less accurate in hypoglycemic levels, blinded monitoring can be useful to identify patterns of glycemic excursions related to specific foods and activity and to identify unawareness or nocturnal hypoglycemia (4).

Typically, postbariatric hypoglycemia is first noted 1 to 3 years after surgery and occurs 1 to 3 hours after eating, especially simple (high glycemic index) carbohydrates (example CGM results, Fig. 1). Hypoglycemia can also occur after activity/exercise and occasionally during overnight hours (*e.g.*, 2:00 to 4:00 AM). Hypoglycemia occurring in the fasting state is not typical of postbariatric hypoglycemia; if fasting

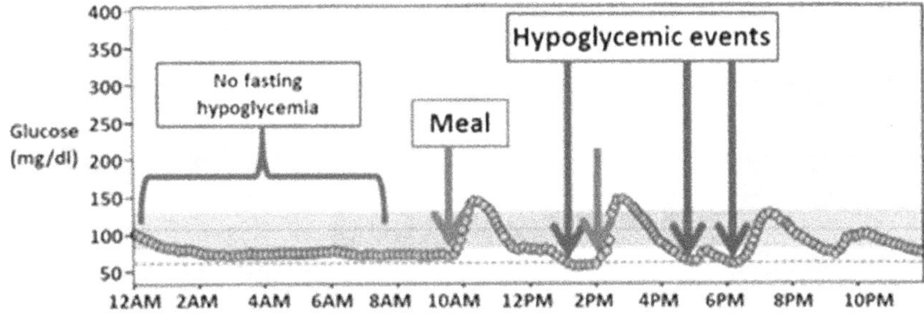

Figure 1. Typical patterns of glycemic excursion in postbariatric hypoglycemia.

hypoglycemia is present, a detailed diagnostic evaluation for autonomous insulin secretion and insulinoma is needed (likely a 72-hour inpatient fast).

If the history is typical for postbariatric hypoglycemia, the next step is to determine whether insulin levels are increased at the time of hypoglycemia. In an ideal world, an analysis of venous glucose and β-cell peptides at the time of a spontaneous episode of hypoglycemia would be optimal. However, this is often not practical; patients may not be able to safely get to a laboratory setting to have blood sampling. Provocative testing, such as glucose or meal tolerance tests, is often considered as an alternative. However, glucose tolerance testing (GTT) is not well tolerated in individuals with a history of bariatric surgery, as the hyperosmolar glucose load often provokes severe dumping syndrome. Moreover, GTT is not advocated for the evaluation of reactive/postprandial hypoglycemia, as 10% of healthy individuals have glucose levels <50 mg/dL during a 4- to 6-hour GTT (5), and low glucose levels during oral GTT do not correlate well with symptoms or electroencephalogram changes (6). Mixed meal testing is preferable. Unfortunately, there is no current standard for meal testing; liquid versus solid and dietary composition vary across practices and clinical studies. Diagnostic criteria are also lacking, but typically postbariatric patients have elevated insulin and C-peptide levels early after the meal and nonsuppressed levels at the time of hypoglycemia (7,8). Such increases in meal-related insulin secretion are likely multifactorial, but a major contributor is very high postprandial levels of the incretin hormone GLP-1, as indicated by clinical studies demonstrating reduction in insulin secretion and partial normalization of glycemia with infusion of GLP1 receptor inhibitors (9,10).

Postbariatric hypoglycemia is characterized by normal suppression of insulin secretion in the fasting state. The question of when/how to rule out autonomous insulin secretion in this setting is often challenging. While postbariatric hypoglycemia is typically postprandial, 22% of insulinomas present with postprandial hypoglycemia only. In my opinion, not every patient needs a prolonged (72 hour) inpatient diagnostic fast. Rather, the approach needs to be individualized for each patient based on risk. If (1) postbariatric [Roux-en-Y gastric bypass (RYGB) or sleeve] patient reports no history of hypoglycemia with fasting, (2) suspicion is low for autonomous insulin secretion, and (3) patient can safely perform an overnight fast at home (does not live alone, can get ride in morning to laboratory, *etc.*), one could consider an overnight fast (after supper) with laboratory testing for glucose, insulin, and C-peptide the next morning. This should be repeated on several occasions and if hypoglycemia progresses or new patterns emerge despite therapy. Diagnostic CGM, although of lower accuracy in the hypoglycemic range, can be used to identify patterns of asymptomatic fasting or nocturnal hypoglycemia that require further testing (4). Prolonged inpatient fasting is essential for patients with documented fasting hypoglycemia or atypical features, or those for whom outpatient testing may not be achieved safely.

In summary, postbariatric hypoglycemia can be diagnosed if the following criteria are met: (1) history of postprandial hypoglycemia occurring >1 year after surgery, (2) documented hypoglycemia (venous glucose <70 mg/dL) at time of symptoms and resolution of symptoms with treatment to raise glucose, (3) elevated insulin and C-peptide at time of hypoglycemia, (4) normal fasting glucose, and (5) no evidence of autonomous insulin secretion, with workup as guided by clinical considerations (see flowchart, Fig. 2).

Treatment

The goal of therapy in postbariatric hypoglycemia is to reduce the frequency and severity of hypoglycemia, improving safety and allowing resumption of activities of daily living. With currently available therapies, the complete elimination of hypoglycemia is unlikely, and ongoing vigilance to diet and nutrition are essential.

The cornerstone of management of postbariatric hypoglycemia is medical nutrition therapy to reduce the stimulus for glycemic spikes and insulin secretion. Our team has recently published practical suggestions for medical nutrition therapy (11). In brief, because simple (high glycemic index) carbohydrates are rapidly digested and absorbed in a postbariatric patient, we advise complete avoidance of high-glycemic-index carbohydrates. Instead, we recommend selecting controlled portions of low-glycemic-index carbohydrates (<30 g per meal, 15 g per snack to begin). Adequate protein and heart-healthy fats provide required caloric needs.

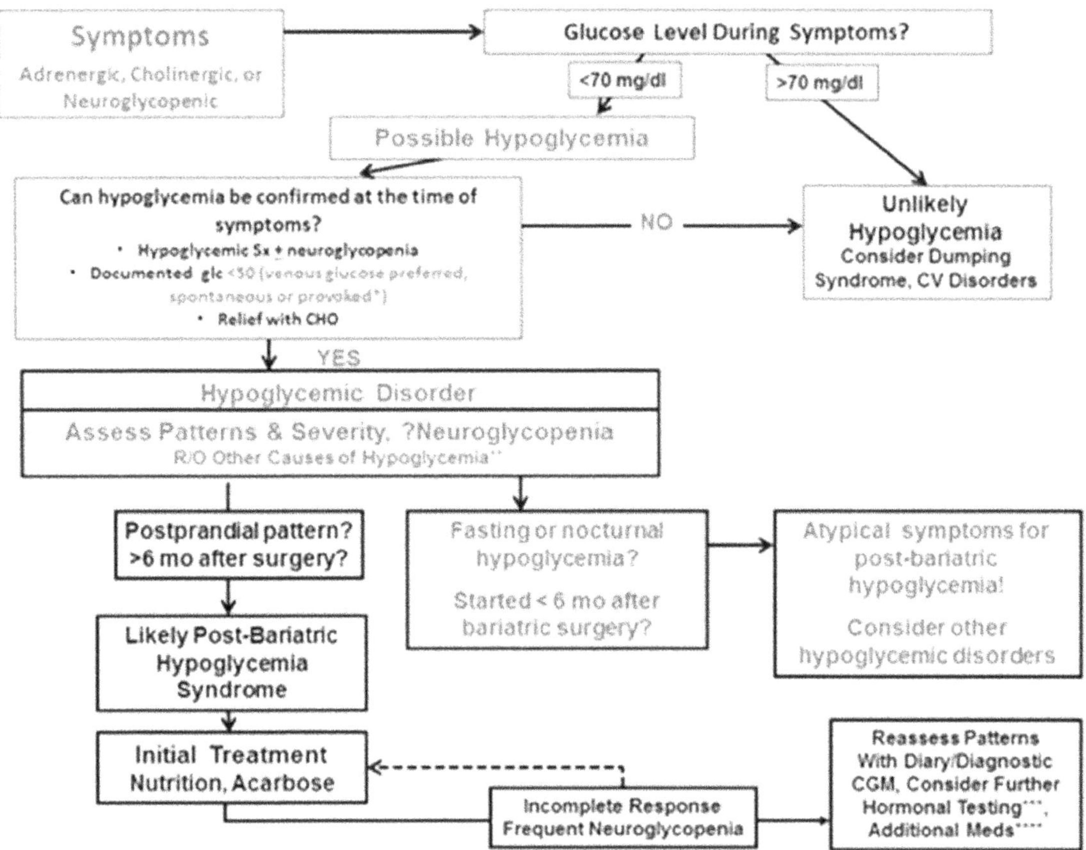

Figure 2. Approach to possible hypoglycemia in a postbariatric patient.

Meal plan composition and carbohydrate content are subsequently adjusted as needed to minimize spikes in individual patients. Additionally, we recommend avoidance of liquids with meals (to minimize dumping-type physiology), avoidance of ethanol and excessive caffeine, and consistent vitamin and mineral intake, guided by laboratory testing.

If medical nutrition therapy is not sufficient to gain control of hypoglycemia, medications can be added. These include acarbose to slow absorption of glucose, reducing glycemic "spikes" and insulin secretion. Although gastrointestinal side effects of gas and abdominal cramping can limit tolerance of acarbose, slow introduction and escalation to a maximal dose of 300 mg/d are often effective. Somatostatin receptor analogues such as octreotide or pasireotide (12) can also reduce incretin and insulin secretion and can be administered at the time of meals (subcutaneous, before each meal, starting dose 25 to 50 μg) or in monthly deep intramuscular (IM) injections (LAR preparation). Octreotide therapy is limited by high cost, as well as side effects, including diarrhea, steatorrhea, and acute hypoglycemia (presumably linked to inhibition of glucagon secretion). Diazoxide, which reduces insulin secretion, can also be helpful in doses of 50 to 100 mg three times per day but can be limited by fluid retention, edema, and headache. Other reports have suggested efficacy of calcium channel blockade and GLP1R agonists, but we have not found these efficacious in our patient population.

Ancillary components of the management strategy include education of the patient and family members about hypoglycemia recognition and treatment, and use of glucose and glucagon to treat established hypoglycemia. CGM can be helpful to allow early detection and treatment of hypoglycemia (4). Sensor low-glucose alarms can allow patients to detect hypoglycemia even when they have unawareness. Moreover, the "rapid drop alarm" allows patients to initiate treatment even when glucose is within target range, before severe hypoglycemia and neuroglycopenia develop.

Additional therapeutic considerations can include the placement of a G-tube for feeding into the bypassed stomach (13). In some patients, continuous feeding into the remnant stomach (either 24 hours or overnight), and minimal oral intake, can reduce the frequency and severity of hypoglycemia, likely due to reduced glycemic excursions and near normalization of incretin and insulin secretion. Although initial reports described partial pancreatectomy for severe postbariatric hypoglycemia (14,15), pancreatic surgery is no longer recommended due to high morbidity and incomplete resolution and/or recurrence of hypoglycemia postoperatively (16). Some patients may benefit from surgical reversal of bariatric surgery, with reduced frequency and severity of symptoms, but results are variable, potentially related to interindividual differences in postsurgical anatomy and surgical team expertise (17–19).

CASES WITH QUESTIONS AND ANSWERS

Case 1

A 60-year-old female had a witnessed generalized seizure. The capillary glucose level obtained by ambulance personnel was 35 mg/dL. Glucose rose after IM glucagon and intravenous dextrose. Central nervous system imaging was negative. The patient has a history of uncomplicated RYGB 5 years previously. Over the last 6 months, she experienced episodic lightheadedness, confusion, and sweating, usually 2 to 3 hours after eating. She was referred to see you in the endocrinology clinic as an outpatient. History was notable for no personal diabetes history (but diabetes in husband), no family history of hypoglycemia or MEN1 components, and recent weight stability. The exam revealed a BMI of 34 kg/m^2 and surgical scars and was otherwise normal. General laboratory testing performed in the fasting state at 8:00 AM was normal, including glucose 82 mg/dL, cortisol 12 μg/dL, and hemoglobin A_{1c} 5.3%.

What are the next best step(s) in diagnostic evaluation? Select all that apply.

A. GTT
B. 72-hour fast
C. Meal tolerance test
D. Food, symptom, and home glucose monitoring diary
E. Venous sample for glucose and β-cell peptides at time of spontaneous hypoglycemia

Answer: C, D, and E

As noted above, an analysis of venous glucose and β-cell peptides at the time of a spontaneous episode of hypoglycemia would be optimal. If this is not practical or safe, provocative testing can be considered. Meal tolerance testing is preferred, as oral glucose is poorly tolerated by postbariatric patients and results do not correlate well with either symptoms or electroencephalogram changes.

The patient was instructed in the use of a home glucose meter to record capillary glucose with symptoms, and completion of a food/activity/symptom log to enable her to identify relationships between specific foods and symptoms. Please note that capillary glucose values should not be used to diagnose hypoglycemia, given that reduced blood flow (as with cold exposure or Raynaud disease) can yield low glucose values not equivalent to central glucose levels. She was given a laboratory slip indicating assays to be checked during a spontaneous episode of hypoglycemia and also scheduled for a mixed-meal tolerance test.

In this case, we were fortunate to be able to "catch" a spontaneous episode. She had a spontaneous hypoglycemic event while at her doctor's office, 2 hours after eating a donut. Venous samples revealed glucose 43 mg/dL, insulin 12 μU/mL (reference range for laboratory 2.0 to 19.6 μIU/mL), and C-peptide 2.2 ng/mL (1.1 to 4.2 ng/mL). These values are typical of postbariatric hypoglycemia, with modest elevations (inappropriately high) in insulin and C-peptide at the time of hypoglycemia.

What should be your next step(s)? Select all that apply.

A. Imaging of pancreas
B. Start meal plan focused on low glycemic carbohydrates in controlled portions
C. Instruction in use of glucagon emergency kit for family members and medical identification bracelet
D. Add hypoglycemia agent screen to blood samples
E. Inpatient fasting

Answer: B, C, and D

History does not suggest fasting hypoglycemia. In the absence of fasting symptoms and/or biochemical evidence of autonomous insulin secretion, both of which are rare in postbariatric patients, anatomical imaging is not indicated. Meal planning to reduce glycemic spikes and thus stimulus for insulin secretion is important. Safety measures should include the education of family members about hypoglycemia and use of glucose and glucagon for rescue and a medical identification bracelet indicating hypoglycemia. It would be important to rule out inadvertent or surreptitious use of sulfonylureas or other hypoglycemic agents.

The question of when/how to safely fast to rule out autonomous insulin secretion is often challenging. While postbariatric hypoglycemia is typically postprandial, recall that 22% of insulinomas present with postprandial hypoglycemia only. Although rare, insulinomas can occur in postbariatric patients (20), and it is essential to identify these as surgical treatment would be needed. In my experience, not every patient needs a prolonged (72 hour) inpatient diagnostic fast. Rather, the approach needs to be individualized for each patient based on clinical risk. If (1) the patient reports no history of hypoglycemia with fasting, (2) suspicion is low for autonomous insulin secretion, and (3) the patient can safely perform an overnight fast at home (does not live alone, can get a ride in morning to laboratory, *etc.*), one could consider an overnight fast (after supper) with laboratory testing for glucose, insulin, and C-peptide the next morning. This should be repeated on several occasions and if hypoglycemia progresses or new patterns emerge despite therapy. Diagnostic CGM, although of lower accuracy in the hypoglycemic range, can be used to identify patterns of asymptomatic fasting or nocturnal hypoglycemia that require further testing. Prolonged inpatient fasting is essential for patients with documented fasting hypoglycemia or atypical features, or those for whom outpatient testing may not be achieved safely.

The patient saw a dietician and initiated a meal plan focused on choosing low-glycemic-index carbohydrates (30 g maximum per meal, 15 g per snack) and no liquids with meals. The frequency of symptoms was reduced, but some moderate hypoglycemia (glucose in 40s, not requiring assistance) persisted.

What is the best next step for treatment?

A. Diazoxide
B. Octreotide
C. Acarbose
D. Calcium channel blocker

Answer: C

The disaccharidase inhibitor acarbose is typically the first pharmacologic therapy for postprandial hypoglycemia as it addresses the major pathophysiologic condition of rapid increases in nutrient absorption. Acarbose slows carbohydrate absorption, reducing peak prandial glucose and reducing both insulin and GLP1 responses to meals (21,22). Common side effects include abdominal gas, bloating, and cramping; these can be reduced by gradual increase in dosing and reduction in carbohydrate intake. The patient was started on acarbose 25 mg with each main meal for 1 week; the dose was increased gradually to 100 mg with each main meal. Hypoglycemic episodes were reduced in frequency and severity.

About 1 year later, neuroglycopenia recurred despite compliance with diet and acarbose. Octreotide was started, initially dosed (by injection) before meals and ultimately IM monthly (LAR). She continues to have mild occasional hypoglycemia.

Case 2

The patient is a 44-year-old female who presented with symptoms of shakiness, blurred vision, lip numbness, cold sweats, and anxiety progressively increasing over 1 month after gastric bypass surgery. The patient had progressive weight gain during adult life, particularly after two pregnancies complicated by gestational diabetes, with peak BMI of 44 kg/m^2. Previous weight loss attempts with commercial weight loss programs (*e.g.*, Jenny Craig and Weight Watchers) were unsuccessful. Evaluation for obesity, hirsutism, and oligomenorrhea led to a diagnosis of polycystic ovarian syndrome. The patient was advised to lose weight with diet and exercise. Metformin was prescribed but discontinued due to symptoms of shakiness and sweating occurring shortly after the first dose. Laboratory testing at the next office visit showed random glucose 88 mg/dL with insulin 50 μU/mL, interpreted as reactive hypoglycemia in association with insulin resistance.

The patient was referred for bariatric surgery due to her severe obesity, hypertension and hyperlipidemia, and underlying insulin resistance. She had an uncomplicated laparoscopic RYGB. While on the recommended postoperative diet, the patient noted symptoms of palpitations, sweating, and lightheadedness, typically after oral intake and occasionally during short walks, and required caloric intake every 3 to 4 hours to prevent symptoms. Capillary glucose levels at the time of symptoms ranged from 30 to 60 mg/dL.

What aspect of this patient's history is an unusual feature of postbariatric hypoglycemia?

A. Hypoglycemia occurring 2 to 3 hours after meals
B. Hypoglycemia starting 1 month after surgery
C. Symptoms of possible hypoglycemia occurring preoperatively

Answer: B

Hypoglycemia typically begins 1 to 3 years postoperatively, but sometimes as late as 10 years postoperatively! This patient was very atypical in that she had worsening of preexisting hypoglycemia immediately postoperatively. This pattern (within the first 6 months postoperative) should raise concern for an alternative diagnosis.

The hypoglycemic symptoms occurring preoperatively have been identified as a potential risk factor for postbariatric hypoglycemia in a survey study (23,24). As with this patient, it is unclear whether nonspecific symptoms, particularly without neuroglycopenia, occurring preoperatively (but not fully evaluated) truly represented hypoglycemia or not. One study evaluating oral glucose tolerance preoperatively showed that patients who developed hypoglycemia postoperatively had lower BMI, fasting glucose, and nadir glucose during GTT and higher β-cell glucose sensitivity preoperatively than those who did not develop hypoglycemia (25). However, all values were within the normal range, making it impossible to distinguish these patients in a clinical setting. Nevertheless, preoperative risk evaluation should include a detailed query for history of possible hypoglycemia. If positive, additional evaluation should be considered to further define the risk of hypoglycemia.

Returning to this patient, endocrine evaluation revealed no other relevant medical history. The family history was important for obesity in her sister and brother and type 2 diabetes in her maternal grandfather. There was no history of neonatal or adult hypoglycemia, or of pancreatic disease or MEN1 component diseases.

Given the atypical nature of hypoglycemia in this postbariatric patient, an assessment of β-cell peptide secretion and its autonomy was necessary. Although her symptoms were typically occurring after meals and with activity, it is important to remember that 22% of insulinomas present with both fasting and postprandial hypoglycemia (26). Given the prominent exercise component, glucose patterns were assessed after an overnight fast and in response to exercise. The patient developed symptoms after 10 minutes of cycling on a stationary bike, with plasma glucose 56 mg/dL. Cortisol, lactate, and pyruvate responses to exercise were normal. With continued fasting over an additional 4 hours, symptoms of neuroglycopenia developed, with minimum glucose 44 mg/dL and inappropriately nonsuppressed insulin (8 μU/mL), C-peptide (1.76 ng/mL), and proinsulin (49 pM) and suppressed β-hydroxybutyrate (0.8 mM). Blood glucose promptly responded to glucagon (1 mg), with increase of glucose of 47 mg/dL at 30 minutes after glucagon.

What do these data suggest is the underlying cause of the patient's hypoglycemia?

A. Postbariatric hypoglycemia syndrome
B. Autonomous insulin secretion
C. Inadequate glycogen stores
D. Exercise-induced hypoglycemia due to MCT1 mutation

Answer: B

Hypoglycemia is confirmed by a low venous glucose at the time of neuroglycopenic symptoms. Inadequately suppressed insulin, C-peptide, and proinsulin at the time of hypoglycemia indicate failure of insulin secretion to be appropriately suppressed, thus defining autonomous insulin secretion. In postbariatric hypoglycemia syndrome, insulin secretion is appropriately suppressed with fasting. (Patients with postbariatric hypoglycemia typically do well if they need to fast for any reason, *e.g.*, surgery or diagnostic testing.)

An increase of >25 mg/dL in glucose after glucagon injection indicates residual glycogen stores (despite fasting), suggesting that insulin-like factors are both causing hypoglycemia and promoting glycogen storage.

Exercise-induced hypoglycemia is associated with a mutation in the MCT1 carrier and can be diagnosed by finding insulin secretion in response to exercise, but not fasting.

Localization of the presumed insulinoma was ultimately achieved using endoscopic ultrasonography with Optison imaging and computed tomography arteriography. Endoscopic ultrasonography–guided fine needle aspiration identified neoplastic epithelioid cells consistent with a well-differentiated, low-grade (grade 1) neuroendocrine tumor. Surgical resection was performed with a minimally invasive approach. Intraoperative localization was achieved by identification of the reaction to the prior needle aspiration and by intraoperative ultrasound.

Given the patient's postbypass hormonal milieu and risk for islet hyperplasia, robot-assisted distal pancreatectomy and splenectomy were performed instead of a pancreas-sparing procedure such as central pancreatectomy or enucleation. Pathologic examination showed a 2.1-cm, well-differentiated neuroendocrine tumor, diffusely immunoreactive for insulin, as well as a second well-circumscribed incidental microadenoma (0.28 cm), which was negative for insulin but positive for synaptophysin. The islets in the background nonneoplastic pancreas showed increased islet density in some areas (mean 197 μm) and a few islets >400 μm in size, possibly representing islet hyperplasia; there were no overt abnormalities in islet cell nuclear size or morphology.

Hypoglycemia resolved postoperatively and has not recurred in follow-up of >2 years. For additional details of a series of postbariatric patients with insulinoma and suggested evaluation, please see Mulla *et al.* (20).

CONCLUSIONS

In summary, postbariatric hypoglycemia results from accelerated delivery of undigested nutrients into the proximal intestine, triggering rapid increases in plasma glucose. In the setting of increased prandial incretin hormone secretion (predominantly GLP1), high glucose levels trigger excessive insulin secretion, rapid reductions in glucose levels, and frank hypoglycemia. Hypoglycemia typically occurs 1 to 3 hours after meals and 1 to 3 years after prior surgery. Although some patients can experience hypoglycemia with activity or nocturnal (2:00 to 4:00 AM) hypoglycemia, morning fasting hypoglycemia is not typical. Not all hypoglycemia postbariatric surgery is symptomatic, potentially due to impaired counterregulatory responses accompanying frequent hypoglycemia or interindividual differences (27).

There are many challenges in the diagnostic workup of postbariatric hypoglycemia. As with any hypoglycemic symptom evaluation, the workup should first confirm (with a venous sample) that symptoms are accompanied by true hypoglycemia, and that symptoms resolve with correction of hypoglycemia. If hypoglycemia is confirmed, further workup should be individualized to define patterns/timing/frequency of hypoglycemia and associated insulin secretion patterns. For those individuals with atypical features or fasting hypoglycemia, prolonged fasting to rule out autonomous insulin secretion is required. If autonomous secretion is defined, imaging to localize the suspected insulinoma is required.

Once postbariatric hypoglycemia is defined, therapeutic approaches include medical nutrition therapy to optimize nutrition, vitamin supplementation, and meal plan focused on controlled portions of complex carbohydrates (30 g per meal, 15 g per snack). If this is not adequate, medications can be added sequentially to nutrition therapy, including acarbose, octreotide, and diazoxide. Pancreatic surgery to reduce islet mass is no longer recommended due to (1) recognition that increased islet mass is not the pathophysiologic defect, (2) high morbidity, and (3) high rates of hypoglycemia recurrence (12). Additional therapeutic strategies are in development for this challenging condition.

REFERENCES

1. Patti ME, Goldfine AB. The rollercoaster of post-bariatric hypoglycaemia. *Lancet Diabetes Endocrinol.* 2016;**4**(2):94–96.
2. Goldfine AB, Patti ME. How common is hypoglycemia after gastric bypass? *Obesity (Silver Spring).* 2016;**24**(6):1210–1211.
3. Patti ME, Li P, Goldfine AB. Insulin response to oral stimuli and glucose effectiveness increased in neuroglycopenia following gastric bypass. *Obesity (Silver Spring).* 2015;**23**(4):798–807.
4. Halperin F, Patti ME, Skow M, Bajwa M, Goldfine AB. Continuous glucose monitoring for evaluation of glycemic excursions after gastric bypass. *J Obes.* 2011;**2011**:869536.

5. Lev-Ran A, Anderson RW. The diagnosis of postprandial hypoglycemia. *Diabetes.* 1981;**30**(12):996–999.
6. Hogan MJ, Service FJ, Sharbrough FW, Gerich JE. Oral glucose tolerance test compared with a mixed meal in the diagnosis of reactive hypoglycemia. A caveat on stimulation. *Mayo Clin Proc.* 1983;**58**(8): 491–496.
7. Goldfine AB, Mun EC, Devine E, Bernier R, Baz-Hecht M, Jones DB, Schneider BE, Holst JJ, Patti ME. Patients with neuroglycopenia after gastric bypass surgery have exaggerated incretin and insulin secretory responses to a mixed meal. *J Clin Endocrinol Metab.* 2007; **92**(12):4678–4685.
8. Salehi M, Gastaldelli A, D'Alessio DA. Altered islet function and insulin clearance cause hyperinsulinemia in gastric bypass patients with symptoms of postprandial hypoglycemia. *J Clin Endocrinol Metab.* 2014;**99**(6):2008–2017.
9. Salehi M, Gastaldelli A, D'Alessio DA. Blockade of glucagon-like peptide 1 receptor corrects postprandial hypoglycemia after gastric bypass. *Gastroenterology.* 2014;**146**(3):669–680.
10. Craig CM, Liu LF, Deacon CF, Holst JJ, McLaughlin TL. Critical role for GLP-1 in symptomatic post-bariatric hypoglycaemia. *Diabetologia.* 2017;**60**(3):531–540.
11. Suhl E, Anderson-Haynes SE, Mulla C, Patti ME. Medical nutrition therapy for post-bariatric hypoglycemia: practical insights. *Surg Obes Relat Dis.* 2017;**13**(5):888–896.
12. de Heide LJ, Laskewitz AJ, Apers JA. Treatment of severe postRYGB hyperinsulinemic hypoglycemia with pasireotide: a comparison with octreotide on insulin, glucagon, and GLP-1. *Surg Obes Relat Dis.* 2014; **10**(3):e31–e33.
13. McLaughlin T, Peck M, Holst J, Deacon C. Reversible hyperinsulinemic hypoglycemia after gastric bypass: a consequence of altered nutrient delivery. *J Clin Endocrinol Metab.* 2010;**95**(4):1851–1855.
14. Service GJ, Thompson GB, Service FJ, Andrews JC, Collazo-Clavell ML, Lloyd RV. Hyperinsulinemic hypoglycemia with nesidioblastosis after gastric-bypass surgery. *N Engl J Med.* 2005;**353**(3):249–254.
15. Patti ME, McMahon G, Mun EC, Bitton A, Holst JJ, Goldsmith J, Hanto DW, Callery M, Arky R, Nose V, Bonner-Weir S, Goldfine AB. Severe hypoglycaemia post-gastric bypass requiring partial pancreatectomy: evidence for inappropriate insulin secretion and pancreatic islet hyperplasia. *Diabetologia.* 2005;**48**(11):2236–2240.
16. Vanderveen KA, Grant CS, Thompson GB, Farley DR, Richards ML, Vella A, Vollrath B, Service FJ. Outcomes and quality of life after partial pancreatectomy for noninsulinoma pancreatogenous hypoglycemia from diffuse islet cell disease. *Surgery.* 2010;**148**(6):1237–1245; discussion 1245–1236.
17. Lee CJ, Brown T, Magnuson TH, Egan JM, Carlson O, Elahi D. Hormonal response to a mixed-meal challenge after reversal of gastric bypass for hypoglycemia. *J Clin Endocrinol Metab.* 2013;**98**(7): E1208–E1212.
18. Shoar S, Nguyen T, Ona MA, Reddy M, Anand S, Alkuwari MJ, Saber AA. Roux-en-Y gastric bypass reversal: a systematic review. *Surg Obes Relat Dis.* 2016;**12**(7):1366–1372.
19. Svane MS, Toft-Nielsen MB, Kristiansen VB, Hartmann B, Holst JJ, Madsbad S, Bojsen-Møller KN. Nutrient re-routing and altered gut-islet cell crosstalk may explain early relief of severe postprandial hypoglycaemia after reversal of Roux-en-Y gastric bypass. *Diabet Med.* 2017;**34**(12):1783–1787.
20. Mulla CM, Storino A, Yee EU, Lautz D, Sawnhey MS, Moser AJ, Patti ME. Insulinoma after bariatric surgery: diagnostic dilemma and therapeutic approaches. *Obes Surg.* 2016;**26**(4):874–881.
21. Moreira RO, Moreira RB, Machado NA, Gonçalves TB, Coutinho WF. Post-prandial hypoglycemia after bariatric surgery: pharmacological treatment with verapamil and acarbose. *Obes Surg.* 2008;**18**(12): 1618–1621.
22. Valderas JP, Ahuad J, Rubio L, Escalona M, Pollak F, Maiz A. Acarbose improves hypoglycaemia following gastric bypass surgery without increasing glucagon-like peptide 1 levels. *Obes Surg.* 2012;**22**(4): 582–586.
23. Lee CJ, Clark JM, Schweitzer M, Magnuson T, Steele K, Koerner O, Brown TT. Prevalence of and risk factors for hypoglycemic symptoms after gastric bypass and sleeve gastrectomy. *Obesity (Silver Spring).* 2015;**23**(5):1079–1084.
24. Lee CJ, Wood GC, Lazo M, Brown TT, Clark JM, Still C, Benotti P. Risk of post-gastric bypass surgery hypoglycemia in nondiabetic individuals: a single center experience. *Obesity (Silver Spring).* 2016;**24**(6): 1342–1348.
25. Nannipieri M, Belligoli A, Guarino D, Busetto L, Moriconi D, Fabris R, Mari A, Baldi S, Anselmino M, Foletto M, Vettor R, Ferrannini E. Risk factors for spontaneously self-reported postprandial hypoglycemia after bariatric surgery. *J Clin Endocrinol Metab.* 2016;**101**(10): 3600–3607.
26. Placzkowski KA, Vella A, Thompson GB, Grant CS, Reading CC, Charboneau JW, Andrews JC, Lloyd RV, Service FJ. Secular trends in the presentation and management of functioning insulinoma at the Mayo Clinic, 1987-2007. *J Clin Endocrinol Metab.* 2009;**94**(4): 1069–1073.
27. Abrahamsson N, Börjesson JL, Sundbom M, Wiklund U, Karlsson FA, Eriksson JW. Gastric bypass reduces symptoms and hormonal responses in hypoglycemia. *Diabetes.* 2016;**65**(9):2667–2675.

Optimizing Outcome Post–Roux-en-Y Gastric Bypass

M43
Presented, March 17–20, 2018

Barbara McGowan, MBBS, PhD. Guy's and St. Thomas' Hospital, London SE1 9RT, United Kingdom, E-mail: barbara.mcgowan@gstt.nhs.uk

SIGNIFICANCE OF THE CLINICAL PROBLEM

Bariatric or metabolic surgery is a highly effective and safe intervention for the treatment of obesity and its complications. The number of worldwide procedures are approaching half a million per year, with the highest number of procedures in the United States and Canada. The most common procedures are Roux-en-Y gastric bypass (RYGB), sleeve gastrectomy (SG), and laparoscopic adjustable gastric band. Many patients who undergo bariatric surgery will have preexisting micronutrient deficiencies presurgery that need to be optimized preoperatively (1, 2). Bariatric surgery compromises the absorption of nutrients to varying degrees and could cause considerable clinical micronutrient deficiencies that require lifelong nutritional and biochemical monitoring.

Obesity medicine specialists, endocrinologists, gastroenterologists, and health care professionals involved in the management of patients after bariatric surgery should be taught to recognize the signs and symptoms of nutrient deficiencies and how to replace them. They should be able to optimize patients postoperatively, including managing patients with type 2 diabetes (T2DM), monitoring changes in blood pressure and other medications, and managing symptoms of hypoglycemia.

BARRIERS TO OPTIMAL PRACTICE

Obesity is a common disease and bariatric surgery now a common procedure. However, few physicians worldwide are trained in obesity medicine and in managing patients pre- and postbariatric surgery, which mostly is left to endocrinologists, diabetologists, and gastroenterologists to manage in secondary care. Therefore, an increasing number of primary care physicians have had little or no training in managing long-term nutritional complications of bariatric surgery. In the United Kingdom, training in obesity and bariatric medicine is now mandatory for trainees specializing in diabetes and endocrinology. However, lack of training in obesity, nutrition, and metabolic medicine continues, which is a major barrier for new physicians in managing the long-term consequences of bariatric surgery.

LEARNING OBJECTIVES

As a result of participating in this session, learners should be able to:

- Identify the most common short- and long-term nutritional deficiencies post-RYGB
- Manage short- and long-term nutritional deficiencies post-RYGB
- Implement annual surveillance post-RYGB
- Manage T2DM post-RYGB

NUTRITIONAL CONSEQUENCES OF OBESITY SURGERY

The mechanisms that contribute to the risk of nutrient deficiencies after bariatric surgery are multifactorial. Preoperatively, deficiencies may be present as a result of obesity itself, poor diet quality, and preoperative weight loss. Postoperatively, deficiencies depend on procedure-specific alterations to digestion and absorption. Mechanisms include reduced food and diet quantity, vomiting, reduced gastric acid secretion, reduced intrinsic factor secretion, altered digestion and absorption, bypass of primary site of absorption, nonadherence to diet and supplements, maladaptive or disordered eating, alcohol or substance abuse, and small intestinal overgrowth.

Preoperative Deficiencies

Obesity has been shown to be associated with a high prevalence of micronutrient deficiencies especially vitamin D (25% to 68%), iron (8% to 18%), vitamin B12 (18%), and thiamine (15% to 29%) (1, 2). Underlying mechanisms may include impaired expression of transporter proteins (*e.g.*, iron as a result of chronic inflammation). Nutritional deficiencies should be investigated and corrected as clinically indicated before surgery. Preoperative blood tests should include the following (3): full blood count, ferritin, folate, vitamin B12, 25 hydroxyvitamin D, bone profile, liver profile, renal profile, fasting glucose and hemoglobin A_{1c} (HbA_{1c}), and lipid profile.

Standard Postoperative Nutritional Replacement

Standard postoperative supplements for RYGB (3, 4) are as follows. (1) A multivitamin and mineral supplement (A to Z), two per day, should include iron, selenium, 2 mg copper (minimum), zinc (ratio of 8 to 15 mg of zinc for each 1 mg copper), folic acid, vitamin K, biotin, thiamine, and vitamin B12. (2) Iron should include 45 to 60 mg from a multivitamin and mineral supplements as well as iron supplements in certain group of patients (200 mg ferrous sulfate, 210 mg ferrous fumarate, or 300 mg ferrous gluconate daily in addition to the multivitamin and mineral supplement). Menstruating women should supplement at least another 100 mg/d iron with regimens that include ferrous sulfate, fumarate, or gluconate (*e.g.*, ferrous sulfate or ferrous fumarate two times per day). Iron should be taken alongside citrus fruits/drinks or vitamin C to aid absorption. Iron and calcium supplements should be taken at least 2 hours apart. (3) Calcium and vitamin D (1200 to 1500 mg/d elemental calcium and 3000 IU/d vitamin D) and (4) vitamin B12 [three monthly 1-mg (IM) injections (oral, subcutaneous, and sublingual also available)].

Postoperative Deficiencies and Replacement

Table 1 summarizes the most common micro/macronutrient deficiencies post-RYGB, their presenting signs and symptoms, routine supplementation regimens, and treatment of deficiencies (3–5). Some of these presentations will be discussed in cases 1 and 2.

Table 1. Blood Tests Required Post-RYGB and SG and Frequency of Monitoring

Blood Test Post-RYGB	Frequency
HbA_{1c} and FBG with preoperative T2DM	Monitor as appropriate
Lipid profile	Monitor in those with dyslipidemia
FBC; renal, liver, and bone profile; PTH; vitamin D; ferritin; folate; and calcium	Three, 6, and 12 mo in first year, annually thereafter
Thiamine	Measure in prolonged vomiting
Vitamin B12	Six and 12 mo in first year, annually thereafter
Zinc and copper	Annually
	Monitor zinc if unexplained anemia, hair loss, or changes in taste
	Monitor copper if unexplained anemia or poor wound healing
Vitamin A	Measure with steatorrhea and symptoms of vitamin A deficiency (*e.g.*, loss of night vision)
Vitamins E and K	Measure vitamin E if unexplained anemia, neuropathy
Selenium	Monitor if unexplained fatigue, anemia, metabolic bone disease, chronic diarrhea, or heart failure

Reproduced with permission from the British Obesity and Metabolic Surgery Society: O'Kane M, Pinkney J, Aasheim ET, et al. BOMSS Guidelines on peri-operative and postoperative biochemical monitoring and micro-nutrient replacement for patients undergoing bariatric surgery, 2014. Accessible at http://www.bomss.org.uk/wp-content/uploads/2014/09/BOMSS-guidelines-Final-version1Oct14.pdf.
Abbreviations: FBC, full blood count; FBG, fasting blood glucose; PTH, parathyroid hormone.

Surveillance Post-RYGB

Patients must be monitored lifelong after bariatric surgery for nutritional micronutrient deficiencies. The type and frequency of biochemical monitoring depends on the bariatric procedure, although this may need to be individualized. Table 2 shows the routine blood tests required post-RYGB ad SG and the frequency of monitoring (3).

Conclusions

Micro/macronutrient deficiencies after RYGB are common and can lead to considerable comorbidity postoperatively unless treated with adequate nutritional replacement. Most obesity physicians must be able to identify and treat these deficiencies and ensure lifelong nutritional monitoring for these patients.

CASE STUDIES

Case 1

A 50-year-old woman presented to the obesity clinic for a consultation. She had undergone a gastric bypass 25 years previously but had not been under formal follow-up. She had lost 71 kg since her operation (158 kg preoperative weight). She had not been taking multivitamins since her operation or other medications. She complained of low energy levels, poor night vision, visual disturbances, and poor memory. She experienced pins and needles in her hands and feet and had sustained two fractures. She had been assessed by several neurologists who had not found a cause for her symptoms of neuropathy. Many health care practitioners believed that there was a psychological component to her symptoms.

In the obesity clinic, the patient was tested for nutritional deficiencies and found to be severely deficient in vitamins A, D, and E; zinc; copper; iron; vitamin B12; and thiamine. She was prescribed multivitamins A to Z, vitamin A (25,000 IU orally for 2 weeks), iron infusions, vitamin B12 injections, and calcium and vitamin D. Her energy levels, neuropathy, and night vision were markedly improved within 1 month of starting treatment.

Discussion

Vitamin A

Vitamin A is a fat-soluble vitamin stored in the liver. It plays an important role in immunological activity and visual acuity. Vitamin A deficiency occurs more commonly after a malabsorptive procedure, such as biliopancreatic diversion where deficiencies of up to 69% have been reported, with up to 11% reported for RYGB (5). Symptoms of vitamin A deficiency include loss of night vision, itching, dry hair, xerophthalmia, and decreased immunity. In severe deficiency with no corneal changes (normal, 1.05 to 2.80 μmol/L), vitamin A should be replaced with 10,000 to 25,000 IU/d or more with night blindness/corneal changes (50,000 to 100,000 IU IM for 3 days followed by 50,000 IU IM for 2 weeks and rechecked 2 to 3 months later).

Table 2. Signs and Symptoms of Macro/Micronutrient Deficiencies Post-RYGB: Suggested Supplementation and Treatment

Macro/ Micronutrient	Signs and Symptoms of Deficiency	Prevention	Treatment
Protein	Fatigue, weakness, brittle hair, peripheral edema, skin rash, recurrent infections	60 to 120 g/d	Enteral/parenteral nutrition in severe deficiency
Calcium	Low bone density, osteoporosis, paraesthesia, muscle contractions, spasms	Oral calcium 80–1200 mg/d	Bisphosphonates if T score <2.5
Magnesium	Muscle contractions, pain, spasms, paraesthesia	Sufficiently contained within multivitamin and mineral supplement	If deficient, replace with magnesium, 300 mg/d orally
Vitamin B1 (thiamine)	Early: anorexia, gait ataxia, paraesthesia, muscle cramps, irritability, memory and concentration problems	Sufficiently contained within multivitamin and mineral supplement	Prolonged vomiting: 200–300 mg/d
	WE (ataxia, ophthalmoplegia, and confusion).		WE: 500 mg/d for 3–5 d followed by 250 mg IV for 3–5 d followed by 100 mg/d until symptoms resolve
	Dry beriberi: convulsions, muscle weakness, pain of lower and upper extremities		
	Wet beriberi: tachycardia or bradycardia, lactic acidosis, dyspnea, leg edema, right ventricular dilatation		
Vitamin B12 (cobalamin)	Macrocytic anemia, pernicious anemia, tingling in fingers and toes, dementia, ataxia, irreversible neuropathy	1000 μg IM every 3 mo	1000–2000 μg/d orally or 1000 μg/wk IM
Folic acid	Macrocytic anemia, palpitations, fatigue, neural tube defects	Sufficiently contained within multivitamin and mineral supplement	1 mg/d for 1–3 mo
		Additional folic acid 5 mg/d in pregnancy	
Vitamin A	Night blindness, itching, dry hair	Sufficiently contained within multivitamin and mineral supplement	No corneal changes: 10,000–25,000 IU/ d orally for 1–2 wk
			With corneal lesions: 50,000–100,000 IU IM for 3 d followed by 50,000 IU IM for 2 wk
Vitamin D	Arthralgia, depression, fasciculations, myalgia	3000 IU/d cholecalciferol	Severe deficiency: 50,000 U one to three times a week to daily until replete
Vitamin E	Anemia, ataxia, motor speech disorder, muscle weakness	Sufficiently contained within multivitamin and mineral supplement	100–400 IU/d
Vitamin K	Bleeding disorder	Sufficiently contained within multivitamin and mineral supplement	10 mg IV
			Chronic malabsorption: 1–2 mg/d orally or 1–2 mg/wk

(Table Continues)

TABLE 2. Signs and Symptoms of Macro/Micronutrient Deficiencies Post-RYGB: Suggested Supplementation and Treatment (Continued)

Macro/ Micronutrient	Signs and Symptoms of Deficiency	Prevention	Treatment
Iron	Microcytic anemia, fatigue, koilonychia, nail changes	45–60 mg from multivitamin and mineral supplements and additional iron supplements [200 mg ferrous sulfate, 210 mg ferrous fumarate, or 300 mg ferrous gluconate one to three times a day (at least twice a day for menstruating women)]	Ferrous sulfate, fumarate, gluconate two to three times a day
			Parenteral iron administration in severe deficiency
Zinc	Skin lesions, poor wound healing, dermatitis, infertility, hair loss, glossitis, pica	Sufficiently contained within multivitamin and mineral supplement	Oral zinc gluconate, sulfate/acetate to provide 8–15 mg elemental zinc
			1 mg copper should be given for each 8–15 mg zinc
Copper	Anemia, altered mental status, unsteady gait, numbness and tingling in hands and feet, painful paraesthesia, poor wound healing	Sufficiently contained within multivitamin and mineral supplement	Oral copper sulfate or gluconate 3–8 mg/d
			Severe deficiency: 2–4 mg/d IV for 6 d
Selenium	Chronic diarrhea, metabolic bone disorder, unexplained cardiomyopathy	Sufficiently contained within multivitamin and mineral supplement	No official recommendation; 80 μg/d orally reported

Reproduced with permission from the British Obesity and Metabolic Surgery Society: O'Kane M, Pinkney J, Aasheim ET, et al. BOMSS Guidelines on peri-operative and postoperative biochemical monitoring and micronutrient replacement for patients undergoing bariatric surgery, 2014. Accessible at http://www.bomss.org.uk/wp-content/uploads/2014/09/BOMSS-guidelines-Final-version1Oct14.pdf.

Vitamin B12

Despite existing recommendations for nutrient supplementation, vitamin B12 deficiency is still, after iron deficiency, one of the most common causes of anemia after biliopancreatic diversion or RYGB with a prevalence of 4% to 62% after 2 years and >19% to 35% after 5 years (5). Hepatic and kidney stores last up to 3 years; hence, patients can present clinically several years after surgery. Signs and symptoms of vitamin B12 include tingling in fingers and toes, dementia, and ataxia. Vitamin B12 deficiency is more common when taking certain medications, including neomycin, metformin, colchicine, proton pump inhibitors, and anticonvulsants. Measurement of methylmalonic acid is a highly sensitive and specific (98%) screening marker for vitamin B12 deficiency, allowing early detection when used in combination with measurements of active vitamin B12. Untreated vitamin B12 deficiency may result in irreversible neuropathy. Supplementation with IM injections of 1 mg vitamin B12 three times a month is recommended post-RYGB.

Symptoms of neuropathy after bariatric surgery should raise the possibility of copper; vitamin E; vitamin B1, B12, and B6; and niacin deficiencies (6). Refer to Table 1 for signs and symptoms and treatment.

Case 2

A 45-year-old woman was brought into the emergency department by her husband with symptoms of confusion, clumsiness, and vomiting. She had undergone an RYGB 6 weeks previously and had experienced intractable vomiting since the operation. She was only able to tolerate sips and soups. She weighed 140 kg preoperatively and had lost weight rapidly to 115 kg within the first week.

On examination, she was confused, dysarthric, and ataxic and displayed nystagmus. She was given intravenous (IV) dextrose to provide calories, after which the patient became drowsy. Wernicke encephalopathy (WE) was suspected, and she was started on IV thiamine replacement (500 mg thiamine IV every 8 hours for 3 days followed by 250 mg IV for 5 days and 100 mg orally). Brain magnetic resonance imaging showed changes consistent with WE. Symptoms improved within 4 weeks, although it took several months for all neurologic deficits to fully resolve.

Discussion

Thiamine

Thiamine is a water-soluble vitamin that undergoes hepatic conversion to thiamine pyrophosphate. It is an essential cofactor for >24 enzymes involved in carbohydrate metabolism and is primarily absorbed in the jejunum and proximal ileum. Mammals cannot synthesize thiamine, and total body stores last 18 to 60 days. Risk factors for deficiency in RYGB include restricted calorie intake, prolonged vomiting, rapid weight loss, and alcohol abuse. Patients can be thiamine deplete without symptoms. Deficiency can lead to WE, which is characterized by ophthalmoplegia; ataxia; neurologic changes such as confusion, apathy, and agitation; and peripheral neuropathy primarily involving the lower extremities.

In most reported cases, admission is within 6 months of surgery with frequent vomiting in 90% of cases lasting a median of 21 days (7). Magnetic resonance imaging of the brain shows characteristic changes of WE in nearly 50% of cases. There is incomplete recovery of neurologic symptoms, including memory deficits and gait difficulties, in nearly 50% of cases (7). IV glucose should be avoided because this can exacerbate thiamine deficiency and symptoms. Treatment should be with thiamine 500 mg IV for 3 to 5 days followed by 250 mg IV for 3 to 5 days, and 100 mg/d orally until symptoms resolve.

Case 3

A 58-year-old woman with a 10-year history of T2DM was referred to the bariatric service for treatment of her multiple comorbidities. She weighed 161 kg preoperatively (body mass index, 70.6 kg/m^2). She had complications of T2DM, including maculopathy, retinopathy, peripheral neuropathy, and diabetic nephropathy. She was insulin resistant and taking metformin 1 g twice a day, NPH insulin 40 U in the morning and 60 U in the evening, and insulin aspart 30 U three times a day. Glycemic control had worsened over several years, and insulin was titrated up accordingly with subsequent weight gain. She did not tolerate incretins because of nausea. Preoperatively, HbA$_{1c}$ was 10%. Other comorbidities were obstructive sleep apnea for which she was on continuous positive airway pressure, ischemic heart disease, and hypertension. The rest of her medications were aspirin, enalapril, furosemide, diltiazem, doxazosin, and atorvastatin.

Before surgery, T2DM was optimized with diet and a sodium-glucose linked transporter 2 inhibitor, which helped to reduce weight preoperatively by 5 kg and achieve a preoperative HbA$_{1c}$ of 8.5%. She underwent an RYGB that required 2 nights in the intensive care unit. Postoperatively, metformin was continued. Within 48 hours of surgery, total insulin requirements were reduced from 190 to 60 U (Insulatard, 15 U twice a day; NovoRapid, 10 U/meal), and within 6 months, total insulin requirements were reduced to 30 U/d, only requiring basal insulin. The patient lost 45 kg in weight at 6 months to 116 kg (body mass index, 50.8 kg/m^2). HbA$_{1c}$ was controlled at 6.5% 6 months postoperatively. Neuropathic pain worsened within the first few weeks of surgery but improved over time. Nephropathy improved postoperatively. Blood pressure improved to 105/60 mm Hg and furosemide and doxazosin were stopped. She was started on multivitamins, calcium and vitamin D, iron supplements, and 3-month vitamin B12 injections.

Discussion

Glycemic control in patients with T2DM should be pre-optimized before metabolic surgery. Reasonable targets for preoperative glycemic control are an HbA$_{1c}$ of ≤6.5% to 7%, a fasting blood glucose of ≤110 mg/dL, and a 2-hour postprandial blood glucose concentration of ≤140 mg/dL (4). These targets are ideal, but in patients in whom glycemic control has been more challenging to achieve, an HbA$_{1c}$ target of 7% to 8% should be the aim, with decisions to operate on patients with an HbA$_{1c}$ >8% based on clinical judgment (4).

In patients with T2DM, the use of all insulin secretagogues (sulphonylureas and meglitinides) should be discontinued, and insulin doses should be adjusted postoperatively (because of low calorie intake) to minimize the risk of hypoglycemia (4). Antidiabetic medication should be withheld postoperatively if T2DM is in remission, but metformin should be continued postoperatively until clinical and biochemical resolution of diabetes is demonstrated (4). Patients on insulin preoperatively may not require insulin postoperatively, although patients with a long duration of diabetes are more likely to need insulin after surgery. For these patients, insulin requirements will decrease substantially. From our bariatric unit, a decrease in insulin requirement to one third of the preoperative insulin dose at the time of discharge has been seen. For patients who do not reach adequate glycemic targets, metformin alongside incretin-based therapies should be considered, although currently, little evidence supports the use of incretins postoperatively (unpublished data).

REFERENCES

1. Ernst B, Thurnheer M, Schmid SM, Schultes B. Evidence for the necessity to systematically assess micronutrient status prior to bariatric surgery. *Obes Surg.* 2009;**19**(1):66–73.
2. Gudzune KA, Huizinga MM, Chang HY, Asamoah V, Gadgil M, Clark JM. Screening and diagnosis of micronutrient deficiencies before and after bariatric surgery. *Obes Surg.* 2013;**23**(10):1581–1589.
3. O'Kane M, Pinkney J, Aasheim E, Barth J, Batterham R, Welbourn R. BOMSS Guidelines on peri-operative and postoperative biochemical monitoring and micronutrient replacement for patients undergoing bariatric surgery, 2014. Available at http://www.bomss.org.uk/wp-content/uploads/2014/09/BOMSS-guidelines-Final-version1Oct14.pdf. Accessed 4 October 2017.
4. Mechanick JI, Youdim A, Jones DB, Garvey WT, Hurley DL, McMahon MM, Heinberg LJ, Kushner R, Adams TD, Shikora S, Dixon JB, Brethauer S; American Association of Clinical Endocrinologists; Obesity Society; American Society for Metabolic & Bariatric Surgery. Clinical practice guidelines for the perioperative nutritional, metabolic, and nonsurgical support of the bariatric surgery patient–2013 update: cosponsored by American Association of Clinical Endocrinologists, the Obesity Society, and American Society for Metabolic & Bariatric Surgery. *Obesity (Silver Spring).* 2013; **21** (Suppl 1): S1–S27.
5. Stein J, Stier C, Raab H, Weiner R. Review article: the nutritional and pharmacological consequences of obesity surgery. *Aliment Pharmacol Ther.* 2014;**40**(6):582–609.
6. Parrish C. Severe micronutrient deficiencies in RYGB patients: rare but potentially devastating. *Pract Gastroenterol.* 2011;**100**:13–27.
7. Aasheim ET. Wernicke encephalopathy after bariatric surgery: a systematic review. *Ann Surg.* 2008;**248**(5):714–720.

ADRENAL

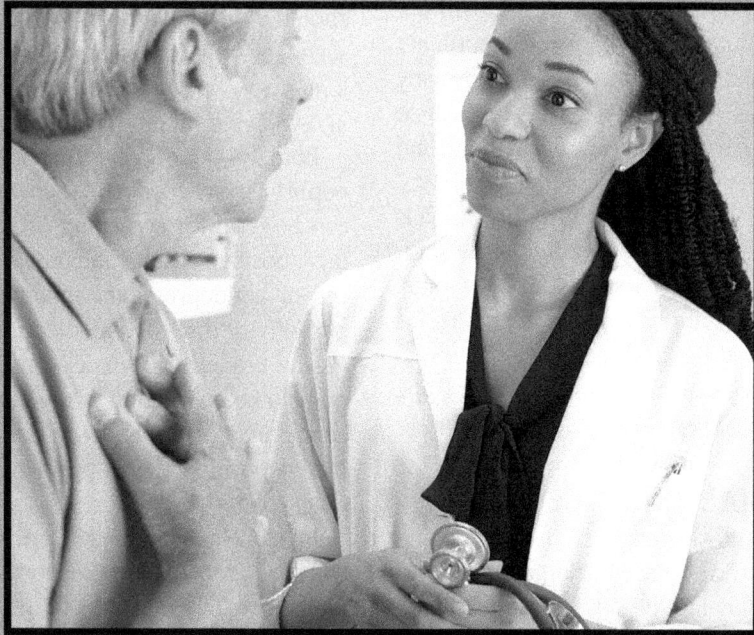

Pheochromocytomas and Paragangliomas

M12
Presented, March 17–20, 2018

Lauren Fishbein, MD, PhD. Department of Medicine, Division of Endocrinology, Metabolism and Diabetes, University of Colorado School of Medicine, Aurora, Colorado 80045, E-mail: lauren.fishbein@ucdenver.edu

SIGNIFICANCE OF THE CLINICAL PROBLEM

Pheochromocytomas (PCCs) and paragangliomas (PGLs) are tumors of the autonomic nervous system that develop within the adrenal medulla (PCC) or at extra-adrenal ganglia (PGL) throughout the body. PCCs/PGLs have high morbidity and mortality if left undiagnosed or untreated. The hypersecretion of catecholamines and metanephrines can lead to hypertension, heart disease, and even death. PCCs/PGLs can be sporadic or inherited. In fact, PCCs/PGLs have the highest degree of heritability of any solid tumor type, with up to 35% to 40% of patients having a germline mutation in a known susceptibility gene and up to 80% of children (1, 2). Despite this, many patients are not referred for clinical genetic testing, which can negatively impact the surveillance for the patient and screening for family members who may be mutation carriers. Up to 20% to 25% of PCCs/PGLs become metastatic, which is defined as evidence of disease in nonchromaffin tissue sites, and metastases can occur even 20 years or more after initial diagnosis. Unfortunately, there are no curative therapies for widely metastatic disease, and the 5-year survival is 50% to 69% (3–5). We have no reliable predictors for metastatic spread; therefore, all patients need lifelong surveillance.

BARRIERS TO OPTIMAL PRACTICE

There are several barriers and challenges to diagnosing and treating patients with PCCs/PGLs. Recognizing and diagnosing the tumor can be challenging, because symptoms vary widely between patients and can mimic many other conditions, and the diagnostic tests can be associated with a high amount of indeterminate results. Referrals for clinical genetic testing are often limited by the perceived expectation of high out-of-pocket expense. However, most genetic testing will be covered by insurance, and knowing the presence of a germline susceptibility gene mutation impacts the surveillance for additional primary PCCs/PGLs, metastatic disease, and other associated tumor types of the patient and his/her family members. Diagnosing and treating metastatic disease can be difficult. There are many imaging options for diagnosis metastatic disease, each with limitations, and unfortunately, there currently are no curative treatments for patients with metastatic PCC/PGL.

LEARNING OBJECTIVES

As a result of participation in this session, learners should be able to:

- Interpret biochemical results to diagnosis PCC/PGL
- Discuss the importance of clinical genetic testing for patients with PCC/PGL
- Evaluate the different imaging options for diagnosing primary and metastatic PCC/PGL

STRATEGIES FOR DIAGNOSIS, THERAPY, AND/OR MANAGEMENT

PCCs/PGLs are known as a "zebra" diagnosis, because they can be difficult to identify. The classic triad of headaches, palpitations, and diaphoresis occurs only in a subset of patients, and these symptoms also overlap with many other more common clinical conditions. Some patients with PCC/PGL can have only atypical symptoms and signs, including, for example, weight changes and hyperglycemia, which make the diagnosis even more difficult. Screening for PCC/PGL also should occur as part of a workup for patients with suspected secondary hypertension, patients with an adrenal incidentaloma (with or without hypertension) (6), and patients with a known susceptibility gene mutation (7) (Table 1).

Both 24-hour urine-fractionated and plasma free metanephrines have over 90% sensitivity for PCC/PGL, and either can be used for screening (8). Many medications can cause false positive results, including acetaminophen, several classes of antidepressants/antianxiolytics, attention deficit hyperactivity disorder medications (stimulants), and certain β- and α-adrenergic blockers (8). These medications should be held before testing. If the medications cannot be stopped, especially for psychotropic medications, and the plasma metanephrine screen is positive, it is appropriate to move on to imaging studies.

Imaging should be performed after a true positive biochemical screen. Cross-sectional imaging with computed tomography (CT) or magnetic resonance imaging (MRI) is the most cost-effective test to pick up primary PCC/PGL. Abdominal imaging is the first place to start, because the vast majority of tumors are in the adrenal gland; ~25% of tumors will be located outside of the adrenal gland, and therefore, if no adrenal mass is seen and clinical suspicion for PCC/PGL is high, imaging of other locations should be done (pelvis, neck, or chest), especially for known susceptibility gene mutation carriers (Table 1).

Functional imaging is not considered the first line to diagnose primary PCC/PGL because of increased cost and radiation exposure. In addition, there are limitations to some of the functional imaging modalities. Nevertheless, functional imaging studies are very helpful in certain circumstances. ^{123}I-metaiodobenzylguanidine (MIBG) is not recommended as the first line, because up to 50% of normal adrenal glands have

Table 1. PCC and PGL Susceptibility Genes

Gene	Syndrome	Tumor Location	Malignancy Rate	Other Associated Tumors
NF1	Neurofibromatosis type 1	Adrenal (bilateral)	12%	Neurofibromas, malignant peripheral nerve sheath tumors, optic gliomas, leukemia
RET	Multiple endocrine neoplasia type 2	Adrenal (bilateral)	<5%	Medullary thyroid cancer, parathyroid adenomas
VHL	von Hippel Lindau	Adrenal (bilateral)	5%	Renal cell carcinoma, pancreatic neuroendocrine tumors, hemangioblastomas, endolymphatic sac tumors
SDHA	Hereditary PGL syndrome	Any location	Possibly intermediate	Renal cell carcinoma, GI stromal tumors
SDHB	Hereditary PGL syndrome	Any location, primarily extra-adrenal	23%	Renal cell carcinoma, GI stromal tumors
SDHC	Hereditary PGL syndrome	Head and neck, can be thoracic	Low	Renal cell carcinoma, GI stromal tumors
SDHD	Hereditary PGL syndrome	Any location, primarily head and neck	<5%	Renal cell carcinoma, GI stromal tumors
SDHAF2 (SHD5)	Hereditary PGL syndrome	Head and neck (multifocal)	Low	Renal cell carcinoma, GI stromal tumors
TMEM127	Familial PGL syndrome	Any location, primarily adrenal	Low	Renal cell carcinoma
MAX	Familial PGL syndrome	Adrenal (bilateral)	Intermediate to high	
EPAS1	Polycythemia PGL syndrome	Any location	Not known	Somatostatinoma
FH	Hereditary leiomyomatosis and renal cell carcinoma	Any location	Possibly high	Cutaneous and uterine leiomyomas, papillary renal cell carcinoma (may have no overlap when PCC/PGL present)
MDH2		Any location	Not known	

Abbreviations: *SDHA, Succinate Dehydrogenase Subunit A*; *SDHB, Succinate Dehydrogenase Subunit B*; *SDHC, Succinate Dehydrogenase Subunit C*; *SDHD, Succinate Dehydrogenase Subunit D*; *SDHAF2* (*SDH5*) *Succinate Dehydrogenase Subunit AF2* (*Succinate Dehydrogenase 5*); GI, gastrointestinal.

increased physiologic uptake, which can lead to false positive results, and up to 60% of PCCs/PGLs are not MIBG avid (9). ^{123}I-MIBG scans can be useful when confirming primary PCC/PGL in the setting of a known mass and indeterminate biochemical results and when considering ^{131}I-MIBG therapy for metastatic PCC/PGL. ^{18}F-fludeoxyglucose (FDG) positron emission tomography (PET)/CT is recommended for diagnosis of metastatic disease, especially for patients with an inherited *Succinate Dehydrogenase Subunit B* (*SDHB*) mutation, because the sensitivity of PET imaging is 74% to 100% (8). Newer functional imaging tests, such as the ^{68}Ga-DOTATATE PET/CT scan, also can be useful for diagnosing metastatic disease. This technique takes advantage of the expression of the Somatostatin Receptor Subtype 2 on many neuroendocrine tissues, because the ^{68}Ga-DOTATATE is a somatostatin analog with a linker to the gallium-68 radionucleotide (10). This imaging modality can be highly sensitive and specific for neuroendocrine tumors as long as the tumor is not dedifferentiated. In the near future, peptide receptor radionucleotide therapy with ^{177}Lu-DOTATATE may be a potential therapeutic option for patients with metastatic PCC/PGL who have avid disease on ^{68}Ga-DOTATATE PET/CT scans. Clinical trials have shown efficacy of this therapy for metastatic gastrointestinal enteropancreatic neuroendocrine tumors, and trials are underway in patients with metastatic PCC/PGL.

A perioperative medical blockade and an experienced anesthesiologist are necessary to reduce morbidity and mortality with surgery in patients with PCC/PGL. The Endocrine Society guidelines (8) recommend phenoxybenzamine, a nonselective, noncompetitive α-blocker, as the first-line treatment and doxazosin, prazosin, or terazosin (competitive selective α1-blockers) with or without a calcium channel blocker as second-line treatment (Table 2). The largest study comparing phenoxybenzamine with competitive selective α1-blockers is retrospective, and it showed that pheonxybenzamine achieved better preoperative and intraoperative blood pressure control but that it was associated with more transient postoperative hypotension, consistent with the mechanism of action of the different medications (11). Metyrosine, a tyrosine hydroxylase inhibitor, may be useful in patients with very high catecholamine production and underlying cardiovascular disease (12). Complete α-blockade usually induces tachycardia and orthostatic hypotension, which should be treated with β-blockade and hydration with high salt intake. Beta-blockers alone can induce a theoretical unopposed α-adrenergic stimulation, leading to a hypertensive crisis, and should not be used until the patient is fully α-blocked. Patients should be screened with plasma metanephrines 4 to 8 weeks postoperatively to ensure complete resection and then annually for life given the potential for additional primary tumors and the long latency of metastatic disease.

Metastatic PCC/PGL is defined by the presence of distant metastases at nonchromaffin tissue sites and occurs in about 10% of PCCs and 20% of PGLs (5). Metastases can occur even 20 years or more after the initial diagnosis, and when present, patients have a 50% to 69% 5-year survival (3–5). Predicting who will develop metastatic disease has proven difficult. There is an increased risk in patients with a germline *SDHB* mutation, but only one-half of patients with metastatic disease have a mutation in this gene (13). Other predictors of metastases include extra-adrenal location, tumor size >4 to 5 cm, and secretion of methyoxytyramine (not yet clinically available in most centers) (5, 14). Pathologic scoring systems of the primary tumor have not been a reliable method to predict metastatic potential given wide inter- and intraobserver variability (15, 16). Therefore, lifelong annual screening with at least plasma metanephrines is recommended for any patient who had a PCC/PGL. Treatments for metastatic disease, such as surgical debulking, chemotherapy with cyclophosphamide, vincristine, and dacarbazine, external beam radiation therapy, or ^{131}I-MIBG treatment, can offer disease control, although they are usually not curative (7). Tyrosine kinase inhibitors are being tested in clinical trials but thus far, show limited efficacy (17, 18). As mentioned above, peptide receptor radionucleotide therapy is also under clinical investigation for patients with metastatic PCC/PGL.

Numerous genes have been associated with an increased risk of PCC/PGL (Table 1) (1). Mutations in three classic tumor suppressor genes, including *NF1*, *VHL*, and *RET*, increase risk of PCC/PGL, leading to Neurofibromatosis type 1, von Hippel Lindau disease, and Multiple Endocrine Neoplasia Type 2, respectively. Mutations in any of the *SDH* genes (*SDHA*, *-B*, *-C*, and *-D*) and the cofactor gene *AF2* are associated with increased risk of PCC/PGL. *SDHx* mutations also increase risk of gastrointestinal stromal tumors and renal cell carcinomas, and they are possibly associated with pituitary adenomas and other tumor types. *SDHB* is the only subunit that carries an increased risk of malignancy, likely around 23% risk in patients who have had a PCC/PGL. Additional genes have been associated with PCC/PGL at a much lower frequency, including *TMEM127*, *MAX*, *EPAS1*, *FH*, and *MDH2* (Table 1). All of the susceptibility gene mutations, except for *EPAS1*, are inherited in an autosomal dominant pattern, meaning that offspring have a 50% chance of inheriting the mutation. *EPAS1* mutations tend to be somatic mosaic. *SDHD* and *SDHAF2* mutations have paternal inheritance, which can complicate the family history taking. One ongoing area of research is to define the penetrance of these mutations in unaffected

Table 2. Perioperative Blockade Medications

Category	Drug	Typical Dosing for PCC/PGL	Common Side Effects
Nonselective, noncompetitive α-blocker	Phenoxybenzamine	10–30 mg given two to three times per day	Orthostatic hypotension, tachycardia, nasal congestion
Selective α1-competitive blocker	Doxazosin	1–16 mg given once day	Orthostatic hypotension, tachycardia
	Prazosin	1–5 mg given two to three times per day	
	Terazosin	1–5 mg given one to two times per daily	
Second-line calcium channel blocker	Nicardipine	30–60 mg two times per day	Edema, headache
	Amlodipine	5–10 mg once daily	
Beta-blocker only after full α-blockade	Metoprolol	25–100 mg given two times per day	Fatigue, dizziness, asthma exacerbation
	Atenolol	25–50 mg given once daily	
Tyrosine hydroxylase inhibitor	Metyrosine	250–500 mg given two to four times per day	Fatigue, dizziness, nausea, vomiting, diarrhea, extrapyramidal side effects

mutation carriers. Initial studies suggested that penetrance for all gene mutations was quite high, but these studies were biased by including index patients. When cohorts exclude index patients, penetrance is often lower than previously appreciated (19).

MAIN CONCLUSIONS

When undiagnosed, PCCs/PGLs carry high morbidity and mortality because of the oversecretion of catecholamines. False positive screening is usually attributed to the presence of an interfering medication, drug, or supplement. Cross-sectional imaging is the most effective tool to find primary PCC/PGL. Functional imaging should be reserved, in most cases, for diagnosis and treatment planning for metastatic disease. Blood pressure management with α-blockade and an experienced anesthesiologist is critical before any surgical procedure. Because 35% to 40% of patients (and 80% of children) with PCC/PGL have a germline mutation in a known susceptibility gene, all patients with PCC/PGL, regardless of family history, should be referred for clinical genetic testing given the implications for the patient and the family members.

CASES

Case 1

A 35-year-old woman with a past medical history of hypothyroidism on levothyroxine presents for evaluation of palpitations and diaphoresis. She also notes increased irritability. Palpitations occur several times a day and last for a few minutes, and they are associated with diaphoresis and sometimes a feeling of not being able to catch her breath. She does not have headaches. She had a recent Holter monitor showing some episodes of sinus tachycardia and a chest CT scan, which showed a homogeneous 1 cm right adrenal nodule with Hounsfield unit (HU) of eight. Aside from the levothyroxine, she takes no other medications except for a few vitamins and supplements from the health food store. There is no known relevant family history. Examination was notable for blood pressure 135/90 mm Hg, heart rate 97 bpm, body mass index 25 kg/m^2, and a mild tremor in her outstretched hands bilaterally. Laboratories show normal thyroid stimulating hormone of 1.9 mIU/mL (normal range 0.5 to 4.5), normal aldosterone/plasma renin activity ratio of 11.4, normal plasma metanephrine (0.25 nmol/L; normal range 0 to 0.49), and elevated plasma normetanephrine (1.35 nmol/L; normal range 0 to 0.89).

Does this woman have a PCC?

Case 2

A 40-year-old man with a past medical history of hypertension for 10 years controlled on two medications presented to his primary care provider, because he was not feeling well and was losing weight. He had a CT scan of the abdomen, which showed a 7-cm retroperitoneal mass. During a biopsy of this lesion, he had a hypertensive crisis and was admitted for observation overnight in the hospital. Pathology showed a PGL. Follow-up 24-hour urinary free metanephrines and catecholamines were checked, and they were >10 times the upper limit of normal, consistent with the diagnosis of a PGL.

What perioperative blockade regimen is best for patients with PCC or PGL? What are the next best steps in following this patient after surgery?

Case 3

A 15-year-old woman with a past medical history of allergic rhinitis presents with a neck mass that did not resolve after a course of antibiotics. Her medical history is notable for her father having an *SDHD* mutation. MRI of her neck revealed a 2-cm carotid body tumor. She is tested for the familial *SDHD* mutation, and she is positive. After discussion, she and her family have elected for surgical resection.

What is the best next step in the care of this patient with a known *SDHD* mutation and carotid body PGL?

DISCUSSION OF CASES AND ANSWERS

Case 1

Does this woman have a PCC?

This patient has some of the classic symptoms and signs of PCC, including palpitations, diaphoresis, and borderline hypertension and tachycardia, making it appropriate to test for the diagnosis. The plasma normetanephrine level returned elevated, which could suggest possible disease, but the results are in the indeterminate range (less than even two times the upper limit of normal for plasma tests). The first thing to check is the list of possible interfering medications, herbs, and supplements that the patient is taking. One supplement that the patient was taking for the last 6 months was an energy booster from the health food store. When the ingredients were investigated, the supplement was found to contain, among other things, cow adrenal gland. This patient agreed to retest after refraining from this supplement for 1 month. The subsequent levels of plasma metanephrines returned normal, and her symptoms resolved.

The adrenal nodule in this case is likely a benign nonfunctioning adrenal cortical adenoma given the small size and the low HU. The precontrast HU on CT scan can be helpful in the differential diagnosis, with low HU under 10 suggesting a benign cortical adenoma. Rapid washout (>50%) on an adrenal protocol CT scan can be suggestive of benign cortical adenomas. MRI showing loss of signal intensity on out-of-phase imaging is suggestive of benign cortical adenomas as well. However, PCCs typically have high HU over 10 on precontrast CT scans, have delayed washout <50% on adrenal protocol CT scans, and maintain signal intensity on out-of-phase imaging on MRI.

Case 2

What perioperative blockade regimen is best for patients with PCC or PGL?

Perioperative α-blockade is critical before any procedure in patients with primary PCC/PGL or metastatic PCC/PGL. The Endocrine Society guidelines (8) recommend first-line therapy with phenoxybenzamine along with hydration and salt loading to help orthostatic hypotension. β-Blockade can be used as needed to treat any tachycardia after full α-blockade is achieved. Most blockades should occur over a 7- to 14-day period before surgery to allow for slow titration of medication to avoid substantial side effects.

What are the next best steps in following this patient after surgery?

All patients with secreting PCC/PGL should have plasma or urine metanephrines checked within 4 to 8 weeks after the operation to ensure complete resection and then annually for life to screen for metastatic disease or additional primary tumors. Because 35% to 40% of patients with PCC/PGL have a mutation in a known germline susceptibility gene, all patients should be referred for clinical genetic testing, because it will affect the screening and surveillance for the patient and any family member with the inherited mutation. Mutation carriers are at higher risk for additional primary PCC/PGL and other associated tumors depending on the syndrome (Table 1). In addition, patients with an *SDHB* mutation are at increased risk of developing malignancy.

Clinical genetic testing showed that this patient carried an *SDHB* mutation as did his 12-year-old daughter. Even if genetic testing could not be performed, this patient has several risk factors for developing metastatic disease, including his young age, the extra-adrenal location, and tumor size over 4 to 5 cm, and he should be followed closely. There are no formal guidelines for following adult *SDHx* mutation carriers, but most experts recommend at least annual biochemical testing and cross-sectional imaging studies of the neck/chest/abdomen/pelvis every 2 years (1). His daughter was screened annually with plasma metanephrines and every 2 years with catecholamines, complete blood count, and full-body MRI per guidelines (20). Unfortunately, 2 years postoperative, the patient developed shoulder pain, and imaging showed a sclerotic lesion in the left scapula. The ^{18}F-FDG PET/CT scan showed multiple bony lesions, and these were found to be ^{123}I-MIBG avid. He was treated with external beam radiotherapy to the scapular lesion for pain control and treated systemically with ^{131}I-MIBG therapy.

Case 3

What is the best next step in the care of this patient with a known *SDHD* mutation and carotid body PGL?

The best first step for this patient is to have screening plasma metanephrines testing. Although most head and neck PGLs are nonsecretory, *SDHD* mutation carriers can develop PCCs/PGLs in any location in the body, and these can be secreting. Before surgery, she needs to be ruled out for a secreting PCC/PGL.

The patient was screened and in fact, had elevated plasma normetanephrine (13.96 nmol/L; normal range 0 to 0.89) and normal plasma metanephrine (0.36 nmol/L; normal range 0 to 0.49). She then had full-body imaging with CT scans of the chest/abdomen/pelvis and was found to have two periaortic masses: 1.9 and 2.5 cm. Given some concern for metastatic disease versus multiple primary tumors, she had an ^{18}F-FDG PET/CT scan, which showed only the three known masses (two abdominal and one carotid body). She was treated with an α-blockade and had resection of the periaortic PGLs. Postoperative, plasma normetanephrine normalized. After recovering, she had surgical resection of the carotid body PGL.

SDHD mutations are autosomal dominant with a paternal inheritance. The daughter's risk of being a mutation carrier even before her symptoms began was 50%, because one of her parents has the mutation; as a mutation carrier, she was at high risk of developing PCC/PGL because of the paternal inheritance (she inherited the mutation from her father). If this patient has biological children in the future, assuming that her partner is unaffected, each child will have a 50% chance of inheriting the mutated *SDHD* allele. Nevertheless, her children would most likely not be at risk for developing PCC/PGL, because the *SDHD* mutations are associated with PCC/PGL only when paternally inherited (with extremely rare exception). However, any of her affected children still would have a 50% chance of passing it along to their children.

REFERENCES

1. Favier J, Amar L, Gimenez-Roqueplo AP. Paraganglioma and phaeochromocytoma: from genetics to personalized medicine. *Nat Rev Endocrinol.* 2015;**11**(2):101–111.
2. Bausch B, Wellner U, Bausch D, Schiavi F, Barontini M, Sanso G, Walz MK, Peczkowska M, Weryha G, Dall'igna P, Cecchetto G, Bisogno G, Moeller LC, Bockenhauer D, Patocs A, Rácz K, Zabolotnyi D, Yaremchuk S, Dzivite-Krisane I, Castinetti F, Taieb D, Malinoc A, von Dobschuetz E, Roessler J, Schmid KW, Opocher G, Eng C, Neumann HP. Long-term prognosis of patients with pediatric pheochromocytoma. *Endocr Relat Cancer.* 2013;**21**(1):17–25.
3. Fishbein L, Ben-Maimon S, Keefe S, Cengel K, Pryma DA, Loaiza-Bonilla A, Fraker DL, Nathanson KL, Cohen DL. SDHB mutation carriers with malignant pheochromocytoma respond better to CVD. *Endocr Relat Cancer.* 2017;**24**(8):L51–L55.
4. Asai S, Katabami T, Tsuiki M, Tanaka Y, Naruse M. Controlling tumor progression with cyclophosphamide, vincristine, and dacarbazine treatment improves survival in patients with metastatic and unresectable malignant pheochromocytomas/paragangliomas. *Horm Cancer.* 2017;**8**(2):108–118.
5. Ayala-Ramirez M, Feng L, Johnson MM, Ejaz S, Habra MA, Rich T, Busaidy N, Cote GJ, Perrier N, Phan A, Patel S, Waguespack S, Jimenez C. Clinical risk factors for malignancy and overall survival in patients with pheochromocytomas and sympathetic paragangliomas: primary tumor size and primary tumor location as prognostic indicators. *J Clin Endocrinol Metab.* 2011;**96**(3):717–725.
6. Zeiger MA, Thompson GB, Duh QY, Hamrahian AH, Angelos P, Elaraj D, Fishman E, Kharlip J; American Association of Clinical Endocrinologists; American Association of Endocrine Surgeons. The American Association of Clinical Endocrinologists and American Association of Endocrine Surgeons medical guidelines for the management of adrenal incidentalomas. *Endocr Pract.* 2009;**15**(Suppl 1):1–20.

7. Fishbein L. Pheochromocytoma and paraganglioma: genetics, diagnosis, and treatment. *Hematol Oncol Clin North Am.* 2016;**30**(1): 135–150.
8. Lenders JW, Duh QY, Eisenhofer G, Gimenez-Roqueplo AP, Grebe SK, Murad MH, Naruse M, Pacak K, Young WF Jr; Endocrine Society. Pheochromocytoma and paraganglioma: an endocrine society clinical practice guideline. *J Clin Endocrinol Metab.* 2014;**99**(6):1915–1942.
9. Mozley PD, Kim CK, Mohsin J, Jatlow A, Gosfield E III, Alavi A. The efficacy of iodine-123-MIBG as a screening test for pheochromocytoma. *J Nucl Med.* 1994;**35**(7):1138–1144.
10. Chang CA, Pattison DA, Tothill RW, Kong G, Akhurst TJ, Hicks RJ, Hofman MS. (68)Ga-DOTATATE and (18)F-FDG PET/CT in paraganglioma and pheochromocytoma: utility, patterns and heterogeneity. *Cancer Imaging.* 2016;**16**(1):22.
11. Weingarten TN, Cata JP, O'Hara JF, Prybilla DJ, Pike TL, Thompson GB, Grant CS, Warner DO, Bravo E, Sprung J. Comparison of two preoperative medical management strategies for laparoscopic resection of pheochromocytoma. *Urology.* 2010;**76**(2):508.e6–508.e11.
12. Wachtel H, Kennedy EH, Zaheer S, Bartlett EK, Fishbein L, Roses RE, Fraker DL, Cohen DL. Preoperative metyrosine improves cardiovascular outcomes for patients undergoing surgery for pheochromocytoma and paraganglioma. *Ann Surg Oncol.* 2015;**22**(Suppl 3):S646–S654.
13. Fishbein L, Merrill S, Fraker DL, Cohen DL, Nathanson KL. Inherited mutations in pheochromocytoma and paraganglioma: why all patients should be offered genetic testing. *Ann Surg Oncol.* 2013;**20**(5): 1444–1450.
14. Eisenhofer G, Lenders JW, Siegert G, Bornstein SR, Friberg P, Milosevic D, Mannelli M, Linehan WM, Adams K, Timmers HJ, Pacak K. Plasma methoxytyramine: a novel biomarker of metastatic pheochromocytoma and paraganglioma in relation to established risk factors of tumour size, location and SDHB mutation status. *Eur J Cancer.* 2012;**48**(11): 1739–1749.
15. Thompson LD. Pheochromocytoma of the Adrenal gland Scaled Score (PASS) to separate benign from malignant neoplasms: a clinicopathologic and immunophenotypic study of 100 cases. *Am J Surg Pathol.* 2002; **26**(5):551–566.
16. Wu D, Tischler AS, Lloyd RV, DeLellis RA, de Krijger R, van Nederveen F, Nosé V. Observer variation in the application of the pheochromocytoma of the adrenal gland scaled score. *Am J Surg Pathol.* 2009; **33**(4):599–608.
17. Ayala-Ramirez M, Chougnet CN, Habra MA, Palmer JL, Leboulleux S, Cabanillas ME, Caramella C, Anderson P, Al Ghuzlan A, Waguespack SG, Deandreis D, Baudin E, Jimenez C. Treatment with sunitinib for patients with progressive metastatic pheochromocytomas and sympathetic paragangliomas. *J Clin Endocrinol Metab.* 2012;**97**(11): 4040–4050.
18. Jasim S, Suman VJ, Jimenez C, Harris P, Sideras K, Burton JK, Worden FP, Auchus RJ, Bible KC. Phase II trial of pazopanib in advanced/ progressive malignant pheochromocytoma and paraganglioma. *Endocrine.* 2017;**57**(2):220–225.
19. Bausch B, Schiavi F, Ni Y, Welander J, Patocs A, Ngeow J, Wellner U, Malinoc A, Taschin E, Barbon G, Lanza V, Söderkvist P, Stenman A, Larsson C, Svahn F, Chen JL, Marquard J, Fraenkel M, Walter MA, Peczkowska M, Prejbisz A, Jarzab B, Hasse-Lazar K, Petersenn S, Moeller LC, Meyer A, Reisch N, Trupka A, Brase C, Galiano M, Preuss SF, Kwok P, Lendvai N, Berisha G, Makay O, Boedeker CC, Weryha G, Racz K, Januszewicz A, Walz MK, Gimm O, Opocher G, Eng C, Neumann HPH; European-American-Asian Pheochromocytoma-Paraganglioma Registry Study Group. Clinical characterization of the pheochromocytoma and paraganglioma susceptibility genes SDHA, TMEM127, MAX, and SDHAF2 for gene-informed prevention. *JAMA Oncol.* 2017; **3**(9):1204–1212.
20. Rednam SP, Erez A, Druker H, Janeway KA, Kamihara J, Kohlmann WK, Nathanson KL, States LJ, Tomlinson GE, Villani A, Voss SD, Schiffman JD, Wasserman JD. Von Hippel-Lindau and hereditary pheochromocytoma/paraganglioma syndromes: clinical features, genetics, and surveillance recommendations in childhood. *Clin Cancer Res.* 2017;**23**(12):e68–e75.

Diagnosis and Treatment of Subclinical Cushing: Who, Why, and How?

M14
Presented, March 17–20, 2018

Irina Bancos, MD. Division of Endocrinology, Metabolism and Nutrition, Mayo Clinic, Rochester, Minnesota 55905, E-mail: bancos.irina@mayo.edu

Antoine Tabarin, MD. Division of Endocrinology and Nutrition, Centre Hospitalier Universitaire Haut Leveque, University of Bordeaux, Bordeaux 33604, France, E-mail: antoine.tabarin@chu-bordeaux.fr

SIGNIFICANCE OF THE CLINICAL PROBLEM

Cushing syndrome is rare and morbid condition (1). It is well established that overt Cushing syndrome is responsible for increased morbidity and mortality (2, 3). Subclinical Cushing syndrome is a misnomer that usually describes a state of autonomous adrenal cortisol secretion resulting in a mild or very mild cortisol excess (mild autonomous cortisol excess [MACE]). Patients with MACE lack physical features of overt Cushing syndrome (*e.g.*, striae, proximal myopathy, and supraclavicular and dorsocervical fat pads) but present with higher rates of metabolic disturbances, osteoporosis and vertebral fractures, and cardiovascular morbidity and mortality (4–6). At this time, MACE is a biochemical diagnosis with multiple combinations of tests assessing the hypothalamic-adrenal (HPA) axis described in the literature and used in practice (5). In endocrinology clinics, MACE is diagnosed in ~15% of patients incidentally discovered with either unilateral or bilateral adrenal tumors (7, 8). Moreover, with active case detection testing, 3% of patients with type 2 diabetes mellitus may be diagnosed with MACE (9, 10).

Endocrinologists face several dilemmas in regard to MACE:

- Who is a candidate for biochemical case detection? What diagnostic tests should be used?
- Among patients with MACE, who are the individuals benefiting from therapeutic intervention (and what is the degree of expected improvement)?
- What is the monitoring approach in patients with MACE who do not undergo surgery?

BARRIERS TO OPTIMAL PRACTICE

- MACE-induced clinical consequences (*e.g.*, obesity, type 2 diabetes mellitus, hypertension, osteoporosis) are common in the general population, but the contribution of MACE is unclear
- Interpretation of biochemical results assessing HPA axis in view of suboptimal assay performance and individual-related factors
- Methodological caveats in studies evaluating the benefits of surgery in adrenal tumors with MACE (small sample size, selection bias, heterogeneity in biochemical and clinical assessments)
- Remaining uncertainties about the natural history of MACE
- Lack of prospective randomized trials evaluating the benefits and harms of adrenalectomy vs aggressive nonsurgical management in patients with MACE

LEARNING OBJECTIVES

As a result of participating in this session, attendees should be able to:

- Appropriately select patients for biochemical case detection of MACE
- Be aware of the limitations in biochemical case detection for Cushing syndrome in patients with type 2 diabetes
- Organize a stepwise evaluation of patients with adrenal tumors to detect MACE according to the international guidelines for management of adrenal incidentalomas
- Describe the evidence on outcomes of adrenalectomy in patients with unilateral or bilateral adrenal tumors associated with MACE
- Organize appropriate longitudinal follow-up of patients with adrenal tumors and MACE not undergoing adrenalectomy

STRATEGIES FOR DIAGNOSIS, THERAPY, AND MANAGEMENT

What Is MACE?

Widely known as and still erroneously called subclinical Cushing syndrome, MACE is a biochemical diagnosis referring to demonstration of abnormal tests for assessment of the HPA axis. Patients with MACE lack classical physical features of overt Cushing syndrome, such as striae, proximal myopathy, supraclavicular and dorsocervical fat pads, easy bruisability, and thinning of the skin. However, patients with MACE are at high risk for developing cortisol-induced metabolic abnormalities such as hypertension, type 2 diabetes mellitus, dyslipidemia, obesity, and fractures (4–6, 11). Although not firmly established, several studies suggest that MACE is associated with reduced life expectancy (4, 12). Thus, the widely used term subclinical is a misnomer. Recent guidelines on management of adrenal incidentalomas have proposed elimination of the term subclinical Cushing syndrome and suggested the term autonomous cortisol secretion to emphasize the most common biochemical abnormality of MACE (7).

Whom Should We Test for MACE?

All patients with incidentally discovered adrenal tumors (adrenal incidentalomas) should undergo evaluation for

MACE. Adrenal tumors are discovered in 4% to 5% of patients undergoing cross-sectional imaging for other reasons (8). MACE is diagnosed in approximately 10% to 15% of patients with adrenal tumors (7, 8).

Another population with higher risk of MACE is comprised by patients with metabolic abnormalities possibly exacerbated by MACE, such as those with type 2 diabetes mellitus. In a study of 993 patients with type 2 diabetes mellitus without features of overt Cushing syndrome, 3.7% of patients were diagnosed with MACE (10). In another large prospective study of 813 patients with type 2 diabetes mellitus, 0.7% were ultimately diagnosed with Cushing syndrome (13). Overall, although systematic evaluation for MACE/Cushing syndrome is not recommended, increased awareness and consideration of hypercortisolism is warranted (9).

Diagnosis of MACE

Current literature reports a variety of approaches and test combinations to diagnose MACE, all targeted at biochemical assessment of abnormalities in the HPA axis. In a recent systematic review and meta-analysis of cardiovascular risk factors in patients with adrenal tumors, 16 unique combinations of tests were reported to have been used by authors of the 26 included studies (n = 1041 patients) (5). These include: abnormal overnight dexamethasone suppression test (DST) with 1, 2, and 8 mg (with morning cortisol cutoffs of 1–5 μg/dL), low adrenocorticotropic hormone (ACTH), loss of circadian rhythm, increased cortisol in 24-hour urine, low dehydroepiandrosterone, and other.

European Society of Endocrinology/European Network for the Study of Adrenal Tumors guidelines on management of adrenal incidentaloma (2016) (7) suggested that the first step should be the 1-mg overnight dexamethasone test in all patients with adrenal incidentaloma. Guidelines propose a cutoff of <1.8 μg/dL (50 nmol/L) to exclude MACE. No complementary investigation is required in this situation. In patients with postdexamethasone cortisol >1.8 μg/dL, guidelines recommend interpreting the results as a continuous rather than categorical variable (the higher the cortisol, the more severe the degree of cortisol secretory autonomy). The DST may be repeated to confirm the abnormality; in addition, other tests may be required to confirm cortisol autonomy (Table 1).

What Are the Consequences/Associated Comorbidities of MACE?

Once MACE is confirmed, it is important to evaluate for associated comorbidities and offer appropriate management of these conditions. These include: hypertension, type 2 diabetes mellitus, dyslipidemia, osteoporosis, and asymptomatic vertebral fractures. Patients with MACE have high baseline prevalence of cardiovascular risk factors (Table 2), and it increases with follow-up.

Incidence of cardiovascular events and increased mortality risk were also reported to be higher in patients with abnormal dexamethasone suppression results (4, 12). In a longitudinal study of 198 patients with adrenal tumors, patients with postdexamethasone cortisol concentrations of 1.8 to 5 μg/dL, especially patients with concentrations >5 μg/dL, had higher incidence of cardiovascular events (6.7% and 16.7%, respectively) (4). Survival rates for all-cause mortality were also lower in patients with MACE, especially cardiovascular mortality (4). In another longitudinal study of 206 patients with an adrenal mass, mortality was higher in patients with postdexamethasone cortisol concentrations >1.8 μg/dL, mainly as a result of cardiovascular (50%) and respiratory infectious (33%) causes (12).

Patients with MACE have higher prevalence of vertebral fractures (for the most part, microfractures) and an increased 2-year incidence of new vertebral fractures. Notably, microfractures may occur despite normal bone mineral density (6).

Who Should Be Offered Adrenalectomy?

Adrenalectomy is an option in any patient with an adrenal mass associated with MACE. The main challenge is to identify patients who do or will manifest MACE-induced comorbidities. Because hypertension, type 2 diabetes mellitus, obesity, dyslipidemia, and osteoporosis are highly prevalent in adults typically diagnosed with adrenal tumors (age 50 to 70 years), it

Table 1. Tests for Assessment of HPA Axis Abnormality and Possible Pitfalls in Interpretation

Test	Result Suggestive of MACE	Possible Pitfalls in Interpretation
1-mg DST (11 PM overnight administration; cortisol measurement at 8 AM)	>1.8 μg/dL (>50 nmol/L)	Assay accuracy at the lower end, concomitant medication use/drug interactions, individual variations in dexamethasone absorption
ACTH (morning measurement)	Low normal/low	Assay accuracy at the lower range
DHEAS	Low normal/low	Differences in the age- and sex-stratified healthy control ranges, assay accuracy
24-hour urine cortisol	Usually normal or mildly increased	Assay differences

DHEAS, dehydroepiandrosterone.

Table 2. MACE-Associated Comorbidities

Comorbidities	Prevalence at Baseline (%)	Improved After Adrenalectomy (%)
Hypertension	68	60.5
Type 2 diabetes mellitus	30	51.5
Dyslipidemia	25.6	24
Obesity	34.6	45
Vertebral fractures	54	30

Data adapted (5, 6, 11).

is difficult to estimate the contribution of MACE to development of these manifestations. Consequently, on an individual level, it is difficult to predict the response to adrenalectomy. Although cardiovascular risk factors are improved in patients with MACE as a group (5), the degree of individual benefit is unclear. This is why the European Society of Endocrinology/European Network for the Study of Adrenal Tumors guidelines on management of adrenal incidentaloma suggest an individualized approach in considering patients with an adrenal mass and MACE and associated comorbidities for adrenalectomy (7). Demographic and clinical factors, such as age, health status, duration and severity of comorbidities, degree of biochemical abnormalities, strong familial history of hypertension/obesity/diabetes, adrenal tumor imaging phenotype, and patient preference, play a role in decision making.

In patients with MACE associated with bilateral adrenal masses, careful consideration of diagnosis (bilateral macronodular hyperplasia vs two contralateral adenomas) is needed if adrenalectomy is considered. Unilateral adrenalectomy of the dominant (bigger) adenoma could be performed in selected patients with bilateral adenomas or macronodular hyperplasia (14, 15). Adrenal vein sampling for cortisol excess (after dexamethasone suppression) (16) or adrenal iodocholesterol scintigraphy (8) is rarely needed (in patients with bilateral adenomas of similar size) to determine whether cortisol secretion is unilateral or bilateral; however, the availability of these procedures is limited to certain centers.

In patients with MACE not undergoing adrenalectomy, annual reassessment of both biochemical and clinical status should be performed (7). If comorbidities such as hypertension, type 2 diabetes, and osteoporosis exist, they should be aggressively treated with lifestyle modifications and medical management. On the basis of the outcome of these evaluations, the potential benefit of surgery should be reconsidered.

CASES WITH QUESTIONS

Case 1

A 65-year-old man was serendipitously discovered to have a 2.9-cm left adrenal mass noted on computed tomography (CT) scan of the abdomen performed for abdominal pain. On unenhanced CT, the adrenal mass was homogeneous, with smooth borders, and demonstrated a density of 5 Hounsfield units. Patient reported no history of malignancy. He is obese (body mass index of 38 kg/m^2). His has type 2 diabetes mellitus and hypertension. For the last 7 years, he has been treated with metformin and lisinopril. Physical examination is negative for any signs suggestive of Cushing syndrome.

What is the best diagnostic approach for MACE?

A. Two late-night salivary cortisol measurements
B. 1-mg DST
C. 24-hour urine collection to measure urinary free cortisol (UFC)
D. No testing, because MACE is unlikely in an adrenal mass of this size

Answer: B.

Prevalence of adrenal tumors increases with age. In CT scan series, adrenal incidentalomas were found in approximately 4% to 5% of patients after the age of 50 years, and their prevalence increases with age, obesity, diabetes, and high blood pressure. In a patient without any symptoms of hormonal excess, adrenal masses <1 cm in size are unlikely to be hormonally active or malignant. Thus, several endocrine societies suggest a cutoff of 1 cm as clinically relevant and necessitating further workup (7, 8, 17). Because this asymptomatic patient has an adrenal mass of 2.9 cm, it is appropriate to proceed with additional investigations for MACE. The hallmark of subclinical secreting adrenal incidentalomas is a state of secretory autonomy that is explored with the 1-mg DST (7). Twenty-four–hour UFC and late-night salivary cortisol tests may lack the sensitivity necessary to diagnose autonomous cortisol secretion.

You have chosen to perform 1-mg DST. Morning cortisol after overnight 1-mg dexamethasone administration was 90 nmol/L (3.3 μg/dL).

Which of the following statement(s) is correct?

A. Adrenal mass can be considered nonfunctioning
B. Results may indicate autonomous cortisol excess
C. Results absolutely suggest autonomous cortisol excess
D. Additional investigations for HPA axis abnormalities will help in making a diagnosis of MACE

Answer: B and D.

According to the recently published recommendations of the European Endocrine Society (7), response to the 1-mg DST should be interpreted as a continuous variable. Possible cortisol secretory autonomy is considered when plasma cortisol after the 1-mg DST is between 50 and 139 nmol/L (1.8 and 5.0 μg/dL) and definitive cortisol secretory autonomy when plasma cortisol is ≥5.0 μg/dL. In the context of possible cortisol secretory autonomy in a patient with comorbidities that may be secondary to mild cortisol excess (hypertension, diabetes), more accurate assessment of the HPA axis is recommended, with complementary biological investigations (24-hour UFC, 8 AM plasma ACTH) and repeat of the 1-mg DST, as well as investigation for additional comorbidities such as osteoporosis and vertebral fractures.

Patient is interested to know whether his type 2 diabetes mellitus will improve with adrenalectomy. You advise that as a group, patients with MACE have ____% chance of improving their disease.

A. 100%
B. 75%
C. 50%
D. 0%

Answer: C.

Unfortunately, no wide-scale prospective randomized study comparing the results of surgical removal of the incidentaloma with those of conservative medical treatment is available. However, currently, a vast majority of retrospective studies indicate that as a group, patients with autonomous mild cortisol excess experience an improvement in hypertension and type 2 diabetes mellitus after surgical excision of the adenoma. A comprehensive systematic review and meta-analysis of published series found that >50% of patients with MACE improve after adrenalectomy, defined as decrease in HbA1C or discontinuation or reduction in the intensity of hypoglycemic therapy (5). However, it is important to note that individual benefit of adrenalectomy is (so far) impossible to accurately predict. This is why decision making regarding adrenalectomy in each patient with MACE and associated comorbidities should be individualized.

Case 2

A 45-year-old overweight man is treated with a combination of metformin and bedtime insulin for type 2 diabetes. He regularly exercises (biweekly biking for 2 hours) and reports that he is compliant with dietary recommendations. His body mass index is stable at 27 kg/m^2. He is treated for hypertension with three drugs, and his blood pressure at the office is 150/80 mmHg. His recent HbA1C is 8.4%. He had a recent cardiovascular workup, which was within normal limits. Patient reports no family history of type 2 diabetes mellitus. Clinical examination does not reveal any features suggestive of overt Cushing syndrome.

Which of the following statement(s) is correct?

A. The probability that the patient has MACE is ~10% to 15%
B. The probability that the patient has MACE is ~3%
C. Biochemical case detection for MACE should be discussed with the patient
D. MACE is secondary to an ACTH-secreting pituitary adenoma is most cases

Answer: B and C

Large systematic screening studies performed mainly in patients with type 2 diabetes mellitus have revealed an unexpectedly high prevalence of undiagnosed MACE or Cushing syndrome (~3%). In most cases, patients are discovered to have an adrenocortical adenoma autonomously secreting cortisol in excess. However, systematic screening of all patients with type 2 diabetes mellitus is only justified if supported by enough evidence of its efficacy and if the benefits outweigh the drawbacks. Evidence to date suggests that the cons exceed the pros; thus, systematic screening for MACE in patients with type 2 diabetes mellitus is not recommended (9). Specifically, in the context of a low pretest probability, biochemical investigations generate more false-positive than true-positive results. Consequently, a case-finding approach is recommended instead (13), as in this case of a relatively young patient with severe hypertension, uncontrolled diabetes, and no familial history of metabolic disease and in whom the pretest probability of MACE is high.

Which is (are) the best next step(s) in case detection of MACE?

A. Abdominal CT for identification of adrenal adenoma
B. 24-hour urinary collection for cortisol
C. Overnight 1-mg DST
D. Case detection for MACE in patients with uncontrolled diabetes mellitus may be difficult

Answer: C and D

In the absence of overt features suggestive of Cushing syndrome, biochemical investigations lack sensitivity (most patients with MACE have normal 24-hour UFC). The 1-mg DST is the screening test of choice in any patient suspected to have MACE. Stress and hypoglycemia are two major stimuli of the HPA axis. Poorly controlled diabetes mellitus (acidoketosis as well as recurrent and profound hyperglycemia) will result in subsequent activation of the HPA axis. Consequently, these patients may demonstrate higher rates of false-positive results during MACE case detection, which is important to consider when deciding on the timing of testing.

REFERENCES

1. Feelders RA, Pulgar SJ, Kempel A, Pereira AM. The burden of Cushing's disease: clinical and health-related quality of life aspects. *Eur J Endocrinol.* 2012;**167**(3):311–326.
2. Clayton RN, Jones PW, Reulen RC, Stewart PM, Hassan-Smith ZK, Ntali G, Karavitaki N, Dekkers OM, Pereira AM, Bolland M, Holdaway I, Lindholm J. Mortality in patients with Cushing's disease more than 10 years after remission: a multicentre, multinational, retrospective cohort study. *Lancet Diabetes Endocrinol.* 2016;**4**(7):569–576.
3. van Haalen FM, Broersen LH, Jorgensen JO, Pereira AM, Dekkers OM. Management of endocrine disease: mortality remains increased in Cushing's disease despite biochemical remission: a systematic review and meta-analysis. *Eur J Endocrinol.* 2015;**172**(4):R143–R149.
4. Di Dalmazi G, Vicennati V, Garelli S, Casadio E, Rinaldi E, Giampalma E, Mosconi C, Golfieri R, Paccapelo A, Pagotto U, Pasquali R. Cardiovascular events and mortality in patients with adrenal incidentalomas that are either non-secreting or associated with intermediate phenotype or subclinical Cushing's syndrome: a 15-year retrospective study. *Lancet Diabetes Endocrinol.* 2014;**2**(5):396–405.
5. Bancos I, Alahdab F, Crowley RK, Chortis V, Delivanis DA, Erickson D, Natt N, Terzolo M, Arlt W, Young WF, Jr, Murad MH. Therapy of

endocrine disease: improvement of cardiovascular risk factors after adrenalectomy in patients with adrenal tumors and subclinical Cushing's syndrome: a systematic review and meta-analysis. *Eur J Endocrinol.* 2016;**175**(6):R283–R295.

6. Chiodini I, Vainicher CE, Morelli V, Palmieri S, Cairoli E, Salcuni AS, Copetti M, Scillitani A. Mechanisms in endocrinology: endogenous subclinical hypercortisolism and bone: a clinical review. *Eur J Endocrinol.* 2016;**175**(6):R265–R282.
7. Fassnacht M, Arlt W, Bancos I, Dralle H, Newell-Price J, Sahdev A, Tabarin A, Terzolo M, Tsagarakis S, Dekkers OM. Management of adrenal incidentalomas: European Society of Endocrinology clinical practice guideline in collaboration with the European Network for the Study of Adrenal Tumors. *Eur J Endocrinol.* 2016;**175**(2):G1–G34.
8. Terzolo M, Stigliano A, Chiodini I, Loli P, Furlani L, Arnaldi G, Reimondo G, Pia A, Toscano V, Zini M, Borretta G, Papini E, Garofalo P, Allolio B, Dupas B, Mantero F, Tabarin A; Italian Association of Clinical Endocrinologists. AME position statement on adrenal incidentaloma. *Eur J Endocrinol.* 2011;**164**(6):851–870.
9. Tabarin A, Perez P. Pros and cons of screening for occult Cushing syndrome. *Nat Rev Endocrinol.* 2011;**7**(8):445–455.
10. Budyal S, Jadhav SS, Kasaliwal R, Patt H, Khare S, Shivane V, Lila AR, Bandgar T, Shah NS. Is it worthwhile to screen patients with type 2 diabetes mellitus for subclinical Cushing's syndrome? *Endocr Connect.* 2015;**4**(4):242–248.
11. Di Dalmazi G, Vicennati V, Rinaldi E, Morselli-Labate AM, Giampalma E, Mosconi C, Pagotto U, Pasquali R. Progressively increased patterns of subclinical cortisol hypersecretion in adrenal incidentalomas differently predict major metabolic and cardiovascular outcomes: a large cross-sectional study. *Eur J Endocrinol.* 2012;**166**(4):669–677.
12. Debono M, Bradburn M, Bull M, Harrison B, Ross RJ, Newell-Price J. Cortisol as a marker for increased mortality in patients with incidental adrenocortical adenomas. *J Clin Endocrinol Metab.* 2014;**99**(12): 4462–4470.
13. Terzolo M, Reimondo G, Chiodini I, Castello R, Giordano R, Ciccarelli E, Limone P, Crivellaro C, Martinelli I, Montini M, Disoteo O, Ambrosi B, Lanzi R, Arosio M, Senni S, Balestrieri A, Solaroli E, Madeo B, De Giovanni R, Strollo F, Battista R, Scorsone A, Giagulli VA, Collura D, Scillitani A, Cozzi R, Faustini-Fustini M, Pia A, Rinaldi R, Allasino B, Peraga G, Tassone F, Garofalo P, Papini E, Borretta G. Screening of Cushing's syndrome in outpatients with type 2 diabetes: results of a prospective multicentric study in Italy. *J Clin Endocrinol Metab.* 2012;**97**(10):3467–3475.
14. Debillon E, Velayoudom-Cephise FL, Salenave S, Caron P, Chaffanjon P, Wagner T, Massoutier M, Lambert B, Benoit M, Young J, Tabarin A, Chabre O. Unilateral adrenalectomy as a first-line treatment of Cushing's syndrome in patients with primary bilateral macronodular adrenal hyperplasia. *J Clin Endocrinol Metab.* 2015;**100**(12): 4417–4424.
15. Perogamvros I, Vassiliadi DA, Karapanou O, Botoula E, Tzanela M, Tsagarakis S. Biochemical and clinical benefits of unilateral adrenalectomy in patients with subclinical hypercortisolism and bilateral adrenal incidentalomas. *Eur J Endocrinol.* 2015;**173**(6): 719–725.
16. Young WF, Jr, du Plessis H, Thompson GB, Grant CS, Farley DR, Richards ML, Erickson D, Vella A, Stanson AW, Carney JA, Abboud CF, Carpenter PC. The clinical conundrum of corticotropin-independent autonomous cortisol secretion in patients with bilateral adrenal masses. *World J Surg.* 2008;**32**(5):856–862.
17. Tabarin A, Bardet S, Bertherat J, Dupas B, Chabre O, Hamoir E, Laurent F, Tenenbaum F, Cazalda M, Lefebvre H, Valli N, Rohmer V; French Society of Endocrinology Consensus. Exploration and management of adrenal incidentalomas. *Ann Endocrinol (Paris).* 2008;**69**(6):487–500.

Management of Adrenocortical Carcinoma*

M35
Presented, March 17-20, 2018

Gary D. Hammer, MD, PhD. University of Michigan Health System, Ann Arbor, Michigan 48109, E-mail: ghammer@umich.edu

Gerard M. Doherty, MD. Brigham & Women's Hospital and Harvard Medical School, Boston, Massachusetts 02115, E-mail: gmdoherty@bwh.harvard.edu

INTRODUCTION

Adrenocortical cancer (ACC) is a rare and typically lethal disease. Management requires careful attention to both the hormonal function of the tumor and the oncologic risk of the malignancy. Given substantial variability in tumor behavior and patient course, as well as the rarity of the tumor and its course, we believe that this is best cared for in specialized centers.

The initial differential diagnosis for small adrenal tumors often includes benign and malignant lesions, such as tumors arising from the adrenal medulla or adrenal cortex, or alternatively, metastatic lesions from other sites. For the typical ACC that presents with a large mass (often >10 cm), alternative diagnoses may include tumors from other organs (*e.g.*, the liver or kidney) or retroperitoneal sarcoma. Although the full evaluation of adrenal masses is beyond the scope of this session, the nature of these masses may become clear with biochemical testing or careful imaging review by an expert radiologist. Biopsy of potentially resectable lesions is contraindicated, because the resulting tumor spill may render resection ineffective.

Resection is the only potentially curative intervention to date. If the patient can have complete resection of all demonstrable tumor, that is generally advisable. Palliative resections to resolve mass effect or severe hormonal syndromes may occasionally be helpful, but are often rendered moot by rapid tumor progression.

There are two key decisions that a clinician must make when confronted with an adrenal tumor: (1) determine the risk of malignancy of the observed lesion and (2) determine any adrenal hormone excess that would support a primary adrenal neoplasm (benign or malignant).

The answers to these questions are essential in the initial work-up of any adrenal lesion and will guide how the endocrinologist, endocrine surgeon, and/or oncologist proceeds with additional diagnostic and/or therapeutic interventions.

This Clinical Case Management session is designed to cover a number of important issues regarding the diagnosis and treatment of adrenocortical carcinoma by discussing several cases seen in our multidisciplinary endocrine oncology clinics. Cases will be presented and discussed.

A few of the topics that will be covered include:

- Is it cancer?
- Treating the primary tumor
- Adjuvant care (to prevent recurrence) once resected
- Treating hormone excess
- Treating recurrence or nonresectable disease

SIGNIFICANCE OF THE CLINICAL PROBLEM

Adrenal tumors are common, affecting 3% to 10% of the population, and the majority are small benign nonfunctional adrenocortical adenomas (ACA) Adrenocortical carcinoma (ACC) is rare, affecting one to two per 1 million adults per year (and 0.2 to 0.3 per 1 million children per year), but difficult to treat with substantial morbidity. Many patients present with a paucity of symptoms despite extensive metastatic disease on initial evaluation. Distinguishing between a benign and a malignant mass in the adrenal is essential but not always straightforward. Most doctors have never seen a case of ACC and/or are not familiar or comfortable with the current multidisciplinary management strategies for the disease. Coordinated care among an endocrinologist, an endocrine surgeon, and a medical oncologist is essential, with additional support from other specialties a frequent necessity.

BARRIERS TO OPTIMAL PRACTICE

- Lack of experience with diagnosis and treatment of ACC—on presentation (diagnosis not entertained)
- Lack of referral to experienced endocrinologist or experienced endocrine surgeon for initial evaluation and treatment
- Inappropriate therapies prior to referral to endocrinologist/endocrine surgeon
- Challenges of mitotane therapy and proper use
- Lack of optimal second- and third-line therapies

LEARNING OBJECTIVES

- To recognize common pitfalls that lead to inaccurate diagnosis or treatment of ACC
- To understand general principles of the management of ACC
- To be comfortable managing associated hormone excess in ACC
- To understand the role of genetics in the biology and management of ACC

STRATEGIES FOR DIAGNOSIS, THERAPY, AND/OR MANAGEMENT

There are three main clinical scenarios in which patients with ACC present. Forty percent to 60% of patients present with symptoms and signs of hormone excess. Another one-third of patients present with nonspecific symptoms such as abdominal or flank pain, abdominal fullness, or early satiety. Lastly, 20% to 30% of ACCs are incidentally diagnosed by imaging procedures for unrelated medical concerns. All adrenal masses must be evaluated for potential hormone excess and possible malignancy. All adrenal masses are evaluated for cortical and medullary hormone excess using standard Endocrine Society guidelines for primary aldosteronism, Cushing's syndrome, and pheochromocytoma. In addition, dehydroepiandrosterone is evaluated. Biochemically or clinically apparent adrenocortical hormone production is evident in 50% to 75% of patients, with Cushing's syndrome being the most common and androgen excess (almost exclusively dehydroepiandrosterone sulfate) the second most commonly observed syndrome in patients (causing rapid-onset male pattern baldness, hirsutism, virilization, and menstrual irregularities in women). Cosecretion of two classes of adrenocortical hormone is most consistent with ACC vs ACA and should be assumed to be ACC until proven otherwise.

Radiologic Evaluation

Routine radiologic evaluation includes an unenhanced computed tomography (CT) scan. Malignant masses (including ACC and metastatic deposit from another primary cancer) can be distinguished from the common lipid-rich ACA, which tend to be small, homogeneous masses that measure <10 HU on unenhanced CT or demonstrate loss of signal on chemical shift magnetic resonance. Homogeneous adrenal tumors exhibiting >10 HU can be benign lipid-poor ACA or nonadenomas. Such lesions can be further characterized using a dedicated adrenal-protocol CT scan. ACAs demonstrate a greater contrast washout than adrenal nonadenomas. Most adrenal masses are benign ACA.

Although most ACCs are diagnosed late in the disease course (*i.e.*, large), it is important to remember that all cancers begin as one cell. Therefore, small masses can still carry a risk of malignancy. The mean stage of ACC diagnosis is as follows: stage I (<5 cm; 14%), stage II (>5 cm; 45%), stage III (local spread or regional lymphadenopathy; 27%), and stage IV (distant metastasis; 24%). The most common metastatic sites are lung (40% to 80%), liver (40% to 90%), and bone (5% to 20%).

Biopsies are only considered when the patient has a current additional nonadrenal primary cancer and additional metastatic disease in the setting of a new adrenal mass. In this case, a biopsy can help determine whether the adrenal mass is a metastatic lesion from the other primary cancer or a new primary adrenal tumor that would necessitate a separate approach.

Pathologic Diagnosis

Pathologic diagnosis relies on review by an endocrine pathologist utilizing the Weiss criteria; these rely on standard histologic parameters that include invasion of tumor into capsule or adjacent vessels, necrosis, increased mitotic rates, and atypical mitotic figures. Tumors with three or more of these features most often behave in a malignant fashion and can be classified as ACC. Moreover, ACCs are considered high grade when >20 mitoses per 50 high-power field (Ki67 >10%) are present and low grade when <20 mitoses per 50 high-power field (Ki67 <10%) are present. There is a high risk of recurrence following resected ACC. Recurrence in high-grade ACC often occurs within the first 3 to 12 months, with distant disease (*e.g.*, liver and lungs) being more common. Low-grade ACC can present with late recurrence (2 to 3 years after resection), often with only local disease at the tumor bed or oligo-metastatic disease in the peritoneum or liver.

Surgical Considerations

Reasons to remove an adrenal mass include autonomous hormone excess and risk of malignancy. Surgical decision making is described below.

Resectable Lesions: Preoperative Considerations

The preoperative evaluation and preparation of the patient for surgery is highly important and includes thorough biochemical evaluation of the adrenal and hypothalamic-pituitary-adrenal axis. Electrolyte abnormalities and hypertension in Conn's or Cushing's syndromes are corrected. Detailed imaging is obtained, most often CT, but magnetic resonance imaging and positron emission tomography CT also have roles. Preoperative evaluation must also consider the cardiac, pulmonary, and nutritional status of the patient. Positron emission tomography CT has been found to be helpful in differentiating benign from malignant tumors in some cases, but specificity is suboptimal; however, this is more often used to try to detect disease beyond the scope of resection prior to operation.

Operative Technique

Open adrenalectomy is the preferred approach for known or suspected ACCs, including those requiring multivisceral resection. The classic anterior approach allows full access to all organs of the peritoneal cavity and chest if necessary. The patient is positioned supine on the table. Incisions can be made in the midline or subcostal, depending on preoperative factors and need for multivisceral resection. Although it is not often required, the thoracoabdominal approach can be useful in patients with large adrenal tumors or those involving the retrohepatic vena cava where visualization would be difficult due to body habitus or prior abdominal surgery. Even very large right adrenal tumors can generally be removed using a subcostal incision with a midline extension and full mobilization of the liver. However, there are some tumors with involvement of the upper abdominal vena cava, particularly inreoperative cases, that are best removed using a thoracoabdominal approach. The patient is placed in semilateral decubitus position on a beanbag with an axillary roll beneath the axilla. The ipsilateral arm is held in place parallel to the contralateral arm with a thoracic arm holder. The pelvis remains flat. An incision is made 2 cm inferior to the ipsilateral scapula and carried from lateral to medial along the eighth intercostal space and then inferiorly along the upper midline of the abdomen to the umbilicus. The diaphragm is incised, allowing access to the chest and abdomen with excellent visualization of the retroperitoneal structures. Recovery can be delayed due to pulmonary issues or recovery of gastrointestinal function, and chronic pain from injury to the neurovascular bundle of the rib can occur.

The first operation is the best and usually the only chance for long-term local control of malignancy, with the goal of a complete (R0) resection in the absence of penetration of the tumor capsule. Poor initial surgical treatment can rarely be corrected, whether by reoperation, radiotherapy, or chemotherapy. Complete removal of the tumor may require concomitant resection of the ipsilateral kidney, liver, spleen, pancreas, stomach, colon, or a portion of the vena cava. This decision should occur early, rather than after handling the tumor to any great extent.

Controversy surrounds the appropriateness of laparoscopic adrenalectomy (LA) for patients with ACC. ACCs can invade through the tumor capsule and are frequently microscopically present at the surface of the gland; application of any pressure to the tumor should be avoided. Some surgeons compromise by initiating adrenalectomies laparoscopically to assess for evidence of intraperitoneal metastasis or invasion of the adrenal gland into other organs; however, this direct exploration of the tumor violates oncologic principles of resection. A recurring argument is that in so-called expert hands, LA may be appropriate for certain malignant adrenal tumors. However, there is no consensus definition of what constitutes adequate expertise. This does not translate to expertise for biologically aggressive, often invasive, larger adrenal cancers. Unfortunately, most ACCs are removed by low-volume and less experienced adrenal surgeons.

Surgical studies should differentiate between local/peritoneal recurrence and distant recurrence for an indication of quality of resection. Type of operative approach probably has less influence on the development of distant metastases compared with local/peritoneal recurrence. A retrospective study from University of Michigan reviewed 88 patients with ACC, 17 of whom underwent LA. Although overall recurrence rates were similar and despite smaller tumors on average in the LA group (7.0 cm) compared with the open adrenalectomy (OA) group (12.3 cm), the LA group had significantly earlier recurrence (9.2 vs 19.2 months). There were more R1 or R2 resections or notation of intraoperative tumor spill (50% vs 18%) in the LA group. These data suggest that although LA may be technically feasible, the use of LA in ACC leads to a shorter disease-free interval and a higher incidence of incomplete resections. These results were confirmed in an extended follow-up study of 110 patients who underwent OA, and 46 who underwent LA. After LA, 30% of patients had positive margins or intraoperative tumor spill compared with 16% of patients who underwent OA, despite larger tumors and more stage III tumors. Overall survival for patients with stage II ACC was significantly longer in those who underwent OA, including a subgroup of those with only R0 resections. Time to visible tumor bed recurrence or peritoneal recurrence in patients with stage II tumors was shorter in patients who underwent LA.

In summary, existing data are inconclusive; more studies are needed to better judge the equivalence of LA and OA. In accordance with the experience gained at the authors' institutions, a conservative approach using an open technique is recommended for all adrenocortical lesions that cannot be classified as benign prior to surgery.

Lymphadenectomy

The role of lymph node sampling or formal regional lymph node dissection in the treatment of ACC remains unknown, and consensus within the field is needed. The impact of regional lymph node metastasis upon overall survival provides impetus for earlier or more aggressive use of additional therapies when disease is present in the lymphatic system. In one retrospective study, performance of locoregional lymph node dissection led to improved oncologic outcome. Some of the improved outcome can be attributed to the upstaging of patients with ACC with lymph node metastasis and subsequent more aggressive treatment. Similarly, more radical surgery in these patients can lead to increased clearance of disease as opposed to a higher rate of positive margins. Nodal basins removed were not clearly reported, and lymph nodes associated with other organs during multivisceral resections were included, thereby leaving the role of prophylactic nodal dissection unknown.

Management of Invasive Tumors

Extirpation of large ACCs can be extremely challenging for even the most experienced surgeon. Adequate visualization can be difficult to achieve. Partial hepatectomy may be required in some patients to achieve en bloc resection. If necessary, the liver can be completely mobilized from the inferior vena cava, affording superb visualization and access to the inferior vena cava should partial resection and reconstruction be necessary, or to facilitate removal of intravascular tumor thrombus. Tumor thrombus is not a contraindication to resection, and removal is indicated when technically feasible. In most cases, venotomy and simple closure suffice for removal of tumor; however, in certain cases, resection of a portion of the vena cava may be required. If the diameter of the vena cava is not decreased by >50%, resection and primary closure are adequate. For cases requiring larger segments of caval resection, autologous tissue is preferred if bowel is also resected or entered during the operation, but prosthetic material may also be used. Vascular control of the vena cava can also be achieved in the chest using a median sternotomy or by a thoracoabdominal approach. In rare circumstances, veno-venous bypass may be useful. For thrombus extending into the right atrium, cardiopulmonary bypass can facilitate complete resection. Transesophageal echocardiography should be used to help identify the level of thrombus extension if it extends into the thorax. If bleeding from the vena cava is encountered, it can be voluminous. However, it is low pressure and can be controlled. In dire situations, various balloon catheters, atriocaval shunts, or Schrock shunts may be useful.

Aorta and Arterial Supply

The need for resection of portions of arteries or their branches is a general but not an absolute contraindication to surgery for ACC. It is not uncommon for the celiac axis and takeoff of the superior mesenteric artery to be partially encased with tumor. If a tumor involves a short segment of the celiac axis or superior mesenteric artery, it is possible to remove this short segment prior to its branching into end arteries. The gastroduodenal artery can supply the liver in a retrograde fashion via supply from the superior mesenteric artery; however, the adequacy of this alternative pathway of hepatic perfusion should be tested.

Diaphragm

En bloc resection of tumor with an accompanying portion of the diaphragm may be required to achieve negative margins. Smaller diaphragmatic defects may be closed primarily using monofilament suture in a running locking or interrupted mattress fashion. For larger defects, various prosthetic materials may be used for closure.

Reoperative Surgery

Extent of disease and tempo of disease progression guide the decision for reoperation in the setting of recurrence. The number of organs involved by tumor at the time of the first metastasis and the length of disease-free recurrence are predictors of survival. Decisions regarding reoperative surgery must be individualized because survival may be prolonged in some patients. Tumor grade can influence the decision for reoperation because patients with low-grade tumors generally have a slower tempo of disease progression. Thus reoperation may be more beneficial in these patients with regard to long-term survival. In contrast, patients with high-grade tumors seem to benefit less, because other sites of disease often appear quickly after resection. It is not uncommon for the authors to wait several months in the setting of questionably resectable tumors or recurrences while treating with systemic therapy to assess for tumor responsiveness and/or tempo of disease progression. If progression is not rapid, surgery may proceed with greater benefit, whereas those with evidence of marked progression of disease do not undergo surgery.

Adjuvant Therapies

For reasons detailed above, adjuvant therapies are often considered. Mitotane, an adrenolytic agent and the only Food and Drug Administration–approved therapy for ACC, has been the most studied adjuvant therapy for ACC. Used most frequently in the setting of resected high-grade ACC, a number of studies have detailed a decrease or delay in recurrence of ACC. Strategies will be discussed.

Radiation therapy for local control is debated. It is used by a few centers in the adjuvant setting and when residual disease, spillage, or positive margins are evident following surgery. Strategies will be discussed.

Definitive Therapies

Nonresectable disease is most often treated with mitotane and/or systemic chemotherapy. The FIRM-ACT trial, in a head-to-head comparison of the most promising regimens, EDPM (etoposide, doxorubicin, cisplatin plus mitotane) vs SM (streptozocin plus mitotane), confirmed the efficacy of chemotherapy and proved the superiority of EDPM, with response rates of 50% when stable disease was included. The median progression-free survival was short (a median of 5 months), underscoring the limitations of chemotherapy for ACC. Radiation therapy is used to treat oligo-metastatic disease in select cases. Strategies will be discussed.

Mitotane is not used for mere hormone control in ACC. Hormone excess is treated with endocrine therapies, most often metyrapone for cortisol excess (ketoconazole is usually ineffective; mifepristone is challenging to implement in this population), mineralocorticoid receptor antagonists for mineralocorticoid excess, and androgen receptor antagonists for androgen excess. Strategies will be discussed.

Genetics

Genetics is increasingly playing a role in the diagnosis, prognosis, and management of cancer. Although more evident in thyroid and neuroendocrine cancers, genetic/genomic data in ACC are emerging and will be discussed.

Although 50% to 80% of pediatric ACC is due to familial mutations in *P53* that result in Li-Fraumeni syndrome, ACC is occasionally seen in Beckwith Wiedemann syndrome due to an imprinting defect in the *IGF2* locus. Germline mutations in *P53* have been found in 10% of adults with ACC, and 3% of adults with ACC have Lynch syndrome due to mutations in mismatch repair genes. Multiple endocrine neoplasia-type 1

(MEN1), familial adenomatous polyposis (FAP), and Carney's Complex have also been associated with ACC in rare cases. All patients with ACC are therefore screened for germline mutations underlying Li-Fraumeni and Lynch syndromes. Evaluations for other cancer risk syndromes are performed only if there is a strong family history.

MAIN CONCLUSIONS

Adrenal masses are common. All masses must be evaluated for hormone excess and assessed for risk of malignancy. ACC is rare. Most cases of ACC are diagnosed due to hormone excess, nonspecific abdominal pain, or incidentally. Surgery is the appropriate front-line approach for resectable disease. Adjuvant therapies, most notably mitotane, are used for treatment of ACC with high risk of recurrence. Systemic therapies, most notably mitotane and EDPM, are used for treatment of nonresectable disease. Hormonal excess is controlled with standard endocrine therapies. Although genetics is increasingly important in cancer care, it is only slowly emerging to enable the development of targeted therapies for ACC.

Cases will be presented to illustrate the challenges and the main teaching points summarized above.

RECOMMENDED READING

Else T, Hammer GD, eds. *Adrenocortical Carcinoma: Basic Science and Clinical Concepts.* New York, NY: Springer; 2011.

Else T, Hammer GD, Rosen C, eds. Adrenocortical carcinoma. In: *Clinical Decision Support: Endocrinology & Metabolism.* New York, NY: Wiley; 2013.

Else T, Kim A, Sabolch A, Raymond V, Kandathil A, Caoili E, Shruti J, Miller BS, Giordano TJ, Hammer GD. Adrenocortical carcinoma. *Endocrine Rev.* 2014;**35**(2):282–326.

Else T, Williams AR, Sabolch A, Jolly S, Miller BS, Hammer GD. Adjuvant therapies, patient and tumor characteristics associated with survival of adult patients with adrenocortical carcinoma. J Clin *Endocrinol Metab.* 2014;**99**(2):455–461.

Hammer GD, Lacroix A, Martin KA, ed. *Treatment of Adrenocortical Carcinoma.* Waltham, MA: Up To Date; 2012.

Miller BS, Gauger PG, Hammer GD, Doherty GM. Resection of adrenocortical carcinoma is less complete and local recurrence occurs sooner and more often after laparoscopic adrenalectomy than after open adrenalectomy. Surgery. 2012;**152**(6):1150–1157.

Zheng S, Cherniack AD, Dewal N, Moffitt RA, Danilova L, Murray BA, Lerario AM, Else T, Knijnenburg TA, Ciriello G, Kim S, Assie G, Morozova O, Akbani R, Shih J, Hoadley KA, Choueiri TK, Waldmann J, Mete O, Robertson AG, Wu HT, Raphael BJ, Shao L, Meyerson M, Demeure MJ, Beuschlein F, Gill AJ, Sidhu SB, Almeida MQ, Fragoso MC, Cope LM, Kebebew E, Habra MA, Whitsett TG, Bussey KJ, Rainey WE, Asa SL, Bertherat J, Fassnacht M, Wheeler DA; Cancer Genome Atlas Research Network, Hammer GD, Giordano TJ, Verhaak RG. Comprehensive pan-genomic characterization of adrenocortical carcinoma. *Cancer Cell.* 2016;**29**:1–14.

*This article is not eligible for CME.

Adrenal Insufficiency: Impact of Patient Education and Choice of Replacement Options

M46
Presented, March 17–20, 2018

Stephanie Hahner, MD. University Hospital of Wuerzburg, 97080 Wuerzburg, Germany, E-mail: hahner_s@medizin.uni-wuerzburg.de

SIGNIFICANCE OF THE CLINICAL PROBLEM

For a long time, it has been assumed that patients with adrenal insufficiency (AI) under established steroid replacement therapy have normal life expectancy and normal daily performance. This presumption has been disproved by more recent studies indicating both an impairment of subjective health status with a negative impact on work life and daily life and increased mortality in a substantial number of patients.

Generally, the burden of illness varies considerably in patients with AI. Although some suffer from neither adrenal crisis (AC) nor impaired subjective health status or fatigue, others are obviously more affected. Long-term management is thus more challenging and goes beyond identification of the correct maintenance dose of corticosteroids. In daily practice, counseling of patients may often be a balancing act between creating hope for a normal life and provision of understanding in case of persistent impairment. Furthermore, possible untoward long-term effects of nonphysiological replacement therapy are an important, as yet unsatisfactorily clarified issue for patients as well as treating physicians.

Mortality from AC is still unacceptably high, and prevention should be of high priority (1–3). Because of the rarity of AI, most physicians are not familiar with this disease. Patients are, however, dependent on adequate management in case of life-threatening AC. To improve patient management, new concepts of replacement therapy along with the importance of educational programs for patients and their social environment as well as emergency equipment are currently discussed, harmonized, and further being developed (4, 5).

BARRIERS TO OPTIMAL PRACTICE

- Current replacement tools are still away from the physiological condition, and replacement needs individual fine tuning, which is difficult because of the lack of objectified parameters.
- Because of the fact that AI is a rare disease, knowledge that physicians have of patient management is often not sufficient.
- Patient education is an important pillar in the treatment and prevention of fatal outcomes as well as the management of daily life. Education is so far neither obligatory nor standardized.

LEARNING OBJECTIVES

As a result of participating in this session, learners should be able to do the following.

- Rate long-term therapeutic challenges in adult patients with AI
- Perform individualized adaptation of corticosteroid replacement
- Use educational and therapeutic strategies for prevention and management of adrenal emergency

STRATEGIES FOR MANAGEMENT

Side Effects

Replacement therapy in AI serves to compensate for the existing deficit, but the standard glucocorticoid (GC) therapy does not fully restore the physiological profile. Because fatigue and reduced subjective health status are frequently reported by the patients (signs of underreplacement), the question arises of what extent GC doses need to be adapted or other steroid regimens need to be implemented. Impairment of glucose tolerance was observed if GCs were administered later during the day compared with circadian administration. Unfavorable effects of current standard replacement regimes on metabolism and bone are a matter of current debate. A recent retrospective review of a large US database revealed an increased prevalence of diabetes mellitus (type 1 or 2, unspecified), hyperlipidemia, and arterial hypertension in patients with AI (6), whereas other analyses did not reveal an increased prevalence of arterial hypertension, hyperlipidemia, obesity, or type 2 diabetes mellitus compared with population-based control cohorts. In terms of bone density, discrepant results have emerged in previous studies, with most studies showing no relevant increase in osteoporosis under currently used standard replacement. Most of the observed discrepancies may thus be explained by differences in the replacement dose. As a consequence, careful individual dose finding is necessary, weighing out the individual risk of under-and overreplacement mainly based on clinical parameters. Analyses assessing patient adherence and their satisfaction with information provided on their disease revealed that patient adherence is generally high. However, in particular, patients were dissatisfied with the information that they received about possible side effects of steroid therapy. Patients can be reassured that classical GC side effects are usually not to be expected in case of adequate replacement.

Quality of Life

High interindividual variability of quality of life (Qol) scores has been observed in different patient cohorts, showing that a subgroup of patients exists that is particularly vulnerable, whereas many others do not differ from average levels in age- and sex-matched controls (7). In cross-sectional analyses, higher GC doses were correlated with worse Qol values. Because of the retrospective nature of these studies, it remains unclear if this observation is the result of overreplacement or rather, if it reflects that treatment doses are more likely to be increased in patients complaining of fatigue and impaired health status. However, these data show that, after a dose increase, the replacement dose should always be re-evaluated.

To improve replacement, technologies that provide more physiological GC replacement have been developed, including subcutaneous hydrocortisone delivery via pumps or galenic modifications of oral hydrocortisone (8). The approved hydrocortisone preparation Plenadren® with two-phase drug release has the advantage of once daily intake and leads to cortisol levels that come closer to the physiological daytime profile compared with conventional hydrocortisone. An improvement of metabolic parameters (reduction of body weight and diastolic and systolic blood pressures as well as hemoglobin A1c) could be shown with a good safety profile (9, 10). Another modified release hydrocortisone preparation is Chronocort®, which is currently investigated in clinical trials. This preparation mimics the physiologic cortisol profile, including the early morning raise in cortisol levels when taken twice daily (8).

In addition to the new oral formulations, a more accurate imitation of the physiologic cortisol profile was studied by continuous subcutaneous (hydrocortisone application via insulin pump, which showed a tendency to improved general condition.

In summary, new formulations for steroid replacement therapy represent interesting developments that facilitate the individual fine tuning of replacement therapy, but they require additional evaluation for their effects on clinical parameters and Qol in larger prospective cohorts. A reduction in the daily GC exposure can frequently be achieved by use of the modified release preparations. The new hydrocortisone formulations can be of particular benefit for patients suffering from impaired Qol, diabetic patients with insufficient control of blood glucose levels, and patients who often forget to take their doses during the day.

Dehydroepiandrosterone

Dehydroepiandrosterone (DHEA) still does not belong to the standard treatment protocol. However, lack of its neuroprotective action and in females, clinical signs and symptoms of androgen deficiency may impact Qol. Beneficial effects assessed by several trials are high interindividual variation with, in general, moderate effects on general wellbeing and depressive symptoms. Because larger-scale phase 3 studies are still lacking, initiation of DHEA replacement is decided on an individual basis, focusing on those patients with impaired wellbeing associated with signs and symptoms of androgen deficiency. Treatment with DHEA is started at a daily morning dose of 25 mg. In some patients, substantially lower doses are needed (*e.g.*, 25 mg three times per week). It is important to communicate to patients that it takes up to several months for beneficial effects of DHEA to be observed. Furthermore, insulin-like growth factor I levels may rise in patients on growth hormone replacement and need to be controlled after initiation of DHEA (11).

Increased Mortality and the Risk for Adrenal Emergencies

Mortality in patients with chronic AI is increased compared with in the general population (12–16). The risk to dying from infectious disease was particularly high, and the clinical course of any emergency in AI patients may be aggravated in the form of an AC. AC results from a mismatch between cortisol needs and supply, especially under conditions of physical and psychological stress. The pathophysiology is not fully understood. Excessive cytokine response (such as interleukin 1 and interleukin 6 as well as tumor necrosis factor-α) because of the lack of immunosuppressive effect of cortisol in the context of infections is hypothesized. In addition, an association with mineralocorticoid and adrenalin deficiency is assumed.

The definition of AC varies, but commonly, it is defined as major acute health deterioration and at least two of the following: hypotension, acute abdominal symptoms, nausea or vomiting, altered mental state, fatigue, fever, and laboratory abnormalities (hyponatremia, hyperkalemia, or hypoglycemia).

Almost every 10th patient suffers an AC during the year, and approximately every 200th patient with AI dies from such a crisis per year (16, 17). Often, these are preventable deaths after delayed or insufficient steroid replacement, even when AI is already known and patients present their emergency card.

Main triggers for AC include infections, gastroenteritis, and surgery. Although history of AC, female sex, primary AI, prevalence of comorbidities, and diabetes insipidus have been found to be associated with a higher risk of AC, every patient needs to be regarded at risk.

The worsening of the clinical condition in the case of AC frequently occurs rapidly. Because an increase in cortisol secretion is an important adaptive mechanism during stress, AC usually occurs in the case of a relative cortisol deficit during stressful events. A quick and sufficient treatment by parenteral GC administration is essential. A retrospective study comparing reported time intervals with time targets recommended by an European expert panel revealed a delay of GC administration by medical professionals in 46% of cases. Only 54% of the patients received GC parenterally within 30 minutes (with a range of 2 to 2400 minutes) after presentation of the emergency card to the medical professional (18). This time interval was even longer in another prospective study (unpublished data), emphasizing the need for improved education of patients.

Treatment of AC is simple and straightforward.

- Intravenous (IV) hydrocortisone should be given as soon as possible (initially 100 mg followed by 100 to 200 mg over 24 hours). Instead of continuous IV hydrocortisone, 50 mg hydrocortisone every 6 hours IV/intramuscularly

Table 1. GC Treatment Options

Preparation	Additional Information
Hydrocortisone	Plasma half-life: 1.5 h
	Typical daily dose 15–25 mg (usually slightly higher doses are needed in primary AI than in secondary AI)
	Distribution of the total daily dose in two to three single doses according to the physiological profile
	Additional situation-adapted intake of smaller amounts (2.5–10 mg; *e.g.*, before physical activity possible)
Modified release hydrocortisone (Plenadren)	Two-phase hydrocortisone preparation with immediate release and sustained release (core)
	Tablets available in 5 and 20 mg; tablets are not divisible
	Single dose, slightly better approximation of physiological cortisol profile compared with conventional hydrocortisone
	Positive effects on Qol and metabolic parameters in previous smaller studies (reduction in weight, hemoglobin A1c, and blood pressure)
Hydrocortisone as continuous subcutaneous infusion via insulin pump (off label)	Experimental off-label therapy, good approximation to physiological profile, tendency to improved Qol parameters documented
	Successful use with poor absorption of oral preparations or otherwise very difficult to adjust diabetes mellitus
Prednisone tablets	Plasma half-life: 5 h; relative potency compared with hydrocortisone: 5–6:1
	Only low mineralocorticoid effect
Tools for emergency management	
Hydrocortisone ampoules	100-mg Hydrocortisone ampoules in combination with syringes and needles should be prescribed
	Available for IV injection by medical professionals or intramuscular or (off-label) subcutaneous self-injection by patients in case of gastroenteritis or other emergencies
	In otherwise healthy patients with AI, subcutaneous and intramuscular administrations show comparable pharmacokinetic profiles
	Systemic availability in obese patients is delayed after subcutaneous administration; thus, intramuscular administration should be preferred
Prednisone suppository	100-mg Prednisolone suppositories can be used as alternative treatment in case of emergency if no vomiting or diarrhea is present
	In case of unavailability of hydrocortisone for parenteral administration, other GCs (*e.g.*, prednisolone) may be given

may also be used. The continuous administration is preferable.

- In case of unavailability of hydrocortisone, any other GC may be used in case of emergency (any GC is better than nothing).
- Rapid infusion of 0.9% saline should be given.

As long as the daily dose of hydrocortisone exceeds 50 mg, no additional mineralocorticoid replacement is necessary.

Patient Education

Patient education is helpful and highly important in several aspects (19). Individualized dosing with adaptation of GC doses to different needs throughout the day may improve performance and Qol. Because many physicians are not familiar with the correct management of AI, leading to dangerous delays in treatment, patients need to be able perform the initial steps of emergency management by themselves to guide health professionals that are not familiar with the disease.

Equipping patients with an emergency card and set (GC ampoules and suppositories) and educating them about dose adaption as well as self-injection of GC are demanded by guidelines (4). To optimize patient training, standardized training programs have been developed at specialized centers, usually consisting of training courses in small groups. These trainings provide background information on the physiological role of the adrenal as well as AI and disease management. Discussion of typical situations that need GC dose adaptation and training in emergency management, including intramuscular or (off-label) subcutaneous self-administration of hydrocortisone, represent the most important part (20). First evaluations show a sustainable increase in knowledge of patients in dealing with their disease and an improvement in the sense of security in dealing with emergency situations. More patients performed

Table 2. Treatment Recommendations for Medical Interventions Based on Expert Opinion

Extensive surgery with short recovery period (for example, caesarean section, knee replacement)	100-mg Hydrocortisone IV (or intramuscularly) before induction of anesthesia followed by continuous hydrocortisone IV (100 mg/24 h)	Continuous hydrocortisone administration IV (100 mg/24 h) until patient is allowed to eat and drink again; then switch to tablets with double oral hydrocortisone dose for 24–48 h and reduce to the normal daily dose
Labor and vaginal birth	At onset of labor, 100 mg hydrocortisone IV (or intramuscularly) followed by continuous hydrocortisone IV (100 mg/24 h)	Continuous hydrocortisone administration IV (100 mg/24 h) until after birth; then switch to tablets with double oral hydrocortisone dose for 24–48 h and reduce to the normal daily dose
Small surgery (*e.g.*, cataract surgery, hernia surgery, laparoscopy), large dental surgeries under general anesthesia	100 mg Hydrocortisone IV (or intramuscularly/subcutaneously) immediately before anesthesia initiation/ anesthesia start	Double oral hydrocortisone dose for 24 h and then reduction to the normal daily dose
Dentistry with local anesthetic (*e.g.*, root canal treatment)	Additional hydrocortisone "morning dose" 1 h before the start of treatment	Double oral hydrocortisone dose for 24 h and then reduction to the normal daily dose
Minor procedures (*e.g.*, small dental procedures, skin biopsies with local anesthetic)	Usually no increase necessary depending on the individual stress or feeling of the patient; if necessary, additional intake of 20 mg hydrocortisone before intervention	Additional hydrocortisone dose (20 mg) when mild signs of cortisol deficiency occur
Bowel examinations with laxatives (*e.g.*, colonoscopy)	Case A: in case of high risk (*e.g.*, older patient, comorbidities, history of AC), hospitalization with IV administration of physiological sodium chloride infusion, 50–100 mg hydrocortisone subcutaneously or intramuscularly during bowel preparation, and 100 mg hydrocortisone IV (or intramuscularly/ subcutaneously) immediately before the start of the examination Case B: low-risk or ambulatory preparation the day before with triple daily hydrocortisone dose (important: 60-min interval between tablet intake and drink solution, drink enough additional water) plus double HC dose in the morning on the day of examination at home and then 50–100 mg hydrocortisone IV (or intramuscularly/subcutaneously) immediately before the start of the examination	Double oral hydrocortisone dose for 24 h and then reduction to the normal daily dose in case of high risk

Data are from the work by Allolio (1), the work by Burger-Stritt and Hahner (21), and the Adrenal Gland, Steroids and Hypertension section of the German Society of Endocrinology (http://www.endokrinologie.net/files/download/hydrocortison-anpassung.pdf).

initial self-medication in the case of emergency to bridge the time until professional help was provided, which clearly shortened the time to sufficient systemic GC levels and seemed to result in better outcomes (unpublished data).

MAIN CONCLUSIONS

Long-term management aims at restoration of Qol and daily performance by individualization of GC replacement adapted to daily needs. New replacement tools better resembling physiological day profiles may be of help. Side effects of GC replacement therapy are generally considered to be minor if adequate individual dose adjustment has been made. Over-replacement and excessively high levels, especially in the afternoon/evening, should be avoided. A routine bone density measurement in all patients with AI is not recommended according to current data and should only be considered individually (*e.g.*, in patients with high GC replacement doses or patients with frequent evening GC intake).

ACs are life-threatening complications of AI, which are triggered in particular by infections, and they require rapid adaptation of GC therapy. In case of vomiting or diarrhea, parenteral GC administration is obligatory. Involvement in training programs (repetition every 6 to 12 months), empowerment, and equipment of patients with emergency GCs and emergency cards should be standard for all patients (Tables 1 and 2).

CASES WITH QUESTIONS AND ANSWERS

Case 1

A 36-year-old female with secondary AI and a hydrocortisone replacement dose of hydrocortisone 20-20-0 mg complains of persistent fatigue and impaired Qol during the day as well as reduced working hours since primary diagnosis 3 years ago.

- Reduce the GC dose?
- Change GC?
- Increase the GC dose?
- Split the dose into three or more daily doses?
- Check comedication?
- Add DHEA to replacement regimen?

Case 2

A 42-year-old male diagnosed with known Addison disease presents with nausea, vomiting, and hypotension. He has already taken 100 mg hydrocortisone as an oral dose.

What is the short-term management? What is the long-term management?

DISCUSSION OF CASES AND ANSWERS

Case 1

The daily GC dose of 40 mg is high. The medication should be checked, because comedication affecting metabolism of cortisol (*e.g.*, inducers of CYP3A1, such as carbamazepine or St. John wort) might increase GC requirement. If increased GC metabolism could be excluded, situations with increased GC should be identified, and more individualized dosing should be targeted. Total daily dose should be reduced as far as is tolerated. Modified release GC treatment in combination with conventional hydrocortisone for coverage of short-term needs may be another option. A trial of 25 mg DHEA could be made. This would ideally be performed at a later time point to evaluate to what extent the respective changes influence general wellbeing.

Case 2

The patient obviously suffers from AC. Absorption of the oral GC dose is not guaranteed. Immediate parenteral administration of GCs (100 mg hydrocortisone IV followed by 100 mg as a continuous IV administration) along with 0.9% saline is necessary. After recovery, training of the patient in emergency management (self-injection of hydrocortisone) needs to be performed.

REFERENCES

1. Allolio B. Extensive expertise in endocrinology. Adrenal crisis. *Eur J Endocrinol.* 2015;**172**(3):R115–R124.
2. Rushworth RL, Torpy DJ, Falhammar H. Adrenal crises: perspectives and research directions. *Endocrine.* 2017;**55**(2):336–345.
3. Puar TH, Stikkelbroeck NM, Smans LC, Zelissen PM, Hermus AR. Adrenal crisis: still a deadly event in the 21st century. *Am J Med.* 2016;**129**(3):339.e1–339.e9.
4. Bornstein SR, Allolio B, Arlt W, Barthel A, Don-Wauchope A, Hammer GD, Husebye ES, Merke DP, Murad MH, Stratakis CA, Torpy DJ. Diagnosis and treatment of primary adrenal insufficiency: an Endocrine Society clinical practice guideline. *J Clin Endocrinol Metab.* 2016; **101**(2):364–389.
5. Husebye ES, Allolio B, Arlt W, Badenhoop K, Bensing S, Betterle C, Falorni A, Gan EH, Hulting AL, Kasperlik-Zaluska A, Kämpe O, Løvås K, Meyer G, Pearce SH. Consensus statement on the diagnosis, treatment and follow-up of patients with primary adrenal insufficiency. *J Intern Med.* 2014;**275**(2):104–115.
6. Stewart PM, Biller BM, Marelli C, Gunnarsson C, Ryan MP, Johannsson G. Exploring inpatient hospitalizations and morbidity in patients with adrenal insufficiency. *J Clin Endocrinol Metab.* 2016;**101**(12): 4843–4850.
7. Burger-Stritt S, Pulzer A, Hahner S. Quality of life and life expectancy in patients with adrenal insufficiency: what is true and what is urban myth? *Front Horm Res.* 2016;**46**:171–183.
8. Mallappa A, Debono M. Recent advances in hydrocortisone replacement treatment. *Endocr Dev.* 2016;**30**:42–53.
9. Johannsson G, Nilsson AG, Bergthorsdottir R, Burman P, Dahlqvist P, Ekman B, Engström BE, Olsson T, Ragnarsson O, Ryberg M, Wahlberg J, Biller BM, Monson JP, Stewart PM, Lennernäs H, Skrtic S. Improved cortisol exposure-time profile and outcome in patients with adrenal insufficiency: a prospective randomized trial of a novel hydrocortisone dual-release formulation. *J Clin Endocrinol Metab.* 2012;**97**(2): 473–481.
10. Nilsson AG, Bergthorsdottir R, Burman P, Dahlqvist P, Ekman B, Engstrom BE, Ragnarsson O, Skrtic S, Wahlberg J, Achenbach H, Uddin S, Marelli C, Johannsson G. Long-term safety of once-daily, dual-release hydrocortisone in patients with adrenal insufficiency: a phase 3b, open-label, extension study. *Eur J Endocrinol.* 2017; **176**(6):715–725.
11. Lang K, Burger-Stritt S, Hahner S. Is DHEA replacement beneficial in chronic adrenal failure? *Best Pract Res Clin Endocrinol Metab.* 2015; **29**(1):25–32.
12. Bergthorsdottir R, Leonsson-Zachrisson M, Odén A, Johannsson G. Premature mortality in patients with Addison's disease: a population-based study. *J Clin Endocrinol Metab.* 2006;**91**(12):4849–4853.
13. Burman P, Mattsson AF, Johannsson G, Höybye C, Holmer H, Dahlqvist P, Berinder K, Engström BE, Ekman B, Erfurth EM, Svensson J, Wahlberg J, Karlsson FA. Deaths among adult patients with hypopituitarism: hypocortisolism during acute stress, and de novo malignant brain tumors contribute to an increased mortality. *J Clin Endocrinol Metab.* 2013;**98**(4):1466–1475.
14. Erichsen MM, Lovas K, Fougner KJ, Svartberg J, Hauge ER, Bollerslev J, Berg JP, Mella B, Husebye ES. Normal overall mortality rate in Addison's disease, but young patients are at risk of premature death. *Eur J Endocrinol.* 2009;**160**(2):233–237.
15. Bensing S, Brandt L, Tabaroj F, Sjöberg O, Nilsson B, Ekbom A, Blomqvist P, Kämpe O. Increased death risk and altered cancer incidence pattern in patients with isolated or combined autoimmune primary adrenocortical insufficiency. *Clin Endocrinol (Oxf).* 2008; **69**(5):697–704.
16. Hahner S, Spinnler C, Fassnacht M, Burger-Stritt S, Lang K, Milovanovic D, Beuschlein F, Willenberg HS, Quinkler M, Allolio B. High incidence of adrenal crisis in educated patients with chronic adrenal

insufficiency: a prospective study. *J Clin Endocrinol Metab.* 2015; **100**(2):407–416.

17. Hahner S, Loeffler M, Bleicken B, Drechsler C, Milovanovic D, Fassnacht M, Ventz M, Quinkler M, Allolio B. Epidemiology of adrenal crisis in chronic adrenal insufficiency: the need for new prevention strategies. *Eur J Endocrinol.* 2010;**162**(3):597–602.
18. Hahner S, Hemmelmann N, Quinkler M, Beuschlein F, Spinnler C, Allolio B. Timelines in the management of adrenal crisis - targets, limits and reality. *Clin Endocrinol (Oxf).* 2015;**82**(4):497–502.
19. Repping-Wuts HJ, Stikkelbroeck NM, Noordzij A, Kerstens M, Hermus AR. A glucocorticoid education group meeting: an effective strategy for improving self-management to prevent adrenal crisis. *Eur J Endocrinol.* 2013;**169**(1):17–22.
20. Hahner S, Burger-Stritt S, Allolio B. Subcutaneous hydrocortisone administration for emergency use in adrenal insufficiency. *Eur J Endocrinol.* 2013;**169**(2):147–154.
21. Burger-Stritt S, Hahner S. Adrenal crisis [in German]. *Internist (Berl).* 2017;**58**(10):1037–1041.

Challenging Hypercalcemia Cases

M48
Presented, March 17–20, 2018

Richard Eastell, MD. Department of Oncology and Metabolism, University of Sheffield, Sheffield S5 7AU, United Kingdom, E-mail: r.eastell@sheffield.ac.uk

SIGNIFICANCE OF THE CLINICAL PROBLEM

Primary hyperparathyroidism (PHPT) is one of the most common endocrine diseases. However, the presence of high serum calcium, high parathyroid hormone (PTH), or both does not always indicate this diagnosis. Even when it does, there can be challenges in patient management.

BARRIERS TO OPTIMAL PRACTICE

- The physician needs to be aware that high calcium or high PTH does not always mean PHPT.
- The physician may need to be aware of the need for medical treatments in PHPT.

LEARNING OBJECTIVES

As a result of participating in this session, learners should be able to:

- Make a differential diagnosis for hypercalcemia
- Appreciate the medical treatments that may be necessary in managing PHPT

STRATEGIES FOR DIAGNOSIS, THERAPY, AND/OR MANAGEMENT

The most common cause of hypercalcemia in clinical practice is PHPT. This disorder is characterized by incompletely regulated, chronic, excessive secretion of PTH from one or more parathyroid glands. Serum calcium is high, and PTH is either high or high-normal in ~12% of cases (1).

The presentation of the disorder has changed over the past 100 years. We commonly saw patients with osteitis fibrosa up to 50 years ago, but now they are rare. With the advent of laboratory automation, high serum calcium often was identified in asymptomatic patients, and the bone complication usually was osteoporosis, with preferential loss of cortical bone (2). During the workup for osteoporosis, we now commonly find high PTH with normal serum calcium, so-called normocalcemic hyperparathyroidism (3).

The diagnosis of PHPT may be considered in two steps. First, are we sure this is PHPT? In this step, we ensure that the serum calcium adjusted for albumin is raised on more than one occasion and that the PTH by second- or third-generation assay is high or high-normal (4). Common causes of low PTH with hypercalcemia are hypercalcemia of malignancy (commonly as a result of high PTH-related protein) or sarcoidosis [as a result of increased active form of vitamin D (1,25-hydroxyvitamin D)]. The most difficult differential diagnosis is familial hypocalciuric hyperparathyroidism (FHH). This is associated with hypercalcemia (usually <12 mg/dL) and high or high-normal PTH, but the urinary calcium excretion rate is low (<100 mg/d), and the fractional excretion of calcium is low (<0.01). If there is doubt, then genetic testing for 1 of the 3 forms of FHH is recommended. Second, the complications of PHTP are sought. The bone mineral density is measured at the lumbar spine, total hip, and one-third forearm (5). If total alkaline phosphatase is raised, then this might signal osteitis fibrosa and merit radiographs of the hand (for subperiosteal erosions) or skull (for pepperpot skull). Vitamin D deficiency is common and should be corrected before surgery and repleted with high-dose vitamin D (6). Kidney stones are commonly asymptomatic and should be sought with imaging (*e.g.*, ultrasound) and a 24-hour urine collection for calcium and creatinine to identify the more than one-third of cases with hypercalciuria.

Management of PHPT usually involves surgery if any complications are present or the criteria for asymptomatic hyperparathyroidism are met and the patient is willing and able to have surgery (7). Indications for surgery in asymptomatic hyperparathyroidism (8) are serum calcium >1 mg/dL above the upper limit of normal, bone mineral density T score at any of the 3 sites below −2.5 or the presence of vertebral fracture, chronic kidney disease stages 3 to 5, hypercalciuria (>400 mg/d), kidney stones or nephrocalcinosis, and age <50 years. There are a number of benefits of surgery, including an increase in bone mineral density, a likely decrease in the risk of vertebral fractures, and a reduction in the risk of kidney stones, and surgery may prevent a decline in renal function (9). The cure rate is 95%, and there are few complications in experienced hands. The complications include damage to the recurrent laryngeal nerve, postoperative hypocalcemia as a result of hypoparathyroidism (low PTH, high phosphate), and hungry bone syndrome (high PTH, low phosphate). There may be recurrence if the PHPT was due to hyperplasia, which can occur in up to 15% of cases; it might indicate the need to search for multiple endocrine neoplasia. Recurrence also may occur after resection of parathyroid cancer; this condition is suspected if the parathyroid tumor is palpable and serum calcium is very high.

If the patient does not undergo surgery, then medical monitoring is recommended. This would include serum calcium testing annually; bone mineral density every 2 years and vertebral fracture assessment, if indicated; and estimated glomerular filtration rate (eGFR) annually. If kidney stones are suspected, then renal imaging and urinary calcium also are recommended.

There are effective medical treatments for PHPT. Cinacalcet reduces PTH and usually returns serum calcium to normal.

However, it has no effect on bone mineral density. Alendronate increases bone mineral density but has little effect on serum calcium (6).

MAIN CONCLUSIONS

Raised PTH and calcium usually indicate PHPT but may indicate FHH. Raised PTH but normal calcium usually indicate secondary hyperparathyroidism but may indicate normocalcemic hyperparathyroidism. Hypocalcemia may follow parathyroidectomy and can be caused by hungry bone syndrome as well as hypoparathyroidism. There is a long differential diagnosis of high calcium and low PTH.

CASES

Case 1

A 52-year-old woman volunteered for a clinical trial and was found to have a calcium level of 10.3 mg/dL (normal, 8.8 to 10.4 mg/dL) and a PTH level of 131 ng/L (normal, <65 ng/L). Vitamin D and eGFR were normal, and she had no other disease or took a drug known to affect mineral metabolism. Is this:

A. PHPT
B. Secondary hyperparathyroidism
C. FHH
D. Normocalcemic hyperparathyroidism

The patient became hypercalcemic after a few years and had accelerated bone loss, but she did not want surgery. Which treatments are effective at preventing bone loss?

A. Denosumab
B. Bisphosphonates
C. Cinacalcet
D. All of the above

Case 2

A 28-year-old women presented to the emergency department with a 1-week history of nausea and fatigue. Her serum calcium was 16.7 mg/dL (4.17 mmol/L); creatinine, 2.5 mg/dL (226 μmol/L); and PTH, 13.2 ng/L (1.4 pmol/L; range, 1.6 to 6.9 pmol/L). What is the most likely diagnosis?

A. Laboratory error
B. PHPT
C. Sarcoidosis
D. FHH

Further investigation revealed that the patient had reticular fibrosis in her lungs and an angiotensin-converting enzyme activity of >150 IU/L. What is the optimal treatment?

A. Bisphosphonates
B. Surgery
C. Prednisone
D. Watch and wait

Case 3

A 30-year-old man was found to have high serum calcium of 15.2 mg/dL (3.8 mmol/L) and high PTH of 350 pg/mL (37 pmol/L). He had successful removal of adenoma. At the postoperative follow-up visit, he was found to have normal serum calcium of 9.0 mg/dL (2.25 mmol/L), high PTH of 316 pg/mL (33.5 pmol/L), undetectable urinary calcium, low vitamin D at 14 ng/mL (35 nmol/L), and high alkaline phosphatase activity at 217 IU/L (normal, <120 IU/L). What is the most likely explanation for these findings?

A. Postoperative hypoparathyroidism
B. Recurrent PHPT
C. Severe vitamin D deficiency
D. Hungry bone syndrome

DISCUSSION OF CASES AND ANSWERS

Case 1

The first answer is D, "Normocalcemic hyperparathyroidism," because the serum calcium is normal and PTH high. These findings also would be present in secondary hyperparathyroidism, but all known causes were ruled out (especially vitamin D deficiency and renal failure). Confirmation of normal serum calcium and raised PTH usually occurs on at least 2 occasions up to 6 months apart to exclude vitamin D deficiency (25-hydroxyvitamin D >20 ng/mL), stage 3 chronic kidney disease (eGFR >60 mg/min/1.73 m^2), drugs known to increase PTH (loop-acting diuretics, antiresorptive drugs, lithium), hypercalciuria, or malabsorption syndrome (4).

The second answer is B, "Bisphosphonates." There are good clinical trial data to support the use of bisphosphonates in PHPT (6). Cinacalcet has no benefit on bone mineral density (surprisingly), and there are no clinical trial data with denosumab.

Case 2

The first answer is C, "Sarcoidosis," which results in high calcium and low PTH. The low PTH rules out PHPT and FHH. Laboratory error is unlikely in that the patient has symptoms consistent with hypercalcemia.

The second answer is C, "Prednisone." Prednisone at a high dose is required (10). The main mechanism for the hypercalcemia is increased calcium absorption as a result of an increase in the active form of vitamin D (1,25-dihydroxyvitamin D), so an inhibitor of bone resorption, such as a bisphosphonate, is unlikely to have much effect, and there is no need for surgery because no parathyroid disease exists. Watching and waiting is dangerous because at these levels of serum calcium, patients become dehydrated and enter a state of disequilibrium hypercalcemia.

Case 3

The answer is D, "Hungry bone syndrome" (11). This condition is most common in patients with osteitis fibrosa before surgery. PTH is high, so the diagnosis cannot be hypoparathyroidism. The serum calcium is low-normal, so the diagnosis is unlikely to be recurrent PHPT. The biochemistry is consistent with severe vitamin D deficiency, except the vitamin D level is in the insufficient range. To have these biochemical changes, we would expect an undetectable (or very low) vitamin D. The recent parathyroid surgery points to hungry bone syndrome.

REFERENCES

1. Fillée C, Keller T, Mourad M, Brinkmann T, Ketelslegers JM. Impact of vitamin D-related serum PTH reference values on the diagnosis of mild primary hyperparathyroidism, using bivariate calcium/PTH reference regions. *Clin Endocrinol (Oxf)*. 2012;**76**(6):785–789.
2. Silverberg SJ, Shane E, de la Cruz L, Dempster DW, Feldman F, Seldin D, Jacobs TP, Siris ES, Cafferty M, Parisien MV, Lindsay R, Clemens TL, Bilezikian JP. Skeletal disease in primary hyperparathyroidism. *J Bone Miner Res*. 1989;**4**(3):283–291.
3. Cusano NE, Silverberg SJ, Bilezikian JP. Normocalcemic primary hyperparathyroidism. *J Clinical Densitom*. 2013;**16**(1):33–39.
4. Eastell R, Brandi ML, Costa AG, D'Amour P, Shoback DM, Thakker RV. Diagnosis of asymptomatic primary hyperparathyroidism: proceedings of the Fourth International Workshop. *J Clin Endocrinol Metab*. 2014;**99**(10):3570–3579.
5. Silverberg SJ, Clarke BL, Peacock M, Bandeira F, Boutroy S, Cusano NE, Dempster D, Lewiecki EM, Liu JM, Minisola S, Rejnmark L, Silva BC, Walker MD, Bilezikian JP. Current issues in the presentation of asymptomatic primary hyperparathyroidism: proceedings of the Fourth International Workshop. *J Clin Endocrinol Metab*. 2014;**99**(10):3580–3594.
6. Marcocci C, Bollerslev J, Khan AA, Shoback DM. Medical management of primary hyperparathyroidism: proceedings of the Fourth International Workshop on the Management of Asymptomatic Primary Hyperparathyroidism. *J Clin Endocrinol Metab*. 2014;**99**(10):3607–3618.
7. Udelsman R, Åkerström G, Biagini C, Duh QY, Miccoli P, Niederle B, Tonelli F. The surgical management of asymptomatic primary hyperparathyroidism: proceedings of the Fourth International Workshop. *J Clin Endocrinol Metab*. 2014;**99**(10):3595–3606.
8. Bilezikian JP, Brandi ML, Eastell R, Silverberg SJ, Udelsman R, Marcocci C, Potts JT Jr. Guidelines for the management of asymptomatic primary hyperparathyroidism: summary statement from the Fourth International Workshop. *J Clin Endocrinol Metab*. 2014;**99**(10):3561–3569.
9. Khan AA, Hanley DA, Rizzoli R, Bollerslev J, Young JE, Rejnmark L, Thakker R, D'Amour P, Paul T, Van Uum S, Sharyyef MZ, Goltzman D, Kaiser S, Cusano NE, Bouillon R, Mosekilde L, Kung AW, Rao SD, Bhadada SK, Clarke BL, Liu J, Duh Q, Lewiecki EM, Bandeira F, Eastell R, Marcocci C, Silverberg SJ, Udelsman R, Davison KS, Potts JT Jr, Brandi ML, Bilezikian JP. Primary hyperparathyroidism: review and recommendations on evaluation, diagnosis, and management. A Canadian and international consensus. *Osteoporos Int*. 2017;**28**(1):1–19.
10. Sandler LM, Winearls CG, Fraher LJ, Clemens TL, Smith R, O'Riordan JL. Studies of the hypercalcaemia of sarcoidosis: effect of steroids and exogenous vitamin D3 on the circulating concentrations of 1,25-dihydroxy vitamin D3. *Q J Med*. 1984;**53**(210):165–180.
11. Brasier AR, Nussbaum SR. Hungry bone syndrome: clinical and biochemical predictors of its occurrence after parathyroid surgery. *Am J Med*. 1988;**84**(4):654–660.

What to Do About Flushing and Sweating Disorders

M54
Presented, March 17-20, 2018

Pierre-Marc Bouloux, BSC, MD, FRCP. Centre for Neuroendocrinology, University College London Medical School, London NW3 2QG, United Kingdom, E-mail: p.bouloux@ucl.ac.uk

SIGNIFICANCE OF THE CLINICAL PROBLEM

Flushing and sweating disorders are frequent causes of referral to an endocrinologist. Flushing describes episodic attacks of redness of the skin together with a sensation of warmth or burning of the face, neck, and less frequently the upper trunk and abdomen. The vasodilatation of flushing can result from the direct action of a circulating vasodilator substance (*e.g.*, histamine) or enhanced vasodilator autonomic neural activity to cutaneous vasculature of face (traveling with the trigeminal nerve), neck, and upper trunk, where flushing is most frequent.

Eccrine sweat glands are innervated by autonomic nerve fibers, and neurally mediated flushing is frequently associated with sweating (wet flushing) as opposed to isolated (dry) flushing secondary to a circulating vasodilator substance. Thus, the presence or absence of sweating may represent an important marker of the flushing mechanism. Flushing attacks are typically transient, in contrast to the persistent erythema of photosensitivity, sunburn, or acute contact reactions. Over time, repeated flushing may however result in telangiectasia or even rosacea.

Flushing and sweating are frequently an exaggeration of a physiological process, and a full biochemical workup of every case is neither practical nor cost-effective. Although a thorough anamnesis frequently identifies an obvious cause (*e.g.*, vasomotor instability in the menopausal years), often the diagnosis is far from obvious, and it becomes incumbent on the practitioner to exclude a potentially serious underlying cause of symptoms, which can have a profound effect on the patient's quality of life.

BARRIERS TO OPTIMAL CLINICAL PRACTICE

The causes of flushing and sweating are potentially myriad, but a careful structured history and examination may yield important diagnostic clues. In an age of defensive medical practice, the attending clinician may (reflexly) perform a bewildering number of complicated and often expensive investigations to rule out rare pathologies. Perseverance and unhurried history taking are essential to eschew this pitfall. Patients with flushing and sweating may reach the endocrinologist "to rule out an endocrine cause," having initially been referred to dermatologists, gastroenterologists, gynecologists, neurologists, neuroendocrine tumor departments, and even psychiatrists without a prior definitive diagnosis. An impoverished patient may present desperate for a diagnosis and treatment, and it behooves the endocrinologist, using common sense and a sound knowledge of internal medicine, to elucidate the diagnosis.

LEARNING OBJECTIVES

- To conduct an appropriate anamnesis
- To appreciate the broad differential diagnosis and unusual causes of these symptoms
- To become familiar with common pathologies and the range of drugs liable to cause flushing/sweating
- To understand the range of possible therapeutic interventions

DIAGNOSTIC EVALUATION OF THE PATIENT WITH FLUSHING/SWEATING

The many characteristics of these symptoms should be elicited prior to embarking on expensive laboratory evaluation. These include the (1) identification of provocative and palliative factors, (2) morphology and distribution of the symptoms, (3) identification of associated features, and (4) temporal characteristics of the symptoms.

Provocative or Palliative Factors

The nature of precipitants (exercise, specific foods, emotion, stress, or anxiety) of a flushing/sweating episode may suggest an etiological underlying systemic disease (*e.g.*, mastocytosis and carcinoid syndrome). Drugs are a particularly common cause of flushing (see Table 1). A recent review has highlighted the fact that some 620 drugs have been associated with flushing!

Morphology of Flush/Distribution of Sweat

- Is it stereotype and does it come and go? Is there photographic evidence?
- Is the redness patchy or confluent?
- What is the color of the flush, and is there cyanosis?
- Is the flushing preceded or followed by pallor?
- Which part(s) of the body is/are affected by sweating?

Associated Features

These include respiratory symptoms (*e.g.*, wheezing), gastrointestinal (GI) symptoms (colicky pain and diarrhea), headache, urticaria, facial edema, hypertension, hypotension, and palpitations.

Temporal Characteristics

What is the frequency and duration of the flush/sweat?

Patients may not have thought carefully about these questions, and important information can be obtained from a

Table 1. Common Drug-Induced Flushing

All vasodilators (*e.g.*, nitroglycerin, prostaglandins)
Calcium channel blockers (nifedipine, *etc.*)
Nicotinic acid (not nicotinamide)
Morphine and other opiates
Amyl nitrite and butyl nitrite
Cholinergic drugs
Bromocriptine used in Parkinson disease
Thyrotropin-releasing hormone
Tamoxifen, clomiphene, goserelin
Cyproterone acetate
Oral triamcinolone
Cyclosporin
Rifampin
Sildenafil citrate, vardenafil, tadalafil

2- to 4-week diary in which the patient records qualitative and quantitative aspects of the flushing/sweating event and lists exposure to all exogenous agents/precipitants. If the diagnosis remains obscure after evaluation of a 2- to 4-week diary, an exclusion diet can be given, paying attention to foods high in histamine, foods and drugs that affect urinary 5-hydroxyindoleacetic acid (5-HIAA) tests, and foods and beverages that cause flushing. If the flushing reactions completely disappear, restoring the excluded items individually (rechallenge) can identify the causative agent. If the flushing/sweating reactions continue unabated, further metabolic workup may be mandated.

SPECIFIC CAUSES OF FLUSHING AND SWEATING

Blushing

Embarrassment or anger may cause blushing in individuals with a low threshold for this response. The reaction itself may be unusually intense. Explanation and reassurance are usually sufficient. If necessary, propranolol or nadolol may be used to alleviate the symptom.

Thermal Stimuli

Heat provokes flushing in many, and overheating can lower the threshold to flushing due to other causes such as menopause. Overheating, such as after exercise or a sauna, and hot drinks can induce physiological flushing due to the action of a rise in blood temperature on the anterior hypothalamic thermoregulatory center. The temperature of hot coffee rather than its caffeine content causes flushing. One useful maneuver for patients faced with a brief thermal exposure is to suck on ice chips carried in an insulated cup, to see if this attenuates flushing.

Menopausal Flushing/Sweating

About 80% of postmenopausal women experience flushing associated with sweating; a similar syndrome may also occur in men with prostate cancer receiving treatment with gonadotropin-releasing hormone analogs such as goserelin. Sixty to seventy percent of postmenopausal women experience hot flushes for 1 to 5 years, 26% for 6 to 10 years, and 10% for >11 years. There is considerable variation in the frequency, intensity, and duration of hot flushes within and among individuals. Typically, a hot flush begins with a sensation of warmth in the head and face, followed by facial flushing that may radiate down the neck and to other parts of the body; it is associated with a slight increase in temperature and pulse rate, followed by a decline in temperature and profuse perspiration over the area of the flush distribution. Visible changes occur in ~50% of women, each flush lasting 1 to 5 minutes. Rapid estrogen withdrawal rather than a low estrogen level *per se* itself induces hot flushes. A pulse of luteinizing hormone appears to be released synchronous with each flush, but not causally so *per se* because the phenomenon persists after hypophysectomy. Rather, synchronization is likely to be with gonadotropin-releasing hormone release. The anterior hypothalamus has estrogen and progesterone receptors, and both hormones can be used effectively to suppress hot flushes. α_2 noradrenergic pathways appear to participate in the pathogenesis of hot flushes because the α_2-adrenergic agonist clonidine attenuates hot flushes by presynaptically suppressing noradrenaline release. A number of drugs can induce a "pharmacological menopause" with associated flushing, including danazol, tamoxifen, clomiphene citrate, and leuprolide.

Certain characteristics suggest the diagnosis of climacteric flushing: drenching perspiration, a prodromal sensation of overheating before the onset of flushing and sweating, and waking episodes at night with the typical symptoms. Alcohol can enhance a menopausal flush. Veralipride, a neuroleptic benzamide dopamine antagonist, attenuates the frequency and intensity of menopausal flushing in premenopausal women pretreated with goserelin (gonadotropin-releasing hormone agonist) for endometriosis, but it has been withdrawn from European markets. Hormone replacement therapy is the most effective at countering menopausal flushing. Micronized progesterone is also helpful, and recently, experimental data has suggested that neurokinin B antagonists may offer an effective nonhormonal way of countering these vasomotor symptoms.

Drug-Induced Flushing

Other drugs include corticotropin-releasing hormone and thyrotropin-releasing hormone, doxorubicin, and niacin (Table 1). Some 5% to 15% of patients taking phosphodiesterase type 5 inhibitors complain of flushing also. Systemic morphine administration can cause histamine-mediated flushing of the face, neck, and upper thorax. Some patients develop facial flushing and/or generalized erythema after epidural or intra-articular administration of triamcinolone; this is counterintuitive, as glucocorticoids are usually vasoconstrictors.

Alcohol-Induced Flushing

Certain Asian genotypes evince extensive flushing in response to modest alcohol intake, due to higher plasma levels of acetaldehyde resulting from deficiency of liver aldehyde dehydrogenase isoenzyme. These patients can be identified using an ethanol patch test, which produces localized erythema. A special type of alcohol flush is also associated with chlorpropamide, a rarely used sulfonylurea compound. Even small amounts of alcohol provoke intense flushing within a few minutes of ingestion. This flushing is not associated with sweating, but in some cases tachycardia, tachypnea, and hypotension may be seen. Alcohol ingestion can trigger flushing in carcinoid tumors, mastocytosis, medullary thyroid carcinoma, and certain lymphoid tumors.

Food-Associated Flushing/Sweating

Spicy or sour foods can induce gustatory facial flushing, due to a neural reflex involving branches of the trigeminal nerve. The flushing may curiously be unilateral. The flushing of monosodium glutamate (MSG; sino-cibal syndrome) is controversial. Oral challenge with MSG often fails to induce flushing in volunteers with a history of MSG flushing, and it may be appropriate to look at other dietary agents, such as red pepper, other spices, nitrites, and sulfites (additives in many foods); thermally hot foods and beverages; and alcohol. Scombroid fish poisoning (tuna and mackerel) is due to the ingestion of fish left in a warm temperature for hours. In addition to flushing, patients with scombroid have sweating, vomiting, and diarrhea. These symptoms are due to intoxication with histamine, which is thought to be generated by histidine decarboxylation by bacteria in spoiled fish.

Carcinoid Syndrome

Manifestations of carcinoid tumors include flushing, bronchoconstriction, GI hypermotility, and cardiac disease. These neuroendocrine tumors can produce a variety of peptides, hormones, and neurotransmitters, many of which are vasoactive. "Carcinoid syndrome" occurs in ~10% of patients with these tumors, and in 75%, episodes of severe flushing are precipitated by exercise, alcohol, stress, and certain foods (spices, chocolate, cheese, avocados, plums, walnuts, red sausage, and red wine). Often, flushing may appear without provocation (Table 2).

Foregut tumors (stomach, lung, and pancreas) are associated with a bright-red "geographic" flush of a more sustained duration, as well as lacrimation, wheezing, sweating, and a sensation of burning. In ileal tumors, the flush is patchier and more violaceous, intermingled with areas of pallor, and does not last as long. Either type may be associated with facial edema that may progress to telangiectasia and even rosacea. Pellagra-like skin lesions (hyperkeratosis; xerosis; scaling of the legs, forearms, and trunk; angular cheilitis; and glossitis) can result from excessive utilization of tryptophan by the carcinoid tumor, leaving little for the daily niacin requirement. Seventy percent of patients also have watery diarrhea, and 35% develop right-sided endocardial fibrosis and pulmonary valve stenosis, leading to right heart failure. Diarrhea and other GI manifestations may precede or coexist with the flushing.

Table 2. Factors Inducing Flushing in Carcinoid Syndrome

Factor
Hot food/beverage
Spicy food
Chocolate
Cheeses
Tomatoes
Avocados
Red plums
Walnuts
Eggplant
Alcohol
Emotional stress
Valsalva maneuver
Straining
Vigorous coughing
Sudden direct pressure on a large carcinoid tumor

Ninety-five percent of all carcinoids are found in the appendix, rectum, or small intestine, the remainder arising outside the intestinal tract (ovary, testis, and bronchus). In general, the larger the primary tumor, the greater the likelihood of metastasis, with prognostic implications. Carcinoids of the appendix and rectum rarely present with the "carcinoid syndrome." Forty to fifty percent of patients with carcinoids of the small intestine or proximal colon have manifestations of the carcinoid syndrome. Tumors that secrete their hormonal product into the portal venous system do not cause flushing because the released amines are inactivated by liver monoamine oxidase. In contrast, liver metastases escape hepatic bioamine inactivation, delivering their product directly into the systemic circulation, triggering flushing. Pulmonary or ovarian carcinoids release pharmacological products directly into the venous circulation, bypassing the portal system, and can therefore cause symptoms without metastasizing to the liver.

Pathophysiology

Foregut carcinoid flushing is caused by histamine release. Flushing seen with ileal carcinoids cannot be explained solely by the production of serotonin. Serotonin may or may not be released into the circulation during flushing, and intravenous (IV) serotonin infusion does not cause flushing. Foregut carcinoids do not generally secrete serotonin but, instead, its precursor, 5-hydroxytryptamine. Screening should therefore seek this product if other metabolites are not elevated. Other potential mediators include prostaglandins and tachykinins. Tachykinins are believed to be mediators of flushing in midgut carcinoids. They exert vasodilation and contraction of various types of smooth muscle. These peptides include substance P, substance K, and neuropeptide K. Urine excretion of histamine is usually increased in patients who have gastric carcinoid.

Diagnosis

Clinical diagnosis is not difficult in patients with flushing episodes associated with systemic symptoms (diarrhea, wheezing, and weight loss) and hepatomegaly. It is more difficult in patients who have occasional flushing without associated symptoms. Only when there is reasonable clinical suspicion should biochemical testing be done, and localization studies must be reserved for those cases proven biochemically.

Provocative Tests

When in doubt, a carcinoid flush can be provoked by alcohol ingestion (4 mL of 45% ethanol) or the infusion of 6 μg noradrenaline, an effect blocked by phentolamine (5 to 15 mg IV). Calcium gluconate, 10 to 15 mg/kg, IV administered over 4 hours, may induce a flush mimicking a spontaneous attack. Epinephrine reverses flushing in patients with mastocytosis but provokes flushing in patients with the carcinoid syndrome. The test must be performed in a controlled environment. A 1 μg/mL solution of epinephrine in normal saline is administered by IV bolus beginning with an initial dose of 0.05 μg. The dose is doubled at intervals of 10 minutes until flushing appears or until a maximum of 6.4 μg is given. When flushing occurs, it usually begins within 60 seconds after epinephrine administration, dissipating after 3 or 4 minutes.

Biochemical Diagnosis

The diagnosis should be confirmed by determining urinary excretion of 5-HIAA, the major metabolite of serotonin, normally 2 to 10 mg (10 to 50 μmol) per 24 hours. A value >150 μmol per 24 hours (30 mg per 24 hours) is usually diagnostic, levels in carcinoid syndrome often exceeding 40 mg per day (sensitivity 75%; specificity nearing 100%). Levels of 5-HIAA do not always correlate with the severity of flushing, suggesting that other vasoactive substances may be at play. Excretion fluctuates, often necessitating repeated measurements. Some patients with carcinoid cannot convert serotonin to 5-HIAA and harbor high circulating levels of serotonin, and have a normal urinary 5-HIAA. Dietary factors are frequent confounders; the patient should therefore receive a diet free of offending items for 3 days before urine collection. Although levels of serotonin in patients with tumors usually far exceed those found after food ingestion, this precaution helps to exclude carcinoid in individuals with borderline high 5-HIAA levels.

Measuring blood serotonin is helpful when urinary 5-HIAA is equivocal. Patients with carcinoid syndrome have very high blood levels of serotonin. Measurement of serotonin and its metabolites permits the detection of >80% of neuroendocrine tumors. Even carcinoids that predominantly secrete 5-hydroxytryptophan are associated with increased urinary 5-HIAA excretion because released 5-hydroxytryptophan is converted to serotonin in other tissues and subsequently metabolized to 5-HIAA. Chromogranin A, a peptide cosecreted with serotonin, is elevated in most patients with carcinoid tumors. In the evaluation of flushing with an equivocal 24-hour urinary 5-HIAA, a normal plasma chromogranin A value suggests nonendocrine causes. This test is sensitive but not specific, and its predictive value in carcinoid is still uncertain. Flushing is associated with a rise in circulating substance P in 80% of patients with gastric carcinoid, and neurokinin A levels are elevated in some patients.

Management

Corticosteroids, phenothiazines, and bromocriptine are sometimes effective in suppressing flushing in patients with bronchial carcinoid tumors, as may cyproheptadine, a serotonin antagonist. Combined administration of H_1 and H_2 receptor antagonists may prevent attacks of flushing in patients with foregut carcinoid tumors that produce histamine. The most researched interferon (IFN) in the treatment of carcinoid disease is IFN-α. Comparable to somatostatin analogs, the most pronounced effects of IFN-α are inhibition of disease progression and symptom relief, with ~75% of patients reporting the resolution of diarrhea or flushing. IFN-α, similar to other IFNs studied in the treatment of carcinoids (*e.g.*, IFN-γ and human leukocyte IFN), has substantial adverse effects, including alopecia, anorexia, fatigue, weight loss, fever, a flu-like syndrome, and myelosuppression; however, IFN-α may show greater antitumor activity than somatostatin analogs.

Because catecholamines are known to precipitate attacks, a trial of clonidine is worthwhile. Long-acting somatostatin analogs such as octreotide/lanreotide are now the agents of choice, producing amelioration of symptoms accompanied by a marked reduction in the urinary excretion of 5-HIAA. Patients should receive an adequate niacin supplement (nicotinamide rather than nicotinic acid, because the latter causes flushing) and should avoid foods, agents, and activities that precipitate symptoms.

In some patients, failure of medical treatment may necessitate carrying out hepatic artery embolization when secondary tumors are evident. This treatment is based upon the dependence of metastatic malignant tissue (but not healthy liver parenchyma) on an intact hepatic arterial blood supply. Antitumor chemotherapy may control the disease, but controlled trials are under way to identify optimal regimens. IFN-α causes symptomatic relief accompanied by lowering of urinary 5-HIAA.

The four radionuclide conjugates most commonly used in the treatment of carcinoid disease are ^{131}I-MIBG (iodine-131-meta-iodobenzylguanidine), ^{111}indium, ^{90}yttrium, and ^{177}lutetium, with the latter three bound to a variety of somatostatin analogs. However, the median tumor response rate for the patients treated with ^{131}I-MIBG is <5%, although the modality appears somewhat more effective in achieving biochemical stability (~50%) or tumor stability (~70%). Although ^{111}In-labeled somatostatin analogs are the most commonly studied radiopeptides to date, largely reflecting their availability, and with therapeutic benefits similar to ^{131}I-MIBG, the most promising advance in radiopeptide therapeutics has been the development of ^{177}Lu-octreotate, which emits both β and γ radiation. In the largest patient series treated to date with lutetium-labeled somatostatin analogs (n = 131; 65 with GI carcinoids), remission rates were correlated positively with high pretherapy octreotide scintigraphy uptake and limited hepatic tumor load. In patients with extensive liver involvement, median time to progression was shorter (26 months) compared with patients who had either stable disease or tumor regression (>36 months).

Prognosis

About one-fifth of patients with the carcinoid syndrome undergo a protracted course. In the remainder, deterioration can be rapid. The mean survival is ~8 years, with some surviving up to 20 years. Mean survival is 36 months after the first flushing episode. Targeted radionuclide therapy may in the future extend the duration of remission in inoperable cases.

Mastocytoses

Etiology

Mastocytoses are benign proliferative disorders of the reticuloendothelial system, and familial cases have been reported. Mastocytoses are due to a hyperplastic rather than a neoplastic process. They are often self-limited, especially in childhood. Mast cells possess the enzyme histidine decarboxylase, which enables them to synthesize and store histamine. Other preformed mediators include tryptase, chymase, and carboxypeptidase. Serotonin has not been detected in human mast cells.

Histopathology

There are increased numbers of normal-looking mast cells in the dermis. These cells may be predominantly perivascular or may show a nodular distribution. The epidermis is normal, apart from increased melanization.

Biochemical Markers

Symptoms of mastocytosis result from the release of products of mast cell activation. Plasma histamine levels are frequently raised in patients with systemic symptoms, and elevated urinary excretion of histamine and its metabolite methyl imidazole acetic acid (MIAA) can also be seen. Plasma tryptase levels can also be elevated. Prostaglandin D_2 (PGD_2) is another product of mast cell activation. Urinary excretion of this substance and its major metabolites can be elevated severalfold in patients with mastocytoses. Urine should be collected within a few hours of an attack.

Clinical Presentation

Episodic bright-red flushing occurs either spontaneously or after rubbing the skin or exposure to alcohol or mast-cell degranulating agents. Attacks may be accompanied by headache, dyspnea, and wheezing, palpitations, abdominal pain, diarrhea, and syncope and may closely resemble the flushing episodes of the carcinoid syndrome, especially the foregut variety, also mediated by histamine. Rosacea may develop rarely. PGD_2 might be associated with the symptoms of flushing and diarrhea. The flushing of cutaneous mastocytosis typically lasts >30 minutes, unlike the typical carcinoid flush, which lasts <10 minutes. In urticaria pigmentosa, the diagnosis is established by demonstrating that gentle rubbing of the lesional skin causes local itching, redness, and whealing (Darier's sign), a reaction due to local histamine release. Darier's sign may also be demonstrated in nonlesional skin. Confirmation of the diagnosis is obtained by skin biopsy. In patients with systemic symptoms, bone marrow biopsy and liver and spleen scans are usually performed. Bone scans should only be carried out in the presence of localized bone symptoms.

Treatment

Treatment of nonlocalized forms of mastocytosis is mainly symptomatic. Patients should avoid known histamine-degranulating agents. Antihistamines remain the preferred treatment of most patients with uncomplicated urticaria pigmentosa. Human skin blood vessels possess H_1 and H_2 receptors, involved in both histamine-induced vasodilation and increased vascular permeability. Thus, combination treatment with an H_1 antihistamine (hydroxyzine, 10 to 20 mg) and H_2 antihistamine (cimetidine, 200 to 500 mg) is logical and sometimes effective at controlling flushing episodes. The mast cell–stabilizing agent disodium cromoglycate has proved effective in some patients. The drug does not decrease urinary excretion of histamine and the histamine metabolite MIAA. Some advocate its use only in patients with systemic mastocytosis suffering from GI symptoms. Photochemotherapy has been reported to cause symptomatic relief as well as objective reduction in the population of mast cells and the urinary excretion of MIAA.

Medullary Thyroid Carcinoma

The range of substances secreted by medullary carcinoma of the thyroid is considerable, whether sporadic or familial. Flushing is the most common symptom after diarrhea, which as in the carcinoid syndrome may be induced by alcohol ingestion. Calcitonin gene–related peptide, an extremely powerful peripheral vasodilator, is the most likely mediator of flushing. Calcitonin stimulates prostaglandin release, which may contribute to the symptoms.

Pheochromocytoma

Flushing is rare in patients with pheochromocytoma and may be caused in some instances by adrenomedullin. If flushing occurs at all, it is seen after a paroxysm of hypertension, tachycardia, palpitations, chest pain, severe throbbing headaches, and excessive perspiration. Pallor is typically present during the attack, and mild flushing may occur after the attack as a rebound vasodilation of the facial cutaneous blood vessels.

Spinal Cord Lesions Above T6

Facial flushing and headache can occur along with sweating of the face, neck, and upper trunk in patients with spinal cord lesions above T6, particularly as an exaggerated response to bowel or bladder distention.

Miscellaneous Causes of Flushing

Other causes are certain pancreatic tumors (VIPomas), insulinoma, and POEMS (polyneuropathy, organomegaly, endocrinopathy, monoclonal proteinemia, and skin changes). Transient flushing of the face, chest, or arms has been noted after neurologic deterioration secondary to rapid rise in intracranial pressure.

Other Endocrine Causes of Hyperhidrosis

Acromegaly, thyrotoxicosis, and hypoglycemia constitute other causes of sweating.

Idiopathic Hyperhidrosis

This may be primary focal (palmar, craniofacial, axillary, or pedal), secondary focal (caused by an underlying condition, such as neuropathy, spinal disease or injury, or compensatory hyperhidrosis), or generalized hyperhidrosis (affecting the entire skin or secondary to other medical conditions, such as tuberculosis, brucellosis, or Hodgkin disease).

Primary Focal Hyperhidrosis

Primary focal hyperhidrosis has at least two of the following characteristics:

- Bilateral and relatively symmetrical
- Impairs daily activities
- Frequency of at least once per week
- Onset before 25 years of age
- Positive family history
- Cessation of local sweating during sleep

It is rarely necessary to perform laboratory tests if the above criteria are met.

Generalized Hyperhidrosis

By contrast, the causes of generalized hyperhidrosis are many and include cardiovascular disorders, respiratory failure, infections, malignancy, endocrine and metabolic causes, and neurologic disorders. Causes of secondary focal hyperhidrosis include neurologic disorders, such as stroke, diabetic autonomic neuropathy, spinal cord lesions, and tumors such as intrathoracic neoplasma (mesothelioma), and gustatory sweating. Treatment depends on the underlying cause. Mercury poisoning may also cause hyperhidrosis. It irreversibly inhibits selenium-dependent enzymes and may also inactivate *S*-adenosyl-methionine, which is necessary for catecholamine catabolism by catechol-*o*-methyltransferase. Due to the body's inability to degrade catecholamines (*e.g.*, epinephrine), a person suffering from mercury poisoning may experience profuse sweating, tachycardia, increased salivation, and hypertension.

Treatment of Primary Hyperhidrosis

For palmar or plantar hyperhidrosis, aluminum salt dusting powder or 20% aluminum chloride hexahydrate in alcohol solution may bring relief. Short courses of 1% hydrocortisone cream may be necessary if skin irritation occurs. Treatment of underlying anxiety may be necessary, including the use of cognitive behavior therapy. Botulinus toxin may be injected into axillae, palms, and plantar surfaces.

Craniofacial hyperhidrosis responds in 70% of cases to endoscopic thoracic sympathectomy.

CASES WITH QUESTIONS

Case 1

A 65-year-old woman was referred with complaints of epigastric discomfort, nausea, dizziness, and episodes of a strong foul taste in her mouth. Upper GI endoscopy was normal, but over the ensuing months, she began to lose weight and to complain of altered smell, nausea, and episodes of recurrent flushing lasting 2 to 3 minutes 10 to 20 times per day and sweating at night. Her blood pressure is 135/70, and there is no goiter. Thyroid function tests, IGF-1, urinary 5-HIAA, and plasma chromogranin A, calcitonin, plasma metanephrines, and vasoactive intestinal polypeptide levels are all normal.

What is your differential diagnosis?

What further investigations are warranted?

Case 2

A 21-year-old female presents with a 5-year history of excessive sweating, involving the face, axillae, and moist palms, which she finds socially and professionally embarrassing. These occur virtually every day. They are partially stress induced. She is on Marvelon. Because of slightly coarsened features, a local endocrinologist conducts a number of investigations and documents normal full blood count and erythrocyte sedimentation rate, blood urea nitrogen, liver function test, C-reactive protein, and thyroid function; normal levels of IGF-1 and growth hormone suppression on oral glucose tolerance test; and normal urinary 5-HIAA, plasma calcitonin, plasma metanephrines, chromogranin A, and serum tryptase.

What is your differentia diagnosis?

What are the management options?

Case 3

A 45-year-old woman is referred because of flushing affecting the face and torso that comes on particularly during exercise and can last up to 30 minutes. She felt that some of the episodes were meal related. During these episodes, she suffers from palpitations and lightheadedness and complains of feeling dizzy. During one provoked episode (10 minutes of brisk walking), her general practitioner reported semi-confluent blotchiness affecting the upper half of the body, a pulse of 140 and blood pressure varying between 130/70 and 160/70. She has been extensively investigated with normal cardiological workup, Holter monitor, urinary free catecholamines and plasma fractionated metanephrines, calcitonin, TFTs, IGF-1, chromogranin A, and serum tryptase of 15 (<20). Basal pulse rate was 68 beats per minute, increasing to 140 on standing. A previous diagnosis of postural orthostatic tachycardia syndrome (POTS) had been made. She was given a therapeutic trial of some drugs, with full resolution of her symptoms.

What is your differential diagnosis?

What drugs controlled her symptoms?

Answers

Diagnoses

1. Temporal lobe epilepsy
2. Idiopathic primary hyperhidrosis
3. Mast cell activation syndrome, controlled by H1 and H2 antagonists

RECOMMENDED READING

Cheung NW, Earl J. Monoamine oxidase deficiency: a cause of flushing and attention-deficit/ hyperactivity disorder? *Arch Intern Med.* 2001; **161**(20):2503–2504.

Corbett M, Abernethy DA. Harlequin syndrome. *J Neurol Neurosurg Psychiatry.* 1999;**66**(4):544.

Dawood MY. Menopause. In: Copeland LJ, ed. *Textbook of Gynecology*, 2nd ed. : W.B. Saunders, 2000.

DeSio JM, Kahn CH, Warfield CA. Facial flushing and/or generalized erythema after epidural steroid injection. *Anesth Analg.* 1995;**80**(3): 617–619.

Dizon MV, Fischer G, Jopp-McKay A, Treadwell PW, Paller AS. Localized facial flushing in infancy. Auriculotemporal nerve (Frey) syndrome. *Arch Dermatol.* 1997;**133**(9):1143–1145.

Drummond PD, Boyce GM, Lance JW. Postherpetic gustatory flushing and sweating. *Ann Neurol.* 1987;**21**(6):559–563.

Fink HA, Mac Donald R, Rutks IR, Nelson DB, Wilt TJ. Sildenafil for male erectile dysfunction: a systematic review and meta-analysis. *Arch Intern Med.* 2002;**162**(12):1349–1360.

Fitzpatrick TB, et al. *Dermatology in General Medicine*, 4th ed. New York: McGraw-Hill; 1993.

Franks AG. Cutaneous manifestations of disorders of the cardiovascular and pulmonary systems. In: Freedberg IM, et al, eds. *Fitzpatrick's Dermatology in General Medicine*, Vol 2, 5th ed. New York: McGraw-Hill; 1999:2064.

Greaves MW. Flushing syndromes, rosacea and perioral dermatitis. In: Champion RH, et al, eds. *Rook/Wilkinson/Ebling Textbook of Dermatology*, Vol 3, 6th ed. New York: Blackwell Scientific; 1998:2099–2104.

Greaves MW. Mastocytoses. In: Champion RH, et al, eds. *Rook/Wilkinson/Ebling Textbook of Dermatology.* Vol. 3, 6th ed. New York: Blackwell Scientific; 1998:2337–2346.

Hornig GW. Flushing in relation to a possible rise in intracranial pressure: documentation of an unusual clinical sign. Report of five cases. *J Neurosurg.* 2000;**92**(6):1040–1044.

Larsen PR, ed. *Williams Textbook of Endocrinology*, 10th ed. New York: W.B. Saunders; 2003.

O'Toole D, Ducreux M, Bommelaer G, Wemeau JL, Bouché O, Catus F, Blumberg J, Ruszniewski P. Treatment of carcinoid syndrome: a prospective crossover evaluation of lanreotide versus octreotide in terms of efficacy, patient acceptability, and tolerance. *Cancer.* 2000;**88**(4): 770–776.

Rubin J, Ajani J, Schirmer W, Venook AP, Bukowski R, Pommier R, Saltz L, Dandona P, Anthony L. Octreotide acetate long-acting formulation versus open-label subcutaneous octreotide acetate in malignant carcinoid syndrome. *J Clin Oncol.* 1999;**17**(2):600–606.

Shakir KM, Jasser MZ, Yoshihashi AK, Drake AJ III, Eisold JF. Pseudo-carcinoid syndrome associated with hypogonadism and response to testosterone therapy. *Mayo Clin Proc.* 1996;**71**(12):1145–1149.

Smith JA, Jr. Management of hot flushes due to endocrine therapy for prostate carcinoma. *Oncology (Williston Park).* 1996;**10**(9): 1319–1322, discussion 1324.

Vercellini P, Vendola N, Colombo A, Passadore C, Trespidi L, Crosignani PG. Veralipride for hot flushes during gonadotropin-releasing hormone agonist treatment. *Gynecol Obstet Invest.* 1992;**34**(2):102–104.

Vinik AI. Neuroendocrine tumors of carcinoid variety. In: DeGroot LJ, ed. *Endocrinology.* Vol. 3, 3rd ed. New York: W.B. Saunders; 1995: 2803–2812.

Wilkin J. Flushing and blushing. In: Moschella SL, Hurley HJ, eds. *Dermatology.* Vol 2, 3rd ed. New York: W.B. Saunders; 1992:2080–2083.

Wilson JD, ed. *Williams Textbook of Endocrinology.* 9th ed. New York: W.B. Saunders; 1998.

BONE AND MINERAL METABOLISM

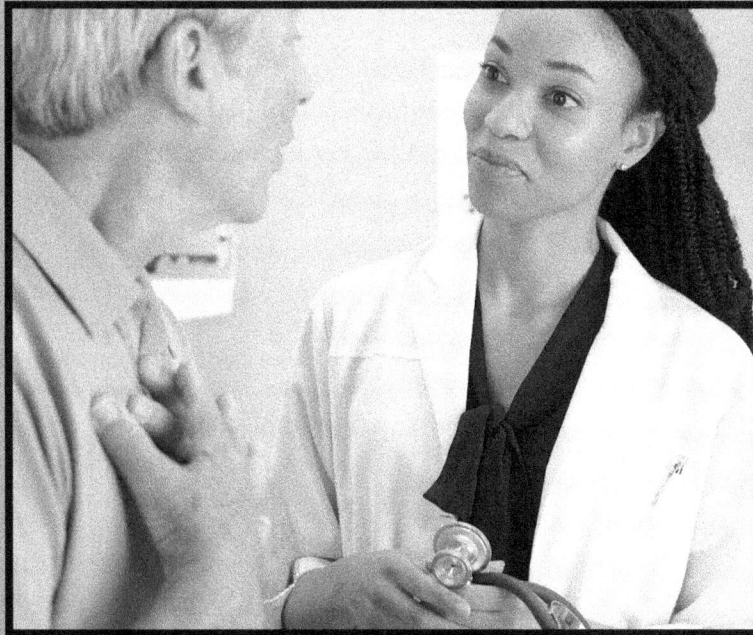

Challenging Hypoparathyroidism Cases

M05
Presented, March 17–20, 2018

Natalie E. Cusano, MD, MS. Bone Metabolism Program, Department of Medicine, Lenox Hill Hospital, New York, New York 10022, E-mail: ncusano@northwell.edu

SIGNIFICANCE OF THE CLINICAL PROBLEM

Hypoparathyroidism is a complex endocrine disorder characterized by low or insufficient parathyroid hormone (PTH) concentrations, hypocalcemia, and hyperphosphatemia (1). There are ~77,000 individuals living with hypoparathyroidism in the United States. The disease has been designated orphan status in the United States and by the European Commission. In 75% of cases, hypoparathyroidism is a postoperative complication from thyroid, parathyroid, or other neck surgery. Of the remaining 25% of cases, autoimmune-mediated damage to the parathyroid glands is the most common etiology. This may occur as an isolated disease or part of autoimmune polyglandular syndrome type 1. Genetic disorders leading to hypoparathyroidism may occur as isolated hypoparathyroidism or part of a syndrome and include *PTH* gene mutations, calcium-sensing receptor (*CASR*) gene mutations, DiGeorge syndrome, and mitochondrial mutations. Identifying the etiology of a patient's hypoparathyroidism may have implications for disease management (2).

Although the acute signs and symptoms of hypoparathyroidism are usually attributable to hypocalcemia, the chronic manifestations may be caused by the underlying disease process or complications of therapy. Complications of hypoparathyroidism include nephrocalcinosis, renal stone disease, renal failure, basal ganglia calcifications, cataracts, anxiety and depression, reduced quality of life, increased risk of infection, and reduced bone remodeling. Management must be personalized to balance symptoms with the risks of treatment (3).

BARRIERS TO OPTIMAL PRACTICE

Because hypoparathyroidism is rare, the average practitioner treats relatively few patients with the disease. There are a number of therapeutic challenges in the management of patients with hypoparathyroidism: blood calcium levels vary during the day; calcium must be taken throughout the day to keep levels stable; it may be difficult to control symptoms completely; and vomiting/diarrhea, infection, anxiety/stress, and excessive exercise as well as other factors can change requirements. In addition, there is a significant risk of complications associated with long-term treatment.

LEARNING OBJECTIVES

- To develop a management plan for the multiple disorders of mineral metabolism that occur in patients with hypoparathyroidism
- To identify patients with hypoparathyroidism that may be candidates for recombinant human parathyroid hormone (1-84) [rhPTH(1-84)] therapy
- To review the initiation of rhPTH(1-84) therapy for a patient with hypoparathyroidism
- To recognize patients with genetic forms of hypoparathyroidism

STRATEGIES FOR DIAGNOSIS, THERAPY, AND/OR MANAGEMENT

Hypoparathyroidism can be diagnosed with concurrent low albumin-corrected serum or ionized calcium and a low or insufficient PTH concentration on at least two occasions separated by at least 2 weeks. Hypo- and hypermagnesemia are the only reversible causes of hypoparathyroidism. Hypoparathyroidism after surgery is considered chronic after 6 months (4).

Conventional therapy of hypoparathyroidism includes calcium and active vitamin D supplementation. Calcium carbonate and calcium citrate contain the most elemental calcium (40% and 21%, respectively). Patients typically require 500 to 1000 mg of elemental calcium three to four times daily. Calcitriol is the active vitamin D analog used in the United States, and the typical dose is 0.25 to 2.0 μg daily. Divided doses are typically recommended if the patient requires >0.75 μg daily. Alfacalcidol is approved outside the United States. It is rapidly converted to calcitriol in the liver, and it is approximately one half as potent as calcitriol, with patients typically requiring 0.5 to 4.0 μg daily. Patients may require supplementation with magnesium and vitamin D_2 or D_3. Thiazide diuretics can be considered for patients with hypercalciuria (3). rhPTH(1-84) was approved by the Food and Drug Administration on January 23, 2015 for the treatment of "patients who cannot be well-controlled on calcium supplements and active forms of vitamin D alone" (3).

There are guidelines for the management of hypoparathyroidism now available from the European Society of Endocrinology (4) and the First International Workshop on the Management of Hypoparathyroidism (5). The primary goals of therapy are to ameliorate symptoms of hypocalcemia and maintain serum calcium in the low normal range. After the primary goals are achieved, secondary goals include maintaining serum magnesium, phosphate, and 25-hydroxyvitamin D levels within or close to the normal range; maintaining the calcium–phosphate product $<55\ mg^2/dL^2$; maintaining urine calcium within sex-specific normal ranges; avoidance of hypercalcemia or relative hypercalcemia; and avoidance of renal and other extraskeletal calcifications. The First International Workshop provides guidance on the management of hypoparathyroidism in patients that may be considered difficult to control with conventional therapy who may be candidates for treatment with rhPTH(1-84) (5).

MAIN CONCLUSIONS

Although hypoparathyroidism may be a rare disease, it places a large burden on patients and their families. The disease can be difficult to manage and may require high doses of calcium and active vitamin D supplementation. Serious complications can occur, including renal and other extraskeletal calcifications. rhPTH(1-84) has been approved for patients with hypoparathyroidism not well controlled on conventional therapy. It is critical to personalize management to balance symptoms with the risks of treatment.

DISCUSSION OF CASES AND ANSWERS

Case 1

T.O. is a 65-year-old man with a history of total thyroidectomy for papillary thyroid cancer 15 years ago complicated by postoperative hypoparathyroidism. He has been managed by his primary care doctor. He has had no evidence of recurrence of thyroid cancer. He complains of 5 days of low-grade fever, congestion, and cough consistent with an upper respiratory infection. He denies perioral or extremity numbness/tingling or other symptoms of hypocalcemia. He has no history of hospitalizations for hypocalcemia.

His past medical history also includes hypertension and gastroesophageal reflux disease. His family and social history are unremarkable.

His current regimen for hypoparathyroidism includes TUMS Ultra 1000-mg tablets (GlaxoSmithKline) twice daily (with food) and calcitriol 0.75 μg twice daily. He rarely has dietary calcium. His other medications include levothyroxine 137 μg daily, hydrochlorothiazide 25 mg daily, and pantoprazole 40 mg daily. He has had no change to his medications in the past year.

Physical examination is notable for body mass index 29.3 kg/m^2, negative Chvostek sign, and a well-healed neck incision with no palpable thyroid tissue; otherwise, it is unremarkable.

He brings a recent laboratory report noting a serum calcium value of 8.0 mg/dL. Evaluation at the time of this visit was significant for

- Calcium 7.2 mg/dL [normal (nl): 8.7 to 10.2; 1.80 mmol/L]; corrected for serum albumin
- PTH 10 pg/mL (nl: 15 to 65; 10 ng/L)
- 25-Hydroxyvitamin D 17.0 ng/mL (nl: >30 ng/mL; 42.4 nmol/L)
- Blood urea nitrogen (BUN)/creatinine 20/1.2 mg/dL [estimated glomerular filtration rate (eGFR) 65 mL/min per 1.73 m^2)
- Phosphorus 5.4 mg/dL (nl: 2.5 to 4.5; 1.74 mmol/L)
- Magnesium 1.3 mg/dL (nl: 1.6 to 2.6; 0.65 mmol/L)
- Thyrotropin 1.54 mIU/mL (nl: 0.27 to 4.20)
- 24-Hour urine calcium 293 mg (nl: 100 to 300; 7.3 mmol)
- Electrocardiogram with normal QTc

Question 1 for Case 1

Does this patient require intravenous calcium?

A. Yes
B. No

Explanation of the Best Answer

Correct Answer: B. Treatment of hypocalcemia in hypoparathyroidism should be guided by not only the absolute calcium value but also the presence of symptoms. This patient is asymptomatic and has a normal QTc with an albumin-adjusted serum calcium value of >7.0 mg/dL. He has been ill for a few days, and his serum calcium is not expected to drop further acutely. Asymptomatic patients with a prolonged QTc or those with a serum calcium ≤7.0 mg/dL should be considered for intravenous calcium infusion because of the risk of laryngeal spasm, bronchospasm, or cardiac arrhythmia seizure that may develop acutely. When needed, a dilute solution of intravenous calcium gluconate should be used, because it is less likely than calcium chloride to cause tissue necrosis if extravasation occurs. Oral calcium and active vitamin D supplementation should also be administered as soon as possible (3).

Question 2 for Case 1

How would you first adjust this patient's regimen at this visit?

A. Increase his dose of calcium carbonate to TUMS 1000 mg three times daily
B. Change calcium carbonate to calcium citrate 600 mg three times daily
C. Increase calcitriol by 0.25 μg daily
D. Start ergocalciferol 50,000 IU weekly
E. Start rhPTH(1-84) 50 μg daily

Explanation of the Best Answer

Correct Answer: B. Acid-reducing medications may cause malabsorption of calcium carbonate. There are reports of severe hypocalcemia occurring in patients with hypoparathyroidism treated with calcium carbonate after initiation of proton pump inhibitors (6–8). Absorption of calcium citrate is not dependent on the presence of acid in the stomach. Substitution of calcium citrate for calcium carbonate should be considered in patients with achlorhydria, those requiring proton pump inhibitors, patients with gastrointestinal symptoms with calcium carbonate, or those unable to take their calcium with meals. Of note, most calcium supplements list as the active ingredient the dose of elemental calcium; however, TUMS lists the active ingredient as the amount of total calcium. This patient's dose of elemental calcium is thus 400 mg twice daily, which is a relatively low dose. The patient is already taking a relatively large dose of calcitriol, and adjustment of his calcium supplementation should be considered before increasing calcitriol further.

Vitamin D_2 or D_3 supplementation is recommended but would be unlikely to increase the patient's serum calcium to goal. Even in patients taking active vitamin D, supplementation with parent vitamin D is recommended, because 25-hydroxyvitamin may have extraskeletal effects. Also, nonrenal expression of 1α-hydroxylase, which is independent of PTH, may activate circulating 25-hydroxyvitamin. Because of its relatively long half-life (14 to 75 days), maintenance of sufficient 25-hydroxyvitamin levels may help provide smoother control (4, 5).

In addition, this patient has hypomagnesemia that should be addressed. Hypomagnesemia may blunt the capacity of the parathyroid glands to secrete PTH. In patients with low but detectable PTH concentrations, the residual capacity of the parathyroid glands to secrete PTH may be improved with magnesium repletion. Sustained release preparations of magnesium minimize renal excretion and have reduced gastrointestinal side effects. The typical requirement is 240 to 1000 mg elemental magnesium in divided doses in a patient with normal renal function (4, 5). Proton pump inhibitors can cause reversible magnesium malabsorption, and a change to an H_2-receptor blocker may be beneficial in this patient (9).

rhPTH(1-84) is indicated for patients with hypoparathyroidism that is difficult to control with conventional therapy. The above changes should be implemented before further consideration of rhPTH(1-84) therapy in this patient.

Question 3 for Case 1

The patient changed his calcium carbonate to calcium citrate 600 mg three times daily and started sustained release magnesium and ergocalciferol 50,000 IU weekly. Calcitriol was continued at 0.75 μg twice daily. The patient began to recover from his upper respiratory infection.

Repeat blood tests 3 days later were significant for
Calcium 8.9 mg/dL (nl: 8.7 to 10.2; 2.23 mmol/L)
Phosphorus 5.1 mg/dL (nl: 2.5 to 4.5; 1.65 mmol/L)
Magnesium 1.7 mg/dL (nl: 1.6 to 2.6; 0.85 mmol/L)

How would you treat this patient's hyperphosphatemia at this time?

A. Titrate down calcitriol
B. Start a low-phosphate diet
C. Start a phosphate binder
D. Increase hydrochlorothiazide to 50 mg daily
E. Start rhPTH(1-84) 50 μg daily

Explanation of the Best Answer

Correct Answer: A. The patient's serum calcium had likely been lower than baseline because of acute illness, and in conjunction with the change in calcium supplementation, his serum calcium increased significantly. Active vitamin D increases intestinal absorption of both calcium and phosphate, whereas calcium may act as a phosphate binder. Increasing calcium supplementation while decreasing active vitamin D can be helpful in reducing hyperphosphatemia (5). In this patient with a robust serum calcium, calcitriol can be titrated down without adjusting calcium supplementation. A low-phosphate diet or a phosphate binder can be considered in certain patients with persistent hyperphosphatemia after making changes to their regimen (4). rhPTH(1-84) can be considered in patients with hyperphosphatemia; however, the first step would be to reduce calcitriol supplementation. Hydrochlorothiazide would not be expected to reduce serum phosphate.

This patient was eventually titrated to calcium citrate 600 mg four times daily and calcitriol 0.5 μg daily, with calcium and phosphate levels maintained at goal.

Case 2

A.L. is a 23-year-old woman with a history of compressive goiter status after total thyroidectomy 1 year ago with postsurgical hypoparathyroidism who is now transferring her care to you. The pathology report from her surgery showed Hashimoto disease with no evidence of cancer; one parathyroid gland was noted. Her postoperative course was complicated by hypocalcemia, requiring hospitalization of almost 1 week. She has had persistent hypoparathyroidism and trouble maintaining her calcium level at goal, requiring six emergency department visits since diagnosis. She reports waking up every day with perioral and extremity numbness and tingling; her symptoms are also intermittent during the day. She reports compliance with all medications.

Her regimen for hypoparathyroidism includes calcium citrate 1200 mg three times daily, calcitriol 1.0 μg twice daily, a serving of yogurt with breakfast, and vitamin D 10,000 IU weekly. Her other medications include levothyroxine 112 μg daily and an oral contraceptive.

Physical examination is unremarkable other than negative Chvostek sign and a well-healed neck incision with no palpable thyroid tissue.

Evaluation at the time of this visit was significant for
Calcium 8.4 mg/dL (nl: 8.7 to 10.2; 2.10 mmol/L); corrected for serum albumin
PTH 5 pg/mL (nl: 15 to 65; 5 ng/L)
25-Hydroxyvitamin D 34.0 ng/mL (nl: >30 ng/mL; 85 nmol/L)
BUN/creatinine 13/0.5 mg/dL (eGFR 154 mL/min)
Phosphorus 4.8 mg/dL (nl: 2.5 to 4.5; 1.55 mmol/L)
Magnesium 1.6 mg/dL (nl: 1.6 to 2.6; 0.80 mmol/L)
24-Hour urine calcium 407 mg (nl: 100 to 250; 10.2 mmol)
Renal ultrasound: negative for nephrocalcinosis or stone

Question 1 for Case 2

How would you adjust her regimen?

A. Make no changes, because serum calcium is within the target range

B. Increase calcitriol by 0.25 μg daily
C. Start hydrochlorothiazide 12.5 mg daily
D. Start PTH(1-34)20 μg daily
E. Start rhPTH(1-84) 50 μg daily

Explanation of the Best Answer

Correct Answer: E. A change in regimen is warranted given the patient's frequent symptoms of hypocalcemia. rhPTH(1-84) was approved by the Food and Drug Administration on January 23, 2015 for the treatment of "patients who cannot be well-controlled on calcium supplements and active forms of vitamin D alone." The First International Workshop on the Management of Hypoparathyroidism (4) provides guidance regarding patients who may fall under this category. The guidelines recommend consideration of rhPTH(1-84) therapy for the following indications: (1) inadequate control of the serum calcium concentration; (2) calcium requirements >2.5 g and/or active vitamin D >1.5 μg daily; (3) hypercalciuria, renal stones, nephrocalcinosis, stone risk, or reduced creatinine clearance or eGFR (60 mL/min); (4) hyperphosphatemia and/or calcium–phosphate product >55 mg^2/dL^2 (4.4 $mmol^2/L^2$); (5) a gastrointestinal tract disorder associated with malabsorption; and/or (6) reduced quality of life. This patient has inadequate control of serum calcium, very high calcium and calcitriol requirements, hypercalciuria, and hyperphosphatemia. The starting dose of rhPTH(1-84) is 50 μg daily and can be titrated to 75 or 100 μg daily as needed (10).

Increasing calcitriol further will likely worsen her hypercalciuria, and she is already taking a high dose of active vitamin D therapy. Hydrochlorothiazide may be helpful for hypercalciuria; however, higher doses are typically needed to reduce urinary calcium excretion. Furthermore, therapy with hydrochlorothiazide would not be expected to ameliorate her symptoms. PTH(1-34) has been studied in patients with hypoparathyroidism, although twice daily dosing is usually necessary to provide control of serum calcium. In addition, use of PTH(1-34)in hypoparathyroidism would be an off-label indication.

Question 2 for Case 2

What information should you give to patients when starting rhPTH(1-84)?

A. Patients must be enrolled in the Risk Evaluation and Mitigation Strategy Program to monitor risk for chondrosarcoma
B. Patients should be instructed to administer rhPTH(1-84) into the thigh
C. Patients should discontinue calcitriol when starting rhPTH(1-84)
D. rhPTH(1-84) is pregnancy category B risk
E. Up to 5.1% of treated patients develop neutralizing antibodies to rhPTH(1-84)

Explanation of the Best Answer

Correct Answer: B. Osteosarcoma, a bone cancer, has been noted in rats given very high doses of PTH(1-34), rhPTH(1-84), and most recently, abaloparatide, a PTH-related peptide analog. Caution should be used in patients at increased risk of osteosarcoma, including patients with a history of radiation therapy and young patients with open epiphyses. There have been no adverse signals of osteosarcoma in humans treated with any form of PTH, and phase 4 studies are ongoing (11, 12). Patients receive rhPTH(1-84) through the NATPARA Risk Evaluation and Mitigation Strategy Program (10). Chondrosarcoma risk has not been elevated in animal models treated with PTH.

rhPTH(1-84) should be administered into the thigh because of pharmacokinetic data showing increased duration of effect over delivery by the subcutaneous route from the abdomen. Patients should be instructed to decrease calcitriol by 50% when starting rhPTH(1-84). Serum calcium should be monitored 3 to 7 days after treatment initiation, with additional titration of supplemental calcitriol or calcium as needed. rhPTH(1-84) is pregnancy category C risk, with animal reproductive studies showing adverse effects but no adequate and well-controlled studies in humans (10).

Across all studies, 14 of 87 (16.1%) patients treated for up to 2.6 years developed low-titer anti-PTH antibodies; three of them were subsequently antibody negative. Only one of these patients (1.1%) developed antibodies with neutralizing activity, although this patient maintained a clinical response to rhPTH(1-84) treatment and had no evidence of adverse reactions related to the immune system. Anti-PTH antibodies had no effect on safety or efficacy during clinical trials; however, whether there is a long-term impact remains unknown (10).

Question 3 for Case 2

The patient is eventually titrated to rhPTH(1-84) 100 μg. She continues to take a serving of yogurt daily and is off all additional supplementation with calcium and calcitriol. She no longer has hypocalcemic symptoms.

Laboratory evaluation was significant for
Calcium 8.4 mg/dL (nl: 8.7 to 10.2; 2.10 mmol/L)
Potassium 3.5 mEq/L (nl: 3.5 to 5.5; 3.5 mmol/L)
Phosphorus 4.6 mg/dL (nl: 2.5 to 4.5; 1.49 mmol/L)
Magnesium 1.6 mg/dL (nl: 1.6 to 2.6; 0.80 mmol/L)
24-Hour urine calcium 307 mg (nl: 100 to 250; 7.7 mmol)

How would you adjust her regimen?

A. Make no changes, because serum calcium is within the target range
B. Increase rhPTH(1-84) to 125 μg daily
C. Start hydrochlorothiazide 25 mg daily
D. Start hydrochlorothiazide 25 mg with amiloride 5 mg daily
E. Change therapy to PTH(1-34) 20 μg three times daily

Explanation of the Best Answer

Correct Answer D. Patients with hypoparathyroidism are at increased risk for nephrocalcinosis, renal stone disease, and renal failure. In one study, the proportion of patients with stages 3 to 5 chronic kidney disease was 2- to 35-fold greater in patients with hypoparathyroidism after adjusting for age compared with the general population using data from the National Health and Nutrition Examination Survey (13). Data from a national patient registry showed that renal insufficiency was threefold higher in postsurgical hypoparathyroidism and sixfold higher in nonsurgical hypoparathyroidism (14–16). The European Society of Endocrinology and the First International Workshop on the Management of Hypoparathyroidism guidelines recommend maintaining urine calcium within the sex-specific normal range to reduce the risk of renal disease associated with hypoparathyroidism.

Thiazide diuretics have been shown to decrease urine calcium in patients with hypoparathyroidism (17). However, high doses (*i.e.*, hydrochlorothiazide 50 mg twice daily) may be needed to significantly reduce urine calcium excretion. Thiazide or thiazide-like diuretics should be used in conjunction with a low-sodium diet for best effect. Given the patient's borderline serum potassium and magnesium, amiloride should also be considered to prevent the development of hypokalemia and hypomagnesemia requiring additional supplementation.

The maximum approved dose of rhPTH(1-84) is 100 μg daily. PTH(1-34) administered by subcutaneous injection has not been shown to reduce urine calcium, although one study using PTH(1-34) administered continuously by pump showed a 59% reduction in urine calcium excretion (18). Use of PTH(1-34) in hypoparathyroidism remains off label.

The patient was eventually titrated up to hydrochlorothiazide 25 mg twice daily and amiloride 5 mg with improvement in urine calcium excretion to within the sex-specific normal range.

Case 3

B.C. is a 20-year-old woman presenting for initial evaluation of a suspected calcium disorder and nephrolithiasis. She had a recent kidney stone that prompted laboratory testing that showed hypocalcemia, low PTH, and hypercalciuria. She has no history of thyroid or other neck surgery. She has no history of seizures. She has no known family history of calcium disorders and no history of consanguinity. She has rare episodes of perioral numbness and tingling, usually after intense exercise.

Examination is unremarkable other than negative Chvostek sign, no mucocutaneous candidiasis, no vitiligo, normal thyroid tissue, no neck scar, and normal nail beds; there were no other syndromic findings.

Evaluation was notable for

Calcium 7.7 mg/dL (nl: 8.7 to 10.2; 1.92 mmol/L)
PTH 14 pg/mL (nl: 15 to 65; 14 ng/L)
25-Hydroxyvitamin D 29.0 ng/mL (nl: >30 ng/mL; 72 nmol/L)
BUN/creatinine 13/0.5 mg/dL (eGFR 167 mL/min)
Phosphorus 4.8 mg/dL (nl: 2.5 to 4.5; 1.55 mmol/L)
Magnesium 1.6 mg/dL (nl: 1.6 to 2.6; 0.80 mmol/L)
24-Hour urine calcium 327 mg (nl: 100 to 250; 8.2 mmol)
Urinary calcium/creatinine 0.21

Question 1 for Case 3

Mutations in all of the following genes are associated with nonsyndromic hypoparathyroidism and can be considered in this patient except

A. *AIRE*
B. *PTH*
C. *CASR*
D. *GNA11*
E. *GCM2*

Explanation of the Best Answer

Best Answer: A. Mutations in the *PTH* and *GCM2* genes have been associated with isolated hypoparathyroidism. Gain-of-function mutations in *CASR* and *GNA11* are associated with autosomal dominant hypocalcemia 1 (ADH1) and ADH2, respectively. Conversely, loss-of-function mutations in these genes are responsible for familial hypocalciuric hypercalcemia 1 and 2, respectively. Mutations in the *AIRE* gene result in autoimmune polyglandular syndrome type 1, consisting of the classic triad of hypoparathyroidism, mucocutaneous candidiasis, and adrenal insufficiency (2).

This patient has mild to moderate hypocalcemia, low but detectable PTH concentrations, hyperphosphatemia, and hypercalciuria. An elevated urinary calcium/creatinine ratio in an untreated patient is highly suggestive of ADH (19). This patient had a mutation in the *CASR* gene and a subsequent diagnosis of ADH1.

Question 2 for Case 3

Patients with ADH1 are at particular risk of which of the following complications with conventional therapy?

A. Basal ganglia calcification
B. Hypercalciuria
C. Posterior subcapsular cataract
D. Dental aplasia
E. Ischemic heart disease

Explanation of the Best Answer

Best Answer: B. Patients with ADH1 (Online Mendelian Inheritance in Man 601198) have an exceptional risk of hypercalciuria, nephrocalcinosis, kidney stones, and renal failure. Treatment should be avoided in asymptomatic patients (19).

In symptomatic patients, cautious repletion with the lowest doses of calcium and active vitamin D can be initiated, with goal calcium levels as low as possible to alleviate symptoms. Thiazide diuretics have been studied in patients with ADH1 and shown efficacy to reduce urinary calcium excretion (19). Twice daily injections of PTH(1-34) were shown to improve serum calcium control in patients with ADH1 but had no effect on urinary calcium excretion (20). No trials investigating PTH(1-84), including the REPLACE Trial (21), enrolled patients with known ADH1.

In this asymptomatic patient with hypercalciuria and nephrolithiasis, hydrochlorothiazide was started with good effect on urinary calcium excretion. Calcium supplementation was recommended only with intense exercise.

REFERENCES

1. Shoback D. Clinical practice. Hypoparathyroidism. *N Engl J Med.* 2008;**359**(4):391–403.
2. Clarke BL, Brown EM, Collins MT, Jüppner H, Lakatos P, Levine MA, Mannstadt MM, Bilezikian JP, Romanischen AF, Thakker RV. Epidemiology and Diagnosis of Hypoparathyroidism. *J Clin Endocrinol Metab.* 2016;**101**(6):2284–2299.
3. Bilezikian JP, Brandi ML, Cusano NE, Mannstadt M, Rejnmark L, Rizzoli R, Rubin MR, Winer KK, Liberman UA, Potts JT Jr. Management of hypoparathyroidism: present and future. *J Clin Endocrinol Metab.* 2016;**101**(6):2313–2324.
4. Brandi ML, Bilezikian JP, Shoback D, Bouillon R, Clarke BL, Thakker RV, Khan AA, Potts JT Jr. Management of hypoparathyroidism: summary statement and guidelines. *J Clin Endocrinol Metab.* 2016; **101**(6):2273–2283.
5. Bollerslev J, Rejnmark L, Marcocci C, Shoback DM, Sitges-Serra A, van Biesen W, Dekkers OM; European Society of Endocrinology. European Society of Endocrinology clinical guideline: treatment of chronic hypoparathyroidism in adults. *Eur J Endocrinol.* 2015;**173**(2):G1–G20.
6. Milman S, Epstein EJ. Proton pump inhibitor-induced hypocalcemic seizure in a patient with hypoparathyroidism. *Endocr Pract.* 2011; **17**(1):104–107.
7. Subbiah V, Tayek JA. Tetany secondary to the use of a proton-pump inhibitor. *Ann Intern Med.* 2002;**137**(3):219.
8. Zaya NE, Woodson G. Proton pump inhibitor suppression of calcium absorption presenting as respiratory distress in a patient with bilateral laryngeal paralysis and hypocalcemia. *Ear Nose Throat J.* 2010;**89**(2):78–80.
9. Epstein M, McGrath S, Law F. Proton-pump inhibitors and hypomagnesemic hypoparathyroidism. *N Engl J Med.* 2006;**355**(17): 1834–1836.
10. Natpara [package insert]. Available at: https://www.accessdata.fda.gov/drugsatfda_docs/label/2015/125511s000lbl.pdf. Accessed 9 November 2017.
11. Andrews EB, Gilsenan AW, Midkiff K, Sherrill B, Wu Y, Mann BH, Masica D. The US postmarketing surveillance study of adult osteosarcoma and teriparatide: study design and findings from the first 7 years. *J Bone Miner Res.* 2012;**27**(12):2429–2437.
12. Cipriani C, Irani D, Bilezikian JP. Safety of osteoanabolic therapy: a decade of experience [published correction appears in *J Bone Miner Res.* 2013;28(4):431]. *J Bone Miner Res.* 2012;**27**(12):2419–2428.
13. Mitchell DM, Regan S, Cooley MR, Lauter KB, Vrla MC, Becker CB, Burnett-Bowie SA, Mannstadt M. Long-term follow-up of patients with hypoparathyroidism. *J Clin Endocrinol Metab.* 2012;**97**(12): 4507–4514.
14. Underbjerg L, Sikjaer T, Mosekilde L, Rejnmark L. Cardiovascular and renal complications to postsurgical hypoparathyroidism: a Danish nationwide controlled historic follow-up study. *J Bone Miner Res.* 2013;**28**(11):2277–2285.
15. Underbjerg L, Sikjaer T, Mosekilde L, Rejnmark L. Postsurgical hypoparathyroidism–risk of fractures, psychiatric diseases, cancer, cataract, and infections. *J Bone Miner Res.* 2014;**29**(11):2504–2510.
16. Underbjerg L, Sikjaer T, Mosekilde L, Rejnmark L. The epidemiology of nonsurgical hypoparathyroidism in Denmark: a nationwide case finding study. *J Bone Miner Res.* 2015;**30**(9):1738–1744.
17. Porter RH, Cox BG, Heaney D, Hostetter TH, Stinebaugh BJ, Suki WN. Treatment of hypoparathyroid patients with chlorthalidone. *N Engl J Med.* 1978;**298**(11):577–581.
18. Winer KK, Zhang B, Shrader JA, Peterson D, Smith M, Albert PS, Cutler GB Jr. Synthetic human parathyroid hormone 1-34 replacement therapy: a randomized crossover trial comparing pump versus injections in the treatment of chronic hypoparathyroidism. *J Clin Endocrinol Metab.* 2012;**97**(2):391–399.
19. McKusick VA, O'Neill MJF. Hypocalcemia, autosomal dominant 1. Online Mendelian Inheritance in Man. Available at: https://www.omim.org/entry/601198 Accessed 9 November 2017.
20. Winer KK, Yanovski JA, Sarani B, Cutler GB Jr. A randomized, crossover trial of once-daily versus twice-daily parathyroid hormone 1-34 in treatment of hypoparathyroidism. *J Clin Endocrinol Metab.* 1998; **83**(10):3480–3486.
21. Mannstadt M, Clarke BL, Vokes T, Brandi ML, Ranganath L, Fraser WD, Lakatos P, Bajnok L, Garceau R, Mosekilde L, Lagast H, Shoback D, Bilezikian JP. Efficacy and safety of recombinant human parathyroid hormone (1-84) in hypoparathyroidism (REPLACE): a double-blind, placebo-controlled, randomised, phase 3 study. *Lancet Diabetes Endocrinol.* 2013;**1**(4):275–283.

Metabolic Bone Disease in Patients With Renal Insufficiency/Failure

M19
Presented, March 17–20, 2018

Peter R. Ebeling, AO. Department of Medicine, School of Clinical Sciences, Monash University, Clayton, Victoria 3168, Australia, E-mail: peter.ebeling@monash.edu

SIGNIFICANCE OF THE CLINICAL PROBLEM

Chronic kidney disease (CKD) is one of the most common medical problems, affecting 20 million Americans. A majority have stage 1, 2, or 3 CKD with estimated glomerular filtration rates (eGFRs) of ≥90 mL/min plus kidney damage, 60 to 89 mL/min plus kidney damage, and 30 to 59 mL/min, respectively (1). However, 300,000 Americans had stage 4 CKD (15 to 29 mL/min) and 452,957 had stage 5 CKD (<15 mL/min) or were on dialysis in 2003 (2). CKD is associated with excess morbidity, mortality, and increased health care costs. CKD–metabolic bone disorder (MBD) occurs in stage 4 and 5 CKD and is characterized by bone (renal osteodystrophy), soft tissue (calcifications), and mineral (phosphate, calcium, fibroblast growth factor 23, calcitriol, sclerostin, and Dikkopf-1) abnormalities. However, the pathological end points of CKD-MBD are increased cardiovascular risk, mortality, and fractures.

Hip fracture incidence increases with age in the general population but is increased at every age for patients with stage 3b, 4, or 5 CKD. Mortality after any fracture is also increased in patients with CKD, being highest in patients with stage 5 CKD. The total annual cost of treating fractures associated with stage 5 CKD is $100 million and is $500 million for non-dialysis CKD.

BARRIERS TO OPTIMAL PRACTICE

Physicians are unsure as to whether conventional anti-osteoporosis drugs are appropriate or effective in patients with CKD. In particular, there is reluctance to measure bone mineral density (BMD) using dual-energy absorptiometry (DXA), because there is concern it may not be as predictive of fractures in patients with CKD as in the general population. There is also reluctance to use antiresorptive drugs, because patients may have low-turnover renal osteodystrophy, so treatment could theoretically worsen skeletal fragility.

BONE DISEASE IN CKD (RENAL OSTEODYSTROPHY)

The TMV classification system exists for CKD and is based on bone turnover, mineralization, and volume; each can be low/absent, normal, or high. The combination of each component can be used to classify the disease; for example, in adynamic bone disease, turnover is low, mineralization is normal, and volume is low, whereas in hyperparathyroidism, turnover is high, mineralization is normal, and volume is low. By contrast, in osteomalacia, turnover is low, mineralization is low, and volume is normal (3).

LEARNING OBJECTIVES

As a result of participating in this session, learners should be able to:

- Understand the epidemiology of CKD and fractures
- Distinguish the CKD-related bone disorders comprising renal osteodystrophy
- Take a case-based approach, including:
- Fracture risk assessment
- Bone disease diagnostic strategies
- Treatment: bisphosphonates, denosumab, teriparatide

CKD-MBD GUIDELINES

Kidney Disease: Improving Global Outcomes Guidelines

Previous Kidney Disease: Improving Global Outcomes (KDIGO) guidelines from 2009 suggested a cutoff for parathyroid hormone (PTH), above which high-turnover renal osteodystrophy would be treated with the calcimimetic drug cinacalcet and the active form of vitamin D. However, the new 2017 KDIGO guidelines state that the optimal PTH level is not known. Instead, there should be a renewed focus on an assessment of both fracture risk and bone turnover in the individual patient with CKD. In patients with high-turnover bone disease, an antiresorptive drug with or without vitamin D should be used, whereas in patients with low-turnover bone disease, an anabolic drug with or without vitamin D should be used instead.

According to the 2017 KDIGO CKD-MBD guideline update, as summarized by Ketteler *et al* (4), the following apply for patients with grade 3a to 5D CKD with evidence of CKD-MBD and/or risk factors for osteoporosis:

- BMD testing is suggested to assess fracture risk if results will affect treatment decisions.
- It is reasonable to perform a bone biopsy if knowledge of the type of renal osteodystrophy will affect treatment decisions.
- The optimal PTH level is not known.
- Use vitamin D_3 supplements for patients with stage 3 CKD to correct vitamin D deficiency.
- Reserve the use of calcitriol or vitamin D analogs for patients with stage 4 or 5 CKD with severe and progressive hyperparathyroidism.
- The antifracture efficacy for any osteoporosis therapy in severe (stage 4 to 5) CKD is lacking.

Review From European Calcified Tissue Society and European Renal Association of Nephrology Dialysis and Transplantation

This alternative guideline (5) suggests there is still value in measuring PTH to differentiate between high- and low-turnover states in renal osteodystropy. The aim of both guidelines is to recommend treatment of renal osteodystrophy based on whether bone turnover is likely to be high or low. The combination of PTH level with the bone formation marker bone-specific alkaline phosphatase (BSAP), which is not affected by renal function, remains the best noninvasive way to divide patients into high- or low-turnover categories. However, in patients with either low PTH levels or low or intermediate levels of BSAP, a bone biopsy may be required to exclude causes of low-turnover renal osteodystropy (adynamic bone disease and osteomalacia; Figs. 1 and 2).

SUMMARY AND CONCLUSION

In CKD-MBD, differentiate and manage accordingly:

- Almost all healthy adults have an age-related decline in renal function.
- Fracture risk and fracture-related complications and costs are higher in patients with CKD.
- DXA T score helps to classify fracture risk in patients CKD but has limitations.
- The combination of PTH and bone turnover markers (particularly BSAP) predicts bone loss and helps guide treatment.
- Bone biopsies are needed when turnover and/or osteomalacia cannot be diagnosed noninvasively.
- An individual and tailored approach to managing bone disease is needed in patients with CKD (Fig. 3).

CASES WITH QUESTIONS

Case 1

A 63-year-old postmenopausal white woman with stage 3 CKD is referred for clinical vertebral fracture (L4, L5).

Medical history:

- Hypertension
- Remote tobacco use

Medication:

- Lisinopril 10 mg once per day

DXA T scores by Fracture Risk Assessment Tool (FRAX):

- Lumbar spine: −1.5; major osteoporotic fracture: 11%
- Total hip: −1.3; hip: 1.9%
- Femoral neck: −2.2
- One-third radius: 0.1

1. What is the patient's diagnosis based on the KDIGO TMV system?
2. Should we measure bone turnover in this patient, and if so, how should it be measured?
3. What treatment would be best for this patient?

Case 2

A 43-year-old woman is referred for low bone density on a knee plain film (osteonecrosis of the knee) and refractory hyperparathyroidism.

- End-stage renal disease (hereditary renal retinal syndrome)
- 1978 to 2003: hemodialysis (HD)
- 2003 to 2007: successful kidney transplant from deceased donor
- 2007: graft failure 2/2 BK virus
- 2007 to present: HD

History:

- Blind
- HD-related neuropathy; walks with unsteady gait
- Menstruating normally
- No tobacco, alcohol, or drugs
- Family history of renal disease (sister with end-stage renal disease)
- Dialysis prescription: Kt/v >1.2 and 2.5-mEq calcium bath (standard)

Medications:

- Prednisone 2.5 to 5 mg since transplantation failure
- Phenobarbitol for seizures
- Never took a bisphosphonate
- Sevelamer 800 mg three times per day with meals
- Paricalcitol 9 μg intravenously on HD days
- Cinacalcet 30 mg once per day for 2 months before visit; dose was increased recently to 60 mg once per day (PTH >400 pg/mL)

Spine X-rays show no fractures. DXA T scores by FRAX were as follows:

- Spine: −0.5 (aortic calcification and end-plate osteosclerosis)
- Total hip: −1.5
- Femoral neck: −2.0
- One-third radius: −3.4 (90% cortical bone)
- Ultradistal radius: −1.7 (80% trabecular bone)

Laboratory tests:

- Calcium (reference range, 8.6 to 10.2 mg/dL): 8.4 mg/dL
- Phosphorus (reference range, 2.5 to 4.5 mg/dL): 5.6 mg/dL
- PTH (reference range, 10 to 65 pg/mL): 545 pg/mL
- 25-hydroxycholecalciferol (25-OHD; reference range, 20 to 100 ng/mL): 20 ng/mL
- Bone alkaline phosphatase (reference range, 4.5 to 16.9 U/L): 32 U/L
- C-terminal telopeptide (CTX; reference range, 40 to 465 pg/mL): 4159 pg/mL

1. What is the patient's diagnosis based on the KDIGO TMV system?
2. Why is there a larger deficit in cortical than trabecular bone?

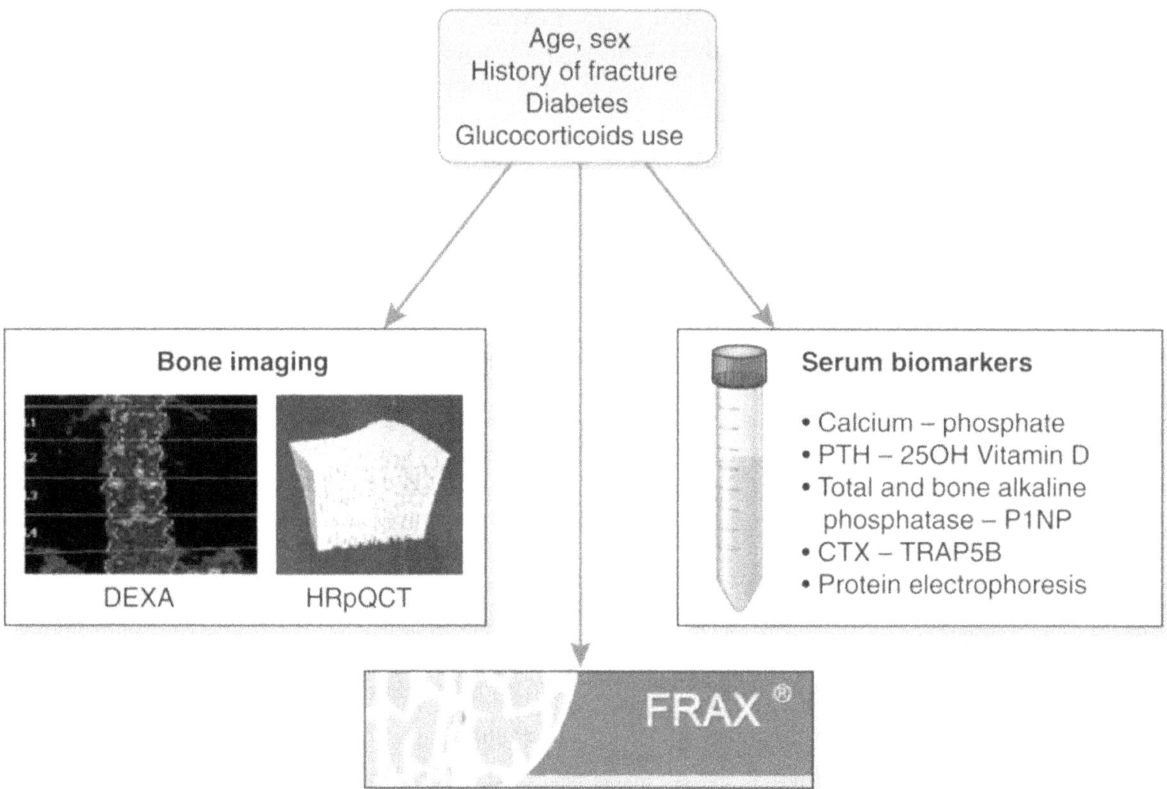

Figure 1. Assessing bone in CKD-MBD. 25-OH, 25-hydroxy; CTX, C-terminal telopeptide; DEXA, dual-energy X-ray absorptiometry; FRAX, Fracture Risk Assessment Tool; HRpQCT, high-resolution peripheral quantitative computed tomography.

3. Should we measure bone turnover in this patient, and if so, how should it be measured?
4. What treatment would be best for this patient?

DISCUSSION

Case 1

In this patient with severe osteoporosis, both BMD and FRAX demonstrate poor sensitivity. In addition, CKD and osteoporosis are coprevalent, with just under 10% of women with an eGFR of <60 mL/min having osteoporosis and 21.3% of women age 70 TO 79 years with osteoporosis having an eGFR <35 mL/min (6, 7).

According to the 2017 KDIGO CKD-MBD recommendations, in patients with stage 3a to 5D CKD with evidence of CKD-MBD and/or risk factors for osteoporosis, BMD testing is suggested to assess fracture risk if results will affect treatment decisions (8).

Limitations of DXA in patients with CKD:

- DXA does not assess microarchitecture or bone strength.
- DXA does not assess turnover, mineralization, or type of renal osteodystrophy.
- Treatment decisions cannot be based on DXA results.

Noninvasive tests, such as PTH and BSAP, can be used to differentiate between low- and non–low-turnover renal osteodystrophy and high- and non–high-turnover renal osteodystrophy, with cutoffs for each available with areas under the curve ranging from 0.70 to 0.76 (9–11).

Bone biopsy is required to guide treatment decisions when:

- Type of renal osteodystrophy is not clear
  1. Low turnover or adynamic bone disease
  2. Osteomalacia
- Unexplained fractures
  1. Normal BMD
  2. No evidence of hyperparathyroidism
  3. GFR <45 mL/min

In this case, the bone biopsy demonstrated:

- Turnover
  1. Low to normal bone formation rate
  2. Rare osteoclasts and osteoblasts
- Mineralization
  1. No defect
- Volume
  1. Cortical thinning (12)
  2. Endosteal trabecularization
  3. Normal trabecular microarchitecture

In a secondary analysis of the FPT (Fracture Prevention Trial) with teriparatide, which contained low numbers of patients with CKD, regardless of whether the eGFR was <80

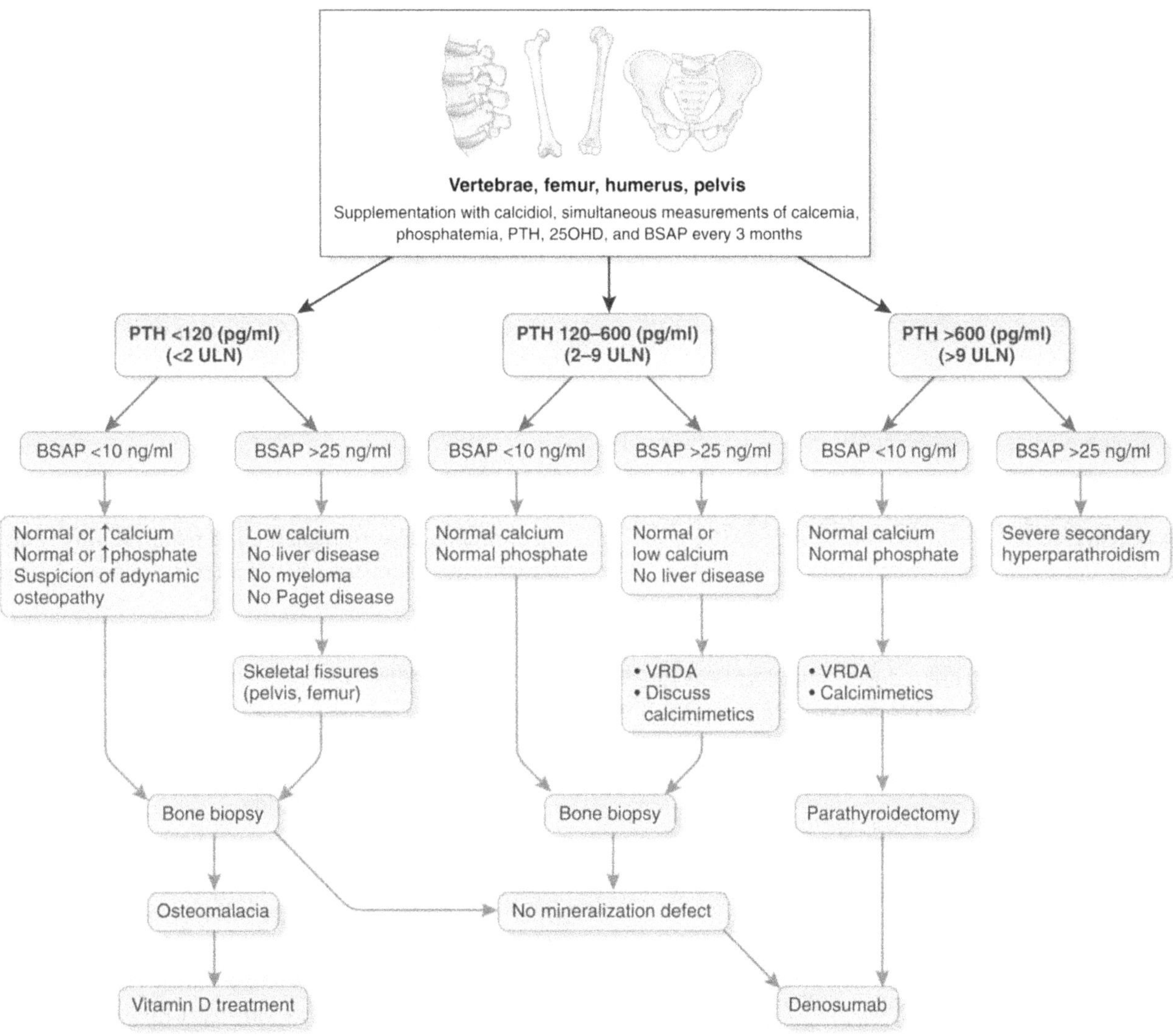

Figure 2. Treatment algorithm in patients with CKD-MBD according to bone turnover. 25-OHD, 25-hydroxycholecalciferol; ULN, upper limit of normal; VRDA, virtual reality dynamic anatomy.

or >80 mL/min, treatment with recombinant human PTH (1-34) increased lumbar spine and femoral neck BMD and reduced the incidence of vertebral and nonvertebral fractures (13). Given this, the patient was treated with teriparatide, because bone formation was low to normal. In the FPT, teriparatide treatment was associated with increased serum calcium in all patients and uric acid in patients with CKD. However, no cases of nephrolithiasis, gout, symptomatic hypercalcemia, or acute rheumatic fever were seen in patients receiving teriparatide.

Repeat DXA 6 months later demonstrated:

- 3% increase in lumbar spine BMD
- 5% increase in femoral neck BMD
- 4% increase in one-third radius BMD

Repeat bone biopsy demonstrated:

- Increased cortical width
- Mild decrease in cancellous bone
- Increase in bone formation rate in the low to normal range

Case 2

This patient has severe secondary hyperparathyroidism, causing cortical osteoporosis. In this situation, the combination of total hip BMD and BSAP is the best at predicting fracture risk (14). Her fracture risk is high given the degree of elevation of BSAP and her increased propensity for falls because of her blindness and peripheral neuropathy. The goal of treatment is to reduce her PTH level to reduce bone remodeling, increase BMD, and reduce fracture risk.

- Increase sevelamer 1600 mg three times per day plus 800 mg with snacks (goal is phosphorus <4.5 mg/dL)
- Maintain 2.5-mEq calcium bath
- Vitamin D_3 repletion (goal is 30 to 40 ng/mL)
- Change phenobarbitol to lamictal to reduce adverse effects on vitamin D and bone
- Paricalcitol: adjust as needed but avoid hypercalcemia
- Cinacalcet: increase dose to 60 mg twice per day but recognize there is limited evidence that this will reduce

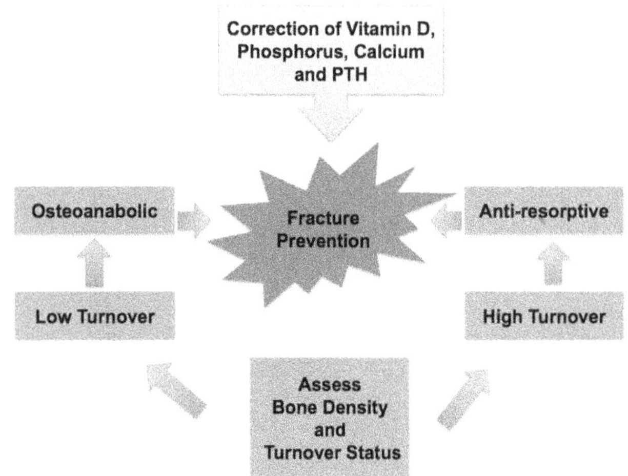

Figure 3. Fracture prevention strategies in patients with CKD-MBD.

fracture risk from EVOLVE (Evaluation of Cinacalcet Hydrochloride Therapy to Lower Cardiovascular Events) trial, where fractures were reduced from 13.2% to 12.2% over 5 years compared with placebo (secondary study outcome) (15)

One year later:

- PTH (reference range, 10 to 65 pg/mL): 413 pg/mL
- 25-OHD (reference range, 20 to 100 ng/mL): 18 ng/mL
- Total alkaline phosphatase (reference range, 33 to 115 U/L): 95 U/L
- CTX (reference range, 40 to 465 pg/mL): 1216 pg/mL

Repeat DXA T scores (% change) (* denotes significant change):

- Spine: −1.0 (−5.6%)*
- Total hip: −1.7 (−3.2%)*
- Femoral neck: −2.0
- One-third radius: −3.6 (−1.9%)*

Medical treatment has been ineffective at preventing bone loss or reducing PTH levels adequately. The best treatment would be parathyroidectomy. In patients with stage 5D CKD matched for age, sex, race, HD duration, and vitamin D dose, parathyroidectomy reduced hip fractures by 32% and any fractures by 31% over 10 years of follow-up. Parathyroid imaging revealed a mildly enlarged right upper parathyroid gland (87 g) and slightly enlarged left lower parathyroid gland (67 g) (16).

However, the patient refused parathyroid surgery, so the dose of cinacalcet was increased to 90 mg twice per day. Deceased donor kidney transplantation was then performed. The post-transplantation immunosuppression regimen comprised:

- Prednisone 5 mg once per day
- Tacrolimus 3 mg twice per day
- MMF 750 mg twice per day
- Immunoglobulin intravenously once every 6 weeks
- Cholecalciferol 1000 IU daily

Post-transplantation tests:

- Estimated glomerular filtration rate eGFR >45 mL/min
- Phosphorous (reference range, 2.5 to 4.5 mg/dL): 3.6 mg/dL
- Calcium (reference range, 8.6 to 10.2 mg/dL): 9.0 mg/dL
- Albumin: 4.0 g/dL
- PTH (reference range, 10 to 65 pg/mL): 267 pg/mL
- 25-OHD (reference range, 20 to 100 ng/mL): 35 ng/mL
- BSAP (reference range, 14.2 to 42.7 U/L): 24.2 U/L
- CTX (reference range, 40 to 465 pg/mL) 1222 pg/mL

Post-transplantation DXA T scores (% change) (* denotes significant change):

- Spine: −1.3 (−3.5%)*
- Total hip: −2.1 (−7.3%)*
- Femoral neck: −2.0
- One-third radius: −4.1 (−6.4%)*

Continuing post-transplantation hyperparathyroidism will increase the risk of fractures if PTH levels are >130 pg/mL.

Treatment options:

- Do nothing (masterly inactivity)
- Vitamin D analog
- Cinacalcet
- Parathyroidectomy
- Antiresorptive
- Anabolic agent teriparatide

Antiresorptive agents (17–20) are the best treatment option, combined with continuing medical management of hyperprathyroidism with cinacalcet, because the patient was still refusing parathyroidectomy.

Both risedronate and denosumab have been shown to reduce vertebral fractures in patients with mild CKD (stage 2 to 4 CKD for risedronate and stage 2 to 3 CKD for denosumab). Data on nonvertebral fracture reduction are lacking. Regardless of renal function, the incidence of adverse events (nonrenal/renal) was similar (serum creatinine, calcium, and phosphorous) in risedronate- and placebo-treated groups. Iliac crest biopsies from risedronate-treated patients with stage 3 or 4 CKD showed a 68% decrease in mineralizing surface and a 54% decrease in activation frequency but no evidence of adynamic bone disease.

Denosumab should be used cautiously in patients with stage 4 CKD, because cases of hypocalcemia have been reported, despite normal serum calcium and vitamin D levels. Its use is probably best avoided in patients with stage 5D CKD.

After 2 years of treatment with risedronate and cinacalcet:

- Creatinine clearance rate: 1.25 mL/min (eGFR: 46 mL/min)
- Phosphorous (reference range, 2.5 to 4.5 mg/dL): 4.2 mg/dL
- Calcium (reference range, 8.6 to 10.2 mg/dL): 8.8 mg/dL
- Albumin: 4.3 g/dL
- PTH (reference range, 10 to 65 pg/mL): 132 pg/mL (down from 168 pg/mL)
- 25-OHD (reference range, 20 to 100 ng/mL): 48 ng/mL
- BSAP (reference range, 4.5 to 16.9 U/L): 10.1 U/L
- CTX (reference range, 40 to 465 pg/mL) 743 pg/mL (down from 1222 pg/mL)

DXA T scores (% change) (* denotes significant change):

- Spine: −0.8 (+5.5%)*
- Total hip: −1.7 (+5.5%)*
- Femoral neck: −1.8
- One-third radius: −3.5 (+8.0%)*

REFERENCES

1. Coresh J, Byrd-Holt D, Astor BC, Briggs JP, Eggers PW, Lacher DA, Hostetter TH. Chronic kidney disease awareness, prevalence, and trends among U.S. adults, 1999 to 2000. *J Am Soc Nephrol.* 2005; **16**(1):180–188.
2. United States Renal Data System (USRDS). 2005 Annual Data Report. Available at: https://www.usrds.org/atlas05.aspx. Accessed 10 January 2018.
3. Cesini J, Cheriet S, Breuil V, Lafage-Proust MH. Osteoporosis: chronic kidney disease in rheumatology practice. *Joint Bone Spine.* 2012; **79**(suppl 2):S104–S109.
4. Ketteler M, Block GA, Evenepoel P, Fukagawa M, Herzog CA, McCann L, Moe SM, Shroff R, Tonelli MA, Toussaint ND, Vervloet MG, Leonard MB. Executive summary of the 2017 KDIGO chronic kidney disease-mineral and bone disorder (CKD-MBD) guideline update: what's changed and why it matters. *Kidney Int.* 2017;**92**(1):26–36.
5. Pimentel A, Ureña-Torres P, Zillikens MC, Bover J, Cohen-Solal M. Fractures in patients with CKD-diagnosis, treatment, and prevention: a review by members of the European Calcified Tissue Society and the European Renal Association of Nephrology Dialysis and Transplantation. *Kidney Int.* 2017;**92**(6):1343–1355.
6. Nickolas TL, McMahon DJ, Shane E. Relationship between moderate to severe kidney disease and hip fracture in the United States. *J Am Soc Nephrol.* 2006;**17**(11):3223–3232.
7. Klawansky S, Komaroff E, Cavanaugh PF Jr, Mitchell DY, Gordon MJ, Connelly JE, Ross SD. Relationship between age, renal function and bone mineral density in the US population. *Osteoporos Int.* 2003; **14**(7):570–576.
8. Yenchek RH, Ix JH, Shlipak MG, Bauer DC, Rianon NJ, Kritchevsky SB, Harris TB, Newman AB, Cauley JA, Fried LF; Health, Aging, and Body Composition Study. Bone mineral density and fracture risk in older individuals with CKD. *Clin J Am Soc Nephrol.* 2012;**7**(7): 1130–1136.
9. Bervoets ARJ, Spasovski GB, Behets GJ, Dams G, Polenakovic MH, Zafirovska K, Van Hoof VO, De Broe ME, D'Haese PC. Useful biochemical markers for diagnosing renal osteodystrophy in predialysis end-stage renal failure patients. *Am J Kidney Dis.* 2003;**41**(5):997–1007.
10. Sprague SM, Bellorin-Font E, Jorgetti V, Carvalho AB, Malluche HH, Ferreira A, D'Haese PC, Drüeke TB, Du H, Manley T, Rojas E, Moe SM. Diagnostic accuracy of bone turnover markers and bone histology in patients with CKD treated by dialysis. *Am J Kidney Dis.* 2016;**67**(4): 559–566.
11. Malluche HH, Mawad HW, Monier-Faugere MC. Renal osteodystrophy in the first decade of the new millennium: analysis of 630 bone biopsies in black and white patients. *J Bone Miner Res.* 2011;**26**(6): 1368–1376.
12. Nickolas TL, Stein EM, Dworakowski E, Nishiyama KK, Komandah-Kosseh M, Zhang CA, McMahon DJ, Liu XS, Boutroy S, Cremers S, Shane E. Rapid cortical bone loss in patients with chronic kidney disease. *J Bone Miner Res.* 2013;**28**(8):1811–1820.
13. Miller PD, Schwartz EN, Chen P, Misurski DA, Krege JH. Teriparatide in postmenopausal women with osteoporosis and mild or moderate renal impairment. *Osteoporos Int.* 2007;**18**(1):59–68.
14. Iimori S, Mori Y, Akita W, Kuyama T, Takada S, Asai T, Kuwahara M, Sasaki S, Tsukamoto Y. Diagnostic usefulness of bone mineral density and biochemical markers of bone turnover in predicting fracture in CKD stage 5D patients–a single-center cohort study. *Nephrol Dial Transplant.* 2012;**27**(1):345–351.
15. Moe SM, Abdalla S, Chertow GM, Parfrey PS, Block GA, Correa-Rotter R, Floege J, Herzog CA, London GM, Mahaffey KW, Wheeler DC, Dehmel B, Goodman WG, Drüeke TB; Evaluation of Cinacalcet HCl Therapy to Lower Cardiovascular Events (EVOLVE) Trial Investigators. Effects of cinacalcet on fracture events in patients receiving hemodialysis: the EVOLVE trial. *J Am Soc Nephrol.* 2015; **26**(6):1466–1475.
16. Rudser KD, de Boer IH, Dooley A, Young B, Kestenbaum B. Fracture risk after parathyroidectomy among chronic hemodialysis patients. *J Am Soc Nephrol.* 2007;**18**(8):2401–2407.
17. Miller PD, Roux C, Boonen S, Barton IP, Dunlap LE, Burgio DE. Safety and efficacy of risedronate in patients with age-related reduced renal function as estimated by the Cockcroft and Gault method: a pooled analysis of nine clinical trials. *J Bone Miner Res.* 2005;**20**(12): 2105–2115.
18. Jamal SA, Bauer DC, Ensrud KE, Cauley JA, Hochberg M, Ishani A, Cummings SR. Alendronate treatment in women with normal to severely impaired renal function: an analysis of the fracture intervention trial. *J Bone Miner Res.* 2007;**22**(4):503–508.
19. Jamal SA, Ljunggren O, Stehman-Breen C, Cummings SR, McClung MR, Goemaere S, Ebeling PR, Franek E, Yang YC, Egbuna OI, Boonen S, Miller PD. Effects of denosumab on fracture and bone mineral density by level of kidney function. *J Bone Miner Res.* 2011;**26**(8): 1829–1835.
20. Broadwell A, Ebeling PR, Franek E, Goemaere S, Wagman RB, Yin X, Yue S, Miller PD. Safety and efficacy of denosumab among subjects with mild-to-moderate chronic kidney disease (CKD) in the "Fracture REduction Evaluation of Denosumab in Osteoporosis every 6 Months" extension study [abstract]. *Arthritis Rheumatol.* 2017; **69**(suppl 10). Abstract 1889.

Metabolic Bone Health in Patients with Cancer

M32
Presented, March 17–20, 2018

Bente L. Langdahl, DMSc. Aarhus University and Aarhus University Hospital, DK-8000 Aarhus C, Denmark, E-mail: bente.langdahl@aarhus.rm

INTRODUCTION

Cancer is very common, with the lifetime risk of cancer being 25%. The most comment metabolic bone health problems in patients with cancer are hypercalcemia because of factors secreted by the cancer, bone metastases, and bone loss caused by treatment of the cancer.

SIGNIFICANCE OF THE CLINICAL PROBLEM

Hypercalcemia has been reported to occur in up to 30% of patients who have malignancy. Hypercalcemia is most common in those who have later-stage malignancy, and it predicts poor prognosis. Patients with hypercalcemia suffer from dehydration, depression, and confusion, and the condition may be life threatening because of cardiac arrhythmias.

Treatment of breast cancer and prostate cancer has improved substantially over the last decades, and many patients live many years beyond the cancer diagnosis and therefore, also have to live with potential long-lasting side effects of cancer treatment. Many women with breast cancer receive treatment with aromatase inhibitors for 5 or more years, and this increases the risk of osteoporosis and fractures. Similarly, men with prostate cancer receive antiandrogen treatment either lifelong or for a limited span of years, and this also increases the risk of osteoporosis and fractures.

BARRIERS OF OPTIMAL PRACTICE

- Symptoms of hypercalcemia are often less clear, and the diagnosis may, therefore, often be delayed
- Patients with breast and prostate cancer are managed in the oncology setting, where many aspects of the disease have to be considered and therefore, bone protection is often not considered

LEARNING OBJECTIVES

- To recognize symptoms of hypercalcemia in cancer patients, exclude other causes of hypercalcemia, and treat the condition
- To understand the pathophysiology underlying cancer treatment–induced bone loss (CTIBL)
- To identify patients with breast cancer in whom prevention of CTIBL should be considered
- To identify patients with prostate cancer in whom prevention of CTIBL should be considered
- To manage prevention and treatment of CTIBL

STRATEGIES FOR DIAGNOSIS, THERAPY, AND/OR MANAGEMENT

Hypercalcemia of Malignancy

The most common causes of malignancy-associated hypercalcemia include humoral hypercalcemia mediated by parathyroid hormone–related peptide (PTHrP), osteolytic cytokine production, and excess 1,25-dihydroxy vitamin D production. The cancers most commonly associated with hypercalcemia are lung cancer, multiple myeloma, renal cell cancer, breast cancer, and colorectal cancer.

Humoral hypercalcemia caused by production of PTHrP by the cancer accounts for ~80% of hypercalcemia in cancer patients (1). PTHrP is structurally similar to parathyroid hormone (PTH) and binds to the PTH receptor, thereby enhancing renal tubular reabsorption of calcium and stimulating osteoblastic production of receptor activator of nuclear factor-κB ligand (RANKL) and bone resorption. Unlike PTH, PTHrP does not stimulate hydroxylation of vitamin D, and therefore, it does not stimulate intestinal calcium absorption (1).

Local osteolytic hypercalcemia accounts for 20% of cases and is usually associated with extensive bone metastases and skeletal tumor burden. It is commonly seen in multiple myeloma, breast cancer, leukemia, and lymphoma (2). The underlying mechanism is primarily release of cytokines that directly or indirectly via RANKL activate osteoclasts; however, release of calcium as a consequence of bone destruction may also play a role (2).

Less than 1% of cases of hypercalcemia in malignancy are caused by production of 1,25-dihydroxy vitamin D by tumors (1); 1,25-dihydroxy vitamin D increases intestinal calcium absorption and osteolytic bone resorption. This is most commonly seen with Hodgkin and non-Hodgkin lymphoma.

The first step in investigation of hypercalcemia in any patient is measurement of intact PTH. If PTH is suppressed, measurement of PTHrP and 1,25-dihydroxy vitamin D will help in distinguishing malignant and benign causes of hypercalcemia. Benign causes of non–PTH-mediated hypercalcemia include sarcoidosis, vitamin D or A intoxication, and very high bone resorptive activity as seen in Paget disease of bone.

Treatment of the underlying cancer is the primary goal of therapy. Additional therapies directed against hypercalcemia are often needed for moderate to severe hypercalcemia. These include a review of concomitant medications; thiazide diuretics and lithium may worsen hypercalcemia and should be discontinued. The patient has increased osteoclastic bone resorption and renal tubular reabsorption. Furthermore, in the case of increased 1,25-dihydroxy vitamin D, intestinal calcium absorption is also increased and treatments should target these mechanisms.

The patients are volume depleted, and the first step is, therefore, rehydration with intravenous or oral fluids: 3 to 4 L/d; this will lead to increased renal excretion of calcium. Patients with known heart failure should be monitored carefully, and the addition of furosemide can be considered. The calciuric effect of furosemide is limited.

The increased bone resorption can be directly inhibited by calcitonin, bisphosphonates, and denosumab. The effect of calcitonin has a rapid onset, but it can only be used for 1 to 2 days because of downregulation of calcitonin receptors. Calcitonin is usually dosed at 4 to 8 IU/kg subcutaneously every 6 to 12 hours or as intravenous infusions.

The effect of bisphosphonates has a slower onset; the effect is not seen until after 2 to 4 days. Zoledronic acid is given as 4 mg intravenously over 15 to 30 minutes; pamidronate pamidronte is given as 60 to 90 mg over 4 to 24 hours. Bisphosphonates are potentially nephrotoxic, and it is, therefore, important that the patient is rehydrated and that the estimated glomerular filtration rate is >30 to 35 mL/min before treatment with a bisphosphonate.

Denosumab has been shown to be more efficacious than zoledronic acid in delaying or preventing hypercalcemia of malignancy in patients with advanced cancers, including breast cancer, other solid tumors, and multiple myeloma (3). Denosumab has also been shown to be effective in patients resistant to bisphosphonates (4). Denosumab is given as 120 mg subcutaneously. A study in patients previously treated with bisphosphonates but still hypercalcemic showed that administration of denosumab as 120 mg on days 1, 8, 15, and 29 lowered plasma calcium in 64% of patients after 10 days (5).

Glucocorticoids (GCs) may also indirectly inhibit bone resorption by inhibiting the release of PTHrP and cytokines by the tumor cells and antagonizing the effects of vitamin D in the case of hypercalcemia caused by increased production of 1,25-dihydroxy vitamin D. Glucocorticoids are given as prednisolone 50 to 100 mg daily or hydrocortisone 200 to 400 mg daily for up to a week, and then, the dose can often be reduced.

Bone Metastases

Circulating breast and prostate cancer cells have an affinity for the bone tissue and marrow microenvironment, but also, other cancer cells may find their way to bone. The cancer cells produce factors that increase the production of RANKL by the osteoblasts and osteocytes. RANKL stimulates recruitment and activation of osteoclasts and thereby, bone resorption. The breakdown of bone matrix releases bone-derived growth factors and cytokines that stimulate proliferation of the cancer cells and their secretion of osteolytic factors. These interactions between the cancer cells and the bone environment contribute to the development of metastases within bone (6).

Treatment of patients with bone metastases requires a multidisciplinary team. The treatment is generally palliative and may include external beam radiotherapy, endocrine treatments, chemotherapy, targeted therapies, radioisotopes, and surgery. These treatments may be complemented by bisphosphonates or denosumab; both have been shown to reduce skeletal morbidity. In patients with bone metastases, denosumab 120 mg every 4 weeks has shown to be superior to zoledronic acid 4 mg every 4 weeks in reducing the overall risk of skeletal-related events (SREs) and delaying the time to first SRE, which reduce the risk of developing moderate/severe pain (7).

CTIBL

Cancer treatment may induce menopause in women and hypogonadism in men. In both sexes, this leads to increased bone loss and subsequently, increased fracture risk. It is, therefore, advised to perform dual energy x-ray absorptiometry (DXA) and evaluate fracture risk based on the DXA and other clinical risk factors; if the fracture risk is high, antiosteoporosis treatment should be considered.

Chemotherapy probably does not have a clinically important toxic effect on bone (8), unless it leads to early menopause in women or hypogonadism in men (9). However, many chemotherapy regimens include high-dose glucocorticoid treatment. It is well documented that chronic glucocorticoid treatment has profound negative effects on bone health (10), but it is less well documented if the same applies to short-term, high-dose treatment regimens (11).

Loss or suppression of ovarian function (OFS) from either chemotherapy or drugs affecting the hypothalamic-pituitary-gonadal axis, such as gonadotropin releasing hormone (GnRH)/luteinizing hormone releasing hormone (LHRH) analogs, causes rapid bone loss that persists for the duration of amenorrhea (12). Some recovery is seen after the treatment is stopped, especially if menses resumes (13). A substudy of the Austrian Breast and Colorectal Cancer Study Group trial-12 (ABCSG-12) Study showed substantial bone loss in women treated with OFS over 3 years. The study also showed partial recovery in the women regaining menses after stopping OFS and that the combination of OFS with aromatase inhibitor led to greater bone loss than the combination of OFS with tamoxifen (14).

Tamoxifen is the most commonly used endocrine drug used in premenopausal women with estrogen receptor (ER)-positive breast cancer. In premenopausal women, tamoxifen acts as an antiestrogen in bone and therefore, causes bone loss (15). When tamoxifen is used in postmenopausal women, it protects against postmenopausal bone loss and reduces fracture incidence compared with placebo (16).

Treatment with aromatase inhibitors (AIs) in postmenopausal women with breast cancer improves disease outcome compared with tamoxifen, but it is associated with bone loss and increased fracture risk (17). Aromatase inhibitors prevent the aromatase-mediated conversion of androgens to estrogen and reduce the serum estradiol profoundly (18). This loss of estrogen leads to a 40% increased fracture risk in comparison with women treated with tamoxifen and less so compared with women treated with placebo (19, 20). Randomized clinical trials including AI for 5 years have suggested an increase in absolute fracture of around 10% (21); however, observational studies have indicated an even higher absolute fracture risk: 18% to 20% (22, 23). When the treatment with aromatase inhibitors is stopped, the bone loss is at least partly recovered (24).

In men with prostate cancer, androgen deprivation therapy (ADT), orchiectomy, or LHRH analog leads to bone loss and increased risk of fracture. The hazard ratio for fragility fracture in men on ADT compared with placebo is 1.65 (25).

Management of CTIBL

The management of CTIBL should comprise both bone-healthy lifestyle and pharmacological intervention. The bone-healthy lifestyle advice includes weight-bearing exercise (26), reduced smoking, moderate alcohol consumption, and adequate intake of calcium and vitamin D (27). There is evidence that antiresorptive therapies, including bisphosphonates and denosumab, prevent CTIBL. The majority of the trials were not designed with a fracture prevention end point; however, data from the osteoporosis setting support the use of BMD improvements as a surrogate for fracture prevention.

Several guidelines on selection of women treated with AI for bone protection have been published over the years (28, 29). None of the existing fracture risk prediction tools have included patients with CTIBL, and these tools underestimate the fracture risk in these patients. It has been suggested that the increased risk in CTIBL patients is similar to the increased risk seen in patients with rheumatoid arthritis (28).

Management of CTIBL in Women With Breast Cancer Treated With AI, Tamoxifen, or OSF

The ABCSG-18 Study is the only study in women treated with aromatase inhibitors with fracture as the primary end point. Denosumab 60 mg subcutaneously twice yearly substantially reduced the risk of clinical fractures by 50% (30). Intravenously administered zoledronic acid 4 mg twice yearly and different orally administered bisphosphonates have been shown to increase bone mass compared with baseline (summarized in ref. 28).

A recent meta-analysis has showed that bisphosphonate treatment in postmenopausal women reduces the incidence of cancer recurrence by 14%, bone recurrence by 28%, and breast cancer–specific mortality by 18% (31). This has led experts to recommend the use of adjuvant bisphosphonate therapy (either intravenous zoledronic acid or oral clodronate) in postmenopausal women with breast cancer and premenopausal women with breast cancer treated with GnRH analogs at intermediate or substantial risk for disease recurrence because of adverse clinical or biological characteristics, such as node-positive disease T2 or above, grade 2/3 breast tumor, or disease found to be ER negative or human epidermal growth factor receptor 2 positive (28).

For postmenopausal women treated with AI and premenopausal women treated with GnRH or tamoxifen not receiving bisphosphonate for recurrence prevention, a bone mineral density (BMD) measurement is advised. Patients with BMD T score >-2 and no other risk factors should be advised to have a bone-healthy lifestyle, and they should be reassessed in 1 to 2 years. Patients with BMD T score <-2 or two or more clinical risk factors for fracture (age >65 years old, BMD T score <-1.5, smoking, body mass index <20, family history of fracture, personal history of fracture >50 years, and oral GC >6 months) should be advised to have a bone-healthy lifestyle and be treated with denosumab or bisphosphonate (28).

Management of CTIBL in Men With Prostate Cancer Receiving ADT

Bisphosphonates and denosumab prevents ADT-induced bone loss (32, 33). Furthermore, denosumab has been shown to prevent vertebral fractures in men with prostate cancer on ADT (32). There has not been similar attention to ADT-induced bone loss as AI-induced bone loss, and therefore, fewer guidelines are available. Generally, it is recommended to treat men on ADT with a BMD T score <-2.5 with zoledronic acid 5 mg yearly, alendronate 70 mg weekly, or denosumab 60 mg every 6 months.

MAIN CONCLUSIONS

Metabolic bone health in patients with cancer may be affected by bone metastases, hypercalcemia, and CTIBL. In all of these scenarios, inhibition of bone resorption by bisphosphonates or denosumab is relevant, because these drugs have been shown to reduce SREs in patients with bone metastases, reduce/normalize plasma calcium in hypercalcemia of malignancy, and prevent CTIBL.

CASES

Case 1

A 73-year-old woman was diagnosed with lung cancer 3 years ago. Surgery with removal of the upper lung segment with the tumor was performed, but cancer cells were seen in some of the lymph nodes in the removed segment. The patient had subsequent chemotherapy. Computed tomography scans of the thorax have been performed annually since the surgical procedure; moderately enlarged lymph nodes had been noticed, but there has been no recurrence of the tumor.

The patient is admitted to the hospital for dehydration and confusion. The husband tells us that he first noticed the symptoms a little over a month ago but that the symptoms have become worse over the last week.

Physical examination showed that the patient is clearly dehydrated and in a state of confusion.

Examination of the lungs reveals lack of ventilation over the lower part of the left thorax. There are no palpable lymph nodes.

Selected biochemistry indicates the following: *p*-ionized calcium: 1.75 mmol/L (1.18 to 1.32 mmol/L), *p*-sodium: 149 mmol/L (137 to 145 mmol/L), and *p*-creatinine: 205 μmol/L (45 to 90 μmol/L).

What would you do next?

A. Additional diagnostic workup, including imaging of the thorax and biochemistry, including PTH and PTHrP
B. Rehydration and new biochemistry in 3 to 6 hours
C. Prednisolone 50 to 100 mg
D. Zoledronic acid 4 to 5 mg intravenously
E. Both C and D

Discussion

Answers A and B are correct.

The most likely cause of hypercalcemia in this patient is her lung cancer, but primary hyperparathyroidism should be ruled out. Rehydration is the most important acute intervention, and it should be initiated before administration of bisphosphonates to protect the kidneys.

After the patient is rehydrated, the need for treatment with glucocorticoids and bisphosphonates should be evaluated based on biochemistry and the condition of the patient.

Case 2

Case 2 is a 56-year-old woman with breast cancer. She had surgery with removal of the left breast, and the treatment decision was 5 years of aromatase inhibitor. Because of the recent meta-analysis showing increased survival in women with breast cancer being treated with zoledronic acid, the patient was treated annually with zoledronic acid 5 mg for 5 years; 4.5 years have passed, and the treating oncologist starts thinking about what to do next. The plan is to stop treatment with aromatase inhibitor and zoledronic acid simultaneously after 5 years.

The oncologist asks for our advice.

A. No need for follow-up; the risk of osteoporosis is low in women with breast cancer
B. Perform DXA
C. Inquire about clinical risk factors for osteoporosis and evaluate the risk/World Health Organization fracture assessment tool: if at risk, perform DXA; if not at risk, there is no need for follow-up
D. Continue treatment with zoledronic acid or another osteoporosis treatment

Discussion

The answer is C.

The risk of osteoporosis is relatively low in women with breast cancer, probably because incidence of breast cancer is associated with relatively high lifelong exposure to estrogen, which will also protect against osteoporosis. Women with breast cancer on average have a higher body weight, which is also associated with reduced risk of osteoporosis. The most rational way forward is, therefore, to focus on those women with breast cancer who have clinical risk factors associated with risk of fractures, including old age, smoking, low body mass index, and previous fractures. In these women, it is recommended to perform DXA, and if osteoporosis is present, osteoporosis treatment should be continued.

Case 3

Case 3 is a 72-year-old man with prostate cancer. Treatment was antiandrogen treatment for 3 years. To prevent CTIBL, he was started on denosumab 60 mg subcutaneously every 6 months. After the 3 years of antiandrogen treatment, testosterone levels were monitored, and denosumab was continued until testosterone was normalized after 3.5 years. The oncologist responsible for this patient asks the following question.

On stopping denosumab treatment, should additional investigations or follow-up be considered?

A. No need for follow-up; testosterone is no longer suppressed
B. Perform a DXA
C. Measure bone turnover markers
D. Continue denosumab
E. Give a single infusion of zoledronic acid

Discussion

We do not know the correct answer. Stopping denosumab treatment in postmenopausal women is associated with substantial increases in bone turnover and bone loss and a possible increased risk of vertebral fractures (case reports). If this is also the case for men with prostate cancer who, on average, have better BMD than postmenopausal women with osteoporosis is currently unknown. We also know that, in postmenopausal women, a single infusion of zoledronic acid is not enough to prevent the increase in bone turnover and bone loss seen after stopping denosumab; if this is the same in men with prostate cancer, we do not know. It could be speculated that, because bone turnover in eugonadal elderly men is lower than that in postmenopausal women, the increase in turnover seen after stopping denosumab could be less and therefore, potentially better controlled with a bisphosphonate, but this is unknown. Although we are waiting for more evidence, a pragmatic way forward could, therefore, be to perform a DXA, and if osteoporosis is found, denosumab treatment should be continued. If it is not found, bone turnover markers should be measured; if they are high or increasing, zoledronic acid should be administered, and bone turnover markers should be followed.

REFERENCES

1. Stewart AF. Clinical practice. Hypercalcemia associated with cancer. *N Engl J Med.* 2005;**352**(4):373–379.
2. Sternlicht H, Glezerman IG. Hypercalcemia of malignancy and new treatment options. *Ther Clin Risk Manag.* 2015;**11**:1779–1788.
3. Diel IJ, Body JJ, Stopeck AT, Vadhan-Raj S, Spencer A, Steger G, von Moos R, Goldwasser F, Feng A, Braun A. The role of denosumab in the prevention of hypercalcaemia of malignancy in cancer patients with metastatic bone disease. *Eur J Cancer.* 2015;**51**(11):1467–1475.
4. Salahudeen AA, Gupta A, Jones JC, Cowan RW, Vusirikala M, Kwong C, Naina HV. PTHrP-induced refractory malignant hypercalcemia in a patient with chronic lymphocytic leukemia responding to denosumab. *Clin Lymphoma Myeloma Leuk.* 2015;**15**(9):e137–e140.
5. Hu MI, Glezerman IG, Leboulleux S, Insogna K, Gucalp R, Misiorowski W, Yu B, Zorsky P, Tosi D, Bessudo A, Jaccard A, Tonini G, Ying W, Braun A, Jain RK. Denosumab for treatment of hypercalcemia of malignancy. *J Clin Endocrinol Metab.* 2014;**99**(9):3144–3152.
6. Weilbaecher KN, Guise TA, McCauley LK. Cancer to bone: a fatal attraction. *Nat Rev Cancer.* 2011;**11**(6):411–425.
7. Stopeck AT, Lipton A, Body JJ, Steger GG, Tonkin K, de Boer RH, Lichinitser M, Fujiwara Y, Yardley DA, Viniegra M, Fan M, Jiang Q, Dansey R, Jun S, Braun A. Denosumab compared with zoledronic acid for the treatment of bone metastases in patients with advanced breast cancer: a randomized, double-blind study. *J Clin Oncol.* 2010;**28**(35): 5132–5139.
8. Vehmanen L, Saarto T, Elomaa I, Mäkelä P, Välimäki M, Blomqvist C. Long-term impact of chemotherapy-induced ovarian failure on bone mineral density (BMD) in premenopausal breast cancer patients. The effect of adjuvant clodronate treatment. *Eur J Cancer.* 2001;**37**(18): 2373–2378.
9. Shapiro CL, Halabi S, Hars V, Archer L, Weckstein D, Kirshner J, Sikov W, Winer E, Burstein HJ, Hudis C, Isaacs C, Schilsky R, Paskett E. Zoledronic acid preserves bone mineral density in premenopausal women who develop ovarian failure due to adjuvant chemotherapy: final results from CALGB trial 79809. *Eur J Cancer.* 2011;**47**(5):683–689.
10. Van Staa TP, Leufkens HG, Abenhaim L, Zhang B, Cooper C. Use of oral corticosteroids and risk of fractures. *J Bone Miner Res.* 2000;**15**(6): 993–1000.
11. Marcocci C, Bartalena L, Tanda ML, Manetti L, Dell'Unto E, Rocchi R, Barbesino G, Mazzi B, Bartolomei MP, Lepri P, Cartei F, Nardi M, Pinchera A. Comparison of the effectiveness and tolerability of intravenous or oral glucocorticoids associated with orbital radiotherapy in the management of severe Graves' ophthalmopathy: results of a prospective, single-blind, randomized study. *J Clin Endocrinol Metab.* 2001;**86**(8):3562–3567.
12. Saarto T, Blomqvist C, Välimäki M, Mäkelä P, Sarna S, Elomaa I. Chemical castration induced by adjuvant cyclophosphamide, methotrexate, and fluorouracil chemotherapy causes rapid bone loss that is reduced by clodronate: a randomized study in premenopausal breast cancer patients. *J Clin Oncol.* 1997;**15**(4):1341–1347.
13. Sverrisdóttir A, Fornander T, Jacobsson H, von Schoultz E, Rutqvist LE. Bone mineral density among premenopausal women with early breast cancer in a randomized trial of adjuvant endocrine therapy. *J Clin Oncol.* 2004;**22**(18):3694–3699.
14. Gnant M, Mlineritsch B, Luschin-Ebengreuth G, Kainberger F, Kässmann H, Piswanger-Sölkner JC, Seifert M, Ploner F, Menzel C, Dubsky P, Fitzal F, Bjelic-Radisic V, Steger G, Greil R, Marth C, Kubista E, Samonigg H, Wohlmuth P, Mittlböck M, Jakesz R; Austrian Breast and Colorectal Cancer Study Group (ABCSG). Adjuvant endocrine therapy plus zoledronic acid in premenopausal women with early-stage breast cancer: 5-year follow-up of the ABCSG-12 bone-mineral density substudy. *Lancet Oncol.* 2008;**9**(9):840–849.
15. Powles TJ, Hickish T, Kanis JA, Tidy A, Ashley S. Effect of tamoxifen on bone mineral density measured by dual-energy x-ray absorptiometry in healthy premenopausal and postmenopausal women. *J Clin Oncol.* 1996;**14**(1):78–84.
16. Fisher B, Costantino JP, Wickerham DL, Cecchini RS, Cronin WM, Robidoux A, Bevers TB, Kavanah MT, Atkins JN, Margolese RG, Runowicz CD, James JM, Ford LG, Wolmark N. Tamoxifen for the prevention of breast cancer: current status of the National Surgical Adjuvant Breast and Bowel Project P-1 study. *J Natl Cancer Inst.* 2005; **97**(22):1652–1662.
17. Coleman R, Body JJ, Aapro M, Hadji P, Herrstedt J; ESMO Guidelines Working Group. Bone health in cancer patients: ESMO Clinical Practice Guidelines. *Ann Oncol.* 2014;**25**(Suppl 3):iii124–iii137.
18. Goss PE, Hadji P, Subar M, Abreu P, Thomsen T, Banke-Bochita J. Effects of steroidal and nonsteroidal aromatase inhibitors on markers of bone turnover in healthy postmenopausal women. *Breast Cancer Res.* 2007;**9**(4):R52.
19. BIG 1-98 Collaborative Group, Mouridsen H, Giobbie-Hurder A, Goldhirsch A, Thürlimann B, Paridaens R, Smith I, Mauriac L, Forbes J, Price KN, Regan MM, Gelber RD, Coates AS. Letrozole therapy alone or in sequence with tamoxifen in women with breast cancer. *N Engl J Med.* 2009;**361**(8):766–776.
20. Cuzick J, Sestak I, Forbes JF, Dowsett M, Knox J, Cawthorn S, Saunders C, Roche N, Mansel RE, von Minckwitz G, Bonanni B, Palva T, Howell A; IBIS-II investigators. Anastrozole for prevention of breast cancer in high-risk postmenopausal women (IBIS-II): an international, double-blind, randomised placebo-controlled trial. *Lancet.* 2014;**383**(9922):1041–1048.
21. Amir E, Seruga B, Niraula S, Carlsson L, Ocaña A. Toxicity of adjuvant endocrine therapy in postmenopausal breast cancer patients: a systematic review and meta-analysis. *J Natl Cancer Inst.* 2011;**103**(17): 1299–1309.
22. Schmidt N, Jacob L, Coleman R, Kostev K, Hadji P. The impact of treatment compliance on fracture risk in women with breast cancer treated with aromatase inhibitors in the United Kingdom [published correction appears in *Breast Cancer Res Treat* 2016;157(2):401]. *Breast Cancer Res Treat.* 2016;**155**(1):151–157.
23. Melton LJ III, Hartmann LC, Achenbach SJ, Atkinson EJ, Therneau TM, Khosla S. Fracture risk in women with breast cancer: a population-based study. *J Bone Miner Res.* 2012;**27**(5):1196–1205.
24. Coleman RE, Banks LM, Girgis SI, Vrdoljak E, Fox J, Cawthorn SJ, Patel A, Bliss JM, Coombes RC, Kilburn LS. Reversal of skeletal effects of endocrine treatments in the Intergroup Exemestane Study. *Breast Cancer Res Treat.* 2010;**124**(1):153–161.
25. Alibhai SM, Duong-Hua M, Cheung AM, Sutradhar R, Warde P, Fleshner NE, Paszat L. Fracture types and risk factors in men with prostate cancer on androgen deprivation therapy: a matched cohort study of 19,079 men. *J Urol.* 2010;**184**(3):918–923.
26. Winters-Stone KM, Dobek J, Nail L, Bennett JA, Leo MC, Naik A, Schwartz A. Strength training stops bone loss and builds muscle in postmenopausal breast cancer survivors: a randomized, controlled trial. *Breast Cancer Res Treat.* 2011;**127**(2):447–456.
27. Yin L, Grandi N, Raum E, Haug U, Arndt V, Brenner H. Meta-analysis: serum vitamin D and breast cancer risk. *Eur J Cancer.* 2010;**46**(12):2196–2205.
28. Hadji P, Aapro MS, Body JJ, Gnant M, Brandi ML, Reginster JY, Zillikens MC, Glüer CC, de Villiers T, Baber R, Roodman GD, Cooper C, Langdahl B, Palacios S, Kanis J, Al-Daghri N, Nogues X, Eriksen EF, Kurth A, Rizzoli R, Coleman RE. Management of Aromatase Inhibitor-Associated Bone Loss (AIBL) in postmenopausal women with hormone sensitive breast cancer: joint position statement of the IOF, CABS, ECTS, IEG, ESCEO IMS, and SIOG. *J Bone Oncol.* 2017;**7**:1–12.
29. Hillner BE, Ingle JN, Chlebowski RT, Gralow J, Yee GC, Janjan NA, Cauley JA, Blumenstein BA, Albain KS, Lipton A, Brown S; American Society of Clinical Oncology. American Society of Clinical Oncology 2003 update on the role of bisphosphonates and bone health issues in women with breast cancer [published correction appears in *J Clin Oncol* 2004;22(7):1351]. *J Clin Oncol.* 2003;**21**(21): 4042–4057.

30. Gnant M, Pfeiler G, Dubsky PC, Hubalek M, Greil R, Jakesz R, Wette V, Balic M, Haslbauer F, Melbinger E, Bjelic-Radisic V, Artner-Matuschek S, Fitzal F, Marth C, Sevelda P, Mlineritsch B, Steger GG, Manfreda D, Exner R, Egle D, Bergh J, Kainberger F, Talbot S, Warner D, Fesl C, Singer CF; Austrian Breast and Colorectal Cancer Study Group. Adjuvant denosumab in breast cancer (ABCSG-18): a multicentre, randomised, double-blind, placebo-controlled trial. *Lancet.* 2015; **386**(9992):433–443.
31. Early Breast Cancer Trialists' Collaborative Group (EBCTCG). Adjuvant bisphosphonate treatment in early breast cancer: meta-analyses of individual patient data from randomised trials. *Lancet.* 2015; **386**(10001):1353–1361.
32. Smith MR, Egerdie B, Hernández Toriz N, Feldman R, Tammela TL, Saad F, Heracek J, Szwedowski M, Ke C, Kupic A, Leder BZ, Goessl C; Denosumab HALT Prostate Cancer Study Group. Denosumab in men receiving androgen-deprivation therapy for prostate cancer. *N Engl J Med.* 2009;**361**(8):745–755.
33. Greenspan SL, Nelson JB, Trump DL, Resnick NM. Effect of once-weekly oral alendronate on bone loss in men receiving androgen deprivation therapy for prostate cancer: a randomized trial. *Ann Intern Med.* 2007;**146**(6):416–424.

Difficult DXAs and When to Use Other Measurement Tools

M38
Presented, March 17–20, 2018

Micol S. Rothman, MD. University of Colorado School of Medicine, Aurora, Colorado 80045, E-mail: micol.rothman@ucdenver.edu

SIGNIFICANCE OF THE CLINICAL PROBLEM

Bone mineral density (BMD) testing by dual-energy X-ray absorptiometry (DXA) has been a part of clinical practice since the 1980s. It remains the gold standard for measuring bone density at the spine and hip. BMD is the bone mineral content in grams per two-dimensional (2D) projected area of bone, which is reported as grams per centimeter^2. In 1994, the World Health Organization defined osteoporosis on the basis of BMD testing by DXA and T score. The T score = (patient's BMD − young normal mean)/standard deviation of young normal. In postmenopausal women and men over 50 years old, a T score of −1.0 and above is considered normal BMD, <-1.0 to -2.5 is defined as low bone mass or osteopenia, and ≤ -2.5 is considered osteoporosis (1). Osteoporosis can also be diagnosed after a low-trauma fracture (fall from a standing height). In younger patients, the Z score is used to compare patients' BMDs with those of others their age. A Z score of <-2.0 indicates an abnormal BMD for age (1, 2).

Osteoporosis is a common bone disease. Fractures affect morbidity and mortality and cost the health care system billions of dollars every year. There are over 2 million fractures in the United States each year, and the risk of having a broken bone after age 50 years old is one in two for women and one in four for men; 20% of women will die in the first year after hip fracture, and 60% of patients never regain their prefracture level of independence. Osteoporosis in men is often underdiagnosed and undertreated, but a man is more likely to die after a hip fracture than a woman (3).

Although DXA is still the most widely used clinical tool to screen for osteoporosis, it has limitations. Additional tools can be used to evaluate fracture risk, because many patients who fracture have bone density scores in the osteopenic or even normal range. Thus, DXA in combination with fracture risk assessment tool (FRAX; https://www.shef.ac.uk/FRAX/) is used as a fracture prediction tool for untreated patients with a diagnosis of osteopenia. FRAX takes into account BMD-independent risks for fracture, including age, glucocorticoid treatment, current tobacco use, parental history of hip fracture, rheumatoid arthritis, and alcohol use of more than three drinks per day. FRAX can be used to calculate fracture risk when BMD is not available as well. Other risk prediction tools include the Garvan calculator, which also incorporates falls, and the osteoporosis self-assessment tool, which looks at body weight and age alone.

Additional imaging techniques and/or measurements of bone quality can be used in patient care in addition to DXA. Trabecular bone score (TBS), a gray-level textural measurement, is now being used in both research and clinical practice (4). TBS can take lumbar spine data from standard DXA testing to noninvasively look at bone microarchitecture. It projects a three-dimensional structure onto a 2D plane and utilizes gray-level variation in images of the lumbar spine to calculate a score. This score has been shown to predict fracture in primary osteoporosis as well as several forms of secondary osteoporosis. Dedicated vertebral imaging via vertebral fracture assessment with DXA or plain films of the spine can also be useful, particularly in adults with osteopenia and additional risk factors for osteoporosis, in whom the finding of a silent fracture would change the recommendations for pharmacologic therapy. Other modalities, such as quantitative computed tomography, can measure volumetric BMD at the spine and hip. Although quantitative computed tomography is thought to be a good measure of bone quality, because of cost and radiation exposure, it is generally used for research only at this time. Bone biopsies give the most direct information about bone microarchitecture, but they are invasive procedures.

BARRIERS TO OPTIMAL PRACTICE

Although BMD testing is widely used, measurements are frequently not reported in concordance with International Society for Clinical Densitometry (ISCD) guidelines. Many clinicians are not familiar with how to interpret DXA images in the face of artifacts and other limitations. Additionally, the use of T scores versus Z scores is often misunderstood. The ISCD suggests that only the lowest site T score be used for a diagnosis (1). That is, one should not report a hip with osteoporosis but a spine with osteopenia. Furthermore, many DXA centers do not have a measurement of least significant change (LSC), which can make it difficult to interpret change in BMD over time.

There are also ongoing controversies about the frequency of DXA for screening and monitoring. Guidelines from national societies give conflicting advice about when to screen and how often to repeat DXA (5). Medicare coverage for screening in some groups differs from what the ISCD and the National Osteoporosis Foundation recommend. Many women who are eligible for screening DXA still do not receive it. In a study of Medicare beneficiaries from 2002 to 2008, 48% of women had no testing done at all; <4% received four or more DXA studies, and thus, undertesting may be more of a problem than overtesting (6).

LEARNING OBJECTIVES

As a result of participating in this session, learners should be able to

- Interpret BMD testing for men and women of all ages
- Use DXA to help guide secondary workup of low BMD or bone loss
- Be familiar with the guidelines (and controversies) regarding DXA screening and follow-up intervals
- Be familiar with the use of TBS and other modalities for vertebral imaging

STRATEGIES FOR DIAGNOSIS, THERAPY, OR MANAGEMENT

The National Osteoporosis Foundation (NOF) Clinician's Guide for 2014 recommends osteoporosis screening for all women over age 65 years old and men over 70 years old. It also advises screening for postmenopausal women and men over 50 years old with other risk factors. In addition, a DXA is suggested after a fracture to define the extent of low BMD. The NOF also suggests that DXA be performed at facilities using accepted quality assurance measures. The US Preventive Services Task Force recommends bone density screening for all women >65 years old (grade B) and women <65 years old whose 10-year risk of fracture as calculated by FRAX is greater than that of a 65-year-old white woman without risk factors (9.3%; grade B) (7). The use of additional vertebral imaging for those with low BMD is also suggested in the following groups: women >70 and men >80 years old with T scores <−1.0, women 65 to 69 and men 70 to 79 years old with T scores <−1.5, and men and women over 50 years old with adult low-trauma fractures, height loss, and glucocorticoid treatment (3). The NOF advises follow-up testing for those on treatment in 1 to 2 years and every 2 years thereafter, but note that certain clinical situations may warrant more or less frequent follow-up.

LSC and precision should be calculated by each technician at a bone density facility. Here, technicians can measure a patient multiple times (15 patients × 3 or 30 patients × 2) to determine their precision and thus, what change in BMD can be interpreted as a true change. There is a formula on the ISCD website (ISCD.org) where patients' data can be entered and precision for each technician can then be calculated. LSC is reported in grams per centimeter^2 for hip and spine. T scores are not used, because they can change with alterations in the database reference population. If a patient's change in BMD does not exceed the LSC, it is not considered an important change. However, even if changes do exceed LSC, this does not mean that they are clinically important. A loss of 1% to 2% per year can be seen with normal aging, and BMD testing done at long intervals may show loss that exceeds LSC but is not considered pathologic.

In the setting of a low T score (or low Z score in a young patient), a workup to rule out secondary causes is advised. This includes looking for common causes of low BMD (renal disease, liver disease, vitamin D deficiency, hyperthyroidism, hyperparathyroidism, hypogonadism, or hypercalciuria) as well as less common causes as clinical suspicion dictates: Cushing syndrome, multiple myeloma, celiac disease, mastocytosis, or osteogenesis imperfecta.

MAIN CONCLUSIONS

BMD should be interpreted using T scores for men >50 years old and postmenopausal women. Younger groups should have Z scores reported.

Low Z scores at any age may indicate the need for a secondary workup of low bone density.

BMD testing should be repeated at a time interval when a change is likely to be important and/or lead to a treatment change. This may vary by patient factors, the treatments used, and other clinical indicators. For those at highest risk, that interval may be 1 to 2 years. For those at lower risk, it can be longer.

Vertebral imaging can help make clinical decisions when bone density is in the osteopenic range in the face of other risk factors.

TBS is a new tool that can help predict fracture risk in many groups. It may be of particular use in populations with BMD that has not historically been low.

CASES

Case 1

A 65-year-old woman with no risk factors for osteoporosis undergoes a screening DXA that shows an L1 to L4 T score of 0.8 and a right femoral neck T score of −1.2.

Which of the following is appropriate to put on the DXA report?

A. "This is a screening study for a 65-year-old woman with no reported risk factors for osteoporosis"
B. "This patient has normal bone density at the lumbar spine and osteopenia at the right hip"
C. "This patient's BMD test does not need to be repeated"
D. "There has been substantial bone loss in this patient"

Case 1: Discussion

The answer is A. The ISCD guidelines specifically note that osteoporosis is a systemic disease, and one unifying diagnosis should be given (not osteopenia at one site and normal at another) (1). Therefore, B is incorrect. Answer D is incorrect, because we do not know in a screening study whether bone loss has occurred. As to answer C, the issue of bone density intervals for monitoring is controversial. In 2012, an article in the *New England Journal of Medicine* by Gourlay *et al.* (8) looked at the use of screening DXA for osteoporosis. They examined a subgroup of women from the Study of Osteoporotic Fractures and looked at the time that it took women with normal BMD or osteopenia to transition to osteoporosis. This time varied with changes in age, estrogen use, and body mass index; <5% of the women with mild osteopenia (which would be the patient in this case) made the transition to osteoporosis over the 15-year period. This article does not support retesting this patient in 1 year, and she is unlikely to have loss that would indicate a need for pharmacologic therapy, but we cannot say at this time that her DXA should never be repeated.

Patient history and risk factors can help determine that interval. The ISCD does suggest that all DXA reports include the following as a minimum: patient demographics, machine manufacturer and model, skeletal sites that were scanned, BMD in grams per centimeter^2 as well as T score and/or Z score where appropriate, World Health Organization criteria for diagnosis, recommendations for the timing of the next study, and risk factors with a statement about fracture risk as well a statement that medical evaluation for causes of low BMD may be indicated.

We will use this case vignette to discuss the guidelines for what should be included on a DXA report as well as controversies surrounding testing intervals.

Case 2

A postmenopausal woman undergoes BMD testing on several occasions. You are concerned that, although the hip BMD is stable, there has been a large decrease in the spine in a rapid timeframe.

What is the next step that you would undertake?

A. Change her oral bisphosphonate to an alternative therapy
B. Add estrogen to her current regimen to increase her spine BMD
C. Order markers of bone turnover to assess for increased osteoclast activity
D. View the images yourself, particularly the spine

Case 2: Discussion

The answer is D. Looking at images for accuracy is a key part of bone density interpretation. Before taking steps that would be costly, such as ordering blood urine tests, or changing to alternative therapies, it is important to view the images. (Thus, A, B, and C are wrong.) As shown here, when the 2016 spine outline was redrawn to match 2015, the changes were no longer important.

This case will highlight the need to view images. Other examples of imaging issues and artifacts will be shown.

Case 3

A 53-year-old man with a history of lung transplant takes 5 mg prednisone daily. His lowest T score is −1.2, and you are concerned that this may not accurately reflect his bone quality.

In thinking about additional imaging, which of the following is true?

A. TBS requires additional images and radiation exposure for the patient
B. Glucocorticoid-treated patients have been shown to have lower TBS, even without changes in BMD
C. Vertebral imaging showing fracture would not change our assessment of his future fracture risk
D. A high TBS indicates poor bone architecture

Case 3: Discussion

The answer is B. TBS is a gray-level textural measurement that uses images already obtained by 2D images (4,9) (A is wrong). A high score is indicative of better microarchitecture (thus, D is wrong), whereas a lower score indicates poor bone architecture. Several studies have shown that TBS can decline with glucocorticoid use, even without changes seen in BMD (10,11). TBS may be particularly useful in this group as well as those with other secondary causes of osteoporosis, in whom BMD may not accurately reflect fracture risk.

This case will serve as a discussion point for talking about the uses and limitations of TBS and other vertebral imaging.

Case 4

A 23-year-old woman with a history of eating disorder is seen for amenorrhea. She has not had menses in 7 months. Recent studies from her primary care provider show a vitamin D level of 35 ng/mL. She brings a bone density with her.

What do you suggest?

A. Begin teriparatide
B. Further assess the amenorrhea and think about a bone mineral–apparent density calculation
C. Add 50,000 IU of vitamin D once a week
D. Begin alendronate based on low T score

Case 4: Discussion

The answer is B. This case brings up the larger issue of how to approach low BMD in younger patients. Often, young patients with low BMD have not reached peak bone mass, and their bone density needs to be interpreted with caution. The use of T scores in men <50 years old and premenopausal women is not appropriate, and in young patients who are not fracturing, we try to avoid pharmacologic therapy (12) (thus, answer D is incorrect). In addition, teriparatide is contraindicated in young patients (answer A), because there can still be concerns for open epiphyses until age 25 years old. With a vitamin D level of 35 ng/mL, additional supplementation is unlikely to help her bone health (thus, C is incorrect). Patients with eating disorders in adolescence may have delayed bone age, and it is important to keep this in mind when thinking about DXA Z scores. In addition, growing patients or those who are smaller stature will have smaller bones. Fracture risk can be overestimated in patients with short stature. A calculation can be done to estimate bone mineral–apparent density and provide more of a volumetric BMD. The term was coined in 1992, and this Web site gives a calculator (https://courses.washington.edu/bonephys/opBMAD.html) (13).

Additional questioning about the amenorrhea and laboratory workup would be appropriate.

We will use this case vignette to talk about the use of T scores and Z scores in young people and when pharmacologic intervention should be considered.

REFERENCES

1. ISCD. 2015 ISCD official positions. Available at: Iscd.org. Accessed 18 December 2017.
2. Lewiecki EM. Bone mineral density measurement and assessment of fracture risk. *Clin Obstet Gynecol.* 2013;**56**(4):667–676.
3. NOF. NOF clinician's guide. Available at: NOF.org. Accessed 18 December 2017.
4. Silva BC, Leslie WD, Resch H, Lamy O, Lesnyak O, Binkley N, McCloskey EV, Kanis JA, Bilezikian JP. Trabecular bone score: a noninvasive analytical method based upon the DXA image. *J Bone Miner Res.* 2014;**29**(3):518–530.
5. Rothman MS, Lewiecki EM, Miller PD. Bone density testing is the best way to monitor osteoporosis. *Am J Med.* 2017;**130**(10):1133–1134.
6. King AB, Fiorentino DM. Medicare payment cuts for osteoporosis testing reduced use despite tests' benefit in reducing fractures. *Health Aff (Millwood).* 2011;**30**(12):2362–2370.
7. Golob AL, Laya MB. Osteoporosis: screening, prevention, and management. *Med Clin North Am.* 2015;**99**(3):587–606.
8. Gourlay ML, Fine JP, Preisser JS, May RC, Li C, Lui LY, Ransohoff DF, Cauley JA, Ensrud KE; Study of Osteoporotic Fractures Research Group. Bone-density testing interval and transition to osteoporosis in older women. *N Engl J Med.* 2012;**366**(3):225–233.
9. Ulivieri FM, Silva BC, Sardanelli F, Hans D, Bilezikian JP, Caudarella R. Utility of the trabecular bone score (TBS) in secondary osteoporosis. *Endocrine.* 2014;**47**(2):435–448.
10. Paggiosi MA, Peel NF, Eastell R. The impact of glucocorticoid therapy on trabecular bone score in older women. *Osteoporos Int.* 2015;**26**(6): 1773–1780.
11. Leib ES, Winzenrieth R. Bone status in glucocorticoid-treated men and women. *Osteoporos Int.* 2016;**27**(1):39–48.
12. Abraham A, Cohen A, Shane E. Premenopausal bone health: osteoporosis in premenopausal women. *Clin Obstet Gynecol.* 2013;**56**(4): 722–729.
13. Carter DR, Bouxsein ML, Marcus R. New approaches for interpreting projected bone densitometry data. *J Bone Miner Res.* 1992;**7**(2):137–145.

Osteoporosis in Men

M58
Presented, March 17–20, 2018

Robert A. Adler, MD. Endocrinology and Metabolism Section, McGuire Veterans Affairs Medical Center, Richmond, Virginia 23249, E-mail: robert.adler@va.gov

SIGNIFICANCE OF THE PROBLEM

As men are now living long enough to fracture, osteoporosis is becoming recognized as a problem that is underdiagnosed, undertreated, and underappreciated. Depending on the population studied, a man at age 50 years has a lifetime risk of osteoporotic fracture of 13% to 25%. Using the National Bone Health Alliance definition of osteoporosis [dual-energy x-ray absorptiometry (DXA) bone mineral density (BMD) T score of less than or equal to −2.5, history of osteoporotic fracture, or Fracture Risk Calculator (FRAX) 10-year hip fracture risk ≥3% or major osteoporotic fracture risk ≥20%], Wright *et al.* (1) estimated that 16% of men over 50 years of age had osteoporosis, rising to 46.3% in the growing group of men aged 80 years or older. There are studies that show that a man who has sustained an osteoporotic fracture or has been placed on chronic glucocorticoids is less likely to receive attention to underlying osteoporosis than a woman. Hip fracture is more deadly in men than in women. In a recent, large observational study (2), DXA screening in men at higher risk (those over age 80 years, on glucocorticoids, or having other key risk factors) actually led to fewer fractures. Men suffer a quarter of the two million osteoporotic fractures that occur in Americans each year. We have to find a way to do better.

BARRIERS TO OPTIMAL PRACTICE

There are not enough endocrinologists and other experts to diagnose and manage osteoporosis in men (and women). Thus, osteoporosis diagnosis and treatment falls to primary care clinicians, already overburdened by symptomatic problems in their aging patients. How many primary care clinicians have read the Endocrine Society Clinical Guideline on Osteoporosis in Men (3)? Osteoporosis is silent until there is a fracture and is thought to be a disorder of postmenopausal women. It is challenging to obtain reimbursement for DXA testing in men, and reimbursement for office-based DXA is less than the cost of the test. Patients diagnosed with osteoporosis are concerned about rare side effects from osteoporosis drugs and may be unwilling to have the diagnosis made because of such fears. The "crisis in osteoporosis" (4) clearly includes men.

LEARNING OBJECTIVES

At the end of the session, participants should be able to:

- Determine which older men should be screened for osteoporosis
- Approach treatment choices based on facts
- Understand the challenges of long-term osteoporosis management

STRATEGIES FOR DIAGNOSIS, THERAPY, AND MANAGEMENT

Osteoporosis is common in men as they age, and estimates of the lifetime fracture risk at age 50 years range from 13% to 25%. In a recent study by Wright *et al.* (1), the prevalence of osteoporosis was estimated by various definitions in American men in the National Health and Nutrition Examination Survey cohort. By DXA T score (less than −2.5) in spine or femoral neck, 3.6% of white men ≥50 years old and 8.9% of white men ≥80 years old had osteoporosis. Using the definition of osteoporosis derived from the FRAX score plus National Osteoporosis Foundation Guidelines (10-year hip fracture risk ≥3% or major osteoporotic fracture risk ≥20%), the prevalence was 13.4% and 37.8% for white men ≥50 and ≥80 years old, respectively. Although having a DXA T score less than −2.5 greatly increases the risk of fracture, it must be remembered that there will actually be more fractures in the so-called osteopenic group simply because there are so many more men with this intermediate bone density. The fracture risk calculator FRAX is one method to determine which of the osteopenic men are likely to fracture. As life expectancy increases for men, more will live long enough to sustain a fracture. Given this information, a strategy for identifying men at risk for fracture can be established.

Diagnosis and Evaluation: BMD

The US Preventive Services Task Force concluded that there was insufficient evidence to recommend for or against general DXA screening in men (5). Although some expert groups have recommended general screening in men (3), until recently there have not been data on which to judge recommendations. In a recent study that encompassed the entire Department of Veterans Affairs (VA) database, Colon-Emeric *et al.* (2) found that general screening of men did not lead to fewer fractures. Some of this may have been due to the poor rate of treatment initiation and adherence. However, when higher-risk men were screened, there were actually fewer fractures captured by the VA and Medicare databases. The following were the higher risk factors: age ≥80 years, chronic glucocorticoid therapy, androgen deprivation therapy for prostate cancer, high fracture risk by FRAX [using body mass index (BMI) as a surrogate for BMD], and, for men over 65 years old, at least one of a list of risks for osteoporosis (low trauma fracture after age 45 years, x-ray evidence of vertebral osteopenia or fracture, hypogonadism, enzyme-inducing antiepileptic medications, gastrectomy, hyperparathyroidism, hyperthyroidism, rheumatoid arthritis, Parkinson disease, stroke, chronic liver disease, chronic lung disease, BMI <25 kg/m^2, excess alcohol consumption, and current smoking). It is true that the men cared for in the VA system tend to be less healthy than the general public, but it is interesting to review a recent study from the generally healthy and educated cohort from the Osteoporotic Fractures in Men Study (MrOS) (6). The following risk factors, when added to the DXA measurement, greatly increased the risk of hip fracture: age ≥75 years, less protein in the diet, any fracture after age 50 years, divorce, tricyclic antidepressants, hypoglycemic agents, height loss, hyperthyroidism, Parkinson disease, inability to do chair stands, decreased executive function, and current smoking. Although not identical, there is considerable overlap between the VA and the MrOS lists of important risk factors. Thus, it is possible to see that history and physical examination can help the clinician choose which older male patients need to undergo DXA testing. Combining the DXA results with other risk factors and with FRAX (now with femoral neck BMD) allows the clinician to identify those men at highest risk and therefore most likely to benefit from therapy. One stumbling block may be the difficulty in obtaining reimbursement for DXA testing in men. At this time, reimbursement is generally available if a man has fractured, is on glucocorticoids, has hyperparathyroidism, or has had substantial height loss. It is hoped that the data from recent studies will lead to a much larger group of men at risk who will be eligible for DXA testing reimbursement.

Diagnosis and Evaluation: Laboratory Testing

Laboratory testing in men at risk for fracture should include a measure of renal function, serum calcium (and albumin), and 25-hydroxyvitamin D. A case can be made to measure a complete blood count because 75% of multiple myeloma patients are anemic and can have fractures that look like osteoporosis. Other testing will be guided by the patient history and physical examination. In the VA population, laboratory testing was very helpful (7); in MrOS, not so much (8). In younger men, a serum testosterone and 24-hour urine calcium can provide clues to middle-aged osteoporosis, which usually presents with vertebral compression fractures or very low spine bone density (9).

Approach to Treatment

Once the diagnosis of osteoporosis or high risk for fracture by FRAX has been made, treatment decisions must be made. In women, calcium and vitamin D can modestly decrease fracture risk, and there is no reason to doubt that such an effect would apply to men as well (10). Oral bisphosphonates (alendronate and risedronate) and the intravenous bisphosphonate zoledronic acid are Food and Drug Administration (FDA) approved for osteoporosis in men. Denosumab, the humanized monoclonal antibody against RANK ligand, and teriparatide, the first 34 amino acids of parathyroid hormone, are also FDA approved to treat osteoporosis in men. Registration trials for osteoporosis drugs are generally performed in women, but all FDA-approved drugs appear to work equally well in women and men. In one trial of zoledronic in men, the primary outcome goal of vertebral fracture risk reduction was met (11), and all surrogates of fracture risk reduction reported in women have been similarly affected in men. Thus, we feel confident that bisphosphonates, denosumab, and anabolic drugs that lower fracture risk in women are very likely to do so in men. Although the magnitude of fracture risk reduction is not empirically established in men, it is assumed that, like women, the risk is decreased by about one-half. Most studies have found that long-term adherence to osteoporosis treatment is as abysmal in men as it is in women. In women, it has been shown that 75% to 80% of oral bisphosphonate doses must be taken (and done so correctly) to demonstrate decreased fracture risk (12). There is no information to suggest that men can "get away with" lower adherence in bisphosphonate use; poor persistence with therapy will likely decrease fracture efficacy.

As stated above, although empiric evidence in men is lacking, all patients need to have adequate dietary calcium, adequate vitamin D (target level somewhat controversial), and, if possible, perform weight bearing exercise on a regular basis. Home safety is important as well as management of any visual deficiency. To these nonpharmacologic modalities, drug treatment is usually indicated for those at augmented fracture risk. In an ideal world, the highest-risk patients would receive anabolic treatment with teriparatide or perhaps abaloparatide (FDA approved for women only at this time). After 1.5 to 2 years of actually building bone, the patients would then be switched to an antiresorptive drug such as a bisphosphonate or denosumab, which would then be continued for some years. The major barrier to this therapeutic paradigm is the cost of anabolic therapy, which is five figures per year, and the nuisance of daily injections. For the moderate or lower-risk patient (and for the higher-risk patient whose insurance or income will only allow bisphosphonate treatment), the usual first choice of treatment is generic alendronate. The dose is 70 mg weekly and, if taken correctly, is generally safe and effective. As in women, oral alendronate must be taken on an empty stomach with 8 ounces of plain water once weekly. The patient should be sitting, standing, or walking over the next half hour and refrain from taking anything else by mouth (including other medications, coffee, breakfast, etc.). It is important to explain to the patient that the reasons for these instructions include the need to prevent esophageal irritation and to eliminate any competition for absorption of the bisphosphonate. The patient also needs to be educated that osteoporosis is a chronic condition and that most patients will be treated for at least 5 years. This should be stressed at every appointment. For those patients who will not or cannot take an oral bisphosphonate (because of gastroesophageal reflux disease not under control, Barrett esophagus, or achalasia, for example), intravenous preparations are available. Of the two intravenous preparations, only zoledronic acid is FDA approved for men. Interestingly, the only study in men in which decreased fracture risk was the primary outcome was done with zoledronic acid. In this 2-year study, men receiving zoledronic acid, compared with placebo had fewer morphometric vertebral fractures (11). The decrease in relative fracture risk reduction was similar to that of studies in women. In other studies of men, the changes in surrogates for fracture (improvement in bone density or changes in bone turnover markers) have been similar to the findings in the registration trials for osteoporosis drugs, which have been conducted in postmenopausal women.

Approach to Long-Term Management

Based on these findings, we can tell our male patients that taking their osteoporosis medications properly and regularly will lower their fracture risk by about half. Nonetheless, there are no long-term studies of osteoporosis treatment in men. The approach to long-term management by expert groups was based on two studies that were extensions of the registration trials for bisphosphonate treatment of postmenopausal osteoporosis (13). The recommendations weighed the potential benefits of fracture risk reduction with the potential harms of osteonecrosis of the jaw and atypical femoral fracture. Most reports of these side effects have described women on bisphosphonates, but the complications have been reported in men as well. It is not known whether the incidence of side effects is the same in men, but we assume that it is. On the other hand, many atypical femoral fractures were reported in active younger postmenopausal women with osteopenia, women who probably would not be treated today. FRAX is very helpful in showing patients that their risk of fracture in the next 10 years is low, so inappropriate use of bisphosphonates has probably diminished. On the other hand, FRAX may keep the man who needs therapy from taking it. Consider the scenario of a 78-year-old man with a femoral neck T score of −2.4, whose 10-year risk of hip fracture is 5%. We would generally treat this man because of the medical and financial consequences of hip fracture. It would not be unusual for the man to say, "Doc, it means I have a 95% chance of not having a hip fracture in the next 10 years." This is the challenge of osteoporosis treatment, complicated by the fact that the treatment will only decrease the fracture risk to half. Add to that the nuisance of taking oral bisphosphonates, the fact that the medications don't make people feel different, and the popular media's depiction of these drugs as poisons. It explains the difficulty of osteoporosis treatment in 2018. Indeed, the crisis of osteoporosis treatment pertains to men as well as women; it may be even worse in men because osteoporosis is considered a disorder of postmenopausal women.

The Role of Testosterone in Male Osteoporosis

Parallel to the decrease in BMD with aging, serum testosterone, particularly free testosterone, also decreases (14). In the MrOS study (15), serum bioavailable estradiol was much more closely correlated with bone density than any measure of testosterone. Of course, the major source of estradiol in men is aromatization of testosterone; in this case, testosterone appears to be a prohormone. Nonetheless, the man with marked testosterone deficiency is likely to have lower muscle mass and may be at higher risk for falling. Without getting into the complicated subject of whether testosterone replacement is safe and effective, it may decrease fall risk if musculature is improved. For men with osteoporosis and hypogonadism, the Endocrine Society Clinical Guideline on Osteoporosis in Men (3) recommends osteoporosis-specific medication to decrease fracture risk because although testosterone clearly increases bone density and more recently has been shown to increase bone strength (16), no studies have been large enough to demonstrate fracture risk reduction. The Guideline states that if the patient has symptoms of hypogonadism, testosterone replacement may be indicated, but the clinician should not expect that it will lower fracture risk.

CONCLUSIONS

Osteoporosis in men is common and the consequences are substantial. An older man with a hip fracture has a 1-year mortality rate of 25% to 35% (17). Despite this, osteoporosis is not on the radar screen of either older men or their clinicians. Targeted screening appears to work, although obtaining a BMD is problematic. Fortunately, if the diagnosis is made, alendronate is inexpensive, and it works in men. Zoledronic acid has become less expensive and is also generally safe and effective. So, there are tools for diagnosis and treatment, but convincing patients that they are at risk for fracture remains challenging. Evaluation also requires obtaining a good history and physical exam, which may lead to a limited number of laboratory tests. The long-term management is completely based on studies in women, but the recommendation of expert groups is to treat men similarly. For the primary clinician focusing on the patient's clinical complaints, attention to fracture risk tends to fall to the bottom of the priority list. Until we find a way to raise awareness, assuage anxieties about treatment, and convince our patients to adhere to treatment, the number of osteoporotic fractures in men is unlikely to decrease.

ILLUSTRATIVE CASES

Case 1

An 84-year-old white man was originally referred at age 79 years, after he suffered an ankle fracture. Evaluation at that time revealed he had fractured his left hip 3 years prior after stepping off a curb; he had received no evaluation or treatment at that time. The patient had hypertension, chronic kidney disease (CKD) 3, neuropathy that affected his balance, and gastroesophageal reflux disease that was controlled with omeprazole. His serum testosterone level was 250 ng/dL.

Bone density at that time showed a spine T score of −1.4, total hip −2, femoral neck −3, and distal 1/3 radius −3.3, all defined by the male normative database. His estimated glomerular filtration rate was 44, and he was started on risedronate. Follow-up bone density 2.5 years later revealed stable readings. Another DXA was done at age 84 years, showing essentially the same bone density (done on the same machine by the same technologist with adequate quality control). His estimated creatinine clearance has now dropped to 28 (Cockcroft-Gault equation), and he still is at risk for falling because of his neuropathy. The femoral neck T score is −2.9 by the male normative database, and by the white female normative database, the T score is −2.7. If he were an untreated patient, his FRAX 10-year major osteoporotic fracture risk would be 18% and 10-year hip fracture risk would be 8.6%.

Questions

1. Would you continue current treatment of this man?

Answer: No. His renal function has deteriorated and his response to risedronate has been minimal. He remains at high risk.

2. Would you consider a different treatment? What would it be?

Answer: Denosumab would be reasonable because of the patient's renal status and one study showing that switching to denosumab from alendronate increased bone density more than staying on alendronate. Although this does not guarantee better fracture risk reduction, it is reasonable to make this switch. It appears that denosumab must be continued indefinitely because of immediate loss of bone after discontinuation and reports of multiple vertebral fractures after discontinuation. Although his testosterone is somewhat low, it is not particularly low for his age. The Endocrine Society Guideline recommends treatment with an osteoporosis-specific drug rather than testosterone.

3. How would you continue to follow him?

Answer: I would continue to do a DXA every 2 years and make sure that all the nonpharmacologic management tools are used. However, I would see the patient at least annually to ask about thigh and bone pain (prodrome to atypical femoral fracture) and dental issues. We look in patients' mouths at each visit, and perhaps with new densitometers able to image the entire femur with a quick single-energy low-radiation scan, it may be reasonable to do this annually

4. What will happen if his renal function deteriorates and he now has CKD 5 and starts hemodialysis?

Answer: As of now, we have little to offer such patients. Whether newer anabolics will work in CKD 5 patients is an important question for a future session. Stay tuned.

Case 2

A 79-year-old man was originally referred for BMD testing at age 65 years after his primary clinician calculated OST (osteoporosis self-assessment tool) for him and found the patient at moderate risk. He was an active man at that time but he had suffered a femur fracture at age 17 years, leading to a 6-month hospitalization and a 1-year period of no ambulation. His DXA at age 65 years showed a spine T score of −4.1, total hip −2.5, and femoral neck of −3.2, all by the male normative database. His evaluation at age 65 years was unrevealing, and he was started on 400 units of vitamin D daily and teriparatide. Two years later, his spine and total hip BMD increases were 9.2% and 4%, respectively. He was started on alendronate 70 mg weekly, which he took for 4 years. He was then lost to Bone Clinic follow-up for 2 years until a bone density was done. His spine had decreased 3.7% but his total hip had increased 4.6%. He was restarted on alendronate and he took it for 1 year. He restarted one more time after a hiatus of ~2 years and continued until 3 months before his latest DXA. Now at age 79 years, his bone density shows a spine T score (continuing with the male database for consistency) of −2.6, total hip −2.2, and the femoral neck −2.9. Over this long period, the patient has been generally healthy, but he has lost 10 pounds in the last year (BMI now 24.8 kg/m^2). He has had some urinary retention and a mild elevation of prostate-specific antigen, but prostate biopsies in the past have been negative. His testosterone level was 200 ng/dL.

Questions

1. Why might this otherwise active, athletic man have such low bone density at age 65 years?

Answer: This case illustrates the importance of attaining peak bone mass. Studies show that men who had delayed puberty have lower bone density than those who went through development at the normal time. In this case, the patient's long-term hospitalization (and presumed immobilization) and prolonged lack of ambulation at a crucial time of life led him to have low bone mass years later. Considering the possible increase in urinary symptoms and rising prostate-specific antigen, I would not consider testosterone in this man at age 79 years. In a younger man with symptoms of hypogonadism and low serum testosterone (and no contraindications), testosterone replacement would increase bone density. At this time, it is not known if fracture risk would be diminished by hormone replacement therapy.

2. Was teriparatide indicated at age 65 years? What would you have chosen instead?

Answer: To my mind, teriparatide was a good choice because the patient had relatively lower bone density in the spine. Sequence of therapy is important, and patients do better if they receive the anabolic treatment first.

3. Has he responded to alendronate?

Answer: Yes, there has been a response to alendronate despite the interruptions in treatment. The patient illustrates that clinicians must stay connected with patients. Even an annual visit helps keep patients on treatment.

4. What to do now?

Answer: Might this be a time to treat the patient with denosumab for a few years and then "maintain" with a bisphosphonate? He would probably increase his hip bone density, and if his renal function remains good, he can switch back to a bisphosphonate (with overlap?) so that the acute loss of bone after discontinuation of denosumab may be mitigated. How will we ever have trials to determine long-term management in patients like this?

REFERENCES

1. Wright NC, Saag KG, Dawson-Hughes B, Khosla S, Siris ES. The impact of the new National Bone Health Alliance (NBHA) diagnostic criteria on the prevalence of osteoporosis in the USA. *Osteoporos Int.* 2017; **28**(4):1225–1232.
2. Colon-Emeric C, Pieper C, Lyles K, VanHoutven C, LaFleur J, Adler R. Primary osteoporosis screening in U.S. male veterans is effective in high risk subgroups but not overall. American Society for Bone and Mineral Research Annual Meeting; September 8–11, 2017; Denver, CO. Abstract LB-SU0373. 2017.
3. Watts NB, Adler RA, Bilezikian JP, Drake MT, Eastell R, Orwoll ES, Finkelstein JS; Endocrine Society. Osteoporosis in men: an Endocrine Society clinical practice guideline. *J Clin Endocrinol Metab.* 2012; **97**(6):1802–1822.
4. Khosla S, Cauley JA, Compston J, Kiel DP, Rosen C, Saag KG, Shane E. Addressing the crisis in the treatment of osteoporosis: a path forward. *J Bone Miner Res.* 2016;**31**(8):1485–1487.
5. U.S. Preventive Services Task Force. Screening for osteoporosis: U.S. Preventive Services Task Force recommendation statement. *Ann Intern Med.* 2011;**154**(5):356–364.
6. Cauley JA, Cawthon PM, Peters KE, Cummings SR, Ensrud KE, Bauer DC, Taylor BC, Shikany JM, Hoffman AR, Lane NE, Kado DM, Stefanick ML, Orwoll ES; Osteoporotic Fractures in Men (MrOS) Study Research Group. Risk factors for hip fracture in older men: the Osteoporotic Fractures in Men Study (MrOS). *J Bone Miner Res.* 2016;**31**(10):1810–1819.
7. Ryan CS, Petkov VI, Adler RA. Osteoporosis in men: the value of laboratory testing. *Osteoporos Int.* 2011;**22**(6):1845–1853.
8. Fink HA, Litwack-Harrison S, Taylor BC, Bauer DC, Orwoll ES, Lee CG, Barrett-Connor E, Schousboe JT, Kado DM, Garimella PS, Ensrud KE; Osteoporotic Fractures in Men (MrOS) Study Group. Clinical utility of routine laboratory testing to identify possible secondary causes in older men with osteoporosis: the Osteoporotic Fractures in Men (MrOS) Study [published correction appears in *Osteoporos Int.* 2017; 28(1):419–420]. *Osteoporos Int.* 2016;**27**(1):331–338.
9. Adler RA. Osteoporosis in men: a review. Bone Res. 2014;2:14001.
10. Weaver CM, Alexander DD, Boushey CJ, Dawson-Hughes B, Lappe JM, LeBoff MS, Liu S, Looker AC, Wallace TC, Wang DD. Calcium plus vitamin D supplementation and risk of fractures: an updated meta-analysis from the National Osteoporosis Foundation [published correction appears in *Osteoporos Int.* 2016;27(8):2643–2646]. *Osteoporos Int.* 2016;**27**(1):367–376.
11. Boonen S, Reginster JY, Kaufman JM, Lippuner K, Zanchetta J, Langdahl B, Rizzoli R, Lipschitz S, Dimai HP, Witvrouw R, Eriksen E, Brixen K, Russo L, Claessens F, Papanastasiou P, Antunez O, Su G, Bucci-Rechtweg C, Hruska J, Incera E, Vanderschueren D, Orwoll E. Fracture risk and zoledronic acid therapy in men with osteoporosis. *N Engl J Med.* 2012;**367**(18):1714–1723.
12. Siris ES, Pasquale MK, Wang Y, Watts NB. Estimating bisphosphonate use and fracture reduction among US women aged 45 years and older, 2001-2008. *J Bone Miner Res.* 2011;**26**(1):3–11.
13. Adler RA, El-Hajj Fuleihan G, Bauer DC, Camacho PM, Clarke BL, Clines GA, Compston JE, Drake MT, Edwards BJ, Favus MJ, Greenspan SL, McKinney R, Jr, Pignolo RJ, Sellmeyer DE. Managing osteoporosis in patients on long-term bisphosphonate treatment: report of a task force of the American Society for Bone and Mineral Research. *J Bone Miner Res.* 2016;**31**(1):16–35.
14. Travison TG, Vesper HW, Orwoll E, Wu F, Kaufman JM, Wang Y, Lapauw B, Fiers T, Matsumoto AM, Bhasin S. Harmonized reference ranges for circulating testosterone levels in men of four cohort studies in the United States and Europe. *J Clin Endocrinol Metab.* 2017; **102**(4):1161–1173.
15. Khosla S, Melton LJ III, Atkinson EJ, O'Fallon WM. Relationship of serum sex steroid levels to longitudinal changes in bone density in young versus elderly men. *J Clin Endocrinol Metab.* 2001;**86**(8): 3555–3561.
16. Snyder PJ, Kopperdahl DL, Stephens-Shields AJ, Ellenberg SS, Cauley JA, Ensrud KE, Lewis CE, Barrett-Connor E, Schwartz AV, Lee DC, Bhasin S, Cunningham GR, Gill TM, Matsumoto AM, Swerdloff RS, Basaria S, Diem SJ, Wang C, Hou X, Cifelli D, Dougar D, Zeldow B, Bauer DC, Keaveny TM. Effect of testosterone treatment on volumetric bone density and strength in older men with low testosterone: a controlled clinical trial. *JAMA Intern Med.* 2017;**177**(4): 471–479.
17. von Friesendorff M, McGuigan FE, Wizert A, Rogmark C, Holmberg AH, Woolf AD, Akesson K. Hip fracture, mortality risk, and cause of death over two decades. *Osteoporos Int.* 2016;**27**(10):2945–2953.

CARDIOVASCULAR ENDOCRINOLOGY

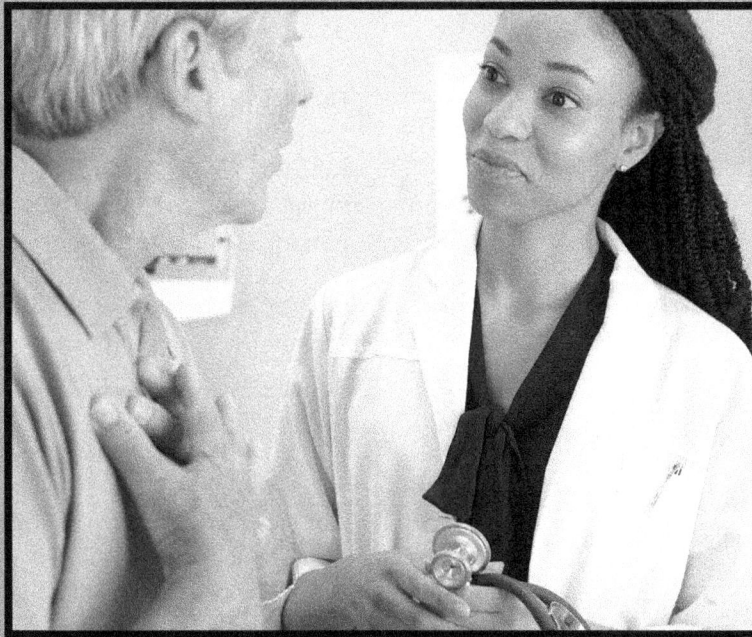

What to Do When Your Patient Has High (or Low) HDL

M13
Presented, March 17–20, 2018

Jeffrey Boord, MD, MPH. Parkview Health System and Indiana University School of Medicine–Fort Wayne, Fort Wayne, Indiana 46845, E-mail: jeffrey.boord@parkview.com

SIGNIFICANCE OF THE CLINICAL PROBLEM

Low high-density lipoprotein cholesterol (HDL-C), especially in the setting of dyslipidemia, is prevalent in adults in the United States. Low HDL-C (<40 mg/dL in men and <50 mg/dL in women), is present in approximately one-third of the adult population. Low HDL has been found to be associated with increased cardiovascular disease (CVD) in men and women in studied populations worldwide (1). HDL-C <20 mg/dL occurs in one in 200 men and one in 400 women (2). Although HDL is a robust biomarker for assessment of cardiovascular risk, its biological role in the development of atherosclerosis is complex and incompletely understood. From an epidemiologic perspective, although high (>60 mg/dL) or very high concentrations (>100 mg/dL) of HDL-C (>60 mg/dL) are uncommon in the US population (16% and 0.7% of men and 32% and 1% of women, respectively), the clinical significance of elevated HDL-C pertaining to atherosclerotic CVD (ASCVD) remains unproven. Current clinical laboratory assessment of HDL through measurement of HDL-C concentration provides little insight into HDL function or its role in atherogenesis for a given individual. There is strong evidence that low-density lipoprotein cholesterol (LDL-C) reduction reduces the burden of ASCVD. However, therapies targeting low HDL-C for the prevention of CVD have largely yielded poor results.

BARRIERS TO OPTIMAL PRACTICE

- HDL function and metabolism are complex and incompletely understood.
- Currently available clinical laboratory assessment of HDL is limited.
- Some secondary causes of low or high HDL-C may be unrecognized.
- Evidence for clinical therapies targeting HDL to improve CVD outcomes is currently limited.

LEARNING OBJECTIVES

At the end of this session, learners will be able to:

- Describe the key metabolic pathways and functions of HDL
- Identify and treat secondary causes of low HDL-C in the clinical setting
- Outline current evidence regarding therapy targeting HDL-C for CVD risk reduction

STRATEGIES FOR DIAGNOSIS, THERAPY, AND MANAGEMENT

HDL particles are macromolecular complexes of lipids and proteins that are largely synthesized in the extracellular space and then later modified in the circulation with the interaction of lipid-transfer proteins, cell-surface proteins, other lipoproteins, and cell-surface receptors (1). HDL is synthesized in the liver and intestine, which both secrete apoprotein A-I (apoA-I). ApoA-I interacts with the cholesterol and phospholipid transporter ATP binding cassette A1 (ABCA1) to acquire lipids and transforms into a nascent HDL particle. HDL acquires additional lipids and apoproteins from hydrolysis of triglyceride-rich apoB-containing lipoproteins. The enzyme lecithin cholesterol acyltransferase (LCAT) acts upon free cholesterol in nascent HDL to generate cholesterol esters in the core of the particle. There are two main pathways for reverse cholesterol transport: (1) direct uptake by the liver or steroidogenic tissues through interaction with scavenger receptor B1 and (2) transfer of cholesterol esters to apoB-containing lipoproteins (in exchange for triglyceride) through the action of cholesterol ester transfer protein (CETP) (3). However, HDL particles have other diverse functions that can modulate atherogenesis, including amelioration of endothelial function, antioxidant effects on LDL, antiapoptosis, macrophage cholesterol efflux stimulation, and anti-inflammatory effects (4).

HDL-C is widely used as a variable in cardiovascular risk prediction models and is essential in calculating non-HDL cholesterol, which estimates the total burden of atherogenic remnant cholesterol (cholesterol content of triglyceride-rich lipoproteins) and LDL-C. Non-HDL cholesterol correlates well with apoB levels and predicts cardiovascular risk better than LDL-C. HDL-C concentration in the clinical setting is measured by homogeneous (*i.e.*, direct) assays, using a variety of methods in virtually all clinical laboratories. These assays generally inhibit or eliminate non-HDL cholesterol with the first reagents and then solubilize HDL particles for measuring cholesterol concentration with the second reagents (5). It is important to note that the HDL-C concentration at any given time is a snapshot of the net state of production, modification, and catabolism of HDL particles but does not provide any measurement of the state of cholesterol transport–mediated flux. The consistent epidemiologic association between low HDL-C and ASCVD in populations and its undisputed utility in prediction of cardiovascular risk led to the classic HDL hypothesis: the concept that HDL-C concentration is directly related to atherosclerosis and that interventions to raise HDL-C concentrations will reduce cardiovascular risk. However, more contemporary genetic studies and clinical trials have greatly challenged this view. Rare Mendelian disorders that lead to very low levels of HDL-C, such as mutations of apoA-I, ABCA1, and LCAT, have not been consistently associated with premature ASCVD. Additionally, mutations of CETP that lead to very high levels of HDL-C have not shown consistent benefit in terms of ASCVD risk (3). Mendelian randomization studies that evaluated single-nucleotide polymorphisms (SNPs) associated with increased HDL-C levels to determine if they were linked to increased risk of myocardial infarction found no significant association for the selected SNPs. In contrast, SNPs associated with high LDL-C levels were correlated with increased risk for myocardial infarction (6). Similarly, genome-wide association studies showed that the effect size of HDL-associated SNPs on HDL-C levels did not correlate with magnitude of effect on coronary heart disease (CHD). In contrast, there was a strong positive relationship between SNPs that increased levels of LDL-C and triglycerides and CHD (4).

HDL-C levels are inversely related to other common CHD risk factors such as obesity, hypertriglyceridemia, increased waist circumference, insulin resistance, diabetes mellitus, tobacco use, and chronic inflammation. Isolated low HDL-C in the population is a rare occurrence (<1%) (1). It is important to recognize other less common causes of low HDL when evaluating patients with dyslipidemia and performing cardiovascular risk assessment. Patients with very low HDL-C (<20 mg/dL) most often have severe hypertriglyceridemia (>500 mg/dL). In the absence of severe hypertriglyceridemia, it is important to consider the differential diagnosis of primary and secondary causes of very low HDL-C. Monogenic primary disorders of HDL metabolism such as apoA-I deficiency, apoA-I structural mutations, homozygous ABCA1 deficiency (Tangier disease), heterozygous ABCA1 deficiency, and LCAT deficiency can cause profoundly low HDL levels but are quite rare in the general population (7). Collaboration with a research or reference laboratory with competency in advanced lipoprotein evaluation techniques, such as two-dimensional gel electrophoresis, evaluation of enzyme mass and function, and cholesterol efflux assays, is essential for definitive diagnosis of primary disorders. Important secondary causes of very low HDL include anabolic androgenic steroids, paradoxical responses to fibrates alone or in combination with thiazolidinediones, and some lymphomas (7). Paraproteinemias can also interfere with common homogeneous HDL-C assays and lead to a falsely low HDL-C concentration.

Regarding pharmacotherapy for HDL, evidence is mixed. The VA-HIT study in male veterans with established coronary artery disease (CAD) and low HDL-C showed that gemfibrozil reduced the primary composite end point death resulting from CAD and nonfatal MI by 22% and stroke by 31%, compared with placebo (8). Gemfibrozil therapy resulted in a modest 6% increase in HDL-C and a 31% reduction in triglycerides. It is important to note that gemfibrozil reduces remnant lipoproteins in addition to increasing HDL-C, which likely accounts for some of its beneficial effects. Additionally, neither the gemfibrozil nor control group received statin therapy in the trial. A number of more contemporary therapy trials targeting HDL-C have failed to show benefits in the setting of concurrent statin therapy. Two large outcome trials using extended-release niacin against a background of statin therapy with optimal LDL control (AIM-HIGH and HPS2-THRIVE) showed no benefit in reducing major adverse cardiovascular events. Furthermore, simvastatin plus niacin/laropiprant therapy in HPS2-THRIVE was associated with an excess of serious adverse events (diabetes complications, bleeding, and infection) compared with simvastatin plus placebo (9). Therefore, niacin should not be used to raise low HDL-C as a target of therapy.

Four separate clinical outcome trials utilizing CETP inhibitors plus statin vs statin plus placebo have been conducted to date. The first trial utilizing torcetrapib was discontinued prematurely because of increased CHD events and total mortality in patients randomly assigned to torcetrapib plus standard statin therapy, despite a 70% increase in HDL-C in the torcetrapib-treated participants (10). Torcetrapib was found to have off-target effects on blood pressure and aldosterone that likely contributed to adverse outcomes. The second trial with the CETP inhibitor dalcetrapib in patients with acute coronary syndrome was also prematurely ended because of futility, with no evidence of benefit despite a 25% mean increase in HDL-C in the treatment group (11). The third CETP inhibitor trial with evacetrapib in patients with high-risk ASCVD demonstrated a 133% increase in HDL-C and 31% reduction in mean LDL-C in the treatment group, compared with controls. However, once again, the trial was terminated early because of lack of efficacy (12). The results of the most recently published phase 3 clinical trial with anacetrapib were rather surprising. Patients with established ASCVD receiving intensive atorvastatin therapy were randomly assigned to anacetrapib or placebo and followed for a median of 4.1 years. Patients in the anacetrapib group achieved a mean 104% increase in HDL-C and 18% reduction in non-HDL cholesterol. The primary outcome of first major coronary event occurred in 10.8% in the anacetrapib group compared with 11.8% in the control group, a relative risk reduction of 9% (13). Given the modest benefit in this trial as well as the negative results of the three prior CETP inhibitor trials, additional studies will be needed to validate this result and better refine the benefits and risks of anacetrapib in the clinical setting.

The studies noted above have led to a paradigm shift from the classic HDL hypothesis to the HDL function hypothesis. It is not HDL-C concentration that drives protection from atherosclerosis, but rather HDL function, which is not discernable with measurement of HDL-C concentration alone. For example, research laboratory methods have been developed that can test the capacity of HDL from a given individual to promote macrophage cholesterol efflux to HDL particles *in vitro*. This HDL cholesterol efflux capacity (CEC) was found in prospective studies in a large multiethnic cohort to be strongly predictive of incident cardiovascular events (14). In a fully adjusted model inclusive of traditional risk factors, there was a 67% reduction in cardiovascular risk in the highest quartile of CEC vs the lowest quartile. Adding CEC to traditional risk factors also improved net discrimination and reclassification indices for cardiovascular risk prediction. There is also evidence supportive of the HDL function hypothesis in evaluation of lifestyle measures that reduce cardiovascular risk. Weight loss through bariatric surgery yields sustained reductions in atherogenic lipoprotein levels, as well as increases in HDL-C. It has also been shown that there is marked improvement in HDL function as measured by CEC in patients 6 months after Roux-en-Y gastric bypass surgery, compared with preoperatively (15). A recent study also demonstrated that consumption of a Mediterranean-type diet, which reduced cardiovascular events in one large randomized clinical trial, also improved CEC and other markers of HDL function in those with increased cardiovascular risk (16). It is hoped that future research and development will lead to useful and cost-effective clinical laboratory assays that will permit evaluation of HDL function as an additional cardiovascular risk biomarker.

MAIN CONCLUSIONS

- HDL-C concentration remains an essential biomarker for the assessment of cardiovascular risk.
- Genetic studies support a direct causal relationship between LDL as well as remnant cholesterol particles and ASCVD. The same is not the case for HDL-C *per se.*
- It cannot be assumed that an intervention that raises HDL-C concentration will reduce cardiovascular risk, and conversely, interventions that reduce HDL-C cannot be assumed to raise cardiovascular risk.
- Niacin should not be considered a therapeutic option for raising HDL-C. Gemfibrozil has been shown to reduce ASCVD events in secondary prevention compared with placebo in patients with low HDL-C. However, no head-to-head clinical outcome trials comparing fibrate therapy to statin therapy have been completed to date.
- Other novel therapeutic approaches such as CETP inhibitors are being investigated to target HDL function, but their utility in reducing ASCVD risk in clinical practice remains to be seen.
- It is important to consider secondary factors that can affect HDL-C concentration as part of cardiovascular risk assessment and treatment.
- An evolving paradigm, the HDL function hypothesis, is a useful concept to understand the complex relationship between HDL-C and ASCVD. It is not HDL-C concentration itself that has a direct effect on atherosclerosis, but rather HDL function.
- HDL function cannot be reliably measured using currently available clinical laboratory methods. It is hoped future research will yield more clinical laboratory tools to aid in assessing HDL function and refining cardiovascular risk assessment in clinical practice.

CASES WITH DISCUSSION AND ANSWERS

Case 1

A 63-year-old man with rheumatoid arthritis and hypertension is referred to you for further evaluation of severe mixed hyperlipidemia. He had been diagnosed with mixed hyperlipidemia ~20 years before presentation and has previously had elevated cholesterol as well as triglyceride levels >600 mg/dL. He has been on and off various lipid-lowering agents over the past 10 years (statin therapy and gemfibrozil). His current medications include: rosuvastatin 5 mg daily, fenofibrate 145 mg daily, atenolol 25 mg daily, hydrochlorothiazide 12.5 mg daily, prednisone 5 mg daily, leflunomide 20 mg daily, alendronate 70 mg weekly, and omeprazole 20 mg twice daily.

He has no prior clinical history of ASCVD, diabetes mellitus, or pancreatitis. He has two siblings with histories of severe hypertriglyceridemia, but there is no known family history of premature ASCVD. He is a nonsmoker.

His physical examination reveals blood pressure of 140/76 mm Hg and body mass index of 30.1 kg/m^2. Neck, cardiac, lung, and abdominal examinations are normal. He has chronic joint changes from his rheumatoid arthritis in his hands.

With rosuvastatin 5 mg daily and fenofibrate 145 mg daily, his cholesterol profile is as follows: total cholesterol, 244 mg/dL; HDL, 31 mg/dL; triglycerides, 369 mg/dL; and LDL, 155 mg/dL. His fasting glucose, thyrotropin, creatinine, and liver function profile are all within normal limits. His calculated 10-year ASCVD risk based on pooled cohort equations is 23%.

You elect to increase his rosuvastatin to 20 mg daily to improve control of his LDL-C. Six months later, he returns for follow-up, and his lipid profile with rosuvastatin 20 mg daily plus fenofibrate 145 mg daily is: total cholesterol, 174 mg/dL; HDL, 13 mg/dL; triglycerides, 263 mg/dL; and LDL, 117 mg/dL.

What would you do next?

A. Continue his current therapy of rosuvastatin 20 mg daily and fenofibrate 145 mg daily
B. Add Niacin 1500 mg daily
C. Obtain an apoA-I lipoprotein level
D. Discontinue fenofibrate
E. Reduce rosuvastatin back to 5 mg daily

Answer: D

This patient has developed a paradoxical response to fenofibrate therapy that has resulted in drug-induced depression in HDL-C concentration. Several drugs can cause extremely low HDL-C (<20 mg/dL), including fibrates, thiazoladinediones, and anabolic steroids (7). Although rare, this idiosyncratic response is completely reversible with discontinuation of fenofibrate. In this case, 2 months after discontinuation of fenofibrate therapy, the HDL-C level improved to 28 mg/dL and has since remained at baseline of 28 to 36 mg/dL with statin monotherapy. Although niacin therapy can increase HDL-C, two prior clinical trials failed to show benefit in ASCVD outcomes when niacin was added to statin therapy (9). Primary apoA-I deficiency can cause very low HDL, but it would not lead to an acquired low HDL-C clinical picture. However, an apoA-I level could be helpful in this setting to help exclude laboratory error in the HDL-C homogeneous (direct) assay method. Rosuvastatin therapy would not be expected to cause a large decrease in HDL-C. In the JUPITER trial, treatment with rosuvastatin increased HDL-C, HDL particle number, and size (17).

Case 2

A 57-year-old man with premature CAD, dyslipidemia, hypertension, and tobacco use presents for evaluation of dyslipidemia. He was diagnosed with CAD at age 48 years when he developed acute coronary syndrome and subsequently underwent three-vessel coronary artery bypass grafting. He has a history of dyslipidemia, with baseline triglyceride level of ~700 mg/dL. He has tried several statin preparations (atorvastatin, pravastatin, simvastatin, and rosuvastatin) but has had intolerable myalgia symptoms with each one. He has been receiving fenofibrate therapy for the last several years and is tolerating it well. He is currently smoking three-fourths of a pack per day. He has no history of diabetes mellitus. He has a strong family history of premature CAD; both his brother and father had onset of CAD before the age of 55 years.

Current medications: aspirin 81 mg daily, fenofibrate 134 mg daily, lisinopril 10 mg daily, and metoprolol-ER 25 mg daily. Physical examination shows blood pressure of 116/66 mm Hg and body mass index of 30.0 kg/m^2 (normal physical examination). His lipid levels with fenofibrate 134 mg daily are as follows: total cholesterol, 164 mg/dL; HDL, 24 mg/dL; triglycerides, 274 mg/dL; and LDL, 85 mg/dL. His thyrotropin, fasting glucose, creatinine, and liver enzymes are all within normal limits.

In addition to recommending appropriate lifestyle measures and smoking cessation, what therapy would you recommend?

A. Add evolocumab 140 mg every 2 weeks
B. Continue fibrate therapy for secondary ASCVD risk reduction
C. Switch fenofibrate to ezetimibe 10 mg daily
D. Switch fenofibrate to omega-3 fatty acids, two capsules daily

Answer: B

Given this patient's history of statin intolerance, fairly severe hypertriglyceridemia, and established CAD, it is reasonable to continue fibrate therapy, based on evidence from the VA-HIT study. Although proprotein convertase subtilisin kexin 9 (PCSK9) inhibitors have been shown to reduce major adverse cardiovascular events when added to statin therapy in high-risk patients, their effect on ASCVD outcomes as monotherapy in statin-intolerant patients is not yet known (18). PCSK9 inhibitors have shown good efficacy and safety in statin-intolerant patients, so it is a reasonable alternative in this case (19). However, the high cost of PCSK9 inhibitors can be a barrier to patient access in clinical practice. Although ezetimibe has been shown to provide additional benefit when added to statin therapy for ASCVD risk reduction, it does not improve hypertriglyceridemia, and its effect on ASCVD outcomes when combined with a fibrate is unknown. Although omega-3 fatty acid supplements can be used to treat severe hypertriglyceridemia, they have not shown any clear benefit in cardiovascular morbidity and mortality in contemporary meta-analyses (20).

Case 3

A 58-year-old white woman with hypertension and anxiety disorder presents to you for a cardiovascular risk assessment. She has no history of diabetes mellitus. She has a 70 pack-year smoking history but quit smoking 12 years ago. Her father had onset of CAD in his early 60s and underwent coronary artery bypass grafting. She recently decided to have a coronary artery calcium screening ~3 months ago after attending a local health fair. Her coronary artery calcium score at that time was elevated at 519 Agatston units, with the majority of this in the left anterior descending coronary artery distribution (495) and a small amount in the left circumflex (24). Her score was in the 99th percentile for age and sex.

Her lipid profile shows: total cholesterol, 161 mg/dL; triglycerides, 59 mg/dL; HDL, 73 mg/dL; and LDL, 76 mg/dL. Current medications: lisinopril 10 mg daily and alprazolam 1 mg daily as needed for anxiety. Her calculated 10-year ASCVD risk based on pooled cohort equations is 2.4%.

What would you recommend?

A. No medication therapy, given her high HDL-C, which acts as a negative risk factor
B. Dietary supplementation with coconut oil to further improve HDL-C levels
C. Consideration of moderate-intensity statin therapy for ASCVD risk reduction
D. Obtain measurement of carotid intima-media thickness to further stratify her cardiovascular risk

Answer: C

This case highlights one of the limitations of HDL-C concentration in assessing HDL function and in global cardiovascular risk. Although her calculated ASCVD risk based upon pooled cohort equations is only 2.4%, her coronary artery calcium score demonstrates a significant burden of CAD, which indicates a higher level of risk than would be predicted based on traditional risk factors alone. The American Heart Association/American College of Cardiology 2013 Cholesterol Treatment Guidelines include the option of considering one or more additional risk factors (*e.g.*, LDL-C ≥ 160 mg/dL, family history of premature ASCVD, high-sensitivity C-reactive protein ≥ 2.0 mg/L, coronary artery calcium score ≥ 300 Agatston units, ankle-brachial index < 0.9, or lifetime ASCVD risk) in primary prevention cases where the initial risk-based decision is unclear (21). This patient's coronary artery calcium score information can be incorporated into her conventional risk factors using the Multi-Ethnic Study of Atherosclerosis (MESA) Risk Score Calculator (available at: https://www.mesa-nhlbi.org/CACReference.aspx). Using this tool, this patient's calculated 10-year risk is 6.1%, which is at a risk threshold where moderate-intensity statin therapy should be considered. Thus, not considering statin therapy for primary prevention would not be appropriate. Carotid intima-media thickness is not recommended in routine clinical practice for risk assessment for a first ASCVD event. Although coconut oil (which contains a high proportion of saturated fat, composed mainly of medium-chain triglycerides) consumption can lead to increases in HDL-C, there is no established cardiovascular benefit from coconut oil supplementation.

REFERENCES

1. Toth PP, Barter PJ, Rosenson RS, Boden WE, Chapman MJ, Cuchel M, D'Agostino RB, Sr, Davidson MH, Davidson WS, Heinecke JW, Karas RH, Kontush A, Krauss RM, Miller M, Rader DJ. High-density lipoproteins: a consensus statement from the National Lipid Association. *J Clin Lipidol.* 2013;**7**(5):484–525.
2. Toth PP, Davidson MH. High-density lipoproteins: marker of cardiovascular risk and therapeutic target. *J Clin Lipidol.* 2010;**4**(5): 359–364.
3. Rader DJ, Hovingh GK. HDL and cardiovascular disease. *Lancet.* 2014;**384**(9943):618–625.
4. Rosenson RS, Brewer HB Jr, Ansell BJ, Barter P, Chapman MJ, Heinecke JW, Kontush A, Tall AR, Webb NR. Dysfunctional HDL and atherosclerotic cardiovascular disease. *Nat Rev Cardiol.* 2016;**13**(1):48–60.
5. Miida T, Nishimura K, Okamura T, Hirayama S, Ohmura H, Yoshida H, Miyashita Y, Ai M, Tanaka A, Sumino H, Murakami M, Inoue I, Kayamori Y, Nakamura M, Nobori T, Miyazawa Y, Teramoto T, Yokoyama S. Validation of homogeneous assays for HDL-cholesterol using fresh samples from healthy and diseased subjects. *Atherosclerosis.* 2014;**233**(1):253–259.
6. Voight BF, Peloso GM, Orho-Melander M, Frikke-Schmidt R, Barbalic M, Jensen MK, Hindy G, Hólm H, Ding EL, Johnson T, Schunkert H, Samani NJ, Clarke R, Hopewell JC, Thompson JF, Li M, Thorleifsson G, Newton-Cheh C, Musunuru K, Pirruccello JP, Saleheen D, Chen L, Stewart A, Schillert A, Thorsteinsdottir U, Thorgeirsson G, Anand S, Engert JC, Morgan T, Spertus J, Stoll M, Berger K, Martinelli N, Girelli D, McKeown PP, Patterson CC, Epstein SE, Devaney J, Burnett MS, Mooser V, Ripatti S, Surakka I, Nieminen MS, Sinisalo J, Lokki ML, Perola M, Havulinna A, de Faire U, Gigante B, Ingelsson E, Zeller T, Wild P, de Bakker PI, Klungel OH, Maitland-van der Zee AH, Peters BJ, de Boer A, Grobbee DE, Kamphuisen PW, Deneer VH, Elbers CC, Onland-Moret NC, Hofker MH, Wijmenga C, Verschuren WM, Boer JM, van der Schouw YT, Rasheed A, Frossard P, Demissie S, Willer C, Do R, Ordovas JM, Abecasis GR, Boehnke M, Mohlke KL, Daly MJ, Guiducci C, Burtt NP, Surti A, Gonzalez E, Purcell S, Gabriel S, Marrugat J, Peden J, Erdmann J, Diemert P, Willenborg C, König IR, Fischer M, Hengstenberg C, Ziegler A, Buysschaert I, Lambrechts D, Van de Werf F, Fox KA, El Mokhtari NE, Rubin D, Schrezenmeir J, Schreiber S, Schäfer A, Danesh J, Blankenberg S, Roberts R, McPherson R, Watkins H, Hall AS, Overvad K, Rimm E, Boerwinkle E, Tybjaerg-Hansen A, Cupples LA, Reilly MP, Melander O, Mannucci PM, Ardissino D, Siscovick D, Elosua R, Stefansson K, O'Donnell CJ, Salomaa V, Rader DJ, Peltonen L, Schwartz SM, Altshuler D, Kathiresan S. Plasma HDL cholesterol and risk of myocardial infarction: a mendelian randomisation study. *Lancet.* 2012;**380**(9841):572–580.
7. Rader DJ, deGoma EM. Approach to the patient with extremely low HDL-cholesterol. *J Clin Endocrinol Metab.* 2012;**97**(10):3399–3407.
8. Bloomfield Rubins H, Davenport J, Babikian V, Brass LM, Collins D, Wexler L, Wagner S, Papademetriou V, Rutan G, Robins SJ; VA-HIT Study Group. Reduction in stroke with gemfibrozil in men with coronary heart disease and low HDL cholesterol: the Veterans Affairs HDL Intervention Trial (VA-HIT). *Circulation.* 2001;**103**(23): 2828–2833.
9. Toth PP, Murthy AM, Sidhu MS, Boden WE. Is HPS2-THRIVE the death knell for niacin? *J Clin Lipidol.* 2015;**9**(3):343–350.
10. Barter PJ, Caulfield M, Eriksson M, Grundy SM, Kastelein JJ, Komajda M, Lopez-Sendon J, Mosca L, Tardif JC, Waters DD, Shear CL, Revkin JH, Buhr KA, Fisher MR, Tall AR, Brewer B; ILLUMINATE Investigators. Effects of torcetrapib in patients at high risk for coronary events. *N Engl J Med.* 2007;**357**(21):2109–2122.
11. Schwartz GG, Olsson AG, Abt M, Ballantyne CM, Barter PJ, Brumm J, Chaitman BR, Holme IM, Kallend D, Leiter LA, Leitersdorf E, McMurray JJ, Mundl H, Nicholls SJ, Shah PK, Tardif JC, Wright RS; dal-OUTCOMES Investigators. Effects of dalcetrapib in patients with a recent acute coronary syndrome. *N Engl J Med.* 2012;**367**(22): 2089–2099.
12. Bowman L, Hopewell JC, Chen F, Wallendszus K, Stevens W, Collins R, Wiviott SD, Cannon CP, Braunwald E, Sammons E, Landray MJ; HPS3/TIMI55–REVEAL Collaborative Group. Effects of anacetrapib in patients with atherosclerotic vascular disease. *N Engl J Med.* 2017; **377**(13):1217–1227.
13. Lincoff AM, Nicholls SJ, Riesmeyer JS, Barter PJ, Brewer HB, Fox KAA, Gibson CM, Granger C, Menon V, Montalescot G, Rader D, Tall AR, McErlean E, Wolski K, Ruotolo G, Vangerow B, Weerakkody G, Goodman SG, Conde D, McGuire DK, Nicolau JC, Leiva-Pons JL, Pesant Y, Li W, Kandath D, Kouz S, Tahirkheli N, Mason D, Nissen SE; ACCELERATE Investigators. Evacetrapib and cardiovascular outcomes in high-risk vascular disease. *N Engl J Med.* 2017;**376**(20):1933–1942.
14. Rohatgi A, Khera A, Berry JD, Givens EG, Ayers CR, Wedin KE, Neeland IJ, Yuhanna IS, Rader DR, de Lemos JA, Shaul PW. HDL cholesterol efflux capacity and incident cardiovascular events. *N Engl J Med.* 2014;**371**(25):2383–2393.
15. Aron-Wisnewsky J, Julia Z, Poitou C, Bouillot JL, Basdevant A, Chapman MJ, Clement K, Guerin M. Effect of bariatric surgery-induced weight loss on SR-BI-, ABCG1-, and ABCA1-mediated cellular cholesterol efflux in obese women. *J Clin Endocrinol Metab.* 2011; **96**(4):1151–1159.
16. Hernáez Á, Castañer O, Elosua R, Pintó X, Estruch R, Salas-Salvadó J, Corella D, Arós F, Serra-Majem L, Fiol M, Ortega-Calvo M, Ros E, Martínez-González MÁ, de la Torre R, López-Sabater MC, Fitó M. Mediterranean diet improves high-density lipoprotein function in high-cardiovascular-risk individuals: a randomized controlled trial. *Circulation.* 2017;**135**(7):633–643.
17. Mora S, Glynn RJ, Ridker PM. High-density lipoprotein cholesterol, size, particle number, and residual vascular risk after potent statin therapy. *Circulation.* 2013;**128**(11):1189–1197.
18. Sabatine MS, Giugliano RP, Keech AC, Honarpour N, Wiviott SD, Murphy SA, Kuder JF, Wang H, Liu T, Wasserman SM, Sever PS, Pedersen TR; FOURIER Steering Committee and Investigators. Evolocumab and clinical outcomes in patients with cardiovascular disease. *N Engl J Med.* 2017;**376**(18):1713–1722.
19. Stroes E, Guyton JR, Lepor N, Civeira F, Gaudet D, Watts GF, Baccara-Dinet MT, Lecorps G, Manvelian G, Farnier M; ODYSSEY CHOICE II Investigators. Efficacy and safety of alirocumab 150 mg every 4 weeks in patients with hypercholesterolemia not on statin therapy: the ODYSSEY CHOICE II study. *J Am Heart Assoc.* 2016;**5**(9):e003421.
20. Jellinger PS, Handelsman Y, Rosenblit PD, Bloomgarden ZT, Fonseca VA, Garber AJ, Grunberger G, Guerin CK, Bell DSH, Mechanick JI, Pessah-Pollack R, Wyne K, Smith D, Brinton EA, Fazio S, Davidson M; American

Association of Clinical Endocrinologists and American College of Endocrinology Guidelines for Management of Dyslipidemia and Prevention of Cardiovascular Disease. American Association of Clinical Endocrinologists and College of Endocrinology guidelines for management of dyslipidemia and prevention of cardiovascular disease. *Endocr Pract.* 2017;**23**(suppl 2):1–87.

21. Stone NJ, Robinson JG, Lichtenstein AH, Bairey Merz CN, Blum CB, Eckel RH, Goldberg AC, Gordon D, Levy D, Lloyd-Jones DM, McBride P, Schwartz JS, Shero ST, Smith SC, Jr, Watson K, Wilson PW, Eddleman KM, Jarrett NM, LaBresh K, Nevo L, Wnek J, Anderson JL, Halperin JL, Albert NM, Bozkurt B, Brindis RG, Curtis LH, DeMets D, Hochman JS, Kovacs RJ, Ohman EM, Pressler SJ, Sellke FW, Shen WK, Smith SC Jr, Tomaselli GF; American College of Cardiology/American Heart Association Task Force on Practice Guidelines. 2013 ACC/AHA guideline on the treatment of blood cholesterol to reduce atherosclerotic cardiovascular risk in adults: a report of the American College of Cardiology/American Heart Association Task Force on Practice Guidelines [published correction appears in *Circulation.* 2015;132(25):e396]. *Circulation.* 2014;**129**(25 suppl 2):S1–S45.

Recently Arrived and Pipeline Drugs for Dyslipidemia

M22
Presented, March 17–20, 2018

Anne Carol Goldberg, MD. Division of Endocrinology, Metabolism, and Lipid Research, Department of Medicine, Washington University School of Medicine, St. Louis, Missouri 63110, E-mail: agoldber@wustl.edu

SIGNIFICANCE OF THE CLINICAL PROBLEM

Several genetic conditions lead to severe dyslipidemia, including familial hypercholesterolemia (FH) and genetic causes of severely elevated triglyceride levels. Statins are first-line therapy for hyperlipidemia and cardiovascular risk reduction. Statins lower low-density lipoprotein (LDL) cholesterol (LDL-C) substantially and decrease rates of fatal and nonfatal coronary heart disease and stroke (1). Evidence suggests that the lower the LDL-C, the better (2). However, some patients have higher-than-desirable LDL levels with maximally tolerated statin therapy, notably patients with FH who are underdiagnosed and undertreated (3). They may not achieve adequate LDL-C reduction, even with the combination of a high-dose statin and a second medication. The approval of a new class of LDL-lowering therapeutics—the proprotein convertase subtilisin/kexin type 9 (PCSK9) inhibitors—makes it possible to obtain substantial LDL-C reductions (4).

Severe hypertriglyceridemia can be due to rare monogenic conditions or to polygenic hyperlipidemias complicated by secondary factors (5–7). Treatment involves diet, weight loss, medication, and the treatment of underlying conditions such as diabetes. However, some patients remain very difficult to treat, including patients with lipoprotein lipase (LPL) deficiency and those with other genetic causes of chylomicronemia and severe hypertriglyceridemia. Patients with chylomicronemia are at risk for developing pancreatitis, which can be a recurrent problem for them and life-threatening.

BARRIERS TO OPTIMAL PRACTICE

- Statins are effective but may not provide adequate LDL reduction in some patients, especially patients with FH.
- The high cost of PCSK9 monoclonal antibodies (mAbs) limits their use.
- Severe hypertriglyceridemia can cause pancreatitis and can be difficult to treat.
- Genetic chylomicronemia syndromes may not respond to lipid-lowering therapies.

LEARNING OBJECTIVES

At the end of this session, attendees will be able to:

- Identify the types of patients who may be candidates for new therapies for severe hypercholesterolemia and hypertriglyceridemia
- Describe the mechanism of action of new therapies to lower LDL-C and triglycerides
- Describe the effects and side effects of new therapies for dyslipidemia

STRATEGIES FOR DIAGNOSIS, THERAPY, AND MANAGEMENT

Hypercholesterolemia

Statins lower LDL-C by 20% to 60%, depending on the statin, dose, and ability of the individual to upregulate LDL receptor function. This therapy is adequate in many patients, but there are patients who need more LDL reduction.

FH is an inherited disorder that causes high LDL levels beginning at birth (3). Left untreated, FH leads to a greatly increased risk of cardiovascular disease in both men and women. The prevalence of heterozygous FH is about 1 in 200 people (8, 9). It is caused by mutations in genes for the LDL receptor or apolipoprotein B (ApoB), or by gain-of-function mutations of PCSK9. LDL-C levels are 160 to 500 mg/dL (4.1 to 13 mmol/L) in heterozygous patients (3).

Diagnosis of FH is made on the basis of LDL-C levels, family history of hyperlipidemia and premature cardiovascular disease, and, if present, physical findings of premature full arcus corneae (before age 40 years) and tendon xanthomas (10). Genetic testing can be done for mutations in the LDL receptor gene, parts of ApoB, and certain PCSK9 gain-of-function mutations. However, not all patients with clinically diagnosed FH have a mutation found on genetic testing.

Treatment of FH involves diet, statins, ezetimibe, bile acid sequestrants, and LDL apheresis. Early diagnosis and treatment decrease the risk of atherosclerotic cardiovascular disease (11).

Mechanism of Action of PCSK9 Inhibitors

The LDL receptor binds to a site on ApoB, the main apolipoprotein on LDL particles. The LDL receptor–LDL complex is internalized by endocytosis in clathrin-coated pits, forming endosomes. A pH change in the endosomes to an acidic environment causes the complex to dissociate, and the LDL particle is then degraded within lysosomes, whereas LDL receptors are recycled to the cell surface. Decreased intracellular cholesterol concentration promotes the upregulation of 3-hydroxy-3-methylglutaryl coenzyme A reductase, causing increased cholesterol synthesis. There is also increased LDL receptor production, which increases LDL uptake. PCSK9 is a secreted protein that limits this process. PCKS9 binds to the LDL receptor, which remains complexed with LDL, and is then degraded (4). Loss-of-function and gain-of-function mutations in the PCSK9 gene can occur. Mutations leading to loss of function are associated with lifelong low LDL-C levels and decreased risk of cardiovascular disease. Gain-of-function mutations lead to increased LDL-C levels and the FH phenotype.

PCSK9 mAbs

mAbs can bind to PCSK9 and prevent it from binding to the LDL receptor, leading to improved LDL receptor function and increased uptake of LDL (4) Two mAbs for PCKS9 have been approved: alirocumab and evolocumab. These agents are given subcutaneously (sc) every 2 to 4 weeks.

In patients with heterozygous FH, LDL-C is reduced by 40% to 70% on top of background therapies. The effect in homozygous FH patients depends on the presence of some LDL receptor function. Receptor-defective patients can have LDL-C reduction of about 23%, whereas PCSK9 mAbs show no effect in receptor-negative patients (12, 13). LDL-C reductions with alirocumab and evolocumab have been shown to persist for over 48 to 78 weeks. Long-term studies showed a trend toward the reduction of cardiovascular events (14, 15). The FOURIER trial demonstrated significant decreases in major cardiovascular events with the addition of evolocumab to standard-of-care treatment in patients with vascular disease (16).

There have not been major issues with side effects. The main side effects are injection site reactions that are generally mild. Very low levels of LDL-C (<25 mg/dL) have not shown greater rates of adverse effects than the generally reported ones in clinical trials.

Alirocumab (75 mg sc or 150 mg sc every 2 weeks or 300 mg sc every 4 weeks) and evolocumab (140 mg sc every 2 weeks or 420 mg sc every 4 weeks) are approved for patients with heterozygous FH or with cardiovascular disease who do not have adequate LDL-C reduction with diet and maximally tolerated lipid-lowering medications. Evolocumab is also approved for homozygous FH (420 mg sc every 4 weeks) and to reduce the risk of myocardial infarction, stroke, and coronary revascularization in adults with established cardiovascular disease. The medications are costly and are not a replacement for statin therapy.

Hypertriglyceridemia

Severe hypertriglyceridemia is multifactorial (5–7). Monogenic causes include LPL deficiency, ApoC2 deficiency, and mutations of ApoA5, GPIHBP1 (glycosylphosphatidylinositol-anchored high-density lipoprotein–binding protein 1), LMF1 (lipase maturation factor 1), and others (7). The lack of functioning LPL causes elevations of chylomicrons, which can manifest as pancreatitis, hepatic and splenic enlargement, lipemia retinalis, eruptive xanthomas, paresthesias, confusion, and dyspnea. The monogenic single-mutation causes are rare. More common are polygenic causes that may interact with secondary factors to produce severe hypertriglyceridemia. The genetic causes of poor LPL function do not respond well or at all to lipid-lowering medications such as statins and fibrates. They require severe dietary restrictions.

One of the new approaches to the treatment of severe hypertriglyceridemia involves decreasing levels of ApoC3. ApoC3 is a 79-amino acid glycoprotein synthesized principally in the liver and enterocytes. It is a component of triglyceride-rich lipoproteins and a potent inhibitor of LPL. Increased ApoC3 adversely affects ApoE-mediated hepatic uptake of triglyceride-rich remnants. This causes an accumulation of very-low-density lipoprotein triglycerides and chylomicrons in plasma and the development of hypertriglyceridemia (17). Carriers of loss-of-function mutations that disrupt ApoC3 functions have a favorable lipid profile and a reduced risk of coronary artery disease (18). Antisense oligonucleotides can be produced that hybridize messenger RNA to reduce the production of a protein. Volanesorsen, an antisense oligonucleotide targeting ApoC3, has been developed for the treatment of severe hypertriglyceridemia. A randomized placebo-controlled phase 2 trial evaluating volanesorsen showed a 31.3% to 70.9% reduction in triglyceride levels among patients with a broad range of baseline triglycerides (19).

Volanesorsen lowers ApoC3 and triglyceride levels in patients with LPL deficiency (20). It can decrease the frequency of attacks of pancreatitis.

Further clinical trials have shown similar efficacy. Side effects have included injection site reactions and thrombocytopenia.

MAIN CONCLUSIONS

New therapies have the potential for treating severe hypercholesterolemia and hypertriglyceridemia. PCSK9 mAbs reduce LDL-C substantially. They are particularly useful in patients with FH. Two PCSK9 inhibitors, evolocumab and alirocumab, have been approved in the United States. Positive cardiovascular outcomes trial data are available for evolocumab. Volanesorsen, an antisense oligonucleotide directed against ApoC3, has been effective in reducing triglyceride levels in patients with severe hypertriglyceridemia. It has not yet been approved or marketed.

CASES

Case 1

A 50-year-old man has had known high cholesterol for many years. Treatment was started at about age 29 years, at which time his baseline LDL-C was 448 mg/dL (11.6 mmol/L). At age 31 years, he developed angina symptoms and was found to have diffuse coronary artery disease. He had coronary artery bypass surgery with six grafts. He has been maintained on high-dose statin and ezetimibe and has not had recurrence of symptoms. His father died at age 53 years of a myocardial infarction. His brother has hyperlipidemia and had bypass surgery at age 36 years. His sister also has elevated cholesterol.

On examination, his blood pressure is normal. His body mass index is 23. He has bilateral Achilles tendon xanthomas. On atorvastatin 80 mg daily and ezetimibe 10 mg daily, his fasting lipid levels are the following: cholesterol 210 mg/dL (5.4 mmol/L), triglycerides 52 mg/dL (0.59 mmol/L), high-density lipoprotein cholesterol (HDL-C) 43 mg/dL (1.1 mmol/L), and LDL-C 195 mg/dL (5.05 mmol/L).

Which of the following is the most reasonable approach to maximally lower his LDL-C?

A. Change atorvastatin 80 mg to rosuvastatin 40 mg daily
B. Add fenofibrate 145 mg daily
C. Add niacin 2000 mg daily
D. Add evolocumab 140 mg every 2 weeks

Answer D. The patient has an elevated LDL-C on maximal-dose statin and ezetimibe and has coronary artery disease. Changing from maximum-dose atorvastatin to maximum-dose rosuvastatin might produce a small further lowering of LDL-C but would not lower it to under 100 mg/dL (2.6 mmol/L). Fenofibrate would likely provide some additional LDL-C lowering, but only about a 10% to 20% further reduction. Niacin would lower LDL-C by about 10% to 20% but has serious potential toxicity. A PCSK9 mAb, either evolocumab or alirocumab, can lower LDL-C by an additional 40% to 70% when added to combination therapy.

In this case, with the addition of evolocumab 140 mg every 2 weeks, lipid levels were the following: cholesterol 152 mg/dL (3.9 mmol/L), triglycerides 85 mg/dL (0.96 mmol/L), HDL-C 55 mg/dL (1.4 mmol/L), and LDL-C 83 mg/dL (2.1 mmol/L).

Case 2

A 20-year-old man has a history of hyperlipidemia known since early childhood. He was diagnosed with LPL deficiency at age 2 years. He has had three episodes of pancreatitis, at ages 17, 18, and 19 years. Neither parent has hyperlipidemia. His older brother and sister both have been diagnosed with LPL deficiency, and both had at least one episode of pancreatitis.

He has a normal physical examination. His body mass index is 21. Fasting lipids are the following: triglycerides 3487 mg/dL (39.3 mmol/L), cholesterol 318 mg/dL (8.2 mmol/L), and HDL-C 22 mg/dL (0.57 mmol/L).

What is the currently available best therapy for him?

A. Fenofibrate 145 mg daily
B. Restriction of fat intake to 10% of daily calories
C. Prescription omega-3 fatty acids 4 g daily
D. Atorvastatin 80 mg daily

Answer B. Fenofibrate and omega-3 fatty acids are not effective in LPL deficiency. Fenofibrate works by increasing LPL activity, which may not be effective in this patient. LDL levels are not elevated in LPL deficiency, and statins are not effective in reducing chylomicron levels. A very low fat diet is needed in LPL deficiency to decrease the production of chylomicrons because they cannot be cleared when LPL does not function.

REFERENCES

1. Baigent C, Blackwell L, Emberson J, Holland LE, Reith C, Bhala N, Peto R, Barnes EH, Keech A, Simes J, Collins R; Cholesterol Treatment Trialists' (CTT) Collaboration. Efficacy and safety of more intensive lowering of LDL cholesterol: a meta-analysis of data from 170,000 participants in 26 randomised trials. *Lancet.* 2010;**376**(9753): 1670–1681.
2. Boekholdt SM, Hovingh GK, Mora S, Arsenault BJ, Amarenco P, Pedersen TR, LaRosa JC, Waters DD, DeMicco DA, Simes RJ, Keech AC, Colquhoun D, Hitman GA, Betteridge DJ, Clearfield MB, Downs JR, Colhoun HM, Gotto AM Jr, Ridker PM, Grundy SM, Kastelein JJ. Very low levels of atherogenic lipoproteins and the risk for cardiovascular events: a meta-analysis of statin trials. *J Am Coll Cardiol.* 2014;**64**(5): 485–494.
3. Nordestgaard BG, Chapman MJ, Humphries SE, Ginsberg HN, Masana L, Descamps OS, Wiklund O, Hegele RA, Raal FJ, Defesche JC, Wiegman A, Santos RD, Watts GF, Parhofer KG, Hovingh GK, Kovanen PT, Boileau C, Averna M, Borén J, Bruckert E, Catapano AL, Kuivenhoven JA, Pajukanta P, Ray K, Stalenhoef AF, Stroes E, Taskinen MR, Tybjærg-Hansen A; European Atherosclerosis Society Consensus Panel. Familial hypercholesterolaemia is underdiagnosed and undertreated in the general population: guidance for clinicians to prevent coronary heart disease: consensus statement of the European Atherosclerosis Society. *Eur Heart J.* 2013;**34**(45):3478–3490.
4. McKenney JM. Understanding PCSK9 and anti-PCSK9 therapies. *J Clin Lipidol.* 2015;**9**(2):170–186.
5. Miller M, Stone NJ, Ballantyne C, Bittner V, Criqui MH, Ginsberg HN, Goldberg AC, Howard WJ, Jacobson MS, Kris-Etherton PM, Lennie TA, Levi M, Mazzone T, Pennathur S; American Heart Association Clinical Lipidology, Thrombosis, and Prevention Committee of the Council on Nutrition, Physical Activity, and Metabolism; Council on Arteriosclerosis, Thrombosis and Vascular Biology; Council on Cardiovascular Nursing; Council on the Kidney in Cardiovascular Disease. Triglycerides and cardiovascular disease: a scientific statement from the American Heart Association. *Circulation.* 2011;**123**(20):2292–2333.
6. Berglund L, Brunzell JD, Goldberg AC, Goldberg IJ, Sacks F, Murad MH, Stalenhoef AF; Endocrine Society. Evaluation and treatment of hypertriglyceridemia: an Endocrine Society clinical practice guideline. *J Clin Endocrinol Metab.* 2012;**97**(9):2969–2989.
7. Hegele RA, Ginsberg HN, Chapman MJ, Nordestgaard BG, Kuivenhoven JA, Averna M, Borén J, Bruckert E, Catapano AL, Descamps OS, Hovingh GK, Humphries SE, Kovanen PT, Masana L, Pajukanta P, Parhofer KG, Raal FJ, Ray KK, Santos RD, Stalenhoef AF, Stroes E, Taskinen MR, Tybjærg-Hansen A, Watts GF, Wiklund O; European Atherosclerosis Society Consensus Panel. The polygenic nature of hypertriglyceridaemia: implications for definition, diagnosis, and management. *Lancet Diabetes Endocrinol.* 2014;**2**(8):655–666.
8. Benn M, Watts GF, Tybjaerg-Hansen A, Nordestgaard BG. Familial hypercholesterolemia in the Danish general population: prevalence, coronary artery disease, and cholesterol-lowering medication. *J Clin Endocrinol Metab.* 2012;**97**(11):3956–3964.
9. de Ferranti SD, Rodday AM, Mendelson MM, Wong JB, Leslie LK, Sheldrick RC. Prevalence of familial hypercholesterolemia in the 1999 to 2012 United States National Health and Nutrition Examination Surveys (NHANES). *Circulation.* 2016;**133**(11):1067–1072.
10. Goldberg AC, Hopkins PN, Toth PP, Ballantyne CM, Rader DJ, Robinson JG, Daniels SR, Gidding SS, de Ferranti SD, Ito MK, McGowan MP, Moriarty PM, Cromwell WC, Ross JL, Ziajka PE. Familial hypercholesterolemia: screening, diagnosis and management of pediatric and adult patients: clinical guidance from the National Lipid Association Expert Panel on Familial Hypercholesterolemia. *J Clin Lipidol.* 2011;**5**(3):133–140.
11. Gidding SS, Champagne MA, de Ferranti SD, Defesche J, Ito MK, Knowles JW, McCrindle B, Raal F, Rader D, Santos RD, Lopes-Virella M, Watts GF, Wierzbicki AS; American Heart Association Atherosclerosis, Hypertension, and Obesity in the Young Committee of the Council on Cardiovascular Disease in the Young; Council on Cardiovascular and Stroke Nursing; Council on Functional Genomics and Translational Biology; Council on Lifestyle and Cardiometabolic Health. The agenda

for familial hypercholesterolemia: a scientific statement from the American Heart Association. *Circulation.* 2015;**132**(22):2167–2192.

12. Raal FJ, Stein EA, Dufour R, Turner T, Civeira F, Burgess L, Langslet G, Scott R, Olsson AG, Sullivan D, Hovingh GK, Cariou B, Gouni-Berthold I, Somaratne R, Bridges I, Scott R, Wasserman SM, Gaudet D; RUTHERFORD-2 Investigators. PCSK9 inhibition with evolocumab (AMG 145) in heterozygous familial hypercholesterolaemia (RUTHERFORD-2): a randomised, double-blind, placebo-controlled trial. *Lancet.* 2015;**385**(9965):331–340.
13. Stein EA, Honarpour N, Wasserman SM, Xu F, Scott R, Raal FJ. Effect of the proprotein convertase subtilisin/kexin 9 monoclonal antibody, AMG 145, in homozygous familial hypercholesterolemia. *Circulation.* 2013;**128**(19): 2113–2120.
14. Robinson JG, Farnier M, Krempf M, Bergeron J, Luc G, Averna M, Stroes ES, Langslet G, Raal FJ, El Shahawy M, Koren MJ, Lepor NE, Lorenzato C, Pordy R, Chaudhari U, Kastelein JJ; ODYSSEY LONG TERM Investigators. Efficacy and safety of alirocumab in reducing lipids and cardiovascular events. *N Engl J Med.* 2015;**372**(16): 1489–1499.
15. Sabatine MS, Giugliano RP, Wiviott SD, Raal FJ, Blom DJ, Robinson J, Ballantyne CM, Somaratne R, Legg J, Wasserman SM, Scott R, Koren MJ, Stein EA; Open-Label Study of Long-Term Evaluation against LDL Cholesterol (OSLER) Investigators. Efficacy and safety of evolocumab in reducing lipids and cardiovascular events. *N Engl J Med.* 2015; **372**(16):1500–1509.
16. Sabatine MS, Giugliano RP, Keech AC, Honarpour N, Wiviott SD, Murphy SA, Kuder JF, Wang H, Liu T, Wasserman SM, Sever PS, Pedersen TR; FOURIER Steering Committee and Investigators. Evolocumab and clinical outcomes in patients with cardiovascular disease. *N Engl J Med.* 2017;**376**(18):1713–1722.
17. Taskinen MR, Borén J. Why is apolipoprotein CIII emerging as a novel therapeutic target to reduce the burden of cardiovascular disease? *Curr Atheroscler Rep.* 2016;**18**(10):59.
18. Jørgensen AB, Frikke-Schmidt R, Nordestgaard BG, Tybjærg-Hansen A. Loss-of-function mutations in APOC3 and risk of ischemic vascular disease. *N Engl J Med.* 2014;**371**(1):32–41.
19. Gaudet D, Alexander VJ, Baker BF, Brisson D, Tremblay K, Singleton W, Geary RS, Hughes SG, Viney NJ, Graham MJ, Crooke RM, Witztum JL, Brunzell JD, Kastelein JJ. Antisense inhibition of apolipoprotein C-III in patients with hypertriglyceridemia. *N Engl J Med.* 2015;**373**(5):438–447.
20. Gaudet D, Brisson D, Tremblay K, Alexander VJ, Singleton W, Hughes SG, Geary RS, Baker BF, Graham MJ, Crooke RM, Witztum JL. Targeting APOC3 in the familial chylomicronemia syndrome. *N Engl J Med.* 2014;**371**(23):2200–2206.

Statin Intolerance

M44
Presented, March 17–20, 2018

Lisa Tannock, MD. University of Kentucky, Lexington VA Medical Center, Lexington, Kentucky 40536, E-mail: lisa.tannock@uky.edu

SIGNIFICANCE OF THE CLINICAL PROBLEM

Patients in the "real world" report statin intolerance to a much greater extent than in the published literature. However, there is robust evidence demonstrating the efficacy of statins in reducing cardiovascular risk. Alternatives to statins are either less effective, have similar side effects, or are extremely expensive, so providers and patients are often faced with challenges managing cardiac risk in patients who report statin intolerance. In this session, we will review the major side effects of statins and safety profiles/risks and discuss approaches to manage patients reporting statin intolerance.

BARRIERS TO OPTIMAL PRACTICE

- Prevalence of statin-associated muscle symptoms (SAMS) is much higher in routine clinical practice than in trials
- Management of SAMS is challenging, but there is robust evidence that statins reduce cardiovascular disease (CVD) events

LEARNING OBJECTIVES

As a result of participating in this session, learners should be able to:

- Discuss adverse effects of statins with both patients and other providers
- Understand the "nocebo" effect
- Develop approaches to managing hyperlipidemia in patients reporting statin intolerance

STRATEGIES FOR DIAGNOSIS, THERAPY, AND/OR MANAGEMENT

The 2013 American College of Cardiology/American Heart Association guidelines identify four groups for consideration of statin therapy:

1. Those with known atherosclerotic CVD
2. Those aged 21 to 75 years with low-density lipoprotein (LDL) ≥190
3. Those aged 40 to 75 years with diabetes
4. Those aged 40 to 75 years with 10-year atherosclerotic CVD risk ≥7.5%

This guideline thus recommends statin use for a large population group. Numerous reports and studies have demonstrated the general safety of this class of medications. However, user reports and the lay literature report the prevalence of statin intolerance, mainly muscle symptoms, to a much greater extent than reported in randomized controlled clinical trials (RCTs). Providers are encouraged to screen patients for CVD risk and indications for statin therapy and prescribe statins to reduce this risk. However, many patients and providers continue to have concern about the tolerability of the statins and struggle to find alternate approaches to reduce CVD risk.

Known Adverse Events With Statins

Serious muscle injury, including rhabdomyolysis, remains one of the most feared adverse events with statin use, yet the occurrence is low, <0.1%. Additional concerns include hepatotoxicity, risk of statin-induced newly diagnosed diabetes, and hemorrhagic stroke.

Rhabdomyolysis and Statin-Induced Myopathy

The terminology used to describe statin adverse events varies; the Food and Drug Administration (FDA)–accepted definition for myopathy is "unexplained muscle pain or weakness accompanied by creatine kinase (CK) elevations >10 times the upper limit of normal (ULN)". Rhabdomyolysis is a severe form of statin myopathy that typically has CK >40 times ULN and often requires hospital admission due to myoglobinuria and risk for acute renal injury. The risk of myopathy attributable to statins is <0.1% relative to placebo in all large long-term RCTs for all currently available statins at approved doses. The risk is greatest in the first year of therapy and/or after a dose increase or addition of another medication that interacts. Overall, the risk of rhabdomyolysis is ~0.01% and can be prevented by immediate discontinuation of the statin. For any individual that has had rhabdomyolysis, statin therapy is generally avoided. Risk factors for rhabdomyolysis and myopathy include patient factors (older individuals, hypothyroidism, renal impairment, preexisting muscle disease, female sex, diabetes, and Chinese ethnicity) and drug factors (polypharmacy with interacting drugs [particularly those metabolized by CYP3A4], statin dose, lipophilicity, bioavailability, and protein binding).

SAMS

However, more common than rhabdomyolysis is SAMS, in which muscle symptoms occur but there is no elevation of CK, or only minor elevations (<5 to 10 times ULN). The prevalence of SAMS is thought to be up to 10% of statin users outside of clinical trials but is not significantly different from placebo in RCTs (1–3). Moreover, numerous studies investigating SAMS have found that the majority of patients reporting muscle aches to statins also have muscle symptoms on placebo when the patient is blinded to drug. For example, Taylor *et al.* (1) evaluated patients with a history of statin intolerance to at least three different statins. The patients were then randomized to simvastatin or placebo in a blinded, crossover design, and only 36% of this group had muscle symptoms only to statin and not to placebo.

Hepatotoxicity

Early animal studies demonstrated hepatic injury with elevations in transaminases with statin therapy, raising concerns about hepatotoxicity. For years, statin prescribing information required measurements of transaminases. However, in 2012, the FDA issued a statement indicating that transaminase measurements are recommended only prior to initiation of therapy, or as clinically indicated. This statement reflects the robust evidence that clinically evident statin toxicity is very rare, and that monitoring transaminase levels has not been shown to prevent hepatotoxicity (2, 3). Although elevations in transaminases are commonly seen in subjects on statins, there is usually another explanation found, such as fatty liver disease or alcohol consumption. Furthermore, there is growing evidence that statins are safe and efficacious in patients with underlying liver disease due to nonalcoholic fatty liver disease or viral hepatitis.

Statin-Induced Diabetes

Although early statin RCTs reported possible protection from the development of diabetes, more recent RCTs have found a higher incidence of newly diagnosed diabetes in statin-treated subjects compared with those randomized to placebo. A meta-analysis reported in 2010 of >91,000 participants found that statin use was associated with a 9% proportional increase in the risk of being diagnosed with diabetes compared with placebo-treated subjects (4). The risk for newly diagnosed diabetes appears to be in patients with multiple preexisting risk factors for diabetes, suggesting that statin therapy leads to these individuals progressing to overt diabetes sooner than they might otherwise have. Importantly, there is no substantial effect of statin therapy on HbA_{1c} or glycemic control in those with existing diabetes. Given the strong evidence that statin therapy significantly reduces CVD risk in patients with and without diabetes, the general thought is that the benefits of statin therapy for CVD risk reduction outweigh any potential harm in onset of newly diagnosed diabetes.

Hemorrhagic Stroke

The ratio of ischemic stroke to hemorrhagic stroke in the US is ~87:13. Clinical trial evidence demonstrates a small absolute increased risk of hemorrhagic stroke in secondary stroke prevention but no increased risk in primary stroke prevention populations.

The Nocebo Effect

The lay literature contains numerous reports of SAMS, which tends to be widely believed. Some of the reports are personal, passionate, and widely shared on social media and other forums. Thus, one challenge providers face is patients with a predisposition to expect harm from statin therapy. The placebo effect (Latin: "I will please") can be summarized as the benefit derived from the belief that a therapy is active or beneficial (when it is not). Similarly, the nocebo effect (Latin: "I will harm") can be summarized as the harm derived from the belief that a therapy is harmful (when it is not). The challenge is that to the individual, these symptoms are real, and may be severe; they are not simply invented symptoms. However, as discussed above, several studies have found that patients who report SAMS to statin therapy cannot distinguish statin from placebo when blinded, and the majority report SAMS to placebo treatment. The power of the nocebo effect can be enhanced when the patient has a prior relationship with a provider who shares their belief that statins are harmful; often in this situation, the provider attempting to prescribe statin therapy cannot overcome a patient's reluctance and a statin may never even be started; thus, the patient may never allow him- or herself the chance to experience the potential benefits or harm of statin therapy.

Management of Patients With SAMS

Coenzyme Q10

The coenzyme Q10 (CoQ10) supplement has been a popular over-the-counter strategy for SAMS. However, in a RCT double-blind crossover study, there was no benefit found, and potential harm (slightly more patients reported muscle pain with CoQ10 than with placebo) (5). However, the use of CoQ10 does not have any impact on the lipid-lowering efficacy of statins, and thus likely does not attenuate the CVD benefit. This author's opinion is that if CoQ10 enables the placebo effect (belief of benefit) to outweigh the nocebo effect (belief of harm), then there is no reason to stop it; however, at present, there is no indication of true reduction in SAMS.

Alternate Statin

Rosuvastatin and pravastatin do not have substantial metabolism through the CYP3A4 pathway (pathway responsible for the metabolism of >50% of pharmacologics), whereas the other statins do. Thus, one strategy for patients experiencing SAMS is to try a different statin, perhaps one that is metabolized through a different hepatic pathway. In addition, the hydrophilicity, bioavailability, and elimination half-lives of different statins differ, and consideration of an alternate agent based on their pharmacokinetic profiles can be useful. It is not entirely clear if the use of an alternate statin due to its different pharmacokinetic profile truly affects SAMS or merely addresses the nocebo effect. However, multiple guidelines recommend that patients reporting SAMS should try at least two to three different agents.

Alternate (Off-Label) Dosing of Statins

Many providers are familiar with patients reporting that they can tolerate a statin for a short period of time, but then SAMS occurs. Several small studies have reported fairly similarly lipid-lowering efficacy (albeit there are no outcome studies) using statin every other day or even one to two doses per week (6). Several of this author's patients report SAMS when they are more active, often on the weekends ("weekend warriors"). I often recommend to these individuals that they take their statin Monday through Friday, and not on the weekends. Anecdotally, this approach has been successful, and there is no evidence of harm with less than daily dosing, perhaps a little reduction in lipid-lowering extent, but in this author's opinion "some statin is better than no statin" for high-CVD-risk individuals.

Combination Therapy

For patients who are able to tolerate a low dose or less than daily dose of statins but remain at high CVD risk due to hyperlipidemia, consideration of combination therapy with another LDL-lowering agent, such as ezetimibe, niacin, PCKS-9 inhibitors, or bile acid–binding resins could be considered. As these agents all work through different pathways and have different metabolism from statins, many patients are able to tolerate them. Furthermore, there is clinical trial evidence for statin plus ezetimibe, statin plus niacin, and statin plus PCSK9 inhibitor therapy that the combination therapy has CVD outcome benefits, likely via the further lowering of LDL cholesterol. Another option exists for patients who fit the subgroup shown to benefit from statin plus fibrate therapy in the Action to Control Cardiovascular Risk in Diabetes (ACCORD) study (those with high triglycerides [TG] and low high-density lipoprotein [HDL] despite statin therapy); however, there is some evidence in the literature suggesting that statin plus fibrate may have higher rates of muscle symptoms than either agent alone.

Alternate Lipid-Lowering Therapy

For patients with a contraindication for statin therapy, or who refuse statin therapy, providers should consider alternate lipid-lowering therapies. For patients with a dyslipidemia comprised predominantly of high TG and low HDL, clinical trial evidence suggests that fibrate monotherapy may provide CVD outcome benefits. Although niacin can be difficult to tolerate itself due to flushing, *etc.*, there is older clinical trial evidence suggesting CVD outcome benefits, at least if sufficient doses can be tolerated. Ezetimibe monotherapy can lower LDL cholesterol up to 25% and should be considered. Although there is no CVD outcome clinical trial evidence to support its use in monotherapy, the LDL lowering would be anticipated to have some benefit. Bile acid–binding resins are often poorly tolerated due to gastrointestinal side effects but should be considered. Finally, PCSK9 inhibitors have potent LDL-lowering properties and are likely to be of benefit even as monotherapy, assuming insurance coverage can be obtained. Finally, there is robust literature demonstrating the CVD benefits of non–lipid-lowering therapies, including some of the newer diabetes drugs, hypertension drugs, and other classes. For a patient unable or unwilling to take statins for CVD risk reduction, therapies aimed at other CVD risk factors should be maximized.

Case

You are asked to evaluate a 57-year-old woman for lipid-lowering therapy. She had essentially no medical care until ~6 years ago when she presented to the emergency room with a foot ulcer. At that time, type 2 diabetes was diagnosed, and over the next few months, she was initiated on several medications, including insulin 70/30 premix and metformin for her diabetes, lisinopril and metoprolol for hypertension, and amitriptyline for neuropathy. Her primary care provider had tried to start statin therapy with atorvastatin or rosuvastatin, but she reported muscle aches to each. Ultimately, her primary care provider was able to convince her to take pravastatin 20 mg/d; she reports that she takes this most days, but about once a month she takes a statin holiday due to increased myalgias. Three years ago, she had a myocardial infarction and was treated with coronary artery bypass graft. She was doing well (with HbA_{1c} in the 7.8% to 8.6% range) since then. She is now referred to you with new-onset exertional angina. Cardiology workup was performed and medical management recommended. Blood pressure is 128/76 mm Hg on her current medications. She does not smoke.

Her current laboratories (on pravastatin 20 mg/d) are as follows: total cholesterol 202 mg/dL, LDL cholesterol 123 mg/dL, HDL cholesterol 42 mg/dL, TG 187 mg/dL, HbA_{1c} 8.2%, thyrotropin 1.2 μIU/mL, and estimated glomerular filtration rate >60 mL/min.

What Is the Best Next Step?

A. Add ezetimibe
B. Add niacin
C. Change to rosuvastatin alternate day therapy
D. Add evolucumab
E. Add liraglutide

DISCUSSION

Correct Answer: Any of the Above That Are Feasible (Cost/Insurance Issues) and Tolerated

This patient has progressive cardiac symptoms despite pravastatin use. She has already had a CVD event, and her 10-year risk for another event is >20%. Per all current guidelines, she should be on a high-intensity statin, but she has not tolerated this in the past. She is a nonsmoker and her blood pressure is well controlled, but her LDL is not adequately lowered on pravastatin, and her diabetes control is less than ideal. The addition of ezetimibe (answer A) or niacin (answer B) would be expected to lower her LDL cholesterol ~25% (predicted LDL on combination would be 93 mg/dL), and each of these agents could and should be tried. Rosuvastatin (answer C) is a high-intensity statin; it is metabolized similarly to pravastatin. Because she is tolerating pravastatin to some extent, changing to rosuvastatin may work. Pravastatin 20 mg/d is expected to lower LDL by ∼25%, whereas rosuvastatin at 20 or 40 mg/d is expected to lower LDL >50% (from baseline); thus, if she was able to tolerate rosuvastatin most days of the week, then her predicted LDL cholesterol would be <75 mg/dL (untreated LDL estimated at 150 mg/dL). The addition of evolucumab would likely lower her LDL >50% in addition to that on statin, and thus could be predicted to achieve an LDL <60 mg/dL. Based on regression analyses correlating achieved LDL with CVD event rate, the lower the LDL the lower her CVD risk would likely be. In this case, the preferred option is answer D, addition of evolucumab. Answer C would be next best, and answers A and B still better than continuing current therapy. However, an alternate option to consider (or additional) would be the addition of another diabetes drug with CVD outcome benefits to her current regimen; thus, the addition of liraglutide (7) (answer E) or empagliflozin (8) (not offered as an answer) would be expected to reduce her CVD risk.

SUMMARY

The approach to patients with statin intolerance does not have a simple answer. Strong communication with the patient, their family, and other care providers is required to discuss the pros and cons of various options. Providers are encouraged to discuss the nocebo effect, but caution must be taken so that patients understand that we are not doubting the reality of their symptoms. The consideration of alternate approaches, often to be taken in a stepwise fashion, may lead to success. Ultimately, it is our patient's choice whether to pursue therapy or not.

REFERENCES

1. Stroes ES, Thompson PD, Corsini A, Vladutiu GD, Raal FJ, Ray KK, Roden M, Stein E, Tokgözoğlu L, Nordestgaard BG, Bruckert E, De Backer G, Krauss RM, Laufs U, Santos RD, Hegele RA, Hovingh GK, Leiter LA, Mach F, März W, Newman CB, Wiklund O, Jacobson TA, Catapano AL, Chapman MJ, Ginsberg HN; European Atherosclerosis Society Consensus Panel. Statin-associated muscle symptoms: impact on statin therapy-European Atherosclerosis Society Consensus Panel Statement on Assessment, Aetiology and Management. *Eur Heart J.* 2015;**36**(17):1012–1022.
2. Cholesterol Treatment Trialists' (CTT) Collaboration, Fulcher J, O'Connell R, Voysey M, Emberson J, Blackwell L, Mihaylova B, Simes J, Collins R, Kirby A, Colhoun H, Braunwald E, La Rosa J, Pedersen TR, Tonkin A, Davis B, Sleight P, Franzosi MG, Baigent C, Keech A. Efficacy and safety of LDL-lowering therapy among men and women: meta-analysis of individual data from 174,000 participants in 27 randomised trials. *Lancet.* 2015;**385**(9976):1397–1405.
3. Collins R, Reith C, Emberson J, Armitage J, Baigent C, Blackwell L, Blumenthal R, Danesh J, Smith GD, DeMets D, Evans S, Law M, MacMahon S, Martin S, Neal B, Poulter N, Preiss D, Ridker P, Roberts I, Rodgers A, Sandercock P, Schulz K, Sever P, Simes J, Smeeth L, Wald N, Yusuf S, Peto R. Interpretation of the evidence for the efficacy and safety of statin therapy. *Lancet.* 2016;**388**(10059): 2532–2561.
4. Sattar N, Preiss D, Murray HM, Welsh P, Buckley BM, de Craen AJM, Seshasai SRK, McMurray JJ, Freeman DJ, Jukema JW, Macfarlane PW, Packard CJ, Stott DJ, Westendorp RG, Shepherd J, Davis BR, Pressel SL, Marchioli R, Marfisi RM, Maggioni AP, Tavazzi L, Tognoni G, Kjekshus J, Pedersen TR, Cook TJ, Gotto AM, Clearfield MB, Downs JR, Nakamura H, Ohashi Y, Mizuno K, Ray KK, Ford I. Statins and risk of incident diabetes: a collaborative meta-analysis of randomised statin trials. *Lancet.* 2010;**375**(9716):735–742.
5. Taylor BA, Lorson L, White CM, Thompson PD. A randomized trial of coenzyme Q10 in patients with confirmed statin myopathy. *Atherosclerosis.* 2015;**238**(2):329–335.
6. Li JJ, Yang P, Liu J, Jia YJ, Li ZC, Guo YL, Wu NQ, Tang YD, Jiang LX. Impact of 10 mg rosuvastatin daily or alternate-day on lipid profile and inflammatory markers. *Clin Chim Acta.* 2012;**413**(1-2): 139–142.
7. Marso SP, Daniels GH, Brown-Frandsen K, Kristensen P, Mann JF, Nauck MA, Nissen SE, Pocock S, Poulter NR, Ravn LS, Steinberg WM, Stockner M, Zinman B, Bergenstal RM, Buse JB; LEADER Steering Committee; LEADER Trial Investigators. Liraglutide and cardiovascular outcomes in type 2 diabetes. *N Engl J Med.* 2016;**375**(4): 311–322.
8. Zinman B, Wanner C, Lachin JM, Fitchett D, Bluhmki E, Hantel S, Mattheus M, Devins T, Johansen OE, Woerle HJ, Broedl UC, Inzucchi SE; EMPA-REG OUTCOME Investigators. Empagliflozin, cardiovascular outcomes, and mortality in type 2 diabetes. *N Engl J Med.* 2015; **373**(22):2117–2128.

How to Prevent Cardiovascular Disease in Diabetes

M47
Presented, March 17–20, 2018

Peter Gaede, DMSc, MD. Department of Cardiology and Endocrinology, Slagelse Hospital, 4200 Slagelse, Denmark, E-mail: phgo@regionsjaelland.dk

SIGNIFICANCE OF THE CLINICAL PROBLEM

During the last decades, numerous studies have identified risk factors for poor outcome in diabetes. Cardiovascular disease (CVD) remains the major cause of morbidity and mortality in diabetes with a risk of CVD twice as high compared with the background population at any age, and being diagnosed with diabetes at the age of 40 years old is associated with a shorter lifespan of around 6 years (1).

Multiple risk factor intervention is the key to successful prevention of complications as clearly shown in the treatment of type 2 diabetes (2, 3). However, even with focus on classical risk factors, residual risk for CVD, and microvascular complications in the kidneys, nerves and eyes remains a clinical problem.

Recent cardiovascular trials of type 2 diabetes have examined the effect of newer glucose-lowering drug classes on diabetes-related complications, and interestingly, some of these have (in subpopulations of patients with type 2 diabetes and known atherosclerotic disease) shown clear benefits on CVD and renal disease beyond classical risk factor intervention (4–6).

Also, new treatment modalities for diabetic dyslipidemia may reduce future CVD markedly (7).

It is critical that diabetes professionals are familiar with use of multiple risk factor intervention and newer drug treatment with regards to indications, contraindications, and common side effects that might interfere with compliance.

BARRIERS TO OPTIMAL PRACTICE

- Poor compliance patterns to both lifestyle intervention and often costly drug therapy and burden of disease may often undermine therapy effectiveness.
- The growing complexity of indications and contraindications of newer diabetes drugs and combination treatment, especially because of impaired renal function, as well as lack of knowledge of newer clinical trials and safety issues might act as a barrier for diabetes professionals to intensify treatment.

LEARNING OBJECTIVES

As a result of participating in this session, learners should be able to do the following.

- Recognize important risk factors for CVD in diabetes
- Discuss optimum management of CVD risk factors based on recent recommendations for individualized treatment of diabetes
- Be aware of the associated comorbidities commonly seen when treating patients with diabetes and their impact on clinical decisions

STRATEGIES FOR DIAGNOSIS, THERAPY, AND/OR MANAGEMENT

Several guidelines focusing on multiple risk factors exist. Table 1 shows the modified treatment recommendations based on guidelines from the American Diabetes Association (8).

MAIN CONCLUSIONS

Strict focus on lifestyle intervention and drug treatment of multiple risk factors as well as use of specific drug classes both reduces the risk for cardiovascular complications and prolongs life in patients with diabetes.

CASES WITH QUESTIONS

Case 1

Case 1 is a 44-year-old single male with no family history of type 2 diabetes. He has no known medical history. During the last 3 to 4 months, he complains of frequent voiding and tiredness.

He has a sedentary lifestyle at both work and home. He "likes all kinds of food" in large amounts. Height is 172 cm, weight is 105 kg, and body mass index is 34.5 kg/m^2.

He smokes 20 cigarettes/d.

His blood pressure is 160/95 mm Hg. Hemoglobin A1c is 10% (86 mmol/mol). Low-density lipoprotein cholesterol is 147 mg/dL (3.8 mmol/L).

He has microalbuminuria and a plasma creatinine of 1.02 mg/dL (90 μmol/L). Estimated glomerular filtration rate is 85 mL/min per 1.72 m^2.

What kind of nonpharmacological steps would you consider?

What would be appropriate risk factor goals for this patient?

What kind of glucose-lowering drugs would you consider?

Would you consider aspirin treatment?

Would you consider other examinations?

Case 2

A 72-year-old female with family history of type 2 diabetes was diagnosed 15 years ago during an admission for a myocardial infarction. Later, she suffered a stroke but has no lasting symptoms.

Table 1. Treatment Guidelines Adapted from the American Diabetes Association's Standards of Medical Care in Diabetes for 2018 (8)

Treatment guidelines
Glucose-lowering therapy
Type 1 DM
Most people with type 1 diabetes should be treated with multiple daily injections of prandial insulin and basal insulin or continuous subcutaneous insulin infusion
Most individuals with type 1 diabetes should use rapid-acting insulin analogs to reduce hypoglycemia risk compared with human insulin
Type 2 DM
Metformin, if not contraindicated and if tolerated, is the preferred initial pharmacologic agent for the treatment of type 2 diabetes
In patients without atherosclerotic CVD, if monotherapy or dual therapy does not achieve or maintain the A1c goal over 3 mo, add an additional antihyperglycemic agent based on drug-specific and patient factors
In patients with type 2 diabetes and established atherosclerotic CVD, antihyperglycemic therapy should begin with lifestyle management and metformin, and it should subsequently incorporate an agent proven to reduce major adverse cardiovascular events (currently, empagliflozin, canagliflozin and liraglutide, and semaglutide) and cardiovascular mortality (currently, empagliflozin and liraglutide) after considering drug-specific and patient factors; in case of HbA1c levels >9.0%, consider initial combination therapy
For patients with type 2 diabetes who are not achieving glycemic goals, drug intensification, including consideration of insulin therapy, should not be delayed
Blood pressure–lowering therapy
Patients with confirmed office-based blood pressure ≥140/90 mm Hg should, in addition to lifestyle therapy, have prompt initiation and timely titration of pharmacologic therapy to achieve blood pressure goals
Patients with confirmed office-based blood pressure ≥160/100 mm Hg should, in addition to lifestyle therapy, have prompt initiation and timely titration of two drugs or a single-pill combination of drugs shown to reduce cardiovascular events in patients with diabetes
Treatment of hypertension should include drug classes shown to reduce cardiovascular events in patients with diabetes (ACE inhibitors, angiotensin receptor blockers, thiazide-like diuretics, or dihydropyridine calcium channel blockers)
Multiple-drug therapy is generally required to achieve blood pressure targets; however, combinations of ACE inhibitors and angiotensin receptor blockers and combinations of ACE inhibitors or angiotensin receptor blockers with direct renin inhibitors should not be used
An ACE inhibitor or angiotensin receptor blocker at the maximal tolerated dose indicated for blood pressure treatment is the recommended first-line treatment of hypertension in patients with diabetes and urinary albumin-to-creatinine ratio ≥300 mg/g creatinine or 30–299 mg/g creatinine; if one class is not tolerated, the other should be substituted
For patients treated with an ACE inhibitor, angiotensin receptor blocker, or diuretic, serum creatinine/estimated glomerular filtration rate and serum potassium levels should be monitored at least annually
Lipid-lowering therapy
For patients of all ages with diabetes and atherosclerotic CVD, high-intensity statin therapy should be added to lifestyle therapy
For patients with diabetes ages <40 years old with additional atherosclerotic CVD risk factors, the patient and provider should consider using moderate-intensity statin in addition to lifestyle therapy
For patients with diabetes ages 40–75 years old and those >75 years old without atherosclerotic CVD and minimal, if any, other ASCVD risk factors, use moderate-intensity statin in addition to lifestyle therapy
In clinical practice, providers may need to adjust the intensity of statin therapy based on individual patient response to medication (*e.g.*, side effects, tolerability, LDL cholesterol levels, or percentage of LDL reduction on statin therapy); for patients who do not tolerate the intended intensity of statin, the maximally tolerated statin dose should be used
For patients with diabetes and atherosclerotic CVD, if LDL cholesterol is ≥70 mg/dL on maximally tolerated statin dose, consider adding additional LDL-lowering therapy (such as ezetimibe or PCSK9 inhibitor) after evaluating the potential for additional atherosclerotic CVD risk reduction, drug-specific adverse effects, and patient preferences; ezetimibe may be preferred because of lower cost
Antiplatelet therapy
Use aspirin therapy (75–162 mg/d) as a secondary prevention strategy in those with diabetes and a history of atherosclerotic CVD
Aspirin therapy (75–162 mg/d) may be considered as a primary prevention strategy in those with type 1 or type 2 diabetes who are at increased cardiovascular risk; this includes most men and women with diabetes ages ≥50 years old who have at least one additional major risk factor (family history of premature atherosclerotic CVD, hypertension, dyslipidemia, smoking, or albuminuria) and are not at increased risk of bleeding

Abbreviations: ACE, angiotensin converting enzyme; ASCVD, atherosclerotic cardiovascular disease; DM, diabetes mellitus; HbA1c, hemoglobin A1c; LDL, low-density lipoprotein; PCSK9, proprotein convertase subtilisin/kexin-type 9.

For full information, see the American Diabetes Association's Standards of Medical Care in Diabetes—2018, published in Diabetes Care 2018; 41(Suppl 1).

She walks the dog every day but is complaining about intermittent claudication. She stopped smoking 5 years ago after the stroke.

Her height is 162 cm, weight is 75 kg, and body mass index is 28.6 kg/m^2.

Blood pressure is 140/65 mm Hg (enalapril/hydrochlorothiazide and amlodipine).

Hemoglobin A1c is 9.0% (75 mmol/L; metformin and glimepiride).

Low-density lipoprotein cholesterol is 104 mg/dL (2.7 mmol/L; atorvastatin 80 mg).

Plasma creatinine is 1.38 mg/dL (105 μmol/L). Estimated glomerular filtration rate is 46 mL/min per 1.72 m^2, and normoalbuminuria is present.

What kind of nonpharmacological steps would you consider?

What would be appropriate risk factor goals for this patient?

What kind of glucose-lowering drugs would you consider?

Would you consider aspirin treatment?

Would you consider other examinations?

A new glucose-lowering drug is added. At a visit 3 months later, creatinine has increased to 1.67 mg/dL (127 μmol/L), and estimated glomerular filtration rate is 36 mL/min per 1.72 m^2.

Will this increase in creatinine change your treatment strategy?

Case 3

Case 3 is a 60-year-old man diagnosed with type 2 diabetes mellitus 10 years ago. Glucose-lowering treatment with metformin 1 g twice daily was used for the first 7 years, and during the last 3 years, this has been combined with liraglutide because of a desire to lose weight.

The patient is now referred because of dysregulation, with an increase in hemoglobin A1c to 10.9% (95 mmol/mol).

There is microalbuminuria but otherwise, no apparent complications. Estimated glomerular filtration rate is 74 mL/min per 1.72 m^2. Electrocardiogram is normal. Weight is 96.9 kg.

Empagliflozin 25 mg was started.

May 9, 2017: 10.9% (95 mmol/mol)

June 29, 2017: 9.4% (79 mmol/mol)

September 27, 2017: 7.3% (56 mmol/mol)

Routine blood samples showed C-peptide level of 1.80 nmol/L (reference: 0.26 to 1.03 nmol/L).

GAD65 antibodies were >25 nmol/L (reference: <0.02 nmol/L).

Would this result change your treatment strategy regarding glucose-lowering treatment?

Similar results were seen but with C-peptide level of 0.180 nmol/L with a plasma glucose of 180 mg/dL (10 mmol/L) and negative GAD65.

Would this result change your treatment strategy regarding glucose-lowering treatment?

REFERENCES

1. Rao Kondapally Seshasai S, Kaptoge S, Thompson A, Di Angelantonio E, Gao P, Sarwar N, Whincup PH, Mukamal KJ, Gillum RF, Holme I, Njølstad I, Fletcher A, Nilsson P, Lewington S, Collins R, Gudnason V, Thompson SG, Sattar N, Selvin E, Hu FB, Danesh J; The Emerging Risk Factors Collaboration. Diabetes mellitus, fasting glucose, and risk of cause-specific death. *N Engl J Med.* 2011; **364**(9):829–841.
2. Gaede P, Lund-Andersen H, Parving HH, Pedersen O. Effect of a multifactorial intervention on mortality in type 2 diabetes. *N Engl J Med.* 2008;**358**(6):580–591.
3. Gæde P, Oellgaard J, Carstensen B, Rossing P, Lund-Andersen H, Parving HH, Pedersen O. Years of life gained by multifactorial intervention in patients with type 2 diabetes mellitus and microalbuminuria: 21 years follow-up on the Steno-2 randomised trial. *Diabetologia.* 2016;**59**(11):2298–2307.
4. Zinman B, Wanner C, Lachin JM, Fitchett D, Bluhmki E, Hantel S, Mattheus M, Devins T, Johansen OE, Woerle HJ, Broedl UC, Inzucchi SE; EMPA-REG OUTCOME Investigators. Empagliflozin, cardiovascular outcomes, and mortality in type 2 diabetes. *N Engl J Med.* 2015; **373**(22):2117–2128.
5. Marso SP, Daniels GH, Brown-Frandsen K, Kristensen P, Mann JF, Nauck MA, Nissen SE, Pocock S, Poulter NR, Ravn LS, Steinberg WM, Stockner M, Zinman B, Bergenstal RM, Buse JB; LEADER Steering Committee; LEADER Trial Investigators. Liraglutide and cardiovascular outcomes in type 2 diabetes. *N Engl J Med.* 2016;**375**(4): 311–322.
6. Neal B, Perkovic V, Mahaffey KW, de Zeeuw D, Fulcher G, Erondu N, Shaw W, Law G, Desai M, Matthews DR; CANVAS Program Collaborative Group. Canagliflozin and cardiovascular and renal events in type 2 diabetes. *N Engl J Med.* 2017;**377**(7):644–657.
7. Sabatine MS, Giugliano RP, Keech AC, Honarpour N, Wiviott SD, Murphy SA, Kuder JF, Wang H, Liu T, Wasserman SM, Sever PS, Pedersen TR; FOURIER Steering Committee and Investigators. Evolocumab and clinical outcomes in patients with cardiovascular disease. *N Engl J Med.* 2017;**376**(18):1713–1722.
8. American Diabetes Association. Standards of medical care in diabetes—2018. *Diabetes Care.* 2018;**41**(Suppl 1):S1–S159.

Sizing up Extreme Triglyceridemia: How to Spot a Coyote in a Wolf's Clothing

M59
Presented, March 17–20, 2018

Richard L. Dunbar, MD, MSTR. Cardiometabolic and Lipid Clinic, Corporal Michael J. Crescenz VA Medical Center, Philadelphia, Pennsylvania 19104, Clinical Research and Development, ICON plc, North Wales, Pennsylvania 19454, E-mail: r.l.dunbar@gmail.com

SIGNIFICANCE OF THE CLINICAL PROBLEM

It's hard to recognize something you aren't familiar with. Triglycerides (TGs) >500 mg/dL constitute severe hypertriglyceridemia (SHTG), and TGs >1000 mg/dL often cause acute pancreatitis (third-leading cause) (1). Patients are often referred for SHTG itself or complicated diabetes. There are two major types of SHTG in which TGs >1000 mg/dL, one common and the other less so. This is one case where it is critical to rule out the so-called zebra immediately, because well-intended usual care could gravely harm patients with the uncommon form or possibly kill them.

Simplistically, the two forms vary by how badly their ability to catabolize TGs is damaged. The rate-limiting step in TG hydrolysis is facilitated by lipoprotein lipase (LPL). For the most part, SHTG involves dysfunctional LPL. In SHTG, TG catabolism can usually be divided neatly into two groups, in which LPL activity is either (1) some but not much or (2) next to none. The most common group is typically a consequence of genetic or acquired causes of overabundant very-low-density lipoprotein (VLDL) and often one or more acquired causes of overproduction or decreased ability to catabolize TGs by LPL and is formally termed polygenic chylomicronemia or type V hyperlipoproteinemia. Once chylomicrons are reduced (*e.g.*, TGs ~1200 mg/dL), these patients might respond to the usual TG-lowering drugs (*e.g.*, fibrates, fish oil, niacin, or even statins), which may reduce VLDL TG levels. The unlucky ones have almost no ability to catabolize TGs, and this less-common cause is termed familial chylomicronemia syndrome (FCS) or type I hyperlipoproteinemia. Familial refers to a critical mutation that results in severe loss of LPL gene expression and/or function and, in turn, severely impaired TG catabolism. Distressingly, the usual drugs often do not work at all for FCS (but seldom harm patients). It makes sense that our usual pharmaceuticals are nontherapeutic, because TG-lowering drugs largely work by reducing VLDL production and/or boosting sluggish TG catabolism. However, they might not work at all when TG catabolism is almost entirely blocked by a mutation that disables LPL.

When patients with chylomicronemia resulting from either FCS or type V initially present, a fat-restricted diet should be instituted; hence, the urgent care approach is similar. Insidiously, treatment diverges during long-term outpatient management. In the common scenario of type V, national guidelines recommend fat restriction as a temporary measure while the chylomicrons are clearing, after which fat intake may be liberalized (2). In contrast, liberalizing fat intake can harm the rare patient with FCS. Long-term adherence to a severely fat-restricted diet is actually the most effective treatment for FCS. Because the long-term dietary recommendations for type V can gravely harm a patient with FCS, a common trap is to back off fat restriction casually without first ruling out FCS.

BARRIERS TO OPTIMAL PRACTICE

"I've seen this a dozen times; I got this."

In contrast to type V, the most effective therapy for FCS is a strictly controlled low-fat diet (*i.e.*, a low-triglyceride diet). There are two interrelated, egregious lapses posing barriers to optimal practice: (1) failing to distinguish FCS from type V, and consequently, (2) encouraging a patient with FCS to back off fat restriction when it may be the only therapy preventing the next bout of pancreatitis. Failed or unattempted diagnosis is all too common, and a contributing factor is that it is harder to distinguish FCS from type V by the usual lipid panel, although clinicians who measure apolipoprotein B (apoB) have a major advantage, because this assay varies between the two (vide infra). Perhaps the more insidious problem is that familiarity with the much more common type V can lull a busy physician into complacency, so precious little thought is given to distinguishing the two causes of SHTG until perhaps the third or fourth bout of pancreatitis.

LEARNING OBJECTIVES

As a result of participating in this session, learners should be able to:

- Understand why failing to distinguish between the types of SHTG could prove harmful
- Learn how to use available clinical laboratory tests to help distinguish between the different types of hypertriglyceridemia (tip: download the ApoB app to your smart phone)
- Discuss how a correct diagnosis can radically change long-term therapy

STRATEGIES FOR DIAGNOSIS, THERAPY, AND MANAGEMENT

"Why aren't the drugs working?"

Table 1. Characteristics of FCS and Type V

Feature	FCS		Polygenic Chylomicronemia
General	Type I hyperlipoproteinemia		Type V hyperlipoproteinemia
Genetics	Monogenic (biallelic, autosomal recessive)		Polygenic, familial clustering observed
Prevalence	1 in 100,000 to 1,000,000	<	Approximately 1 in 600
Disease onset	Childhood/adolescence > adulthood		Mostly adulthood
Clinical features	Abdominal pain		Abdominal pain
	Eruptive xanthomas	>>	Eruptive xanthomas (rare)
	Lipemia retinalis	>>	Lipemia retinalis (rare)
	Pancreatitis	>>	Pancreatitis (~10%)
	Hepatosplenomegaly		
Response to fibrate or fish oil	None to marginal	<<	Robust
CVD risk	None to minimal risk	<<	Evidence of increased risk
Lipoprotein profile*			
Major lipoproteins	Chylomicrons		Chylomicrons and VLDL
Features of chylomicronemia	TGs >1000 mg/dL	>>	TGs >1000 mg/dL
	Latescent plasma	>	Latescent plasma
	TGs/TCs >5 mg/dL	>	TGs/TCs >5 mg/dL
	TGs/apoB ≥8.8 mg/dL	>	TGs/apoB ≥8.8 mg/dL
ApoB	<75 mg/dL	<	≥75 mg/dL

Abbreviations: CVD, cardiovascular disease; TC, total cholesterol.
*Recommend ApoB app for smart phone for all lipid cases.

Diagnosis

Table 1 compares and contrasts FCS and type V. The diagnostic problem is evident by extensive overlap in general features, where FCS often differs by greater intensity rather than pathognomonic characteristics. For example, FCS tends to present earlier in life, with higher TGs and more physical stigmata and greater frequency of recurrent pancreatitis. Those relying on the usual lipid panel will find little help from the laboratory. The gold-standard diagnostic is lipoprotein electrophoresis or ultracentrifugation (3), but these are cumbersome and have longer reporting times. In contrast, apoB is a cheap, well-validated, and readily available lipid assay that can help distinguish FCS from type V. Unlike in FCS, apoB is characteristically elevated in type V (4–6), which naturally led several authorities to advocate apoB to distinguish FCS from type V (4, 7). A practical disadvantage of apoB seems to be that it often does not appear on the pick list in the electronic medical record, making it hard to order, and exceptionally shoddy insurance plans might not pay the extra $20 (even the Veterans Administration pays for this).

Both FCS and type V can have TG >1000 mg/dL, and the impaired TG clearance causes alimentary TGs to accumulate in the form of chylomicrons, causing chilled plasma to appear creamy. TG concentrations are much higher than total cholesterol, yielding a TG:total cholesterol ratio >5 mg/dL and especially >10 mg/dL (4). Because each TG-rich lipoprotein (TRL) has only one apoB, plasma apoB is a proxy for the prevalence of TRL counts. When chylomicron TG catabolism is impaired, the chylomicrons accumulate, and there is more TG per apoB molecule. Thus, when apoB is ordered, this is easily detected as a high ratio of TG:apoB (≥8.8 mg/dL), a feature of both FCS and type V. Fortuitously, FCS involves isolated chylomicronemia absent an increase in total apoB, whereas the mechanism of type V also involves increased apoB. Thus, when apoB is evaluated, it can discriminate between the two, because apoB will be elevated in type V but suppressed in FCS (*e.g.*, <75 to 100 mg/dL) (4, 7).

Therapy and Management

Frustratingly, FCS is minimally responsive to chronic use of TG-lowering drugs such as fibrates and fish oil, and this is actually an important clue that a patient has the defective LPL function that typifies FCS (2, 4, 8). Severe restriction of dietary fat intake is the only reliable initial treatment of FCS at this point. (2, 8, 9)

To ward off pancreatitis in a patient with FCS, restrict dietary fat to <15% of total energy intake (2, 8, 9). Specifically, patients with FCS should limit fat to 10% to 15% of calories, with 60% from carbohydrates and 25% to 30% from protein, preferably avoiding concentrated simple carbohydrates and alcohol (9). On average, 10% to 15% fat works out to 20 to 30 g/d. To put this into context, a tablespoon of olive oil has 12 g of fat. Restriction of fat and TGs retards chylomicron accumulation, bringing patients closer to the target TG level of <500 mg/dL with an approximate TG decrease of 20% to 25% daily. For example, patients should avoid fried and fast foods, whole-fat dairy products, fatty meats, and baked desserts. Patients should refrain from using fats, including all vegetable oils, butter, margarine, and full-fat salad dressings.

A Dangerous Trap Awaits You

In the long term, the FCS diet contrasts with the usual recommendation for type V, insofar as FCS requires a lifelong commitment to a severely fat-restricted diet, whereas patients with type V may loosen the fat restriction with more of an emphasis on lowering carbohydrates. Indeed, after the chylomicronemia resolves, many patients with type V do well with usual medications and a diet more focused on carbohydrate control. Superficially, advising a patient with FCS to direct his or her energies toward a low-carbohydrate diet may sound harmless enough. However, patients' efforts to restrict carbohydrates often end up increasing fat intake. Thus, the well-intended and seemingly ubiquitous public health harangue that "carbs are bad" may unwittingly shame a patient with FCS into eradicating carbohydrates, prompting an insidious rise in fat and TG intake, culminating in pancreatitis. Optimal care of the patient with FCS should include rigorous efforts to counteract these general messages and instead relentlessly emphasize severe fat restriction. This is best initiated with the help of a dietician skilled in FCS, but in any case, it requires long-term reinforcement and much coaching. Successful fat restriction usually improves xanthomas, hepatosplenomegaly, and abdominal pain and lessens the risk of acute pancreatitis (10). Unfortunately, this dietary regimen is unpalatable and difficult to maintain. Hence, long-term compliance is poor in many patients, underscoring the desperate need for novel therapeutics for FCS.

Emerging Pharmacotherapy

Several developers have been exploring novel therapeutics that promise to treat FCS, overcoming the lackluster to absent effects of current pharmacotherapy. The quadrants of Fig. 1 organize these attempts according to dominant mechanism of action. Because the defect of FCS is obstructed TG catabolism, most efforts focus on unblocking TG catabolism, yielding four new approaches. Two disinhibit LPL by inhibiting LPL inhibitors (apoC3 and ANGPTL3 inhibitors), and two fortify compounds that boost LPL activity (apoC2 mimetic and LPL gene replacement therapy). An apoE mimetic would hasten TRL catabolism. On the other side are approaches that retard TG synthesis (DGAT inhibition) or TRL synthesis (MTP inhibition).

Status of Emerging Approaches

Not all of these are clinically or commercially viable. For example, several DGAT inhibitors were abandoned because of insurmountable gastrointestinal obstacles and LPL gene replacement therapy because of insurmountable commercial obstacles. The MTP inhibitor is approved for familial hypercholesterolemia, but off-label use for SHTG risks serious adverse effects. The apoC2 and apoE mimetics are in early-stage development. However, apoC3 and ANGPTL3 inhibitors are further along and seem clinically viable. For each, the best-validated mechanism of action is inhibiting a protein that inhibits LPL activity; thus, these drugs disinhibit LPL, thereby accelerating TG catabolism. It was surprising that this approach would help FCS, because it was presumed that residual LPL activity was effectively nil, so the drugs should not have worked.

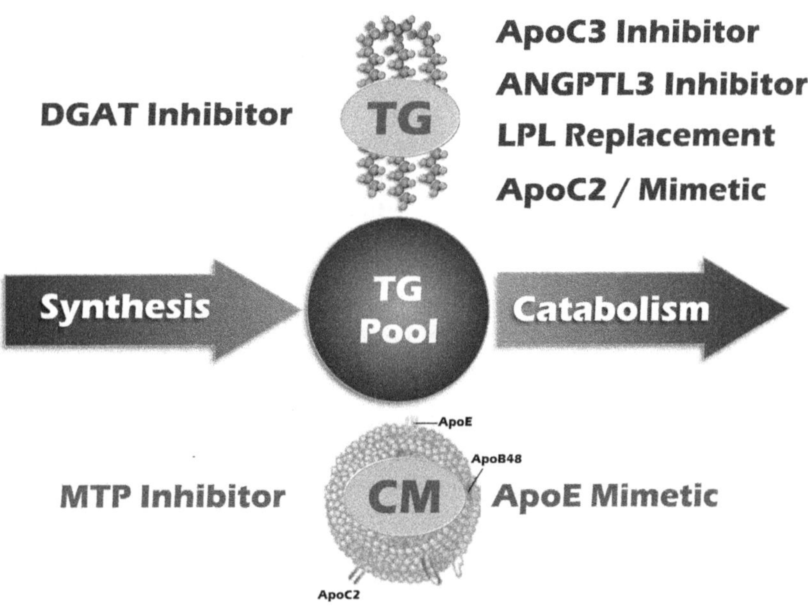

Figure 1. Strategies to treat FCS with novel therapeutics. CM, chylomicron.

Demonstrable efficacy could mean even undetectable LPL activity is remediable by knocking out LPL inhibitors. However, another mechanism independent of LPL could be in play.

Not only is apoC3 an endogenous LPL inhibitor, but it also disrupts the role of apoC2 as an LPL cofactor (Fig. 2). Carriers of loss-of-function (LOF) *APOC3* mutations have lower fasting and postprandial TG levels, supporting apoC3 as a target for drug development. Encouragingly, *APOC3* LOF carriers are also far less prone to *coronary heart disease* (CHD) events (odds ratio, 0.60; 95% confidence interval, 0.47 to 0.75) (12). An antisense oligonucleotide was developed that successfully suppresses apoC3 synthesis. In turn, apoC3 inhibition provoked profound drops in TGs (−70%), well beyond those produced by usual TG-lowering drugs (13). Plausible mechanisms include: accelerating TRL clearance by abolishing apoC3-mediated LPL inhibition and liberating apoC2 as an LPL cofactor, or retarding VLDL production. Shockingly, apoC3 inhibition lowered TGs by 56% to 86% in three patients with FCS (14). This signals a breakthrough, because current therapy is effectively useless in FCS. Moreover, for the first time, each patient with FCS reached his or her TG target of <500 mg/dL. Among patients with diabetes, the profound drop in TGs resulting from apoC3 inhibition was accompanied by significantly improved glucose control by HgbA1c and insulin sensitivity by hyperinsulinemic-euglycemic clamp (15). A new drug application was filed this year.

ANGPTL3 also inhibits LPL function among other lipases. Conversely, people with homozygous *ANGPTL3* LOF mutations have hyperactive LPL activity (16). The latter bestows familial combined hypolipidemia, so these patients enjoy lower LDL cholesterol and TG levels (17). Encouragingly, *ANGPTL3* LOF carriers are far less prone to CHD events (odds ratio, 0.59; 95% confidence interval, 0.41 to 0.85) (18), with results strikingly similar to the CHD benefits of *APOC3* LOF. Both a monoclonal antibody and an antisense oligonucleotide were developed to suppress ANGPTL3. A single dose of the former profoundly reduced TG levels in dyslipidemic patients (−76%) (18), again well beyond that produced by usual TG-lowering drugs. Presently, both apoC3 inhibition and ANGPTL3 inhibition are the most promising approaches for further development, because several of the approaches in Fig. 1 are defunct or far behind. The surprisingly consonant results from apoC3 and ANGPTL3 inhibition suggest relieving LPL inhibition could be broadly beneficial, with the potential to not only lower fasting and postprandial TGs but also improve carbohydrate metabolism or perhaps even prevent CHD.

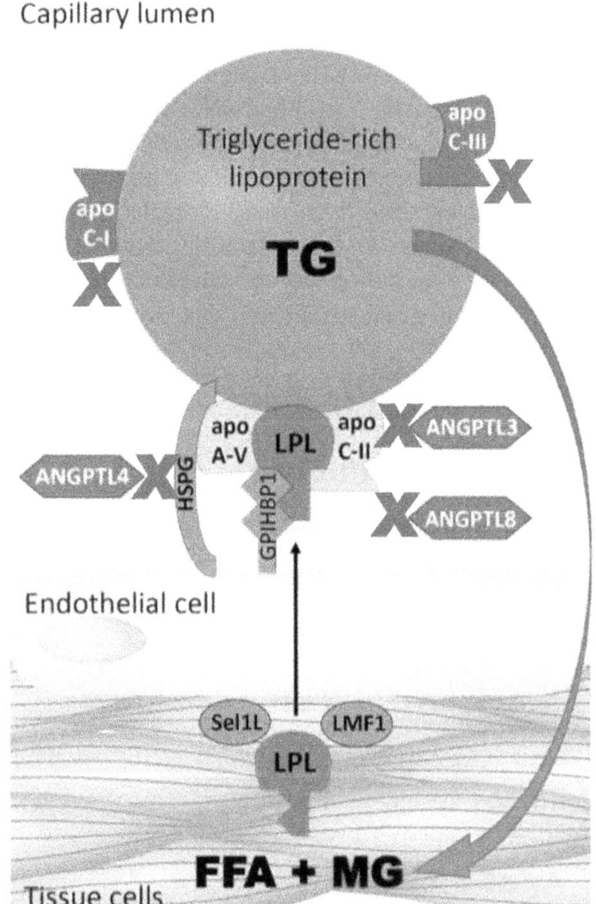

Figure 2. Factors that modify LPL activity. Endogenous LPL inhibitors indicated by X. Open source figure by Wolska *et al* (11).

Molecular Diagnosis To Refine Therapy

If FCS is the likely diagnosis, at some point during the course of treatment, pursuit of a genetic diagnosis should be considered. Table 2 lists several genes coding proteins that influence LPL function, including LPL itself. A homozygous LOF mutation in one of these would effectively rule in a diagnosis of FCS, as would compound heterozygosity. Absence of a mutation does not rule out FCS physiology, because an unknown mutation could be present, and with autoimmune disease, antibodies may inactivate LPL (*e.g.*, systemic lupus erythematosus). In the latter, FCS is technically a misnomer, but the distinction is academic, because the approach to therapy overlaps. An important reason to pursue a genetic diagnosis is that at least one of the mutations, apoC2 deficiency, opens up an important therapeutic option (11). ApoC2 appears in sufficient quantities in normal plasma that apoC2-deficient patients benefit from plasma transfusion. This can help shorten intensive care unit and total hospital stays for acute pancreatitis and can even be used as an outpatient therapy to keep apoC2-deficient patients out of the hospital. Thus, determining whether a patient with FCS has apoC2 deficiency could have a major impact on his or her outcome. The major practical limitation to genetic testing is that most insurance providers would rather pay for a series of prolonged intensive care unit stays than a one-time laboratory test and therefore refuse to pay for testing.

Table 2. Mutations Causing FCS

Gene	Effect on LPL-Dependent Lipolysis
LPL	Key enzyme that hydrolyzes TGs
LMF1	Chaperone protein of LPL, required for maturation and transport
GPIHBP1	Important protein in LPL tethering, dimerization, and stabilization to the endothelium
APOC2	Activating cofactor of LPL
APOA5	Stabilizing cofactor of LPL and apoC2 and modulator of hepatic TG metabolism

MAIN CONCLUSIONS

- SHTG is a semiurgent condition because of the risk of pancreatitis, regardless of the cause; treatment that lowers TGs can avert pancreatitis.
- Failing to distinguish FCS within SHTG early on can unnecessarily delay definitive treatment; thus, one must be on the lookout for FCS, regarding it as the proverbial coyote in a wolf's clothing.
- The diagnosis is hard enough with usual laboratory work; spend the extra $20 for the apoB assay, and use the free ApoB app to determine the lipid classes.
- Take care not to tell all patients with SHTG they should eradicate carbohydrates, because this can unwittingly result in patients with FCS increasing their fat intake, to their peril.
- If FCS is the likely diagnosis, special steps are advised:
  1. Recommend a strictly low-fat diet featuring 10% to 15% of calories from fat per day (on average, 20 to 30 g of fat/d).
  2. Consider genotyping to confirm FCS, and determine whether the patient has apoC2 deficiency.
  3. Consider enlisting the help of a dietician.
  4. Consider referring the patient to a regional center with expertise in FCS, because such a center may be able to perform genotyping and/or offer experimental therapeutics under research protocols.

OVERVIEW OF FCS CASES

Three siblings presented with SHTG/chylomicronemia in their teens, and their maximum TGs ranged from 5000 to 7200 mg/dL. They include a set of fraternal twins and their older brother. In their 20s, they were diagnosed with type I hyperlipoproteinemia at the National Institutes of Health. Accordingly, the National Institutes of Health advised a severely fat-restricted diet, and this lowered their TGs substantially. Regrettably, after several decades of care in their community, their TG levels spiraled out of control because the diet was not reinforced, and they returned to a more typical fat-laden American diet. The twin brother had the worst control and was actually attempting to lower his TGs with a low-carbohydrate diet, the higher fat content of which was probably worsening his TGs and provoking pancreatitis more frequently. The older brother was the most disciplined of the three and was able to adhere to a low-fat diet consistently and had far fewer episodes of pancreatitis over his lifetime. They visited our clinic in their 50s for a second opinion on management of worsening TG control and recurrent pancreatitis (Table 3; Fig. 3).

Table 3. Clinical Features of Case Studies

Clinical Feature	Female Twin	Male Twin	Older Brother
Age at onset, years	13	17	18
Maximum TGs, mg/dL	7200	6000	6000
Minimum TGs, mg/dL	700	774	321
Pancreatitis episodes	4 times/year	4 times/year	2 times/lifetime
Eruptive xanthoma	Never	Never	Never
Lipemia retinalis	Yes	Yes	NA
Hepatomegaly	No	No	No
Maximum TG:TC ratio	14:1	20:1	11:1
Maximum TG:apoB ratio	>59.2:1	>96.1:1	>47.1:1
Minimum apoB, mg/dL	<40	<40	<40
LPL activity, method 1: normal, 34.8 μmol/L/min; range, 22–47.6 μmol/L/min (% of reference)	4.8 (13.8%)	2.5 (7.2%)	NA
LPL activity, method 2 (% of reference)	NA	0 (0%)	0 (0%)
LPL activity, method 3: normal, 378.11 nmol/mL/min (% of reference)	NA	134.99 (35.7%)	146.08 (38.6%)
LPL mass, ng/mL (% of reference)	NA	112 (39.9%)	87.9 (31.3%)

Abbreviations: NA, not applicable; TC, total cholesterol.

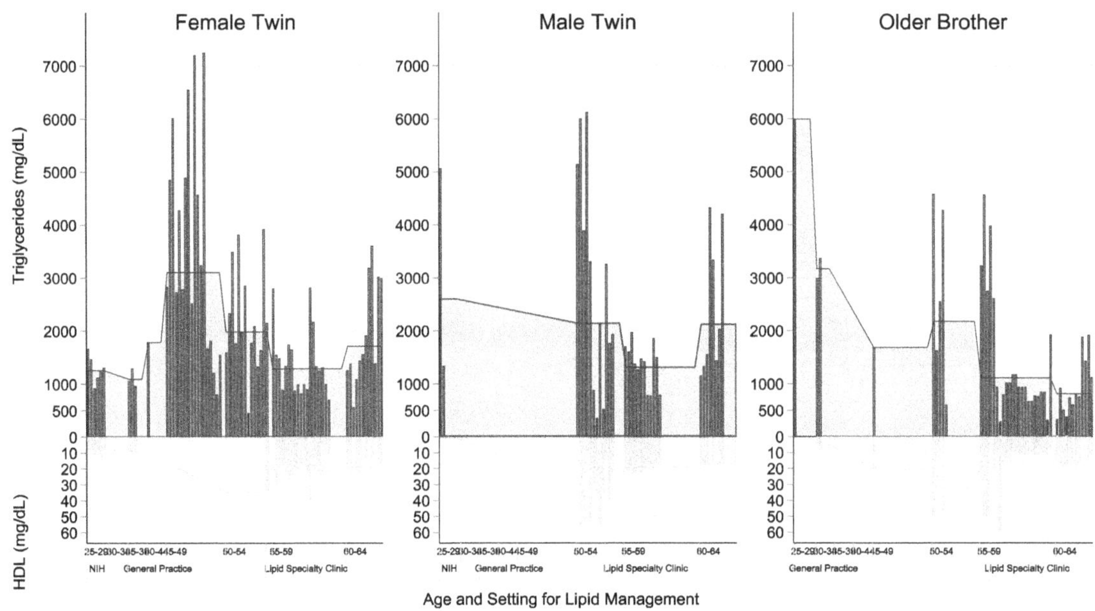

Figure 3. Lipid management in case studies. HDL, high-density lipoprotein.

Specialized Laboratory Investigations

The twins had extremely reduced LPL activities: the sister's was 4.8 mmol/L/min, and her twin brother's was 2.5 mmol/L/min (reference range, 22 to 47.6 mmol/L/min). By a separate assay, the two brothers were assessed as having zero activity. We determined all three siblings to have a homozygous variant, c.617T>C p.V206A in *LPL*, the first reported cases of homozygosity. Concurrent sequencing of other FCS- and HTG-related genes *APOC2*, *APOA5*, *LMF1*, *GPIHBP1*, and *GPD1* revealed no other potentially pathogenic variants. The results of both reduced LPL functional studies and genotyping in all three siblings confirmed the diagnosis of FCS as a result of the LOF LPL mutation, leading to LPL deficiency.

Response to Current Treatment Options

We reacquainted them with an extremely low-fat diet with the help of a dietician and regularly reinforced the dietary advice during their follow-up care. Adjunctive therapies were also prescribed, but they were not as effective. They did much better with the diet, with fewer episodes of pancreatitis. Although improved, their TGs generally settled in the range of 2000 to 3000+ mg/dL. Thus, optimal therapy still left them short of the goal of TGs <500 mg/dL.

Response to Novel Therapeutics in Development

I enrolled the twins in a randomized, double-blinded clinical experiment, wherein the sister received a single dose of an experimental ANGPTL3 inhibitor and her twin brother received placebo. ANGPTL3 inhibition brought her TGs from 3020 mg/dL to a nadir of 1509 mg/dL 36 days postdose (~50% reduction). Her TG levels remained suppressed for up to 150 days postdose, indicating a durable TG suppression from only a single dose. This is especially encouraging because approved TG-lowering drugs do little to nothing by comparison. In contrast, with placebo, her twin brother had typical wide swings in his TG levels, ranging from −38% to +89% from the baseline of 2030 mg/dL. Although overall study results have not been published, the experience of this set of twins encourages the notion that ANGPTL3 inhibition can lower TGs in FCS. The female twin qualified for another study, receiving multiple doses of an experimental apoC3 inhibitor, which lowered her TGs from 3447 mg/dL to as low as 201 mg/dL (−94%).

DISCUSSION OF CASES AND ANSWERS

Although SHTG is not uncommon, our case of three siblings illustrates the importance of distinguishing FCS from type V SHTG. Patients with FCS may fall short of goals because of a lack of familiarity with the disease in their community. After dietary counseling, the siblings gained a better understanding of FCS and have done well. Until more effective TG-lowering medications become available for FCS, dietary fat restriction is critical to prevent recurrent pancreatitis. Referral to a lipid specialist and a registered dietitian is advisable. Novel therapeutics may offer the ability to reduce TGs to much lower levels and better prevent pancreatitis.

This presentation and case study were adapted from a manuscript and presentation to the National Lipid Association Scientific Sessions 2017 authored by Ueda *et al* (19).

REFERENCES

1. Dunbar RL, Rader DJ. Demystifying triglycerides: a practical approach for the clinician. *Cleve Clin J Med.* 2005;**72**(8):661–666, 670–672, 674–675 passim.

2. Jacobson TA, Maki KC, Orringer CE, Jones PH, Kris-Etherton P, Sikand G, La Forge R, Daniels SR, Wilson DP, Morris PB, Wild RA, Grundy SM, Daviglus M, Ferdinand KC, Vijayaraghavan K, Deedwania PC, Aberg JA, Liao KP, McKenney JM, Ross JL, Braun LT, Ito MK, Bays HE, Brown WV, Underberg JA; NLA Expert Panel. National lipid association recommendations for patient-centered management of dyslipidemia: part 2 [published correction appears in J Clin Lipidol. 2016;10(1): 211]. *J Clin Lipidol.* 2015;**9**(6, suppl):S1–S122.e1.
3. Beaumont JL, Carlson LA, Cooper GR, Fejfar Z, Fredrickson DS, Strasser T. Classification of hyperlipidaemias and hyperlipoproteinaemias. *Bull World Health Organ.* 1970;**43**(6):891–915.
4. Stroes E, Moulin P, Parhofer KG, Rebours V, Löhr J-M, Averna M. Diagnostic algorithm for familial chylomicronemia syndrome. *Atheroscler Suppl.* 2017;**23**:1–7.
5. Sniderman AD, Ribalta J, Castro Cabezas M. How should FCHL be defined and how should we think about its metabolic bases? *Nutr Metab Cardiovasc Dis.* 2001;**11**(4):259–273.
6. Sveger T, Nordborg K. Apolipoprotein B as a marker of familial hyperlipoproteinemia. *J Atheroscler Thromb.* 2004;**11**(5):286–292.
7. de Graaf J, Couture P, Sniderman A. A diagnostic algorithm for the atherogenic apolipoprotein B dyslipoproteinemias. *Nat Clin Pract Endocrinol Metab.* 2008;**4**(11):608–618.
8. National Cholesterol Education Program (NCEP) Expert Panel on Detection, Evaluation, and Treatment of High Blood Cholesterol in Adults (Adult Treatment Panel III). Third report of the National Cholesterol Education Program (NCEP) expert panel on detection, evaluation, and treatment of high blood cholesterol in adults (Adult Treatment Panel III) final report. *Circulation.* 2002;**106**(25):3143–3421.
9. Williams L, Wilson DP. Editorial commentary: dietary management of familial chylomicronemia syndrome. *J Clin Lipidol.* 2016;**10**(3): 462–465.
10. Brahm AJ, Hegele RA. Chylomicronaemia—current diagnosis and future therapies. *Nat Rev Endocrinol.* 2015;**11**(6):352–362.
11. Wolska A, Dunbar RL, Freeman LA, Ueda M, Amar MJ, Sviridov DO, Remaley AT. Apolipoprotein C-II: new findings related to genetics, biochemistry, and role in triglyceride metabolism. *Atherosclerosis.* 2017;**267**:49–60.
12. Musunuru K, Pirruccello JP, Do R, Peloso GM, Guiducci C, Sougnez C, Garimella KV, Fisher S, Abreu J, Barry AJ, Fennell T, Banks E, Ambrogio L, Cibulskis K, Kernytsky A, Gonzalez E, Rudzicz N, Engert JC, DePristo MA, Daly MJ, Cohen JC, Hobbs HH, Altshuler D, Schonfeld G, Gabriel SB, Yue P, Kathiresan S. Exome sequencing, ANGPTL3 mutations, and familial combined hypolipidemia. *N Engl J Med.* 2010;**363**(23): 2220–2227.
13. Gaudet D, Alexander VJ, Baker BF, Brisson D, Tremblay K, Singleton W, Geary RS, Hughes SG, Viney NJ, Graham MJ, Crooke RM, Witztum JL, Brunzell JD, Kastelein JJ. Antisense inhibition of apolipoprotein C-III in patients with hypertriglyceridemia. *N Engl J Med.* 2015;**373**(5):438–447.
14. Gaudet D, Brisson D, Tremblay K, Alexander VJ, Singleton W, Hughes SG, Geary RS, Baker BF, Graham MJ, Crooke RM, Witztum JL. Targeting APOC3 in the familial chylomicronemia syndrome. *N Engl J Med.* 2014;**371**(23):2200–2206.
15. Digenio A, Dunbar RL, Alexander VJ, Hompesch M, Morrow L, Lee RG, Graham MJ, Hughes SG, Yu R, Singleton W, Baker BF, Bhanot S, Crooke RM. Antisense-mediated lowering of plasma apolipoprotein C-III by volanesorsen improves dyslipidemia and insulin sensitivity in type 2 diabetes. *Diabetes Care.* 2016;**39**(8):1408–1415.
16. Arca M, Minicocci I, Maranghi M. The angiopoietin-like protein 3: a hepatokine with expanding role in metabolism. *Curr Opin Lipidol.* 2013;**24**(4):313–320.
17. Musunuru K, Pirruccello JP, Do R, Peloso GM, Guiducci C, Sougnez C, Garimella KV, Fisher S, Abreu J, Barry AJ, Fennell T, Banks E, Ambrogio L, Cibulskis K, Kernytsky A, Gonzalez E, Rudzicz N, Engert JC, DePristo MA, Daly MJ, Cohen JC, Hobbs HH, Altshuler D, Schonfeld G, Gabriel SB, Yue P, Kathiresan S. Exome sequencing, ANGPTL3 mutations, and familial combined hypolipidemia. *N Engl J Med.* 2010;**363**(23): 2220–2227.
18. Dewey FE, Gusarova V, Dunbar RL, O'Dushlaine C, Schurmann C, Gottesman O, McCarthy S, Van Hout CV, Bruse S, Dansky HM, Leader JB, Murray MF, Ritchie MD, Kirchner HL, Habegger L, Lopez A, Penn J, Zhao A, Shao W, Stahl N, Murphy AJ, Hamon S, Bouzelmat A, Zhang R, Shumel B, Pordy R, Gipe D, Herman GA, Sheu WHH, Lee IT, Liang KW, Guo X, Rotter JI, Chen YD, Kraus WE, Shah SH, Damrauer S, Small A, Rader DJ, Wulff AB, Nordestgaard BG, Tybjærg-Hansen A, van den Hoek AM, Princen HMG, Ledbetter DH, Carey DJ, Overton JD, Reid JG, Sasiela WJ, Banerjee P, Shuldiner AR, Borecki IB, Teslovich TM, Yancopoulos GD, Mellis SJ, Gromada J, Baras A. Genetic and pharmacologic inactivation of ANGPTL3 and cardiovascular disease. *N Engl J Med.* 2017;**377**(3):211–221.
19. Ueda M, Burke F, Walters L, Lalic D, Sikora T, Greene H, Der-Ohannessian S, McIntyre A, deGoma E, Hegele R, Rader D, Dunbar R. Familial chylomicron syndrome: importance of discerning the rare among the common. *J Clin Lipidol.* 2017;**11**(3):818–819.

DIABETES MELLITUS AND GLUCOSE METABOLISM

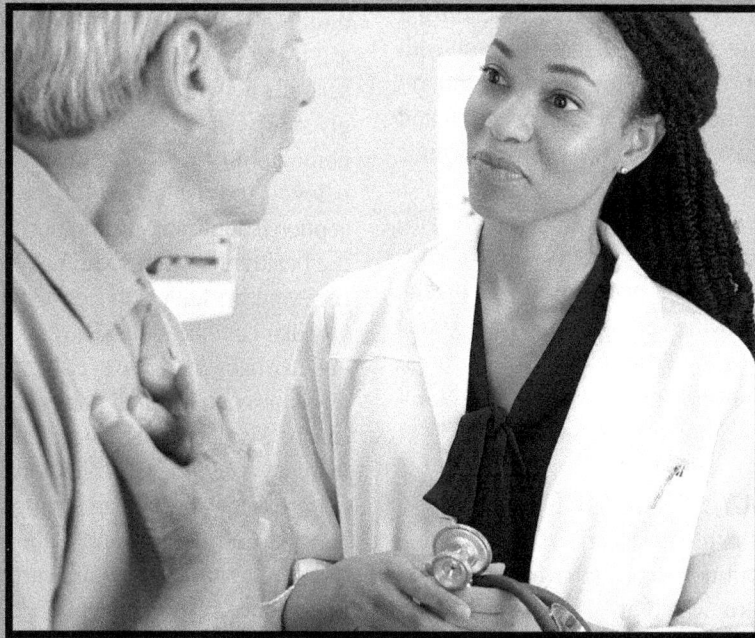

Management of Diabetes in Pregnancy: The Importance of Preconception Care

M02
Presented, March 17–20, 2018

Susan E. Kirk, MD. University of Virginia Health System, Charlottesville, Virginia 22908, E-mail: sek4b@virginia.edu

SIGNIFICANCE OF THE CLINICAL PROBLEM

With the continued changing health demographics of the US population, particularly the unhealthy trends of increasing obesity and metabolic disorders in adolescent females and reproductive-aged women, health care professionals continue to witness an increase in the number of pregnancies complicated by diabetes. This includes gestational diabetes mellitus, overt diabetes, pregestational type 1 diabetes mellitus, and pregestational type 2 diabetes mellitus. Although many issues must be considered in the management of such pregnancies, this session focuses on one specific area: maximizing the health and glycemic control of the female patient with pregestational diabetes before conception. This session reviews current technology for both the delivery of insulin and the monitoring of blood glucose levels and discusses glycemic targets both before and during pregnancy.

As health care professionals who care for women with diabetes, providing optimal care to women who are contemplating pregnancy can lead to a positive impact on the health of both the mother with diabetes and her fetus. Despite that this tenet is widely accepted, not all women with diabetes receive preconception counseling or heed it when they do.

BARRIERS TO OPTIMAL PRACTICE

- In many communities, the greatest barriers to providing optimal diabetes care continue to be high treatment costs and limited access to care, which are especially true for some of the newer or more sophisticated management tools, including insulin pumps and continuous glucose monitors (CGMs). In addition, the successful treatment of women with diabetes during pregnancy depends on their compliance with management strategies. Similar to those patients with diabetes who are not pregnant, this remains a major obstacle to ideal practice in diabetes and pregnancy.
- Randomized controlled trials (RCTs) to identify ideal glycemic targets, effective pharmacologic agents, and optimal management strategies are scarce; therefore, in the area of diabetes and pregnancy, evidence-based recommendations often are weak and instead are the result of expert consensus opinion.

LEARNING OBJECTIVES

As a result of participating in this session, learners should be able to:

- Know the issues that complicate pregnancy in women with diabetes that should be addressed before conception
- Understand the glycemic targets for the preconception period
- Understand that not all women respond positively to preconception counseling and to know which conversations may help women to delay their pregnancy until glycemic targets are obtained

STRATEGIES FOR PRECONCEPTION COUNSELING IN WOMEN WITH DIABETES

All postpubertal adolescents and women of reproductive age should receive preconception counseling. This discussion should occur in some form at each visit and include at a minimum the type of contraception the woman or her partner are using if pregnancy is not being actively planned. If she is sexually active, the patient should be reminded of the specific glycemic target to achieve before conception [in most cases a hemoglobin $A_{1c} < 6.5\%$ or as close to normal as possible (see below)] and a plan should be reviewed for ceasing contraception if applicable. In addition, the risks to her health as well as the health of her fetus and baby posed by pregnancy should be reviewed, including the development or worsening of microvascular complications. The patient should be reminded that she and her baby might be at risk for complications even if excellent glycemic control is maintained, although if achieved, those risks can be significantly reduced. Therefore, the engagement of a team of health care professionals, including obstetricians experienced in the management and delivery of diabetic pregnancies, nutritionists, and diabetes educators, is important.

Despite that most health care professionals understand the importance of preconception planning and recognize that it can improve maternal and fetal outcomes, less than one half of pregnancies complicated by diabetes are planned (1). Perhaps more realistically, even though the majority of women have discussed the importance of optimizing their glycemic control and overall health before conception with their health care provider, glycemic targets and health goals often are abandoned before they are realized (2). Women with diabetes who plan their pregnancies are more likely to have higher income and education levels and private health insurance, to have received care from an endocrinologist, to be married and white, and to have received encouragement from their health care provider. Moreover, women were less likely to heed advice about delaying conception until glycemic targets are reached if they believed that they were being discouraged or judged by their health care provider. When discussing pregnancy with a patient who might be contemplating pregnancy, it is important to emphasize that with good glycemic control, management of comorbidities, and the assistance of a multidisciplinary team, odds are in her favor for delivering a healthy baby and remaining healthy herself. This strategy was effective in helping some women with diabetes to plan their pregnancies compared with other women who did not plan their pregnancies (2).

GLYCEMIC TARGETS FOR THE PRECONCEPTION PERIOD AND PREGNANCY AND THE USE OF NEWER TECHNOLOGY TO ACHIEVE THEM

Maternal hyperglycemia has a negative impact on fetal, neonatal, and maternal outcomes. The Hyperglycemia and Adverse Pregnancy Outcomes study suggested that there may be no lower limit of glucose during pregnancy below which adverse events can be avoided (3). Likewise, the teratogenicity of higher maternal serum glucose values is well established, but an RCT studying the thresholds of maternal glucose values either before conception or during the first trimester would be difficult (if not unethical) to carry out. The current recommendation by the American Diabetes Association is for conception be delayed in women with pregestational diabetes until hemoglobin A_{1c} levels are <6.5% and ideally <6% without inducing problematic hypoglycemia (4). The highest risk for severe hypoglycemia during pregnancy in women with diabetes appears to be in those who have a history of hypoglycemia unawareness or prior episodes of severe hypoglycemia. Specifically, 10% of women carry 60% of the risk (5). Special counseling about strategies to monitor for and avoid hypoglycemia should be given to this group of women. Average blood glucose values that would correspond to a hemoglobin A_{1c} in the range of ≤7% have been associated with a risk of fetal congenital malformations equal to that of nondiabetic populations (~2%). However, there is evidence that hemoglobin A_{1c} levels that are below this level but still mildly elevated early in pregnancy may be associated with an increased risk of macrosomia (6).

In women with type 1 diabetes, no RCTs have shown a clear advantage to the use of continuous subcutaneous insulin infusion (CSII) over multiple daily injections (MDIs); however, few RCTs have adequately studied this question. In nonpregnant patients with diabetes, CSII has demonstrated an advantage of allowing patients to achieve lower hemoglobin A_{1c} levels with a lower risk of hypoglycemia (7). Theoretically, this would be advantageous in the preconception period. However, the absolute degree of glycemic control rather than the method used to achieve it likely affects maternal, fetal, and neonatal outcomes. The woman and her health care provider should discuss the optimal method in terms of both lifestyle and cost well before conception to avoid any increased risk of hyper- or hypoglycemia during the transition from one method to another if attempted during pregnancy. Until recently, most self-glucose monitoring in pregnant women with diabetes was done with glucose monitors and capillary blood. The frequency and timing of such testing with regard to preventing both maternal and fetal complications was found to be inconclusive according to a comprehensive review of studies addressing this topic (8). Likewise, studies examining the use of CGM, both intermittent and continuous, have shown inconclusive results regarding the lowering of risks other than reduction of hemoglobin A_{1c} (8). Studies are limited and, in some cases, do not reflect current daily use of CGM devices or self-monitoring of blood glucose in pregnant women with diabetes. Moreover, an analysis by Hernandez and Barbour (9) examined some of the factors that may have confounded the results. They concluded that the conditions under which data were collected, variables of interest defined, and methods to deal with incongruous prospective data often were lacking. Finally, it is reasonable to expect in the near future the use of artificial pancreas systems during pregnancy (10). Artificial pancreas systems use mathematical algorithms with CGM and CSII to automatically adjust insulin infusion depending on glucose levels. Currently, there are no published data regarding their use during pregnancy, but now that one prototype is commercially available (MiniMed 670G; Medtronic, Edgewater, MD), it is logical to assume that health care providers may encounter their use in pregnant patients.

ADDRESSING COMPLICATIONS AND COMORBIDITIES IN THE PRECONCEPTION PERIOD

Pregnancy can exacerbate both acute and chronic complications of diabetes. Comorbidities, if not properly managed, can worsen risks to both the mother and her baby. Therefore, it is important to systematically plan for their assessment and treatment before conception. Of note, like studies on optimal management for glycemic control, very few or no RCTs have addressed these issues.

Retinopathy

Pregnancy affects the progression of diabetic retinopathy, and the cause is likely to be multifactorial. Retinopathy is more likely to occur if diabetes has been present for >10 years. In most cases, changes revert to baseline after delivery, although generally not for several months. In cases of severe proliferative retinopathy, progression may lead to permanent deterioration in vision (11). Therefore, recommendations that are based on expert consensus or nonanalytic studies include a retinal examination 3 to 6 months before conception or, when pregnancy is unplanned, in the first trimester. Whether to repeat a retinal examination in the second or third trimester should depend on the level of diabetic retinopathy detected in the preconception period or first trimester (11). Laser photocoagulation is the treatment of choice for severe nonproliferative diabetic retinopathy or proliferative diabetic retinopathy. Anti–vascular endothelial growth factor medications should be avoided. Very few data on the treatment of macular edema during pregnancy exist, but one study suggested that it can be deferred until after delivery (12).

Nephropathy

Like retinopathy, mild disturbances in renal function, such as microalbuminuria, frequently progress during pregnancy, with return to baseline after delivery. An abnormal microalbumin:creatinine ratio in the preconception period is associated with an increased risk of both pregnancy-induced hypertension and preeclampsia. Patients with known renal insufficiency are at an increased risk for a permanent decrease in glomerular filtration rate (GFR), including the need for renal replacement therapy (13). Because both angiotensin-converting enzyme (ACE) inhibitors and angiotensin receptor blockers (ARBs) are contraindicated during pregnancy, women who are planning to conceive and who are taking these medications as renal protective agents and for the treatment of hypertension should be transitioned to antihypertensive agents that are safe for use during pregnancy. Women with microalbuminuria who are normotensive should discontinue ACE inhibitors and ARBs through the end of pregnancy and lactation.

Neuropathy

In general, neuropathy does not worsen appreciably during pregnancy; however, gastroparesis can be associated with severe nausea and vomiting, especially during the first trimester. Conservative therapy, including prevention of dehydration and hypoglycemia, is optimal. Many antiemetics, including ondansetron, are associated with risks to the fetus and should be avoided unless the benefits clearly outweigh the risks.

Cardiovascular Disease

There are few reviews about the incidence or prevalence of coronary artery or other macrovascular complications of diabetes during pregnancy, and most information is in the form of case reports. However, one article that addressed myocardial infarction in women with type 1 diabetes during pregnancy or the peripeural period noted a very high maternal and fetal mortality rate (14). Although no RCTs have addressed this issue, the Pregnancy Summary of Evidence and Consensus Recommendations for Care recommend screening with a resting electrocardiogram for women with diabetes >35 years of age or for those who are of reproductive age with symptoms or signs of cardiovascular disease during a careful history or physical examination (15).

Hyperlipidemia

The use of statins is contraindicated during pregnancy. Moreover, normal maternal cholesterol levels are elevated during pregnancy independent of baseline levels or comorbidities such as diabetes. However, a baseline lipid panel should be obtained in the preconception period to identify any woman with very-high levels of triglycerides (>1000 mg/dL) so that treatment of hypertriglyceridemia can be optimized before conception (16).

Thyroid Disease

Screening for and treatment of thyroid disease will be discussed separately in this session.

SUPPLEMENTS/MEDICATIONS FOR THE PRECONCEPTION PERIOD

Women with diabetes who are planning to conceive should begin taking folic acid supplements. Although folic acid is known to reduce the risk of neural tube defects, the optimal dose has not been determined in RCTs. Many practitioners recommend 600 to 800 μg/d, although the 400 μg found in prenatal vitamins likely is effective. The US Preventive Services Task Force recommends the use of low-dose aspirin (75 mg) during pregnancy in women at high risk for preeclampsia (17). Because women with pregestational diabetes have an increased risk of preeclampsia, low-dose aspirin should be started in the preconception period or at the first antenatal visit. Finally, because of the increased risk of hypoglycemia, especially during the first trimester, the use of glucagon should be reviewed and prescriptions renewed during a preconception or first antenatal visit.

MAIN CONCLUSIONS

Optimizing glycemic control for women in the preconception period remains challenging for several reasons, including noncompliance or nonadherence to management recommendations. Moreover, few RCTs have assessed optimal glycemic targets, insulin delivery systems or regimens, or methods for monitoring glucose. Health care providers depend on the consensus opinions from the Endocrine Society, American Diabetes Association, and American Congress of Obstetricians and Gynecologists to aid in management decisions. Moreover, not all patients have access to all treatments, with the more expensive and technologically advanced therapies and devices often being restricted to those who are well-resourced or well-insured. Health care providers should discuss maternal and fetal risks of pregnancy in a way that is compassionate and culturally sensitive to maximize adherence. Finally, achieving glycemic targets alone is insufficient preparation for pregnancy. Complications of diabetes should be screened, and comorbidities should be stabilized before conception to increase the likelihood for positive outcomes for the mother and her infant.

CASES

Case 1

You have been caring for a 34-year-old woman with a 16-year history of type 1 diabetes. At a routine visit, she tells you that she would like to try to become pregnant. She uses both an insulin pump and a CGM. Three months ago, her hemoglobin A_{1c} was 8.0%. Eighteen months ago, she was the driver in a single-car motor vehicle accident that was believed to be due to a severe hypoglycemic episode. Six months ago, she had two other episodes of hypoglycemia at work where she required the assistance of another person. To reduce both maternal and fetal risks, your advice to the patient includes

A. No changes to her regimen at this time; maintain her hemoglobin A_{1c} at 8%
B. Attempt to lower her hemoglobin A_{1c} to ≤6% but to cease driving
C. Change from insulin pump to MDIs with neutral protamine Hagedorn (NPH) and insulin lispro
D. Lower her hemoglobin A_{1c} to <7% and ideally <6.5% if she has no further episodes of severe hypoglycemia
E. Attempt to lower her hemoglobin A_{1c} to ≤6.0% but not until she has obtained a service dog that detects hypoglycemia

Case 2

One of your patients with a history of well-controlled type 1 diabetes for 15 years (most recent hemoglobin A_{1c} = 6.2%) tells you that she would like to become pregnant. She is 32 years old and has a history of very mild background retinopathy (rare microaneurysms occasionally reported by her ophthalmologist, the most recent being 4 months ago) and a urine albumin:creatinine ratio between 25 and 35 at most visits (normal ≤ 30). She is normotensive and takes lisinopril 10 mg/d. You advise her to

A. Avoid becoming pregnant until her hemoglobin A_{1c} is <5.5% so that further progression of her microvascular complications can be avoided
B. Avoid pregnancy because of the high likelihood of permanent vision loss or decrease in her GFR
C. Stop lisinopril
D. Stop lisinopril and begin labetalol 100 mg twice a day
E. Stop lisinopril and begin losartan 25 mg daily

Case 3

You are comanaging with the maternal-fetal medicine group a patient with type 2 diabetes who is now in her ninth week of pregnancy. She had been seen by a general obstetrician who transferred her care to you. Because of treatment failure with oral agents several years ago, the patient has controlled her diabetes with twice daily insulin detemir and premeal insulin aspart. At her first visit 2 weeks ago, her hemoglobin A_{1c} was 6.4%. The obstetrician had given her glucose targets of <90 mg/dL fasting and <120 mg/dL 2 hours postprandially. Her glucose log shows fasting values between 95 and 105 mg/dL, occasional postprandial dinner values of 130 to 135 mg/dL, and frequent moderate hypoglycemia between meals (45 to 60 mg/dL). In addition, the patient reports that her partner had to call the emergency medical technicians one morning when she could not be awakened from sleep. A capillary glucose measurement shortly thereafter was 28 mg/dL. The single best change in her management at this point is which of the following:

A. Change her insulin management to MDIs using NPH and regular insulin
B. Increase her glycemic targets slightly such that hypoglycemia is avoided
C. Increase her overnight insulin detemir dose to lower the incidence of fasting hyperglycemia
D. Increase her dinner bolus to lower the incidence of postprandial hyperglycemia
E. Prescribe a CGM

DISCUSSION OF CASES AND ANSWERS

Case 1

The correct answer is D, "Lower her hemoglobin A_{1c} to <7% and ideally <6.5% if she has no further episodes of severe hypoglycemia." When answering this question, one should remember that no RCTs have specifically addressed this issue and that weighing risks and benefits often is important for the individual patient. Answer A is incorrect because maintaining a hemoglobin A_{1c} of 8% places the fetus and infant at risk for congenital malformations and macrosomia, which lead to additional maternal complications during delivery. This patient is at risk for a serious hypoglycemic episode with her history of a motor vehicle accident and hypoglycemia unawareness. As her health care provider, it is prudent to realize the specific risks that she may have when driving. However, traumatic accidents as a result of a serious hypoglycemic event are not limited to those that occur when driving; therefore, answer B is also incorrect. Because the use of CSII may allow for more-intensive control with less risk for a severe hypoglycemic episode compared with MDIs, answer C would not be correct. Although service dogs that detect hypoglycemia can be a useful adjunct in the prevention of serious episodes and are currently popular, limited data support their use. In addition, answer E is not an option that would be widely available to all patients because of financial or practical constraints. The guidelines from most major organizations target a hemoglobin A_{1c} < 6.5% or as close to normal as possible in the preconception period if hypoglycemia can be avoided. In this patient with known serious hypoglycemia and a history of morbidity as a result, a hemoglobin A_{1c} < 7% may be more desirable (16).

Case 2

The correct answer is C, "Stop lisinopril." Women with mild background retinopathy and/or microalbuminuria are likely to experience progression of their microvascular disease during pregnancy; however, in nearly all cases, these conditions will revert to baseline after pregnancy. If, however, microvascular complications are advanced, such as proliferative diabetic retinopathy or a decreased GFR, the patient is at risk for permanent worsening of her condition. There is no evidence that lowering hemoglobin A_{1c} to the nondiabetic range in the preconception period will have an impact on microvascular complications in the short term; therefore, answer A is incorrect. Likewise, because this patient's microvascular disease is mild, answer B is also incorrect. For women who have microalbuminuria but are normotensive, current guidelines suggest that medications used to prevent progression of renal disease, such as ACE inhibitors and ARBs, can be stopped without substituting another therapy unless hypertension develops during pregnancy. Therefore, answer C is correct, as opposed to D and E. Answer E is also incorrect because ARBs, like ACE inhibitors, are contraindicated during pregnancy.

Case 3

The correct answer is B, "Increase her glycemic targets slightly such that hypoglycemia is avoided." Although answers C and D ultimately may be beneficial in helping this patient to maintain acceptable glucose control during pregnancy, her greatest risk of immediate harm is due to her history of hypoglycemia during the first trimester, including a severe episode; therefore, the correct answer is B. She should be counseled that moderation of her glucose targets might be acceptable, especially for the short term, because she is already meeting the target for pregnancy in women with diabetes (hemoglobin $A_{1c} < 6.5\%$) and at the lowest risk for congenital malformations in the fetus (hemoglobin $A_{1c} < 7.0\%$). On the other hand, hypoglycemia with traumatic injury could bring harm to both her and her fetus. There is no evidence that NPH is superior to insulin analogs for the prevention of hypoglycemia; therefore, answer A is incorrect. There are very limited data about the use of CGM in patients with type 2 diabetes and inconclusive data about their prevention of hypoglycemia during pregnancy. Although answer E may be a correct choice in the future, at this time not enough evidence warrants it as an option for this patient.

REFERENCES

1. Wahabi HA, Alzeidan RA, Bawazeer GA, Alansari LA, Esmaeil SA. Preconception care for diabetic women for improving maternal and fetal outcomes: a systematic review and meta-analysis. *BMC Pregnancy Childbirth.* 2010;**10**(1):63.
2. Holing EV, Beyer CS, Brown ZA, Connell FA. Why don't women with diabetes plan their pregnancies? *Diabetes Care.* 1998;**21**(6): 889–895.
3. Metzger BE, Lowe LP, Dyer AR, Trimble ER, Chaovarindr U, Coustan DR, Hadden DR, McCance DR, Hod M, McIntyre HD, Oats JJ, Persson B, Rogers MS, Sacks DA; HAPO Study Cooperative Research Group. Hyperglycemia and adverse pregnancy outcomes. *N Engl J Med.* 2008;**358**(19):1991–2002.
4. American Diabetes Association. 13. Management of diabetes in pregnancy. *Diabetes Care.* 2017;**40**(Suppl 1):S114–S119.
5. Ringholm L, Pedersen-Bjergaard U, Thorsteinsson B, Damm P, Mathiesen ER. Hypoglycaemia during pregnancy in women with Type 1 diabetes. *Diabet Med.* 2012;**29**(5):558–566.
6. Rey E, Attié C, Bonin A. The effects of first-trimester diabetes control on the incidence of macrosomia. *Am J Obstet Gynecol.* 1999;**181**(1): 202–206.
7. Bode BW, Steed RD, Davidson PC. Reduction in severe hypoglycemia with long-term continuous subcutaneous insulin infusion in type I diabetes. *Diabetes Care.* 1996;**19**(4):324–327.
8. Moy FM, Ray A, Buckley BS, West HM. Techniques of monitoring blood glucose during pregnancy for women with pre-existing diabetes. *Cochrane Database Syst Rev.* 2017;**6**:CD009613.
9. Hernandez TL, Barbour LA. A standard approach to continuous glucose monitor data in pregnancy for the study of fetal growth and infant outcomes. *Diabetes Technol Ther.* 2013;**15**(2):172–179.
10. Kovatchev B, Tamborlane WV, Cefalu WT, Cobelli C. The artificial pancreas in 2016: a digital treatment ecosystem for diabetes. *Diabetes Care.* 2016;**39**(7):1123–1126.
11. Morrison JL, Hodgson LAB, Lim LL, Al-Qureshi S. Diabetic retinopathy in pregnancy: a review. *Clin Experiment Ophthalmol.* 2016;**44**(4): 321–334.
12. American Academy of Ophthalmology Retina/Vitreous Panel. Preferred Practice Guidelines. Available at: https://www.aao.org/clinical-statement/screening-diabetic-retinopathy. Accessed 1 November, 2017.
13. Biesenbach G, Stöger H, Zazgornik J. Influence of pregnancy on progression of diabetic nephropathy and subsequent requirement of renal replacement therapy in female type I diabetic patients with impaired renal function. *Nephrol Dial Transplant.* 1992;**7**(2): 105–109.
14. Gordon MC, Landon MB, Boyle J, Stewart KS, Gabbe SG. Coronary artery disease in insulin-dependent diabetes mellitus of pregnancy (class H): a review of the literature. *Obstet Gynecol Surv.* 1996;**51**(7): 437–444.
15. Kitzmiller JL, Block JM, Brown FM, Catalano PM, Conway DL, Coustan DR, Gunderson EP, Herman WH, Hoffman LD, Inturrisi M, Jovanovic LB, Kjos SI, Knopp RH, Montoro MN, Ogata ES, Paramsothy P, Reader DM, Rosenn BM, Thomas AM, Kirkman MS. Managing preexisting diabetes for pregnancy: summary of evidence and consensus recommendations for care. *Diabetes Care.* 2008;**31**(5):1060–1079.
16. Feldman AZ, Brown FM. Brown FM. Management of type 1 diabetes in pregnancy. *Curr Diab Rep.* 2016;**16**(8):76–90.
17. US Preventive Services Task Force. Final recommendation statement: low-dose aspirin use for the prevention of morbidity and mortality from preeclampsia: preventive medication. Available at: www.uspreventiveservicestaskforce.org/Page/Document/RecommendationStatementFinal/low-dose-aspirin-use-for-the-prevention-of-morbidity-and-mortality-from-preeclampsia-preventive-medication. Accessed 1 November, 2017.

Designing a Treatment Plan for Patients With T2DM

M25
Presented, March 17–20, 2018

Jane E. B. Reusch, MD. Department of Medicine, Division of Endocrinology, Metabolism and Diabetes, University of Colorado School of Medicine, Aurora, Colorado 80045, E-mail: jane.reusch@ucdenver.edu

Jack Leahy, MD. Department of Medicine and Division of Endocrinology, University of Vermont College of Medicine, South Burlington, Vermont 05403, E-mail: jleahy@uvm.edu

SIGNIFICANCE OF THE CLINICAL PROBLEM

Diabetes is estimated to affect 30.3 million people in the United States and 422 million people worldwide. Prediabetes is estimated to affect ~80 million people in the United States (1). The staggering increase in the prevalence of diabetes is a consequence of changes in society favoring high-caloric density, poor-quality food and decreased physical activity and increased sedentary behavior. As such, many individuals presenting with type 2 diabetes mellitus (T2DM) have a predominant contribution from a lifestyle that could be termed "diabetogenic." The profound increase in diabetes in the United States and worldwide presents a major burden to those with the disease, their families, and the economies in which they live. Diabetes is currently the leading cause of blindness, amputation, end-stage renal disease, and foot ulcer in the United States (1). In addition, despite significant improvements in cardiovascular outcomes overall, diabetes still imparts a two- to fourfold increase in cardiovascular disease (CVD) risk. The estimated cost of diabetes in the United States in 2012 was $214 billion.

Effective treatment of diabetes requires a multifactorial focus on blood glucose control, blood pressure control, cholesterol treatment, and psychosocial support. Individuals with diabetes and their families need to be fully engaged in strategies for the prevention or treatment of diabetes. Specifically, most individuals who have had diabetes for greater than a few years will require medications for glucose, blood pressure, and cholesterol. For the health care provider treating patients with diabetes and other, concomitant medical conditions, helping to enable a patient to effectively manage all aspects of their diabetes care can be daunting. One of the most challenging barriers—perhaps the most challenging—is to provide resources to patients in order to support them for behavior change related to lifestyle. The health care provider needs to understand the resources within their medical system, in terms of dietitian and Certified Diabetes Educator® (CDE) support, as adjuvants to the traditional patient–provider interaction. One of the most useful strategies is to work with patients and their families to educate them on the cause and consequence of diabetes-related complications, to establish goals, and to discuss the tools and behaviors that will be necessary to accomplish these goals. It is then possible for the provider and the patient to lay out a series of steps, sometimes using a milestone approach, to achieve the agreed-on goals and to measure outcomes. The tactics that are first laid out to achieve these goals may not be successful; both the provider and the individual with diabetes may need to revise the plan to get to goal and prevent diabetes-related complications. The main aim of this presentation is to present a series of typical patients with T2DM, and to present strategies (and alternatives) for successful management.

BARRIERS TO OPTIMAL PRACTICE

- Diabetes management requires engagement by the patient and substantial patient-executed diabetes self-management. Behavior change is difficult, particularly in terms of lifestyle in which there are many barriers to change including habitual low physical activity and poor nutrition. In addition, T2DM carries a social stigma that may interfere with diabetes self-management choices such as glucose monitoring and insulin injection outside of the home.
- Simultaneous treatment of blood glucose, blood pressure, cholesterol, and other comorbid conditions is commonly related to polypharmacy, high cost, side effects, and lack of self-efficacy. Patients are often labeled noncompliant despite taking 10 to 12 medicines as directed and attempting complex glucose-management strategies.

LEARNING OBJECTIVES

As a result of participating in this session, learners should be able to

- Have an effective discussion with the patient about strategies to increase physical activity and improve high-quality nutrition, even on a budget
- Understand the interaction between family history and obesity.
- Appreciate the impact of physical activity on glucose metabolism, CVD risk, and all-cause mortality
- Have a strategy to use all resources within their health care system to provide support for changes in diet and augmentation of physical activity
- Use dietitians and CDEs to support physical activity and dietary recommendations
- Encourage creativity in patient-centered tactics and resources to optimize behavior change

- Respect the interaction of socioeconomic status and depression with adherence to lifestyle recommendations
- Appreciate the critical importance of multifactorial CVD risk prevention in adults and youth with diabetes and the use of preclinic screening tools to identify CVD risk assessments and interventions needed for each individual
- Identify opportunities for risk factor modification using the electronic medical record to assess interventions and outcomes
- Own the importance of lifestyle as a seminal component of aggressive CVD risk factor reduction

STRATEGIES FOR DIAGNOSIS, THERAPY, AND/OR MANAGEMENT

The following is based on the American Diabetes Association (ADA) 2017 standards of care (2, 3).

The initial evaluation of an individual that is newly diagnosed with diabetes includes a medical history, a physical examination, and a laboratory evaluation (2). This information allows the clinician to have a well-informed conversation with the patient about the priorities and goals of treatment. Any important findings from a comprehensive diabetes evaluation will be addressed with the primary care provider. For the purpose of this book, we will focus on a simple, uncomplicated patient and on step-wise management.

COMPONENTS OF THE COMPREHENSIVE DIABETES MEDICAL EVALUATION

Medical History

- Age and characteristics of onset of diabetes (*e.g.*, diabetic ketoacidosis, asymptomatic laboratory finding)
- Eating patterns, nutritional status, weight history, sleep behaviors (pattern and duration), and physical activity habits; nutrition education; and behavioral support history and needs
- Complementary and alternative medicine use
- Presence of common comorbidities and dental disease
- Screen for depression, anxiety, and disordered eating using validated and appropriate measures (3)
- Screen for diabetes distress using validated and appropriate measures (3)
- Screen for psychosocial problems and other barriers to diabetes self-management, such as limited financial, logistical, and support resources
- History of tobacco use, alcohol consumption, and substance use
- Diabetes education, self-management, and support history and needs
- Review of previous treatment regimens and response to therapy (A1C records)
- Assess medication-taking behaviors and barriers to medication adherence
- Results of glucose monitoring and patient's use of data
- Diabetic ketoacidosis frequency, severity, and cause
- Hypoglycemia episodes awareness, frequency, and causes
- History of increased blood pressure, abnormal lipids
- Microvascular complications: retinopathy, nephropathy, and neuropathy (sensory, including history of foot lesions; and autonomic, including sexual dysfunction and gastroparesis)
- Macrovascular complications: coronary heart disease, cerebrovascular disease, and peripheral arterial disease
- For women with childbearing capacity, review contraception and preconception planning

Physical Examination

- Height, weight, and body mass index (BMI); growth and pubertal development in children and adolescents
- Blood pressure determination, including orthostatic measurements when indicated
- Examination of teeth and gums (should have formal dental examination)
- Fundoscopic examination (should have referral for formal retinal screening)
- Thyroid palpation
- Skin examination (*e.g.*, for acanthosis nigricans, insulin injection, or infusion set insertion sites)
- Comprehensive foot examination: inspection, palpation of dorsalis pedis and posterior tibial pulses, presence/absence of patellar and Achilles reflexes
- Neurologic examination: determination of proprioception, vibration, and monofilament sensation

Laboratory Evaluation

- A1C, if the results are not available within the past 3 months
- If not performed/available within the past year:
  - Fasting lipid profile, including total low- and high-density lipoprotein cholesterol and triglycerides, as needed
  - Liver function tests
  - Spot urinary albumin–to–creatinine ratio
  - Serum creatinine and estimated glomerular filtration rate
  - Thyroid antibodies (this is a cost-effective replacement from the ADA recommendation of thyroid-stimulating immunoglobulin)

PATIENT-CENTERED CARE

Lifestyle Management

In people predisposed to the development of T2DM, the most common precursor is a lifestyle involving excess calories plus a combination of sedentary behavior and limited physical activity. Based on the relationship between lifestyle and the development of diabetes, there is a certain blame or guilt associated with T2DM. It is crucial for the patient to understand that improving lifestyle will offer critical benefits for metabolic control, CVD risk, and longevity, as well as increase the responsiveness of glucose, blood pressure, and cholesterol to medicines. It is our opinion that a patient's feelings of guilt related to causing one's own diabetes must be discussed formally and set aside. It is helpful for the patient to understand that it is the interaction between genetics and lifestyle that led to the diabetes. It is also crucial, early in a trusting patient–provider relationship, to outline the progressive nature of T2DM, even in the context of highly effective changes in diet and physical activity. In addition, it should be emphasized that early adoption of effective changes in diet and physical activity will make the management of diabetes more straightforward for the rest of the patient's life.

Diabetes Self-Management Education and Support

Making alterations in diet and exercise is a fundamental aspect of overall diabetes care. This is perhaps the most difficult aspect of diabetes management and the least well executed. There are 8760 hours in a year. Most patients see a provider four times a year for up to an hour (0.04566% of the year). This calculation illustrates that it is unrealistic for a provider to expect outstanding outcomes unless individuals with diabetes are motivated or engaged in managing their diabetes. The terms diabetes self-management education (DSME) and diabetes self-management support (DSMS) refer to strategies that enable effective and persistent diabetes self-management. The initial step is an open conversation between the patient and the provider to assess the patient's beliefs, goals, resources, medical literacy, and ability to actively engage in self-management. The next step in DSME/DSMS is to provide patients with the tools they will need to be "in charge" of their own diabetes.

The formal recommendations for DSME/DSMS include a recommendation that all people with diabetes participate in a DSME/DSMS program that will "facilitate the knowledge, skills, and ability necessary for diabetes self-care and in diabetes self-management support to assist with implementing and sustaining skills and behaviors needed for ongoing self-management, both at diagnosis and as needed thereafter (Level B)" (3). The literature suggests that effective DSME/DSMS should enable the patient to have improved quality of life and health status. There is excellent evidence that patient-centered DSME/DSMS is more effective when it is respectful and responsive to individual patient preferences and values. It would follow, based on improved outcomes, that DSME/DSMS should reduce costs and improve outcomes (3). Based on cost effectiveness, a new benefit under Medicare supports DSME/DSMS for diabetes prevention; however, DSME/DSMS for people with diabetes is variably available and inconsistently reimbursed. It is recommended that DSME/DSMS be (1) provided to patients at diagnosis, (2) reassessed at an annual visit, and (3) reintroduced at transition of care and if a new complication occurs that alters life and self-efficacy.

Medical Nutrition Therapy

One of the burning questions on the mind of most people with diabetes is What should I eat? The valid answer is that there is no specific "diabetic diet." The lack of a specific diabetic diet is both empowering and overwhelming to people with diabetes and providers. The central message is that people with a lifetime ahead of them with diabetes have choices, and that no food item is bad or not allowed. The obesity literature is replete with behavioral data indicating that negative messaging about food and strict low-calorie diets designed for weight loss are not sustainable without considerable support. Based on the weight-loss literature and a series of different diabetic diets over the last decades, the messaging around food has moved to common sense: Eat food with high nutritional value that is not processed and with portion control. Or, to quote Michael Pollan's nondiabetes book *In Defense of Food: An Eater's Manifesto* (4), "Eat food, not so much, mainly plants." Food, as described by Pollan, is something your grandmother would recognize (*i.e.*, not processed).

General Rules for Medical Nutrition Therapy for Individuals With Diabetes

The overall objective is to facilitate improved nutritional status using nonjudgmental messaging and reinforcing moderate and sustainable behavior change (3).

Promote healthy eating habits
- Eat nutrient-dense foods (vegetables, fruits, whole grains, nuts, and lean meats)
- Replace refined sugars with natural ones (fruits)
- Understand portion sizes and use strategies to minimize overeating

Emphasize the benefits of individualized nutrition therapy
- Healthy body weight
- Appropriate glycemic, lipids, and blood pressure
- Prevent/delay diabetic complications

Consider individual nutritional needs based on
- Personal preferences
- Cultural/religious/familial norms
- Socioeconomic status
- Health literacy
- Access to a variety of healthy foods
- Willingness to change diet and behavioral habits
- Willingness of family/friends to help with behavioral/dietary changes

Address other health issues
- Nondietary unhealthy habits (smoking, alcohol consumption, drug use)
- Use one-on-one interactions with the patient and family to address not only nutrition but all aspects of lifestyle

The next critical step in medical nutrition therapy is to provide robust education around carbohydrates and portion control. Useful additional guidance might regard carbohydrate intake through whole grains and not sugar-sweetened foods, and the consideration of a Mediterranean-based or DASH (Dietary Approaches to Stop Hypertension)-based diet. If overweight, the patient should aim to start losing 5% to 10% of body weight using calorie restriction.

Physical Activity

Physical activity is a cornerstone of diabetes management. Physical activity is defined as vigorous, moderate, light, standing, and sitting. In the exercise literature, these definitions are aligned with certain metabolic equivalents, or energy utilization per unit time. Interventional studies such as the Diabetes Prevention Program (DPP) have demonstrated that increasing physical activity in combination with dietary changes that reduce bodyweight by 3% to 5% can prevent diabetes. Across the United States and around the world, there is inadequate engagement in physical activity. People with prediabetes and diabetes most commonly have very low levels of physical activity at diagnosis. As such, the introduction of physical activity as an effective behavior change requires support and education. The DPP study, which was conducted in individuals with impaired glucose tolerance, engaged in a number of tactics including coaching, formal opportunities for supervised exercise, group exercise activities, and rewards. Importantly, Medicare has recently approved a DPP-based intervention for people with prediabetes. It is unfortunate that similar health plan–covered services to support a physical activity lifestyle change are not routinely available for people with diabetes. Encouragement and coaching to increase safe and effective increases in physical activity fall under the rubric of DSME/DSMS.

The Physical Activity Guidelines for Americans endorse the following activity levels for people with or without diabetes:

- Youth: Children and adolescents with type 1 diabetes mellitus (T1DM), T2DM, and prediabetes should engage in 60 min/d or more of moderate- or vigorous-intensity aerobic activity, with vigorous muscle-strengthening and bone-strengthening activities at least 3 d/wk.
- Adults: Most adults with T1DM, T2DM, and prediabetes should engage in 150 minutes or more of moderate- to vigorous-intensity physical activity per week, spread over at least 3 d/wk, with no more than 2 consecutive days without activity. Shorter durations (minimum of 75 min/wk) of vigorous-intensity or interval training may be sufficient for younger and more physically fit individuals. Adults with T1DM, T2DM, and prediabetes should engage in two to three sessions per week of resistance exercise on nonconsecutive days. Flexibility training and balance training are recommended two to three times per week for older adults with diabetes.
- Sedentary behavior: All people with T1DM, T2DM, and prediabetes should decrease sedentary behavior, specifically by limiting screen time, interrupting sitting, and increasing standing time.

Cardiorespiratory Fitness Predicts Cardiovascular and All-Cause Mortality

An additional argument for interventions to augment physical activity and cardiorespiratory fitness in people with prediabetes and diabetes comes from the epidemiological literature. In people with and without diabetes, cardiorespiratory fitness is a primary prognosticator of cardiovascular and all-cause mortality. Our research group and others have demonstrated a 20% to 30% decrease in cardiorespiratory fitness in sedentary people with diabetes compared with individuals without diabetes matched for physical activity, weight, and age (5–8). Simply stated, diabetes *per se* leads to an impairment in cardiorespiratory fitness that is observed in youth and adults with T1DM and T2DM. Cohort studies in both T1DM and T2DM indicate a positive relationship between cardiorespiratory fitness and outcomes. Interventional studies have yet to demonstrate a benefit on cardiovascular outcomes but have demonstrated improvements in cognition, functional status, diabetes self-efficacy, and, in most cases, metabolism.

Pharmacologic Therapy

The main focus of this presentation is nonpharmacologic strategies for prediabetes and T2DM. However, optimal care also usually requires a discussion with the patient regarding the many diabetes drugs that are available, helping them choose what decision points are most important to them. In addition, diabetes treatment guidelines around the world are being adjusted to incorporate new information about the effectiveness, side effects and safety profiles, cost, and prevention of diabetes end-organ complications related to the various agents.

Effectiveness

On average, oral medications tend to be less effective at lowering A1C levels (usually <1% reduction) than injection medications [both insulin and glucagon-like peptide-1 (GLP-1) receptor agonists, alone or in combination]. Not only do these injectable medications result in much larger reductions in A1C depending on the baseline A1C level, but basal insulin and GLP-1 receptor agonists are reasonably similar in terms of A1C lowering when used as the first injectable. Thus, with an A1C level of mid to high 7s, adding an oral medication is reasonable. With A1C values of 8% and above, adding one of the injection medications makes the most sense, although occasionally, adding two or more oral medications can bring a high A1C level to goal.

Weight Effect

The traditional diabetes medications of sulfonylurea, thiazolidinediones, and insulin are often associated with weight gain. A particularly desirable feature for many patients is choosing a "weight-sparing" medication such as a GLP-1 receptor agonist or sodium-glucose cotransporter-2 (SGLT2) inhibitor.

Risk of Hypoglycemia

This issue came to the forefront when the DPP-4 inhibitor agents became available, as a differentiating feature from sulfonylureas. The higher death rate in the intensively treated group of the ACCORD trial, which was initially assumed to be based on the hypoglycemia incidence, furthered the concern over drug-induced hypoglycemia. Many subsequent epidemiologic studies have linked a higher rate of hypoglycemia in persons with diabetes to a variety of poor or dangerous clinical outcomes, as well as a higher use of emergency room and hospital services. The consequence is a widely agreed-on goal that safe diabetes therapy minimizes as much as possible the risk of hypoglycemia. This feature is most closely linked to DPP-4 inhibitors, GLP-1 receptor agonists, and SGLT2 inhibitors, although their protective effect is minimized when any of these agents is used in combination with "high-risk hypoglycemia agents" such as sulfonylureas and insulin. Also, a lowered risk of hypoglycemia is the major differentiating feature of analog insulins, especially the newer ultra-long analog insulins, vs human insulin.

Side Effects

The major fear of many patients when adding medication is the occurrence of an unpleasant, and occasionally serious, side effect. This concern is often worsened with relatively new agents when the amount of time they have been on the market or the prescriber's experience with that agent is minimal. In reality, we learn a lot about drug safety with a longer clinical experience, and unexpected side effects do pop up—important examples are the increased risk of congestive heart failure with some DPP-4 inhibitors and the heightened frequency of bone fractures in postmenopausal women with thiazolidinediones. In addition, the fear that some patients have over new drugs is often worsened by lawyer advertisements that focus on whatever infrequent side effect they can find (real or imagined), portraying it as medical malpractice. Current examples are pancreatitis with incretin agents and amputations with canagliflozin. This fear can cause patients not to fill a prescription or to stop it. As such, health care providers need to be fully up-to-date on the known side effects of the various agents, their relative frequencies, and what patient groups are most at risk.

Prescribing Guidelines

Allowable drugs and appropriate dosages are often based on a patient's health issues such as renal and cardiac function. Renal function is one of the most important, with DPP-4 inhibitors (at proper doses) and some of the GLP-1 receptor agonists allowable, even in patients with severe renal dysfunction. In contrast, SGLT2 inhibitors and metformin have specific renal function guidelines. Again, the health care provider must be familiar with the positive and negative effects of the various diabetes agents on various organ pathophysiologies (renal, cardiac, nonalcoholic steatohepatitis, gastrointestinal) to help the patient choose the most effective drug regimen.

Cost

The concept of factoring cost into the choice of drug therapy is easy to understand but, in practice, can be extremely complex unless the provider is working within a fully transparent system with easy-to-understand costs to the patient. A general rule of thumb is older drugs are cheaper than newer drugs. In reality, however, drug formularies, discount coupons, deductibles, and insurance types (Medicare, Medicaid, Veterans Affairs, private) all have important effects on a drug's cost, often making it hard to identify the most cost-effective agent for any patient. This means that health care providers (or someone in their office settings) must be aware of the formulary and costs of the common insurers in their area and may have to help the patient weigh the financial aspects of a therapy along with the health aspects.

Cardiovascular and Renal Protection

Perhaps the most discussed (and important) recent topic regarding drug therapy for T2DM relates to the CVD safety outcome trials for recent diabetes drugs (9). The U.S. Food and Drug Administration mandated in 2008 that all new diabetes medications in the United States must undergo dedicated and appropriately powered studies in persons at high risk for CVD to confirm cardiac safety. Essentially, the concept is that an increased risk of cardiac disease [typically considered a composite of new myocardial infarction, new stroke, or cardiac death, called a three-point major adverse cardiovascular event (3-point MACE)] is not an acceptable trade-off, no matter how good the diabetes drug otherwise is. These trials are intended to show cardiac *safety*; that is, the lack of a worsened CVD outcome vs a placebo or active comparator. However, the hope of the diabetes specialty community has been that a drug or a class of drugs that lowers cardiac risks will be identified; that is, cardiac *protection*. However, it is crucial to point out that few studies are powered for cardiac protection (only for CVD safety), and the results are relevant only to the studied population of persons with a high risk of CVD that is usually based on preexisting CVD. Recent studies have shown CVD safety (but not protection) with insulin glargine (ORIGIN trial) (10) and insulin degludec (DEVOTE trial) (11), as well with the GLP-1 receptor agonist lixisenatide (ELIXA trial) (12). Trials of DPP-4 inhibitors have also shown CVD safety based on the usual composite outcomes (*i.e.*, saxagliptin in the SAVOR-TIMI trial (13), alogliptin in the EXAMINE trial (14), and sitagliptin in the TECOS trial) (15), although the saxagliptin trial (13) and possibly the alogliptin trial showed a higher hospitalization rate for congestive heart failure.

Things changed dramatically in 2015, with the first trials not only showing cardiac safety but also causing stabilization of renal function in patients who had some element of nephropathy (16–18). As such, the treatment paradigm is rapidly changing toward using these agents in patients with preexisting CVD and/or nephropathy.

SGLT2 Inhibitors

1. The EMPA-REG OUTCOME trial randomized 7020 patients, all with known CVD, to placebo or one of two doses of empagliflozin for a median 3.1 years (19). It observed a 14% reduction in the composite 3-point MACE, with the main finding of dramatic reductions in CVD death and all-cause death. Also, unexpectedly, a 35% reduction in hospitalization for congestive heart failure was observed. These improvements were observed within a few weeks of starting empagliflozin. The EMPA-REG OUTCOME study also showed a stabilization of kidney disease in persons with preexisting modest chronic kidney disease with or without albuminuria (17).
2. The CANVAS and CANVAS-R trials compared canagliflozin vs placebo in persons with preexisting CVD (66%) or a high risk of CVD based on age and CVD risk factors. It noted a 14% reduction in 3-point MACE, although no single component of MACE dominated (16). Also observed was a 33% reduction in hospitalization for heart failure and a 40% reduction in a composite renal disease outcome. In contrast, an unexpected outcome was a twofold higher incidence of amputation (mostly toes or partial foot amputation, typically in patients with prior amputations or a known history of peripheral vascular disease) that had not been documented in trials with other SGLT2 inhibitors.
3. The CVD-REAL study is a real-world trial of SGLT2 inhibitor therapy (canagliflozin, dapagliflozin, and empagliflozin) vs other diabetes drugs in six countries (the United States, Denmark, Norway, Sweden, Germany, and the United Kingdom) (18). The major finding was a 40% reduction in heart failure and a 50% reduction in all-cause death with the SGLT inhibitors.
4. In summary, a class effect of SGLT2 inhibitors appears to be a dramatic and rapid reduction in clinically important heart failure, as well as the onset and progression of chronic renal disease in persons with T2DM and preexisting end-organ disease. Also likely is an important reduction in overall death. Importantly, the relevance of these effects in patients without preexisting CVD or renal disease is unknown.

GLP-1 Receptor Agonists

1. The ELIXA trial showed cardiac safety but failed to show cardiac protection with the short-acting GLP-1 receptor agonist lixisenatide (12). It is unknown whether this failure to show protection was impacted by the trial's patient population, which was at particular high risk for additional CVD.
2. The LEADER trial randomized 9340 patients with known CVD (81%) or risk factors for CVD to liraglutide or placebo for a median of 3.8 years (20). It observed a 13% reduction in the composite 3-point MACE with liraglutide. In contrast to SGLT2 inhibitors, there was no reduction in hospitalization for congestive heart failure. In addition, CVD protection was seen for a much longer period as compared with SGLT2 inhibitors (12 to 18 months), suggesting that the mechanism is a reduction in the atherosclerosis pathogenesis. Like SGLT2 inhibitors, a 22% lowering in a composite renal outcome was seen with liraglutide, with the major effect being a reduction in new-onset microalbuminuria (21).
3. The SUSTAIN 6 trial randomized 3297 T2DM patients with known CVD or high risk of CVD to placebo or two doses of semaglutide for a median of 2 years (22). Unlike the other trials, this is not a dedicated CVD outcome trial with the requisite number of CVD events, but is a combination of phase 3 registration trials for semaglutide. Also, semaglutide is an unusually potent GLP-1 receptor agonist in terms of weight loss and A1C lowering, so there were large differences in these outcomes between the semaglutide and placebo groups. Trial investigators reported a 26% reduction in a 3-point MACE outcome with semaglutide, with the most dramatic effect being a 39% reduction in nonfatal stroke, as well as a 36% reduction in new or worsened nephropathy. In contrast, a 76% increase in retinopathy was observed in the semaglutide group, believed (based on the potency of this agent) to reflect the well-known effect of rapidly improving glycemia to transiently worsen preexisting retinopathy.
4. The EXSCEL trial randomized 14,752 T2DM patients with known CVD (73%) or high risk of CVD to placebo or weekly exenatide for a median of 3.2 years (23). It reported a 9% reduction in a 3-point MACE outcome with exenatide, but this rate barely missed statistical significance, so this was a negative safety trial.
5. In summary, some but not all GLP-1 receptor agonists have been shown to lower CVD risks and nephropathy. Whether or not this is a class effect is unclear. In contrast to SGLT2 inhibitors, this effect takes much longer to occur (more than a year), and there has been no observed protection against heart failure.

MAIN CONCLUSIONS REGARDING EFFECTIVE NONPHARMACOLOGIC THERAPY FOR PREDIABETES AND T2DM

These should be congruent with the learning objectives.

1. Diabetes represents a lifelong disease that requires effective and reinforced education and support for diabetes self-management.
2. The systemic sequelae of diabetes, including microvascular and macrovascular complications, requires a

multifaceted intervention consisting of strategies to manage glucose, cholesterol, hypertension, and lifestyle.

3. Effective support of lifestyle interventions requires rigorous education and reinforcement in nutrition, the safe and effective augmentation of physical activity, and decreases in sedentary time.
4. Regardless of the stage of diabetes or the medications required for glucose control, people with diabetes need a lifelong focus on diabetes self-management, medical nutrition therapy, and physical activity.
5. Providers and systems of care need to support dietitians, CDEs, and exercise physiologists to enable the successful execution of effective lifestyle management for diabetes.

MAIN CONCLUSIONS REGARDING EFFECTIVE PHARMACOLOGIC THERAPY FOR T2DM

1. T2DM involves the progressive loss of β-cell function and insulin resistance, which, in most people with over 10 years of diabetes mellitus, will require medications for optimal glucose control.
2. The need for medications is not a failure on the part of the patient or the provider.
3. There is compelling evidence that early intensive blood glucose control in uncomplicated T2DM confers long-term benefit.
4. Personalized care is needed due to the increased number of medications that have differing glucose-lowering efficacies, weight effects, risks of hypoglycemia, costs, and cardiovascular benefits.
5. Combination therapy, using agents with different mechanisms of action, is effective and durable and should be considered in people with A1C levels >8%.
6. Allowing glucose control to deteriorate before adding another agent is ineffective and should be avoided.
7. Having a CDE or other provider support a patient in the initiation and titration of GLP-1 receptor agonists and insulin is crucial for patient acceptance and long-term adherence.

CASES WITH QUESTIONS AND ANSWERS

Case 1

27-year-old Spanish-American female
Fasting blood sugar (FBS) 135 mg/dL
Past medical history: G2P2 9 lb 2 oz, 10 lb 1 oz, with no mention of gestational diabetes or glucose
Family history of hypertension, diabetes mellitus with end-stage renal disease, and congestive heart failure
126/77, 88, 18 (99% room air), BMI 32
A1C 7.2%

Where do we start?

A. Diet and physical activity
B. Diet and physical activity plus basal insulin
C. Diet and physical activity plus metformin
D. Diet and physical activity plus basal/bolus insulin
E. Diet and physical activity plus prandial insulin

First 2 years:
Began walking with a neighborhood group for 45 minutes three times per week (reinforced by a pedometer).
Took a cooking class at the ADA.
Became a community wellness volunteer.
Switched from 12- to 8-inch dinner plate (no refills).
BMI 29; FBS 88 mg/dL; A1C 6.2%.

Point

When baseline behavior is diabetogenic, doable, minor behavior changes work very well.

Case 2

62-year-old African-American Banker presents after a community screen reveals FBS 198; A1C 7.8; total cholesterol 210; high-density lipoprotein 30; triglycerides 250; low-density lipoprotein 130; microalbumin-to-creatinine ratio 41.
Past medical history: hypertension (hydrochlorthiazide average blood pressure 130/75); degenerative joint disease–nonsteroidal anti-inflammatory drugs
Social history: married 4 children, occasional alcohol consumption, no tobacco use
Lifestyle: works out five times per week and diet is excellent (spouse had coronary artery bypass graft 3 years ago)

Point

Diabetes is a progressive disease that will require medication plus lifestyle changes.

What is next?

A. Lifestyle
B. Lifestyle plus basal/bolus insulin
C. Lifestyle plus insulin and GLP-1 receptor agonist
D. Lifestyle plus insulin pump
E. Lifestyle plus metformin

REFERENCES

1. National Diabetes Statistics Report, 2017: Estimates of diabetes and its burden in the United States. National Center for Chronic Disease Prevention and Health Promotion, Division of Diabetes Translation, Centers for Disease Control and Prevention. https://www.cdc.gov/diabetes/pdfs/data/statistics/national-diabetes-statistics-report.pdf.
2. American Diabetes Association. Comprehensive medical evaluation and assessment of comorbidities. Sec. 3 in Standards of Medical Care in Diabetes—2017. *Diabetes Care.* 2017;**40**(Suppl 1):S25–S32.
3. American Diabetes Association. Lifestyle management. Sec. 4 in Standards of Medical Care in Diabetes—2017. Diabetes Care. 2017; **40**(Suppl 1):S33–S43.
4. Pollan M. *In Defense of Food: An Eater's Manifesto.* New York, NY: Penguin Press; 2008.
5. Brandenburg SL, Reusch JE, Bauer TA, Jeffers BW, Hiatt WR, Regensteiner JG. Effects of exercise training on oxygen uptake kinetic

responses in women with type 2 diabetes. *Diabetes Care.* 1999; **22**(10):1640–1646.

6. Regensteiner JG, Bauer TA, Reusch JE-B, Brandenburg SL, Sippel JT, Vogelsong AM, Smith S, Wolfel EE, Eckel RH, Hiatt WR. Abnormal oxygen uptake kinetic responses in type II diabetes mellitus. *J Appl Physiol.* 1998;**85**(1):310–317.
7. Nadeau KJ, Zeitler PS, Bauer TA, Brown MS, Dorosz JL, Draznin B, Reusch JEB, Regensteiner JG. Insulin resistance in adolescents with type 2 diabetes is associated with impaired exercise capacity. *J Clin Endocrinol Metab.* 2009;**94**(10):3687–3695.
8. Nadeau KJ, Regensteiner JG, Bauer TA, Brown MS, Dorosz JL, Hull A, Zeitler P, Draznin B, Reusch JEB. Insulin resistance in adolescents with type 1 diabetes and it relationship to cardiovascular function. *J Clin Endocrinol Metab.* 2010;**95**(2):513–521.
9. Abdul-Ghani M, DeFronzo RA, Del Prato S, Chilton R, Singh R, Ryder REJ. Cardiovascular disease and type 2 diabetes: has the dawn of a new era arrived? *Diabetes Care.* 2017;**40**(7):813–820.
10. ORIGIN Trial Investigators. Basal insulin and cardiovascular and other outcomes in dysglycemia. *N Engl J Med.* 2012;**367**(4):319–328.
11. Marso SP, McGuire DK, Zinman B, Poulter NR, Emerson SS, Pieber TR, Pratley RE, Haahr PM, Lange M, Brown-Frandsen K, Moses A, Skibsted S, Kvist K, Buse JB; DEVOTE Study Group. Efficacy and safety of degludec versus glargine in type 2 diabetes. *N Engl J Med.* 2017; **377**(8):723–732.
12. Pfeiffer MA, Claggett B, Diaz R, Dickstein K, Gerstein HC, Køber LV, Lawson FC, Ping L, Wei X, Lewis EF, Maggioni AP, McMurray JJV, Probstfield JL, Riddle MC, Solomon SD, Tardif J-C; ELIXA Investigators. Lixisenatide in patients with type 2 diabetes and acute coronary syndrome. *N Engl J Med.* 2015;**373**:2447–2457.
13. Scirica BM, Bhatt DL, Braunwald E, Steg PG, Davidson J, Hirshberg B, Ohman P, Frederich R, Wiviott SD, Hoffman EB, Cavender MA, Udell JA, Desai NR, Mosenzon O, McGuire DK, Ray KK, Leiter LA, Raz I; SAVOR-TIMI 53 Steering Committee and Investigators. Saxagliptin and cardiovascular outcomes in patients with type 2 diabetes mellitus. *N Engl J Med.* 2013;**369**(14):1317–1326.
14. White WB, Cannon CP, Heller SR, Nissen SE, Bergenstal RM, Bakris GL, Perez AT, Fleck PR, Mehta CR, Kupfer S, Wilson C, Cushman WC, Zannad F; EXAMINE Investigators. Alogliptin after acute coronary syndrome in patients with type 2 diabetes. *N Engl J Med.* 2013; **369**(14):1327–1335.
15. Green JB, Bethel MA, Armstrong PW, Buse JB, Engel SS, Garg J, Josse R, Kaufman KD, Koglin J, Korn S, Lachin JM, McGuire DK, Pencina MJ, Standl E, Stein PP, Suryawanshi S, Van de Werf F, Peterson ED, Holman RR; TECOS Study Group. Effect of sitagliptin on cardiovascular outcomes in type 2 diabetes. *N Engl J Med.* 2015;**373**(3):232–242.
16. Neal B, Perkovic V, Mahaffey KW, de Zeeuw D, Fulcher G, Erondu N, Shaw W, Law G, Desai M, Matthews DR; CANVAS Program Collaborative Group. Canagliflozin and cardiovascular and renal events in type 2 diabetes. *N Engl J Med.* 2017;**377**(7):644–657.
17. Wanner C, Inzucchi SE, Lachin JM, Fitchett D, von Eynatten M, Mattheus M, Johansen OE, Woerle HJ, Broedl UC, Zinman B; EMPA-REG OUTCOME Investigators. Empagliflozin and progression of kidney disease in type 2 diabetes. *N Engl J Med.* 2016;**375**(4): 323–334.
18. Kosiborod M, Cavender MA, Fu AZ, Wilding JP, Khunti K, Holl RW, Norhammar A, Birkeland KI, Jørgensen ME, Thuresson M, Arya N, Bodegård J, Hammar N, Fenici P; CVD-REAL Investigators and Study Group*. Lower risk of heart failure and death in patients initiated on sodium-glucose cotransporter-2 inhibitors versus other glucose-lowering drugs: the CVD-REAL Study (Comparative Effectiveness of Cardiovascular Outcomes in New Users of Sodium-Glucose Cotransporter-2 Inhibitors). *Circulation.* 2017;**136**(3):249–259.
19. Zinman B, Wanner C, Lachin JM, Fitchett D, Bluhmki E, Hantel S, Mattheus M, Devins T, Johansen OE, Woerle HJ, Broedl UC, Inzucchi SE; EMPA-REG OUTCOME Investigators. Empagliflozin, cardiovascular outcomes, and mortality in type 2 diabetes. *N Engl J Med.* 2015; **373**(22):2117–2128.
20. Marso SP, Daniels GH, Brown-Frandsen K, Kristensen P, Mann JF, Nauck MA, Nissen SE, Pocock S, Poulter NR, Ravn LS, Steinberg WM, Stockner M, Zinman B, Bergenstal RM, Buse JB; LEADER Steering Committee; LEADER Trial Investigators. Liraglutide and cardiovascular outcomes in type 2 diabetes. *N Engl J Med.* 2016;**375**(4): 311–322.
21. Mann JFE, Ørsted DD, Brown-Frandsen K, Marso SP, Poulter NR, Rasmussen S, Tornøe K, Zinman B, Buse JB; LEADER Steering Committee and Investigators. Liraglutide and renal outcomes in type 2 diabetes. *N Engl J Med.* 2017;**377**(9):839–848.
22. Marso SP, Bain SC, Consoli A, Eliaschewitz FG, Jódar E, Leiter LA, Lingvay I, Rosenstock J, Seufert J, Warren ML, Woo V, Hansen O, Holst AG, Pettersson J, Vilsbøll T; SUSTAIN-6 Investigators. Semaglutide and cardiovascular outcomes in patients with type 2 diabetes. *N Engl J Med.* 2016;**375**(19):1834–1844.
23. Holmann RR, Bethel MA, Mentz RJ, Thompson VP, Lokhnygina Y, Buse JB, Chan JC, Choi J, Gustavson SM, Iqbal N, Maggioni AP, Marso SP, Ohman P, Pagidipati NJ, Poulter N, Ramachandran A, Zinman B, Hernandez AF; EXSCEL Study Group. Effects of once-weekly exenatide on cardiovascular outcomes in type 2 diabetes. *N Engl J Med.* 2017; **377**:1228–1239.

Hypoglycemia in Diabetes

M30
Presented, March 17–20, 2018

Elizabeth R. Seaquist, MD. Division of Diabetes and Endocrinology, Department of Medicine, University of Minnesota, Minneapolis, Minnesota 55455, E-mail: seaqu001@umn.edu

SIGNIFICANCE OF THE CLINICAL PROBLEM

Hypoglycemia is the limiting factor that prevents patients with type 1 and advanced type 2 diabetes from obtaining optimal glycemic control. The consequences of hypoglycemia can range from inconvenience to confusion, seizures, and death. Up to 10% of the deaths in patients with type 1 diabetes are estimated to be attributable to hypoglycemia (1). More than one third of patients with type 1 diabetes experience at least 1 episode of severe hypoglycemia (defined as an event of hypoglycemia that requires the assistance of another) each year (2, 3). Approximately 10% of patients with type 2 diabetes experience severe hypoglycemia each year, and clinical trials have repeatedly demonstrated that such an event predicts an increased risk for mortality in subsequent months (4).

Hypoglycemia in diabetes is the consequence of treatment with insulin and/or insulin secretagogues. When prescribing such therapies, clinicians must ensure that their patients understand how to anticipate, recognize, and treat hypoglycemia. Recurrent episodes of hypoglycemia can blunt the counterregulatory response to a subsequent episode of hypoglycemia in the next few days. As a result of this blunting, patients must reach a lower and lower glucose concentration before eliciting the catecholamine release that leads to the adrenergic symptoms that trigger the patient's recognition of hypoglycemia (5). If the glucose level at which this response is elicited falls below that which causes neuroglycopenia, the first symptom of hypoglycemia the patient experiences may be unconsciousness. Impaired awareness of hypoglycemia may occur in up to one third of all patients with type 1 diabetes (6, 7), which puts many at risk for accidents and injury.

To optimize diabetes control without hypoglycemia requires caregivers to be aware of which patients are at risk for hypoglycemia and to be knowledgeable about how to mitigate this risk. Particular attention must be paid to recognizing and managing patients with impaired awareness of hypoglycemia. These knowledge gaps are addressed in this session.

BARRIERS TO OPTIMAL PRACTICE

One of the major barriers to managing hypoglycemia in diabetes is a lack of time to adequately review the patient's glucose records and integrate them with the history of medication doses taken, food eaten, and exercise/activity performed. A second barrier is that not all patients will remember to report episodes of hypoglycemia to their clinician, and many do not realize that they have impaired awareness of hypoglycemia. Clinicians need a systematic approach to determining whether their patients have impaired awareness of hypoglycemia.

LEARNING OBJECTIVES

As a result of participating in this session, learners should be able to:

- Identify factors that contribute to hypoglycemia in patients with diabetes
- Recognize impaired awareness of hypoglycemia in patients with diabetes
- Develop treatment regimens that minimize the risk of hypoglycemia in patients with diabetes
- Assist patients with diabetes and impaired awareness of hypoglycemia to regain their awareness of hypoglycemia

STRATEGIES FOR DIAGNOSIS, THERAPY, AND MANAGEMENT

Diagnosis

The diagnosis of impaired awareness of hypoglycemia in patients with diabetes is made by determining whether the patient has symptoms of a low blood sugar when they have a value <70 mg/dL. Although healthy people can have blood sugar levels <70 mg/dL without symptoms, this level of glucose should be viewed as an alert value in patients who take insulin or secretagogues and additional questions should be asked. The 2013 American Diabetes Association and Endocrine Society Hypoglycemia Workgroup report included a patient questionnaire that can be used to determine the hypoglycemia risk of any given patient (8). The following questions are particularly helpful for identifying patients with impaired awareness of hypoglycemia: To what extent can you tell by your symptoms that your blood sugar is low (never, rarely, sometimes, often, or always)? In a typical week, how many times will your blood glucose go below 70 mg/dL? How many times have you had a severe hypoglycemic episode (where you needed someone's help and were unable to treat yourself) since the last visit and in the past year?

Therapy and Management

When hypoglycemia becomes a problem, the diabetes health care provider should review the risk factors commonly associated with hypoglycemia (9), which are listed below. While working with the patient, the provider should make adjustments in the treatment regimen to ensure that euglycemia is achieved by a combination of insulin/insulin secretagogue taken, food eaten, and activity performed. A referral to a comprehensive diabetes education program also should be made for patients with new problems with hypoglycemia.

Health care providers should be alert to identifying patients with diabetes who may have impaired awareness of hypoglycemia. The questions listed above from the Hypoglycemia Workgroup should be asked of all patients at risk for hypoglycemia during the clinic visit. In addition, patients with a history of previous episodes of severe hypoglycemia, absolute insulin deficiency as is seen in long-duration type 1 diabetes, and overly aggressive A1C targets may be at particular risk for the development of impaired awareness of hypoglycemia (9). Restoring awareness of hypoglycemia often is difficult, and referral to a structured diabetes education program should be mandatory for such patients (10). Reevaluation of treatment goals and drugs used to manage diabetes also should be done to ensure that the regimen best meets the needs of the patient.

Risk Factors for Hypoglycemia

- Doses of insulin or insulin secretagogue excessive or ill timed
- Amount of carbohydrates eaten without consideration of the anticipated effect of insulin or insulin secretagogue taken
- Activity increased without a change in food eaten or insulin/insulin secretagogue taken
- Sensitivity to insulin increased, such as with weight loss or improved glucose control
- Alcohol ingestion (impairs hepatic glucose production)
- Insulin clearance reduced, such as in renal failure

MAIN CONCLUSIONS

Hypoglycemia is a common occurrence in patients with diabetes treated with insulin or insulin secretagogues. Because of the dangers associated with hypoglycemia, care must be taken to help patients to avoid low blood sugar, which is best done by educating the patient about how to anticipate, detect, and treat hypoglycemia as well as by ensuring that the drugs and treatment goals are appropriate for the patient. Impaired awareness of hypoglycemia occurs in patients with recurrent episodes of hypoglycemia over a short period. Because such patients experience loss of consciousness as their first symptom, it is imperative that clinicians identify patients with impaired awareness in their practice. Structured educational programs to reduce hypoglycemia may be particularly helpful in reversing impaired awareness of hypoglycemia in patients with diabetes.

CASES WITH QUESTIONS

Case 1

A 78-year-old woman with 30-year history of type 2 diabetes is brought to your office by her daughter because of concerns about hypoglycemia. The daughter stopped by to visit at 2:00 PM the previous day and found her mother unresponsive on the couch. The paramedics were called, and the patient's blood glucose was found to be 32 mg/dL. The patient does not know what happened but remembers sitting down to watch television at 9:30 AM. Today, the patient is fine, but she is angry that her daughter does not believe that she should live alone any longer. The patient's medical history is notable for atherosclerotic cardiovascular disease, with a stent placed 3 years ago. Current medications are clopidogrel, atorvastatin, lisinopril, glyburide 5 mg twice a day, metformin 2000 mg every day, and sitagliptin 100 mg every day.

What additional information do you need to assist the patient in her diabetes management?

A. Log book of home blood glucose levels
B. History of content and timing of meals/snacks ingested in the past week
C. Record of activity done in the past week
D. All of the above

Case 2

A 49-year-old man with type 1 diabetes since age 11 years needs assistance with diabetes management. His wife is concerned because the patient had a seizure at night last week from low blood sugar. He has always strived to maintain good glycemic control, but his hemoglobin A_{1c} values have ranged from 8.1% to 9.7% over the past several years. The patient has had severe hypoglycemia in the past, but the last episode was >1 year ago. He checks his sugar before meals and at bedtime and has averaged 197 mg/dL over the past month. He usually feels when his sugar is low if it is ≤50 mg/dL. The patient's current medications are glargine 21 U in the morning, lispro 1 U for every 7 g of carbohydrate plus a 1:50 correction with a target of 100 mg/dL, lisinopril, simvastatin, and aspirin.

Which of the following information tells you that the patient currently has impaired awareness of hypoglycemia?

A. He is striving for good glycemic control.
B. He had an episode of severe hypoglycemia >1 year ago.
C. He does not recognize low blood sugar until it is ≤50 mg/dL.
D. He has had type 1 diabetes for >30 years.

Which of the following recommendations would most likely restore his awareness of hypoglycemia?

A. Enroll in a comprehensive diabetes education program that focuses on adjusting insulin doses to meet the metabolic needs of the moment
B. Switch from insulin injections to a pump
C. Eat a bedtime snack every night
D. Switch from U100 glargine to U300 glargine

DISCUSSION OF CASES AND ANSWERS

Case 1

The correct answer is D, "All of the above." Glycemia at any point in time is determined by the medication taken, food ingested, and activity performed in the preceding hours. When patients present with a history of severe hypoglycemia, it is critical to determine the factors that led to the episode so that the patient's regimen can be altered to prevent future episodes. In addition, the clinician must examine how the patient's glycemia has responded to changes in food, medication, and activity in the home setting, which is best done by examining a record of home glucose values, medications taken, food ingested, and activities performed.

Case 2

The correct answer to the first question is C, "He does not recognize low blood sugar until it is ≤50 mg/dL," which means that the patient has a blunted counterregulatory response to hypoglycemia. Striving for good glycemic control has put patients in clinical trials at greater risk of hypoglycemia, but achieving optimal control in the absence of hypoglycemia will not impair the counterregulatory response. Having severe hypoglycemia in the past is a risk factor for subsequent episodes of severe hypoglycemia but does not necessarily mean that the patient has impaired awareness of hypoglycemia. Patients with long-duration type 1 diabetes are at greater risk for hypoglycemia, but most do not have impaired awareness of hypoglycemia.

The answer to the second question is A, "Enroll in a comprehensive diabetes education program that focuses on adjusting insulin doses to meet the metabolic needs of the moment." A structured diabetes education program has been demonstrated to be effective in restoring awareness of hypoglycemia in some but not all patients with type 1 diabetes and impaired awareness of hypoglycemia (10). Changes in the mode of insulin administration or the type of insulin or the addition of a bedtime snack by themselves are not likely to restore impaired awareness of hypoglycemia in this patient.

REFERENCES

1. Skrivarhaug T, Bangstad HJ, Stene LC, Sandvik L, Hanssen KF, Joner G. Long-term mortality in a nationwide cohort of childhood-onset type 1 diabetic patients in Norway. *Diabetologia*. 2006; **49**(2):298–305.
2. Pedersen-Bjergaard U, Pramming S, Heller SR, Wallace TM, Rasmussen AK, Jørgensen HV, Matthews DR, Hougaard P, Thorsteinsson B. Severe hypoglycaemia in 1076 adult patients with type 1 diabetes: influence of risk markers and selection. *Diabetes Metab Res Rev*. 2004;**20**(6): 479–486.
3. Donnelly LA, Morris AD, Frier BM, Ellis JD, Donnan PT, Durrant R, Band MM, Reekie G, Leese GP; DARTS/MEMO Collaboration. Frequency and predictors of hypoglycaemia in type 1 and insulin-treated type 2 diabetes: a population-based study. *Diabet Med*. 2005;**22**(6): 749–755.
4. Heller SR, Choudhary P, Davies C, Emery C, Campbell MJ, Freeman J, Amiel SA, Malik R, Frier BM, Allen KV, Zammitt NN, Macleod K, Lonnen KF, Kerr D, Richardson T, Hunter S, McLaughlin D; UK Hypoglycaemia Study Group. Risk of hypoglycaemia in types 1 and 2 diabetes: effects of treatment modalities and their duration. *Diabetologia*. 2007;**50**(6): 1140–1147.
5. Cryer PE. Mechanisms of hypoglycemia-associated autonomic failure in diabetes. *N Engl J Med*. 2013;**369**(4):362–372.
6. Geddes J, Schopman JE, Zammitt NN, Frier BM. Prevalence of impaired awareness of hypoglycaemia in adults with type 1 diabetes. *Diabet Med*. 2008;**25**(4):501–504.
7. Jordan LV, Robertson M, Grant L, Peters RE, Cameron JT, Chisholm S, Voigt DJ, Matheson L, Kerr EJ, Maclean K, Macalpine RR, Wilson E, Mackie AD, Summers NM, Vadiveloo T, Leese GP. The Tayside insulin management course: an effective education programme in type 1 diabetes. *Int J Clin Pract*. 2013;**67**(5):462–468.
8. Seaquist ER, Anderson J, Childs B, Cryer P, Dagogo-Jack S, Fish L, Heller SR, Rodriguez H, Rosenzweig J, Vigersky R. Hypoglycemia and diabetes: a report of a workgroup of the American Diabetes Association and the Endocrine Society. *Diabetes Care*. 2013;**36**(5): 1384–1395.
9. Cryer PE, Axelrod L, Grossman AB, Heller SR, Montori VM, Seaquist ER, Service FJ; Endocrine Society. Evaluation and management of adult hypoglycemic disorders: an Endocrine Society Clinical Practice Guideline. *J Clin Endocrinol Metab*. 2009;**94**(3):709–728.
10. Yeoh E, Choudhary P, Nwokolo M, Ayis S, Amiel SA. Interventions that restore awareness of hypoglycemia in adults with type 1 diabetes: a systematic review and meta-analysis. *Diabetes Care*. 2015;**38**(8): 1592–1609.

Inpatient Management of Diabetes: Goals, Challenges, and Implications

M39
Presented, March 17–20, 2018

Guillermo E. Umpierrez, MD, CDE, FACP, FACE. Emory University School of Medicine, Atlanta, Georgia 30307, E-mail: geumpie@emory.edu

SIGNIFICANCE OF THE CLINICAL PROBLEM AND LIMITATIONS

There are over 8.5 million hospital admissions for patients with diabetes in the United States. About 20% to 30% of patients have a prior history of diabetes. The prevalence of hyperglycemia is even higher and reported in 38% of patients in community hospitals (1), in 41% of critically ill patients with acute coronary syndromes (2), and in 80% of patients after cardiac surgery (3). Diabetes imposes a substantial economic burden on society. The total estimated cost of diagnosed diabetes in 2012 in the United States was $245 billion, of which $76 billion (41%) represented inpatient medical care (4).

Extensive data from observational and randomized controlled trials indicate that inpatient hyperglycemia, in patients with or without a prior diagnosis of diabetes, is associated with an increased risk of complications and mortality (1, 5, 6). It is also well established that improvement in glucose control with goal-directed insulin regimens reduces hospital complications and mortality in critically ill patients, as well as in general medicine and surgery patients. Recent studies and meta-analyses have shown that intensive insulin therapy is associated with increased risk of hypoglycemia, which has been independently associated with increased morbidity and mortality in hospitalized patients.

This lecture will (1) review the results of recent randomized control studies in intensive care unit (ICU) and non-ICU patients with hyperglycemia and diabetes, (2) discuss the role of computer-guided insulin algorithms in the ICU, and (3) present easy-to-follow insulin- and noninsulin-based treatment regimens for the management of inpatient hyperglycemia.

HYPERGLYCEMIA IN ICU SETTING

There is substantial observational evidence linking hyperglycemia in critically ill patients (with and without diabetes) to higher rates of hospital complications, longer hospital stay, higher health care resource utilization, and greater hospital mortality. Intravenously (IV) administered insulin is most beneficial to critically ill patients with or without a history of diabetes (7). Because of the short half-life of circulating insulin, IV delivery allows rapid dosing adjustments to address alterations in patient status. Insulin infusion is ideally administered via validated written or computerized protocols that allow for predefined adjustments to the insulin infusion rate according to glycemic fluctuations and insulin dose. For most critically ill patients, a starting threshold of no higher than 180 mg/dL is recommended. Once IV insulin is started, the glucose level should be maintained between 140 and 180 mg/dL. Glucose targets <110 mg/dL and >180 mg/dL are not recommended because of risk of hypoglycemia and hospital complications, respectively.

Previous randomized controlled trials have provided conflicting evidence when comparing intensive [blood glucose (BG) <110 mg/dL] vs. conventional glucose management (BG target <180 to 200 mg/dL). The Leuven surgical trial at the turn of the century demonstrated a reduction in mortality, shorter ICU stay, decreased need of prolonged ventilation, and lower risk of sepsis of critically ill patients treated with intensive glucose control compared with conventional glucose management (8). In contrast, the Normoglycemia in Intensive Care Evaluation and Surviving Using Glucose Algorithm Regulation (NICE-SUGAR) trial investigators found that intensive glucose control increased mortality in medical and surgical ICU patients (9). More recently, several randomized controlled trials have reported (3) no substantial differences in the composite of complications between intensive (100 to 140 mg/dL) and conservative groups (BG target 140 to 180 mg/dL) in cardiac surgery patients. However, there is substantial heterogeneity in treatment effect according to diabetes status, with no differences in complications among patients with diabetes treated with intensive or conservative regimens, but a substantially lower rate of complications in patients without diabetes treated with an intensive compared with a conservative treatment regimen

HYPERGLYCEMIA IN NON-ICU SETTINGS

In the general medical and surgical non-ICU patient, observational and randomized controlled trials have also shown a strong association between hyperglycemia and poor clinical outcomes, including prolonged hospital stay, infection, disability after hospital discharge, and death (10). The basal bolus insulin regimen with basal analogs (glargine or detemir) or intermediate acting insulin [neutral protamine Hagedorn (NPH)] given once or twice a day in combination with regular or rapid-acting insulin analogs (lispro, aspart, or glulisine) administered prior to meals is considered the physiologic approach. In insulin-naïve patients, a starting insulin dose of 0.3 to 0.5 U/kg/d is recommended. Elderly patients or those with renal insufficiency (estimated glomerular filtration rate <60 mL/min) should be started on a total daily dose ≤0.3 U/kg (Fig. 1).

Basal Bolus Insulin Regimen

In patients with adequate oral intake, the basal bolus approach is the preferred regimen as it addresses the three components

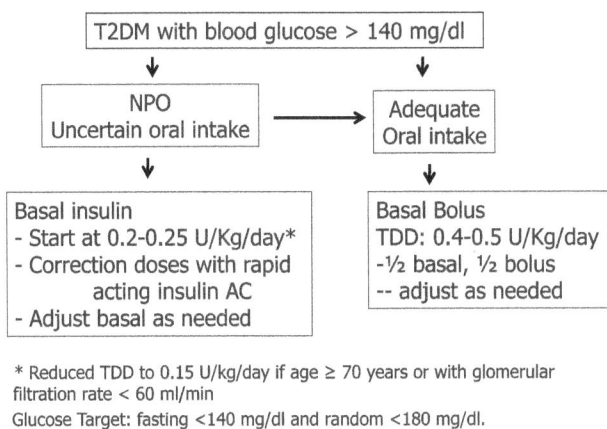

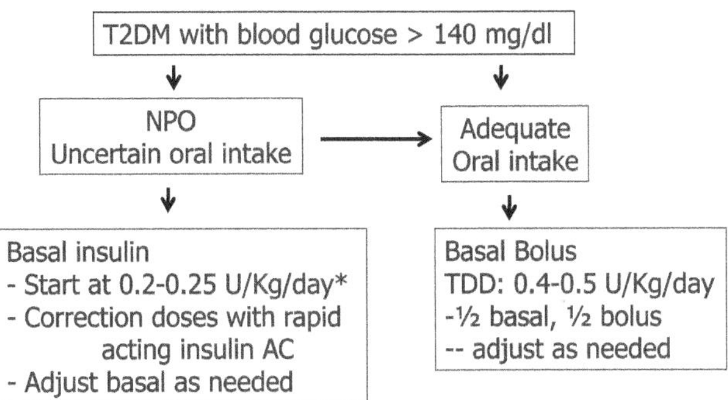

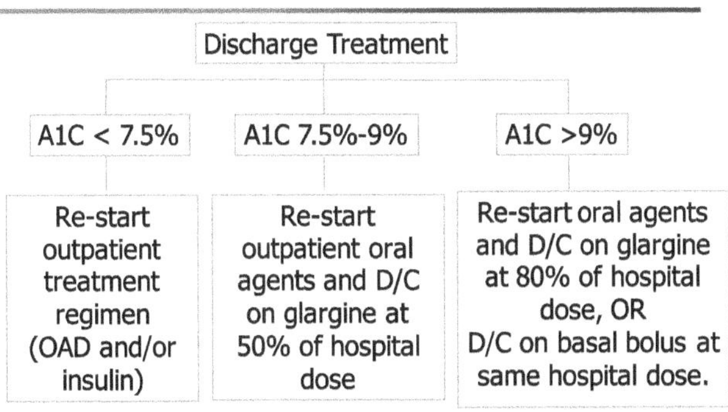

Figure 1. Initial insulin treatment in non-ICU.

of insulin requirement: basal, nutritional, and correctional doses (11). The use of basal bolus insulin had greater improvement in BG control than sliding scale alone (12). In general surgery patients, the basal bolus regimen resulted in substantial improvement in glucose control and a reduction in the frequency of the composite of postoperative complications, including wound infection, pneumonia, respiratory failure, acute renal failure, and bacteremia (13).

The use of multidose human NPH and regular insulin has been compared with basal bolus treatment with insulin analogs in two open-label controlled trials in medical patients with type 2 diabetes (14, 15). One study compared detemir once daily and aspart before meals to NPH and regular insulin given twice daily, two-thirds of the total daily dose given in the morning prebreakfast and one-third in the evening (14). A more recent study compared a basal bolus regimen with glargine once daily and glulisine before meals to NPH given twice daily and regular insulin before meals (15). Both studies reported that treatment with human NPH and regular insulin resulted in similar improvements in glycemic control and hospital length of stay, with lower rates of severe hypoglycemia.

Many patients in the hospital have reduced total caloric intake due to lack of appetite, acute illness, medical procedures, or surgical interventions. In such patients, the recent Basal Plus Trial (16) randomized patients with type 2 diabetes to receive a standard basal bolus regimen with glargine once daily and glulisine before meals and a single daily dose of glargine and supplemental doses of glulisine for correction of hyperglycemia (>140 mg/dL) per sliding scale (16). This study reported that the basal plus correction approach resulted in similar improvement in glycemic control and in the frequency of hypoglycemia compared with the basal bolus regimen. Current guidelines recommend that the basal plus correction insulin regimen is the preferred treatment of patients with poor oral intake or who are taking nothing by mouth. In contrast, an insulin regimen with basal, nutritional, and correction components (basal bolus) is the preferred treatment of patients with good nutritional intake (17).

Noninsulin Therapies

The use of oral antidiabetic agents is generally not recommended in hospitalized patients due to the limited data available on their safety and efficacy. Potential adverse effects, including hypoglycemia associated with insulin secretagogues, can also increase the risk of complications and mortality in acutely ill patients (5). In addition, the slow onset of action of some agents precludes their use for achieving rapid glycemic control and dose adjustments often required in hospitalized patients (1, 2). The safety and efficacy of dipeptidyl peptidase 4 (DPP-4) inhibitors for the management of inpatient hyperglycemia is an area of active research. Three studies recently reported that DPP-4 inhibitors in patients with mild to moderate hyperglycemia (<200 mg/dL) treated with diet, oral antidiabetic agents, or a low daily insulin dose (≤0.4 U/kg/d) experience a similar improvement in glycemic control with lower frequency of hypoglycemia compared with the basal bolus insulin regimen (18, 19). However, patients with an admission glucose >180 to 200 mg/dL treated with sitagliptin alone had higher mean daily BG compared with patients treated with basal bolus or sitagliptin plus glargine.

Clinical guidelines recommend holding metformin and other oral agents the day of surgery. Because of a recent report of diabetic ketoacidosis in patients treated with SGLT2 inhibitors after surgery and stress, these agents should be stopped 48 to 72 hours before surgery (20).

MANAGEMENT OF HYPERGLYCEMIA AFTER HOSPITAL DISCHARGE

Transition to an outpatient setting requires planning and coordination. Although insulin is used for most patients with diabetes in the hospital, many patients do not require insulin after discharge. The recent Endocrine Society inpatient guidelines for the management of non-ICU patients with diabetes (10) recommended that patients with diabetes and hyperglycemia should have their HbA_{1c} measured to assess preadmission glycemic control and to tailor the treatment regimen at discharge. Patients with acceptable diabetes control could be discharged on their prehospitalization treatment regimen (oral agents and/or insulin therapy) if there are no contraindications to therapy. Patients with suboptimal control should have intensification of therapy, either by addition or increase in oral agents, addition of basal insulin, or a more complex insulin regimen as warranted by their admission glucose control. Our preliminary experience indicates that measurement of HbA_{1c} on admission is useful in assessing metabolic control on admission and to guide treatment regimen at the time of hospital discharge in patients with type 2 diabetes (21). Patients admitted with an HbA_{1c} <7% can be discharged on the same preadmission diabetes therapy (oral agents or insulin). Those with HbA_{1c} between 7% and 9% can be discharged on oral agents plus basal insulin at 50% of the hospital basal insulin, and patients with HbA_{1c} >9% should be discharged on basal bolus insulin or the combination of metformin (contingent on renal function and patient tolerance) plus basal insulin at 80% of hospital dose.

CASE DISCUSSION

Case 1

Case Presentation: General Medicine Patient With Diabetes and Pneumonia

A 48-year-old male with an 8-year history of diabetes was admitted with a 3-day history of fever, cough, and right lower lobe pneumonia on chest x-ray. He was previously treated with metformin and sulfonylurea.

Laboratory results are as follows: BG 264 mg/dL, creatinine 1.4 mg/dL, and HbA_{1c} = 8.4%.

Questions

Given this patient's history and laboratory values, what is the best treatment option for glycemic management?

- Continue oral antidiabetic agents?
- Split-mixed regimen?
- Basal bolus regimen?

Case 2

Case Presentation: Diabetes and Ischemic Heart Disease and Heart Failure

A 62-year-old female with a 10-year history of type 2 diabetes treated with metformin 500 mg two times per day and sitagliptin 100 mg/dL. The patient has a history of coronary artery disease and an acute myocardial infarction in 2016. She was admitted with increasing shortness of breath, paroxysmal nocturnal dyspnea, and orthopnea.

A physical exam showed +S3 and 2+ pedal edema. A chest x-ray was consistent with congestive heart failure. Laboratory results are as follows: BG 214 mg/dL, creatinine 1.2 mg/dL, and HbA_{1c} = 8.0%.

Questions

What is the best treatment option for glycemic management?

- Basal bolus or basal alone?
- Glucagon-like peptide 1 agonist?
- Continue DPP-4 inhibitor?

Case 3

Case Presentation: Diabetes and General Noncardiac Surgery

A 62-year-old male with chronic knee osteoarthritis is referred for a "tune-up" of glycemic control prior to knee replacement surgery. The patient has a 6-year history of type 2 diabetes treated with metformin 1 g two times per day and glargine 24 U at bedtime.

Laboratory results are as follows: BG 244 mg/dL, creatinine 1.2 mg/dL, and HbA_{1c} = 8.2%.

Questions

Should we delay surgery until glucose and HbA_{1c} levels are close to target goals?

What is the best treatment option for glycemic management in uncomplicated surgery?

Case 4

Case Presentation: Diabetes and Corticosteroid Therapy

A 55-year-old female was admitted with chronic obstructive pulmonary disease exacerbation with increasing shortness of breath, dyspnea on exertion, and wheezing for 3 days. Physical exam revealed tachypnea and wheezing. The chest x-ray was consistent with chronic obstructive pulmonary disease. The patient has a 4-year history of type 2 diabetes treated with metformin. The patient received bronchodilators and 40 mg of methylprednisolone. She is scheduled to receive prednisone 40 mg/daily for ~5 days.

Laboratory results are as follows: HbA_{1c} = 7.6%, BG prior to steroid = 144 mg/dL, and BG the following morning = 188 mg/dL.

Questions

What is the best treatment option for glycemic management?

- Sliding scale?
- Basal bolus or basal alone?
- NPH or premixed insulin?

Case 5

Case Presentation: Diabetes and Nutrition Support

A 60-year-old female was admitted with a 14-year history of type 2 diabetes with poor oral intake after abdominal aortic aneurysm repair surgery. She is to be started on nutrition support with enteral feedings with a goal of 1,500 calories/day. She is currently treated with regular insulin per sliding scale.

Laboratory results are as follows: HbA_{1c} = 8.2%, mean fasting BG 198 mg/dL, and before meal BG 184 mg/dL.

Questions

What is the best treatment option for glycemic management?

- Sliding scale?

- Basal alone?
- NPH or premixed insulin two times or three times per day?

REFERENCES

1. Umpierrez GE, Isaacs SD, Bazargan N, You X, Thaler LM, Kitabchi AE. Hyperglycemia: an independent marker of in-hospital mortality in patients with undiagnosed diabetes. *J Clin Endocrinol Metab.* 2002; **87**(3):978–982.
2. Kosiborod M, Inzucchi SE, Spertus JA, Wang Y, Masoudi FA, Havranek EP, Krumholz HM. Elevated admission glucose and mortality in elderly patients hospitalized with heart failure. *Circulation.* 2009;**119**(14): 1899–1907.
3. Umpierrez G, Cardona S, Pasquel F, Jacobs S, Peng L, Unigwe M, Newton CA, Smiley-Byrd D, Vellanki P, Halkos M, Puskas JD, Guyton RA, Thourani VH. Randomized controlled trial of intensive versus conservative glucose control in patients undergoing coronary artery bypass graft surgery: GLUCO-CABG Trial. *Diabetes Care.* 2015;**38**(9): 1665–1672.
4. American Diabetes Association. Economic costs of diabetes in the U.S. in 2012 [published correction appears in *Diabetes Care.* 2013;36(6): 1797]. *Diabetes Care.* 2013;**36**(4):1033–1046.
5. Kotagal M, Symons RG, Hirsch IB, Umpierrez GE, Dellinger EP, Farrokhi ET, Flum DR; SCOAP-CERTAIN Collaborative. Perioperative hyperglycemia and risk of adverse events among patients with and without diabetes. *Ann Surg.* 2015;**261**(1):97–103.
6. Falciglia M, Freyberg RW, Almenoff PL, D'Alessio DA, Render ML. Hyperglycemia-related mortality in critically ill patients varies with admission diagnosis. *Crit Care Med.* 2009;**37**(12):3001–3009.
7. Moghissi ES, Korytkowski MT, DiNardo M, Einhorn D, Hellman R, Hirsch IB, Inzucchi SE, Ismail-Beigi F, Kirkman MS, Umpierrez GE; American Association of Clinical Endocrinologists; American Diabetes Association. American Association of Clinical Endocrinologists and American Diabetes Association consensus statement on inpatient glycemic control. *Diabetes Care.* 2009;**32**(6):1119–1131.
8. van den Berghe G, Wouters P, Weekers F, Verwaest C, Bruyninckx F, Schetz M, Vlasselaers D, Ferdinande P, Lauwers P, Bouillon R. Intensive insulin therapy in critically ill patients. *N Engl J Med.* 2001; **345**(19):1359–1367.
9. Finfer S, Chittock DR, Su SY, Blair D, Foster D, Dhingra V, Bellomo R, Cook D, Dodek P, Henderson WR, Hébert PC, Heritier S, Heyland DK, McArthur C, McDonald E, Mitchell I, Myburgh JA, Norton R, Potter J, Robinson BG, Ronco JJ; NICE-SUGAR Study Investigators. Intensive versus conventional glucose control in critically ill patients. *N Engl J Med.* 2009;**360**(13):1283–1297.
10. Umpierrez GE, Hellman R, Korytkowski MT, Kosiborod M, Maynard GA, Montori VM, Seley JJ, Van den Berghe G; Endocrine Society. Management of hyperglycemia in hospitalized patients in non-critical care setting: an endocrine society clinical practice guideline. *J Clin Endocrinol Metab.* 2012;**97**(1):16–38.
11. King AB, Armstrong DU. Basal bolus dosing: a clinical experience. *Curr Diabetes Rev.* 2005;**1**(2):215–220.
12. Umpierrez GE, Smiley D, Zisman A, Prieto LM, Palacio A, Ceron M, Puig A, Mejia R. Randomized study of basal-bolus insulin therapy in the inpatient management of patients with type 2 diabetes (RABBIT 2 trial). *Diabetes Care.* 2007;**30**(9):2181–2186.
13. Umpierrez GE, Smiley D, Jacobs S, Peng L, Temponi A, Mulligan P, Umpierrez D, Newton C, Olson D, Rizzo M. Randomized study of basal-bolus insulin therapy in the inpatient management of patients with type 2 diabetes undergoing general surgery (RABBIT 2 surgery). *Diabetes Care.* 2011;**34**(2):256–261.
14. Umpierrez GE, Hor T, Smiley D, Temponi A, Umpierrez D, Ceron M, Munoz C, Newton C, Peng L, Baldwin D. Comparison of inpatient insulin regimens with detemir plus aspart versus neutral protamine Hagedorn plus regular in medical patients with type 2 diabetes. *J Clin Endocrinol Metab.* 2009;**94**(2):564–569.
15. Bueno E, Benitez A, Rufinelli JV, Figueredo R, Alsina S, Ojeda A, Samudio S, Cáceres M, Argüello R, Romero F, Echagüe G, Pasquel F, Umpierrez GE. Basal bolus regimen with insulin analogs versus human insulin in medical patients with type 2 diabetes: a randomized controlled trial in Latin America. *Endocr Pract.* 2015;**21**(7):807–813.
16. Umpierrez GE, Smiley D, Hermayer K, Khan A, Olson DE, Newton C, Jacobs S, Rizzo M, Peng L, Reyes D, Pinzon I, Fereira ME, Hunt V, Gore A, Toyoshima MT, Fonseca VA. Randomized study comparing a basal-bolus with a basal plus correction insulin regimen for the hospital management of medical and surgical patients with type 2 diabetes: Basal Plus Trial. *Diabetes Care.* 2013;**36**(8):2169–2174.
17. American Diabetes Association. Standards of medical care in diabetes-2015 abridged for primary care providers. *Clin Diabetes.* 2015;**33**(2): 97–111.
18. Pasquel FJ, Gianchandani R, Rubin DJ, Dungan KM, Anzola I, Gomez PC, Peng L, Hodish I, Bodnar T, Wesorick D, Balakrishnan V, Osei K, Umpierrez GE. Efficacy of sitagliptin for the hospital management of general medicine and surgery patients with type 2 diabetes (Sita-Hospital): a multicentre, prospective, open-label, non-inferiority randomised trial. *Lancet Diabetes Endocrinol.* 2017;**5**(2):125–133.
19. Garg R, Schuman B, Hurwitz S, Metzger C, Bhandari S. Safety and efficacy of saxagliptin for glycemic control in non-critically ill hospitalized patients. *BMJ Open Diabetes Res Care.* 2017;**5**(1):e000394.
20. Handelsman Y, Henry RR, Bloomgarden ZT, Dagogo-Jack S, DeFronzo RA, Einhorn D, Ferrannini E, Fonseca VA, Garber AJ, Grunberger G, LeRoith D, Umpierrez GE, Weir MR. American Association of Clinical Endocrinologists and American College of Endocrinology position statement on the association of Sglt-2 inhibitors and diabetic ketoacidosis. *Endocr Pract.* 2016;**22**(6):753–762.
21. Umpierrez GE, Reyes D, Smiley D, Hermayer K, Khan A, Olson DE, Pasquel F, Jacobs S, Newton C, Peng L, Fonseca V. Hospital discharge algorithm based on admission HbA1c for the management of patients with type 2 diabetes. *Diabetes Care.* 2014;**37**(11):2934–2939.

New Onset Diabetes After Transplantation

M45
Presented, March 17–20, 2018

Jaime A. Davidson, MD. The University of Texas Southwestern Medical Center, Dallas, Texas 75230, E-mail: jaime.davidson@utsouthwestern.edu

SIGNIFICANCE OF THE CLINICAL PROBLEM

New onset diabetes after transplantation remains greatly underestimated in the literature. One of the most important reasons in the past was the definition of "insulin requirement." The natural history of new onset diabetes after transplantation seems to be similar to type 2 diabetes mellitus. It may take years before clinical symptoms appear; therefore, follow up over time is essential (1). In many cases, the diagnosis is made soon after the transplant. The incidence rates reported by Medicare recipients among 11,659 patients were 9.1%, 16.0%, and 24.0% at 3, 6, and 36 months, respectively (2).

BARRIERS TO OPTIMAL PRACTICE

New onset diabetes after transplantation has been known for decades. The lack of proper follow-up led to the idea that patients who developed type 2 diabetes after transplantation were immune to both the microvascular and macrovascular complications of type 2 diabetes. Another important factor was diagnostic criteria, from insulin requirements to fasting glucose levels > 200 mg/dL, and finally, the lack of long-term follow-up.

Opportunities to change are available. Adding an endocrinologist to the transplant team when possible could lead to better outcomes; however, data are not available. Pretransplant evaluation regarding risk factors is of utmost importance. Proper interventions for each risk factor in the pre- and posttransplantation periods, plus long-term follow-up, are essential. It is also important not to delay treatment once the diagnosis is made. Treatment needs to be more than just glucocentric, because usually hyperglycemia does not present by itself. Hyperglycemia usually has bad company such as hypertension and hyperlipidemia, which are part of the metabolic syndrome problem. Treating all three conditions is a must (3).

There are potentially modifiable and nonmodifiable risk factors, which include weight, pretransplantation-impaired fasting, and/or postprandial glucose. Some reports of hypomagnesaemia exist, but the number of cases is so small that magnesium replacement is not likely to be generally useful. Another risk factor is hepatitis C virus. Nonmodifiable risk factors include minorities and/or ethnicity (*e.g.*, African American and Hispanic); male recipient; family history of diabetes; HLA A30, B27, and B42 plus HLA mismatches; deceased and/or male donor; and a previous acute rejection (4).

LEARNING OBJECTIVES

As a result of participating in this session, learners should be able to describe the following:

- Important aspects of the epidemiology of new onset diabetes after transplantation
- Predictive factors for the development of diabetes in patients who are transplant recipients
- Different aspects in the pre- and posttransplantation management of patients with new onset diabetes after transplantation
- Proper interventions for glucose lowering, hypertension, and lipid management

STRATEGIES FOR DIAGNOSIS, THERAPY, AND/OR MANAGEMENT

The diagnosis of type 2 diabetes is well documented and agreed upon by all organizations dealing with the problem, including the American Association of Clinical Endocrinologists, American Diabetes Association, Endocrine Society, as well as the World Health Organization. Screening and management of patients pre- and posttransplantation can minimize the risk of developing diabetes (4). The recommendation is to include patients with glucose intolerance (defined as fasting plasma glucose levels between 100 mg/dL and 125 mg/dL and postprandial levels between 140 mg/dL and 199 mg/dL). If initial glucose levels are within normal limits, it does not ensure that the patient will remain normoglycemic in the future. The guidelines recommend close follow-up and based on risk factors, sooner better than later. We must follow present recommendations. Once the patient is diagnosed with diabetes, early treatment is the present recommendation. Patients and their relatives should be educated on every aspect of diabetes care, *i.e.*, nutrition, hygiene (including oral care), physical activity, self-glucose monitoring, *etc.* If a certified diabetes educator and registered nutritionist are available, they should provide the patient with knowledge on new onset diabetes after transplantation. We must remember that patients with new onset diabetes after transplantation have a lot more to do than a regular patient with diabetes. So we should expect to spend more time and several sessions on education. The general diabetes care guidelines by different organizations have more similarities than in years past.

There are risk factors to look for, such as obesity and/or ectopic fat (abdominal, hepatic, *etc.*), a family history of diabetes, and, in females, a history of gestational diabetes or having delivered babies > 9 lbs.

THERAPY CONSIDERATIONS

In addition to nonpharmacological management, it is important to consider pharmacological intervention from day 1 if possible. In a recent study by Baggesen *et al.* (5) in patients with type 2 diabetes, those who were treated early with metformin and who responded well (*i.e.*, with a large initial HbA1c reduction and achievement of near-normal HbA1c within 6 months after metformin initiation) were associated with having a lower risk of cardiovascular events and death. In addition, several trials in patients with type 2 diabetes and either previous cardiovascular events and/or high-risk factors have shown a decrease in future events and even mortality (6–8).

A problem in patients with new onset diabetes after transplantation is the lack of long-term studies with specific medications. Insulin and metformin were mainly used in the past. Now, although they were small trials, there are data on DPP4i, pioglitazone, and GLP1RA. No trials have been conducted with SGLT2i, but the class with two positive cardiovascular outcome trials could be a welcome option for patients with new onset diabetes after transplantation. SGLT2 inhibitors is a class of antihyperglycemic medications, including canagliflozin, dapagliflozin, and empagliflozin. These are relatively new, and no proper clinical trials have been conducted in patients with new onset diabetes after transplantation (NODAT). Sulfonylureas are not recommended due to the risk of hypoglycemia, weight gain, poor durability, and the possibility of increasing cardiovascular events.

In 2013, a randomized placebo-controlled clinical trial with DPP4i and pioglitazone showed no interaction with immunosuppressant medications, demonstrated safety, and improved glucose control (9). GLP-1RA has been reported to have good results, including glucose lowering, blood pressure improvements, and weight reduction (10).

There is no single pharmacological intervention that is 100% safe for all patients. Therefore, it is important to follow the recommendations and to individualize therapies for each patient. Although endocrinologists are not in charge of managing immunosuppression, they can make suggestions to the transplant team. For example, one could taper the dose of steroids earlier and, when possible, avoid the administration of tacrolimus. It should never be forgotten that the number one goal in a patient who is a transplant recipient is to maintain a good graft without rejection. Good glucose control, as well as management of hypertension and lipids, is part of the treatment plan.

MAIN CONCLUSIONS

New onset diabetes is a major complication of transplantation and, if untreated or poorly treated, has substantial negative consequences. It seems to have a high incidence and until recently, guidelines were not available. With new guidelines, we at least have a common ground for action. Whenever possible, preventing diabetes is the goal; without the presence of diabetes, the risk of micro- and macrovascular complications is diminished and the overall cost of care is much lower. Screening for diabetes is extremely important not only in the pretransplantation period, but also in the posttransplantation stage on an ongoing basis. If diabetes is diagnosed, educating and treating the patient immediately will result in a better future for the transplant recipient. The treatment is not just glucocentric—it also involves treating hypertension and hyperlipidemia because all three conditions are important in the prevention of cardiovascular events. Tailoring the immunosuppressive regimen when possible will help with the prevention of diabetes and its undesirable consequences.

DISCUSSION OF CASE AND ANSWER

Case 1

Medical History

M.L. is a 53-year-old woman. She was referred by the transplant team for diabetes evaluation. She was diagnosed in her early 30s with polycystic kidney disease. She was treated for hypertension for several years but never achieved a blood pressure of 130/80 mm Hg. Several different agents were used, as well as a combination of two agents. During her late teens and early twenties, she smoked 10 to 20 cigarettes/d until she was diagnosed with polycystic kidney disease and the doctor asked her to stop. In addition to antihypertensive medications, she was taking a multivitamin. Her kidney functions continued to deteriorate, and she was placed on the wait list for kidney transplant. Her family history was positive for type 2 diabetes. Her father died as the result of renal failure in his late fifties due to polycystic kidney disease after years of undergoing dialysis. M.L. was matched, but her donor was not a live donor. She is on a routine immunosuppressive plan that includes taking steroids and tacrolimus.

Physical Examination

M.L. is an overweight woman with no fundi abnormalities, and her thyroid appeared normal. Her lungs were clear, and her pulse was 84 beats/min. Her blood pressure was 148/92 mm Hg. The rest of the physical examination was unremarkable, except for her surgical scar.

Laboratory results prior to her endocrinology appointment showed that her blood glucose level was 142 mg/dL. On reviewing previous laboratory data, her fasting blood glucose level was in the range of 104 to 107 mg/dL before the transplantation and continued to increase over time. Four months prior to the visit, one of her nonfasting glucose levels was 205 mg/dL.

Question 1

To begin with, which of the following would you have recommended for her polycystic kidney disease? (1) Recommend increasing fluid intake; (2) include caffeinated drinks (coffee); (3) control blood pressure to at least 130/80 mm Hg; (4) all of the above; (5) 1 and 2; or (6) 1 and 3.

Explanation of the best answer: The most important recommendation is to increase fluid intake, but not with caffeinated drinks or alcohol. The second most important recommendation is to achieve a blood pressure of 130/80 mm

Hg or slightly lower. Nothing else is recommended for polycystic kidney disease except follow-up; 50% of patients develop end-stage renal disease by the age of 50 years, and the likelihood increases with age. Signs and symptoms are usually noticed by the age of 30 to 40 years and include back or side pain, increased abdominal size, hematuria, recurrent urinary tract infections, and hypertension. Polycystic kidney disease is the fourth leading cause of kidney failure. It occurs equally in women and men, and it affects all races (11).

Question 2

Which of the following are risk factors for developing new onset diabetes after transplantation: (1) family history of type 2 diabetes; (2) high triglyceride levels and elevated high-density lipoprotein; (3) family and/or properly matched donor; (4) use of steroids; (5) 1, 2, and 4; or (6) 1 and 4?

Explanation of the best answer: There are many risk factors that increase the risk for developing new onset diabetes after transplantation, but a family history of type 2 diabetes and use of steroids are the correct answers. M.L. was treated with high-dose steroids plus tacrolimus, and she also had a family history of type 2 diabetes and a high body mass index. Other risk factors include ethnicity (*e.g.*, Hispanic) and race (*e.g.*, black), low high-density lipoprotein and high triglyceride levels, deceased donor, and male donor. Tacrolimus is also a risk factor; if hyperglycemia develops, other agents such as cyclosporine should be considered.

Question 3

What should M.L.'s target glucose levels be? (1) A1c < 8%; (2) A1c < 7%; (3) A1c < 6.5%; (4) A1c < 6.5% plus FPG < 110 mg/dL and PPG < 140 mg/dL; or (5) none of the above.

Explanation of the best answer: The closer to normal without hypoglycemia and/or weight gain, the better. To achieve an A1c < 6.5%, the patient needs to work on fasting and postprandial targets. Thus, self-monitoring of blood glucose is important to achieve such targets (12). The clinical data show that metformin, pioglitazone, and DPP4 inhibitors or a combination are the best choices today. No hypoglycemia is an important factor, and there is no weight gain with metformin and/or DPP4i.

Question 4

Which pharmacological intervention would you recommend if M.L.'s A1c was 7.7%, her fasting blood glucose was in the 130 to 140 mg/dL range, and her postprandial blood glucose was in the low 200 mg/dL levels? What else do you need to know before deciding? The estimated glomerular filtration rate (eGFR) was 79 mL/min/1.73 m^2. M.L. was not anemic (hemoglobin, 14.2 g/dL). Because all rejection parameters looked ideal, the transplant team preferred to continue with the present immunotherapy and will consider tapering the steroids. Pharmacological interventions: (1) sulfonylurea monotherapy; (2) metformin plus pioglitazone; (3) metformin plus DPP4i; (4) metformin plus GLP1RA; (5) SGLT-2i; or (6) insulin.

Explanation of the best answer: The patient A1c is not at target. Ideally, an A1c of 6.5% or less without hypoglycemia or other unwanted side effects such as weight gain will be best. Therefore, SUs are not a good choice because of the potential side effects of weight gain and hypoglycemia. Insulin sometimes is the choice, but with an A1c of 7.7%, other options are better, because insulin will have the same potential side effects of weight gain and hypoglycemia. Metformin, if the eGFR allows it, should be used. Because titration is a must due mainly to gastrointestinal side effects, AACE recommends dual therapy. In NODAT, we have literature to support pioglitazone, DPP-4i, and GLP-1RA. No data on SGLT-2s as of December 2017 are available. Therefore, metformin and a DPP-4i or metformin and pioglitazone will be good oral choices without hypoglycemia. To minimize edema and weight gain, start pioglitazone at 15 mg daily and increase to 30 mg if necessary. If injectable is not an issue and it shouldn't be, a GLP-1 is a good alternative as well. There should be no weight gain, and in some patients there could be weight loss, some improvements in blood pressure, and a small increase in pulse. Monitoring glucose to adjust dosing is best medical practice in NODAT.

REFERENCES

1. Davidson JA, Wilkinson A; International Expert Panel on New-Onset Diabetes after Transplantation. New-Onset Diabetes after Transplantation 2003 International Consensus Guidelines: an endocrinologist's view. *Diabetes Care.* 2004;**27**(3):805–812.
2. Kasiske BL, Snyder JJ, Gilbertson D, Matas AJ. Diabetes mellitus after kidney transplantation in the United States. *Am J Transplant.* 2003; **3**(2):178–185.
3. Professional Practice Committee. *Diabetes Care.* 2017;**40**(Suppl 1):S3.
4. Davidson J, Wilkinson A, Dantal J, Dotta F, Haller H, Hernández D, Kasiske BL, Kiberd B, Krentz A, Legendre C, Marchetti P, Markell M, van der Woude FL, Wheeler DC; International Expert Panel. New-onset diabetes after transplantation: 2003 International Consensus Guidelines. Proceedings of an international expert panel meeting. Barcelona, Spain, 19 February 2003. *Transplantation.* 2003;**75**(10 Suppl):SS3–SS24.
5. Svensson E, Baggesen LM, Johnsen SP, Pedersen L, Nørrelund H, Buhl ES, Haase CL, Thomsen RW. Early glycemic control and magnitude of HbA1c reduction predict cardiovascular events and mortality: population-based cohort study of 24,752 metformin initiators. *Diabetes Care.* 2017;**40**(6):800–807.
6. Zinman B, Wanner C, Lachin JM, Fitchett D, Bluhmki E, Hantel S, Mattheus M, Devins T, Johansen OE, Woerle HJ, Broedl UC, Inzucchi SE; EMPA-REG OUTCOME Investigators. Empagliflozin, cardiovascular outcomes, and mortality in type 2 diabetes. *N Engl J Med.* 2015; **373**(22):2117–2128.
7. Marso SP, Daniels GH, Brown-Frandsen K, Kristensen P, Mann JF, Nauck MA, Nissen SE, Pocock S, Poulter NR, Ravn LS, Steinberg WM, Stockner M, Zinman B, Bergenstal RM, Buse JB; LEADER Steering Committee; LEADER Trial Investigators. Liraglutide and cardiovascular outcomes in type 2 diabetes. *N Engl J Med.* 2016;**375**(4): 311–322.
8. CANVAS program. In: Proceedings of the European Association for the Study of Diabetes; September, 2017; Lisbon, Portugal.
9. Werzowa J, Hecking M, Haidinger M, Lechner F, Döller D, Pacini G, Stemer G, Pleiner J, Frantal S, Säemann MD. Vildagliptin and pioglitazone in patients with impaired glucose tolerance after kidney

transplantation: a randomized, placebo-controlled clinical trial. *Transplantation.* 2013;**95**(3):456–462.

10. Sadhu AR, Schwartz SS, Herman ME. The rationale for use of incretins in the management of new onset diabetes after transplantation (NODAT). *Endocr Pract.* 2015;**21**(7):814–822.
11. Shivaswamy V, Boerner B, Larsen J. Post-tranplant diabetes mellitus: causes, treatment, and impact on outcomes. *Endocr Rev.* 2016;**37**(1): 37–61.
12. Garber AJ, Abrahamson MJ, Barzilay JI, Blonde L, Bloomgarder ZT, Bush MA, Dagogo-Jack S, DeFronzo RA, Einhorn D, Fonseca VA, Garber JR, Garvey WT, Grunberger G, Handelsman Y, Hirshch IB, Jellinger PS, McGill JB, Mechanick JI, Rosenblit PD, Umpierrez GE. Consensus statement by the American Association of Clinical Endocrinologists and American College of Endocrinology on the comprehensive type 2 diabetes management algorithm: 2018 executive summary. *Endocr Pract.* 2018;**24**(1):91–120.

Management of Diabetes in the Athlete

M49
Presented, March 17–20, 2018

Anne Peters, MD. Keck School of Medicine of USC, Los Angeles, California 90033, E-mail: momofmax@mac.com

SIGNIFICANCE OF THE CLINICAL PROBLEM

Athletes with diabetes have a different set of challenges compared with those who do not. In the past decade, more people with diabetes are competing at high levels of sport. Many physicians do not know how to manage athletes with diabetes or how to access the resources needed to help them with their care. This workshop will review approaches to dealing with these individuals. A patient athlete will be part of the workshop to discuss his own strategies for training and competing with type 1 diabetes (T1D).

BARRIERS TO OPTIMAL PRACTICE

- Lack of an understanding of exercise physiology in people with T1D
- Limited experience with the management of insulin, devices, and nutrition in the management of the athlete with T1D

LEARNING OBJECTIVES

As a result of participating in this session, learners should be able to the following.

- Assess the metabolic requirements of an athlete with diabetes
- Create a regimen involving insulin adjustments, carbohydrate intake, and use of continuous glucose monitoring to help with management of the athletes with diabetes

STRATEGIES FOR DIAGNOSIS, THERAPY, AND/OR MANAGEMENT

Two recent articles explain the management of exercise in people with diabetes. An American Diabetes Association position statement on exercise is an excellent, fairly broad review of physical activity in people with diabetes (1). More details for how to manage a T1D athlete are found in an article in *The Lancet Diabetes & Endocrinology* (2). Some of the key learning points are provided below.

Exercise Challenges for Individuals With Diabetes

- Varying workouts—type/duration/intensity
- Different responses to training versus competition
- Unpredictability
- Risk for hypoglycemia
- Impact of hyperglycemia on performance
- Physical factors (sweat/water/heat/cold)
- Everything else that impacts individuals without diabetes

Blood Glucose Level at Start of Exercise (2)

Starting Glycemia Below Target (<90 mg/dL)

- Ingest 10 to 20 g of glucose before starting exercise
- Delay exercise until blood glucose level > 90 mg/dL and monitor closely for hypoglycemia

Starting Glycemia Near Target (90 to 124 mg/dL)

- Ingest 10 g of glucose before starting aerobic exercise
- Anaerobic exercise and high-intensity interval training sessions can be started

Starting Glycemia at Target Level (124 to 180 mg/dL)

- Aerobic exercise can be started

Table 1. CHO Intake Before, During, and After Exercise

Situation	Endurance Exercise Performance in Athletes
Meal (low fat, low glycemic index) consumed before exercise	A minimum of 1 g CHO per 1 kg body weight according to exercise intensity and type
Meal or snack consumed immediately before exercise (high glycemic index)	No CHO required for performance, unless BG below target
Meal consumed after exercise	1–1.2 g CHO per 1 kg body weight
Exercise (up to 30 min)	No CHO required for performance unless low
Exercise (30- to 60-min duration)	Small amounts of CHO (15–30 g/h) could enhance performance
Exercise (60- to 150-min duration)	30–60 g CHO/h
Exercise (>150 min); mixture of CHO sources	60–90 g CHO per hour spread across the activity (*e.g.*, 20–30 g CHO every 20 min); use CHO sources that use different gut transporters (*e.g.*, glucose and fructose)

Abbreviations: BG, blood glucose; CHO, carbohydrate.

From Riddell MC, Gallen IW, Smart CE, et al. Exercise management in type 1 diabetes: a consensus statement. *Lancet Diabetes Endocrinol.* 2017;5:377–390.

Table 2. Insulin Adjustments

Dose	Prolonged Endurance Exercise (Mainly Aerobic)
Bolus insulin dose reduction at the meal before exercise	Advised when exercise occurs within ~120 min of bolus dose; the magnitude of reduction varies according to timing, type, duration, and intensity of exercise
Before exercise, basal insulin dose reduction (of ~20%) in patients on MDI	Useful especially if exercise is done less than every 3 d or if the frequency of exercise is high throughout the day
Basal nocturnal insulin dose reduction (of ~20%) after exercise in patients on MDI or pumps to avoid night lows	Particularly important if the exercise was done in the afternoon or early evening
Temporary basal rate change (for pumpers)	Basal rate can be suspended during exercise, but keeping some basal delivery is preferred; to take into account insulin pharmacokinetics, a basal rate reduction should occur before exercise (up to 90 min); resume normal basal rate at the end of exercise or later in recovery depending on glucose trends

Abbreviation: MDI, multiple daily injection.

From Riddell MC, Gallen IW, Smart CE, et al. Exercise management in type 1 diabetes: a consensus statement. *Lancet Diabetes Endocrinol.* 2017;5:377–390.

- Anaerobic exercise and high-intensity interval training sessions can be started, but glucose concentrations could rise

Starting Glycemia Slightly Above Target (180 to 270 mg/dL)

- Aerobic exercise can be started
- Anaerobic exercise and high-intensity interval training sessions can be started, but glucose concentrations could rise

Starting Glycemia Above Target (>270 mg/dL)

- If the hyperglycemia is unexplained, check blood ketones. If ketones are modestly elevated (0.6 to 1.4 mmol/L), limit exercise to a light intensity for a brief duration (<30 minutes). A small pre-exercise corrective dose of insulin might be needed. If blood ketones are >1.5 mmol/L, exercise is contraindicated, and glucose management should be initiated rapidly by the patients diabetes health care team (Tables 1 and 2).

MAIN CONCLUSIONS

A detailed history of the patient is vital with regard to training and competition schedules and other details to understand the sport and the patient's metabolic requirements. An individualized plan should be created for the athlete on how adjust insulin and carbohydrate intake as well as how to use real-time information from a continuous glucose monitor to adjust glucose levels and keep them in a safe range.

CASE

The case will be an actual patient who will discuss his training regimen and how he deals with his diabetes during competition. He sets up diabetes running groups around the country and will be able to answer questions regarding how to help athletes in your community.

REFERENCES

1. Colberg SR, Sigal RJ, Yardley JE, Riddell MC, Dunstan DW, Dempsey PC, Horton ES, Castorino K, Tate DF. Physical activity/exercise and diabetes: a position statement of the American Diabetes Association. *Diabetes Care.* 2016;**39**(11):2065–2079.
2. Riddell MC, Gallen IW, Smart CE, Taplin CE, Adolfsson P, Lumb AN, Kowalski A, Rabasa-Lhoret R, McCrimmon RJ, Hume C, Annan F, Fournier PA, Graham C, Bode B, Galassetti P, Jones TW, Millán IS, Heise T, Peters AL, Petz A, Laffel LM. Exercise management in type 1 diabetes: a consensus statement. *Lancet Diabetes Endocrinol.* 2017; **5**(5):377–390.

ENDOCRINE DISRUPTION

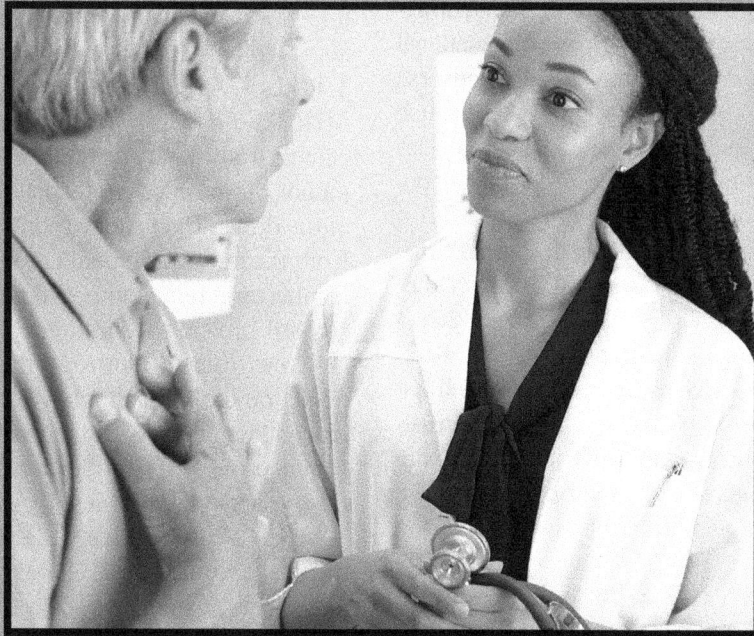

Endocrine Immune-Related Adverse Events

M50
Presented, March 17–20, 2018

Ramona Dadu, MD. Department of Endocrine Neoplasia and Hormonal Disorders, University of Texas MD Anderson Cancer Center, Houston, Texas 77030, E-mail: rdadu@mdanderson.org

SIGNIFICANCE OF THE CLINICAL PROBLEM

Checkpoint blockade immunotherapy has revolutionized the treatment of cancer, with impressive clinical benefit. To date, six immune checkpoint inhibitors are approved by the US Food and Drug Administration: anti–cytotoxic T-lymphocyte antigen 4 (CTLA-4) antibody (ipilimumab), anti–programmed cell death-1 (PD-1) antibodies (pembrolizumab, nivolumab), and anti–programmed cell death-1 ligand (PD-L1) antibodies (atezolizumab, durvalumab, avelumab). Despite achieving great clinical success, the challenges and limitations of immunotherapy when used as monotherapy or in various combinational strategies include the development of immune-related adverse events (irAEs). The two more common endocrine irAEs include acute hypophysitis resulting in pituitary hormonal deficiencies (central hypothyroidism, central adrenal insufficiency, hypogonadotropic hypogonadism), especially with anti–CTLA-4 drugs, and thyroid disease or abnormalities in thyroid function tests (TFTs), especially with anti–PD-1/PD-L1 drugs. Other endocrinopathies, such as primary adrenal insufficiency, hypogonadism, hypercalcemia, primary hypoparathyroidism, and type 1 diabetes mellitus, have been reported as well but are rare. Consensus recommendations on identification, treatment, and monitoring of patients with irAEs, including endocrinopathies, were recently published (1). More evidence-based data should be obtained to guide the best clinical decision making.

BARRIERS TO OPTIMAL PRACTICE

- Lack of criteria for diagnosis of immune-related hypophysitis (IH)
- Lack of evidence-based data to guide appropriate treatment and long-term follow-up for hypophysitis
- Lack of guidelines to provide recommendations to manage thyroid abnormalities resulting from the use of immunotherapy

LEARNING OBJECTIVES

As a result of participating in this session, learners should be able to:

- Name the most common endocrine irAEs resulting from anti–CTLA-4 and anti–PD-1/PD-L1 antibodies
- Recognize the clinical presentation and natural course of the two most common endocrine irAEs (hypophysitis and thyroiditis)
- Apply appropriate management strategies for hypophysitis and thyroiditis cases

STRATEGIES FOR DIAGNOSIS, THERAPY, AND MANAGEMENT

Immune checkpoint inhibitors act by restoring the ability of the immune system to detect and destroy cancer cells. In normal conditions, T cells require two signals to become fully activated: one, the T-cell receptor interacts with peptide-HMC molecules on the membrane of antigen-presenting cells; and two, CD28 binds to B7. CTLA-4 was the first described immune checkpoint. It is present on activated T cells and binds B7 with greater affinity and avidity than CD28, thus enabling it to outcompete CD28 for its ligands. This interaction inhibits the proliferation and recruitment of more T cells. However, in the presence of anti–CTLA-4 antibody, these protective interactions are lost, resulting in enhanced T-cell activation. Several other immune checkpoints have been described (PD-1/PD-L1, LAG3, TIM3, KIR, VISTA, CD-40, OX-40, CD-137, GITR), and agonistic or antagonistic antibodies are used in clinical trials. Many of the irAEs are driven by the same immunologic mechanisms responsible for the therapeutic effects of the drugs. The toxicity profiles of these drugs are different from those of traditional cytotoxic chemotherapies or molecular targeted agents. irAEs typically have a delayed onset and prolonged duration compared with adverse events resulting from chemotherapy, and effective management depends on early recognition and prompt intervention. Skin, gut, endocrine, lung, and musculoskeletal irAEs are relatively common, whereas cardiovascular, hematologic, renal, neurologic, and ophthalmologic irAEs occur much less frequently.

There is considerable variation in definitions of irAEs and their severity, as well as variation in symptoms and signs that may be attributable to other irAEs. Currently, there are no good predictors for either response to or toxicity resulting from immunotherapy. Therefore, identification of patients at risk, consistent communication between patients and medical teams, and frequent monitoring for and early recognition and treatment of irAEs are critical in optimizing treatment outcomes. Additionally, in all patients receiving immune checkpoint inhibitors, routine monitoring for clinical signs and symptoms of endocrinopathies, in addition to patient education, is recommended. All patients should be tested before starting immunotherapy for thyroid [thyrotropin (TSH) and free T4], adrenal [early-morning adrenocorticotropin (ACTH) and cortisol], and glycemic control (glucose and HbA1c). Before each cycle, thyroid testing (TSH and free T4) should be repeated, along with a baseline metabolic panel to allow monitoring of glycemic trends. Routine monitoring with early-morning ACTH and cortisol levels should be considered (every month for 6 months, then every 3 months for 6 months, then every 6 months for 1 year).

Here, we present the clinical course and proposed management of the two most common endocrine irAEs (hypophysitis and thyroiditis).

IH

Because of the lack of strict definitions, there is difficulty in obtaining accurate data on incidence and prevalence of this disorder based on clinical trials. Therefore, prevalence varies greatly, from 1% to 17%. Additionally, several reports focusing on endocrine irAEs (each case evaluated by an endocrinologist) have reported IH prevalence as 8% to 11% (2–5). None of these studies used strict criteria for the definition of IH.

IH occurs mainly in patients treated with anti–CTLA-4 antibodies (ipilimumab and tremelimumab) alone or in combination with other checkpoint inhibitors and remains rare in patients treated with single-agent anti–PD-1 or –PD-L1 antibodies. The median time from starting ipilimumab to diagnosis of IH is 8 to 9 weeks or after third dose of ipilimumab. Headache and fatigue are most commonly seen and can occur in 85% and 65% of patients, respectively. Visual changes are uncommon. However, some patients remain asymptomatic. Clinical suspicion is frequently raised when routine TFT monitoring (as recommended in the package insert) shows evidence of central hypothyroidism, leading to further testing. The most common hormone deficiency seems to be central hypothyroidism (>90%), followed by central adrenal insufficiency (75%) and hypogonadism (70%). In our experience, involvement of all three pituitary axes occurs in half of patients. Prolactin level has been low in >50% of patients, but high levels have also been reported. Hyponatremia occurs in 55% of patients. No cases of diabetes insipidus have been reported to date. Magnetic resonance imaging (MRI) findings may be mild and may not be readily apparent without comparison with a baseline scan. In my experience, 90% of patients had increased height of the gland when compared with baseline scans. Other MRI abnormalities include stalk thickening (70%), suprasellar convexity (48%), and heterogeneous enhancement of the pituitary gland (37%) (6). Resolution of pituitary enlargement is common, with all cases resolved on follow-up scans at 2 months (3, 7–9).

There are no good predictors to help identify patients at risk. Interestingly, a progressive decline in TSH level has been noted before the onset of symptom or IH diagnosis. Also, on MRI of the sella, pituitary enlargement can precede the development of clinical and biochemical evidence of IH (3).

Strict criteria for diagnostic confirmation of IH are not currently available. On the basis of previous retrospective data and clinical experience, proposed confirmation criteria of IH include ≥ one pituitary hormone deficiency (TSH or ACTH deficiency required) combined with an MRI abnormality, or ≥ two pituitary hormone deficiencies (TSH or ACTH deficiency required) in the presence of headache and other symptoms.

Management of confirmed IH includes replacement of deficient hormones (physiologic doses of steroids and thyroid hormone). High doses of steroids may be necessary in the setting of severe headaches, vision changes, or adrenal crisis, rarely noted. In a small prospective study, treatment with higher doses of steroids did not seem to improve pituitary function recovery compared with physiologic doses of steroids (10, 11). Similarly, in my and others' experience, most patients were successfully symptomatically treated with physiologic glucocorticoid replacement instead of a high-dose steroid regimen (1, 7–9, 12).

Both adrenal insufficiency and hypothyroidism seem to represent long-term sequelae of hypophysitis, and lifelong hormonal replacement is needed in most cases (1, 4, 8–10). Recovery of thyroid and gonadal axes was noted in a small percentage of patients. Continuous monitoring with clinical assessment and repeat biochemical evaluation aimed at testing for recovery is needed to appropriately treat these patients. We recommend periodic assessment, such as every 3 months in the first year and every 6 months thereafter.

Thyroid Dysfunction

The reported prevalence of thyroid dysfunction described as hypothyroidism, hyperthyroidism, or thyroiditis ranged from 6% to 20% in large phase 3 clinical trials.

Thyrotoxicosis may occur secondary to thyroiditis or Graves disease. Thyroiditis is the most common cause of thyrotoxicosis, commonly seen with anti–PD-1/PD-L1 drugs or combinations. Graves disease (manifested as hyperthyroidism or Graves orbitopathy only) is a rare cause of immunotherapy-induced hyperthyroidism, reported with anti–CTLA-4 antibodies only (13). Several cases of immune-related thyroiditis and its natural course have been reported (2, 14–17). Immunotherapy-related thyroiditis is a unique entity characterized by rapid development of asymptomatic thyrotoxicosis followed by a quick transition to hypothyroidism. Thyrotoxicosis phase occurs after an average of 1 month after starting immunotherapy, but it can occur as early as 4 days. A majority of patients are asymptomatic (painless thyroiditis), and routine laboratory monitoring reveals thyrotoxicosis. It may also present with weight loss, palpitations, heat intolerance, tremors, anxiety, diarrhea, and other symptoms of hypermetabolic activity, although these symptoms may be masked if the patient is taking beta-blockers. Conservative therapy with beta-blockers and close monitoring during the thyrotoxicosis phase of thyroiditis are sufficient. Additional tests can be undertaken when thyroiditis is suspected, primarily to rule out other causes of thyrotoxicosis, such as Graves disease. These include thyroid-stimulating hormone receptor antibody or thyroid-stimulating immunoglobulin and thyroid peroxidase as well as images when feasible, including radioactive iodine uptake scan or technetium-99m (pertechnetate) thyroid scan if recent iodinated contrast was used. Thyroiditis is a self-limiting process and leads to permanent hypothyroidism after an average of 1 month after the thyrotoxicosis phase and 2 months from initiation of immunotherapy. Repeat thyroid hormone levels should be performed every 2 to 3 weeks and thyroid hormone replacement initiated at the time of hypothyroidism diagnosis (1, 8, 9, 12). Immunotherapy hold is only required for patients with severe symptoms limiting self-care and when hospitalization is indicated for life-threatening consequences. In most cases, immunotherapy can be continued.

CASES

Case 1: Anti–CTLA-4 Antibody–Related Hypophysitis

A 65-year-old man with metastatic prostate cancer receiving androgen-deprivation therapy was treated with ipilimumab 3 mg/kg every 3 weeks. Routine laboratory evaluation before his fourth ipilimumab infusion showed low free T4 (0.44 ng/dL) and low TSH (0.04 nIU/mL) levels, low total testosterone (<20 ng/dL) level, and normal sodium level. He is scheduled for his fourth dose of ipilimumab later today. He is referred to you for evaluation of abnormal TFT before receiving his infusion. He describes a mild headache and fatigue that started 1 week before. On physical examination, his vital signs were normal, with no orthostasis.

Question: What would you recommend next?

A. Continue immunotherapy as planned and start thyroid hormone at a dose of 1.6 μg/kg/d and repeat TFT in 6 to 8 weeks
B. Stop immunotherapy and never restart and hospitalize the patient for administration of high doses of steroids
C. Continue immunotherapy as planned and monitor closely without treatment
D. Hold immunotherapy until you perform additional testing to include AM cortisol and ACTH and MRI of the sella

Answer: D.

Discussion

The patient has laboratory evidence of central hypothyroidism after three doses of ipilimumab, raising a high suspicion for IH. Hypophysitis occurs more frequently in patients treated with anti–CTLA-4 antibodies (ipilimumab or tremelimumab). The median time from starting ipilimumab to diagnosis of hypophysitis is 8 to 9 weeks or after the third dose of ipilimumab. Symptoms commonly include headache (85%) and fatigue (66%); visual changes are uncommon. Clinical suspicion of hypophysitis is frequently raised when routine TFT shows low TSH with low free T4, suggestive of a central etiology. Patients have various degrees of anterior pituitary hormonal deficiency, with central hypothyroidism being most commonly seen (>90%), followed by central adrenal insufficiency, which is also found in a majority of patients. Both central hypothyroidism and adrenal insufficiency occur in two thirds of patients. The recommended approach for patients with high clinical suspicion of hypophysitis is to hold immunotherapy until workup is completed and appropriate hormone replacement is started. All patients with suspected hypophysitis based on clinical findings (headache, fatigue) or biochemical evaluation (routine TFT showing low free T4 with low/normal TSH) should undergo further testing for diagnostic confirmation, such as evaluation of adrenal function (ACTH, cortisol, or 1-μg cosyntropin stimulation test), gonadal hormones, and MRI of the sella. If central adrenal insufficiency is confirmed, start physiologic steroid replacement with hydrocortisone of approximately 10 mg/m^2 (hydrocortisone 15 mg in the AM, 5 mg at 3 PM). For severe/life-threatening symptoms such as adrenal crisis, severe headache, or visual field deficiency, hospitalize as appropriate and start high-dose corticosteroid (equivalent of prednisone 1 mg/kg/d) in the acute phase, followed by tapering over 1 month. If the patient has central hypothyroidism, replace thyroid hormone after corticosteroids have been initiated.

Case 2: Anti–PD-1 Antibody–Related Thyroiditis

A 54-year-old woman with metastatic non–small-cell lung cancer has received treatment with nivolumab 240 mg every 2 weeks. Before her fourth dose of nivolumab, routine TFT monitoring shows a low TSH level of 0.09 mIU/mL and a low free T4 level of 0.45 ng/dL. She is referred for endocrine consultation for abnormal TFT. The patient is asymptomatic at this time. On review of her prior testing, you note that she had normal baseline TFTs, with free T4 of 1.28 ng/dL and TSH of 1.96 mIU/mL; before her second nivolumab infusion, her TSH was 0.1 mIU/mL and free T4 was 1.9 ng/dL; and before her third nivolumab infusion, her TSH was 0.01 mIU/mL and free T4 was 3.65 ng/dL.

Question: What would you do next?

A. Patient has evidence of central hypothyroidism, and additional pituitary hormonal testing to include adrenal and gonadal axes and MRI of sella are needed
B. Stop immunotherapy and never restart; start high doses of steroids (equivalent of prednisone 1 to 2 mg/kg/d)
C. Continue immunotherapy and start thyroid hormone replacement
D. Stop immunotherapy and start methimazole

Answer: C.

Discussion

This case describes a typical case of immunotherapy-mediated thyroiditis, occurring after 1 month from initiation of therapy with anti–PD-1 antibody. It is more commonly associated with anti–PD-1 drugs used either alone or in combination with anti–CTLA-4. Thyrotoxic phase occurs after an average of 1 month after starting immunotherapy and leads to permanent hypothyroidism after an average of 1 month after thyrotoxic phase and 2 months from initiation of immunotherapy.

Patients are usually asymptomatic, and thyrotoxicosis is diagnosed based on abnormal routine testing (TFT monitoring before each dose is recommended based on package insert). This case highlights an important clinical scenario with transition to hypothyroidism based on low free T4; however, it is too early for TSH to rise after the thyrotoxic phase. The combination of low free T4 with low TSH is commonly mistaken as central hypothyroidism, leading to unnecessary pituitary hormonal evaluation and MRI of the sella to rule out hypohysitis. The first step is to review prior TFTs, which clearly show a thyrotoxicosis episode. Conservative therapy during thyrotoxic phase of thyroiditis is sufficient, followed by treatment with thyroid hormone when hypothyroidism is confirmed. Immunotherapy can be continued. High doses of steroids (equivalent of prednisone 1 to 2 mg/kg/d) for anti-inflammatory effect are not needed. Treatment with antithyroidal drugs is not appropriate. Although few cases of Graves disease in patients receiving anti–CTLA-4 antibody have been reported, this patient does not have clinical evidence of Graves disease, and he was treated with anti–PD-1 antibody.

REFERENCES

1. Puzanov I, Diab A, Abdallah K, Bingham CO III, Brogdon C, Dadu R, Hamad L, Kim S, Lacouture ME, LeBoeuf NR, Lenihan D, Onofrei C, Shannon V, Sharma R, Silk AW, Skondra D, Suarez-Almazor ME, Wang Y, Wiley K, Kaufman HL, Ernstoff MS; Society for Immunotherapy of Cancer Toxicity Management Working Group. Managing toxicities associated with immune checkpoint inhibitors: consensus recommendations from the Society for Immunotherapy of Cancer (SITC) Toxicity Management Working Group. *J Immunother Cancer.* 2017;**5**(1):95.
2. Ryder M, Callahan M, Postow MA, Wolchok J, Fagin JA. Endocrine-related adverse events following ipilimumab in patients with advanced melanoma: a comprehensive retrospective review from a single institution. *Endocr Relat Cancer.* 2014;**21**(2):371–381.
3. Faje A. Immunotherapy and hypophysitis: clinical presentation, treatment, and biologic insights. *Pituitary.* 2016;**19**(1):82–92.
4. Faje AT, Sullivan R, Lawrence D, Tritos NA, Fadden R, Klibanski A, Nachtigall L. Ipilimumab-induced hypophysitis: a detailed longitudinal analysis in a large cohort of patients with metastatic melanoma. *J Clin Endocrinol Metab.* 2014;**99**(11):4078–4085.
5. Corsello SM, Barnabei A, Marchetti P, De Vecchis L, Salvatori R, Torino F. Endocrine side effects induced by immune checkpoint inhibitors. *J Clin Endocrinol Metab.* 2013;**98**(4):1361–1375.
6. Shah K, Ahmed S, Cabanillas M, Dadu R, Pitteloud M, Waguespack S. Imaging findings of cancer immunotherapy induced hypophysitis. In: Proceedings of the 53rd Annual Meeting of the American Society of Neuroradiology; April 25–30, 2015; Chicago, IL.
7. Pitteloud M, Dadu R, Cabanillas ME, Shah K, Hu MI, Habra M, Waguespack SG. Hypophysitis in the age of cancer immunotherapy: experience in a large cancer center. In: Proceedings of the 97th Annual Meeting of the Endocrine Society, March 5–8, 2015, San Diego, CA.
8. Byun DJ, Wolchok JD, Rosenberg LM, Girotra M. Cancer immunotherapy - immune checkpoint blockade and associated endocrinopathies. *Nat Rev Endocrinol.* 2017;**13**(4):195–207.
9. Cukier P, Santini FC, Scaranti M, Hoff AO. Endocrine side effects of cancer immunotherapy. *Endocr Relat Cancer.* 2017;**24**(12):T331–T347.
10. Min L, Hodi FS, Giobbie-Hurder A, Ott PA, Luke JJ, Donahue H, Davis M, Carroll RS, Kaiser UB. Systemic high-dose corticosteroid treatment does not improve the outcome of ipilimumab-related hypophysitis: a retrospective cohort study. *Clin Cancer Res.* 2015;**21**(4):749–755.
11. Honegger J, Buchfelder M, Schlaffer S, Droste M, Werner S, Strasburger C, Störmann S, Schopohl J, Kacheva S, Deutschbein T, Stalla G, Flitsch J, Milian M, Petersenn S, Elbelt U; Pituitary Working Group of the German Society of Endocrinology. Treatment of primary hypophysitis in Germany. *J Clin Endocrinol Metab.* 2015;**100**(9):3460–3469.
12. Dadu R, Zobniw C, Diab A. Managing adverse events with immune checkpoint agents. *Cancer J.* 2016;**22**(2):121–129.
13. Cabanillas ME, Waguespack SG, Pitteloud M, Roman-Gonzalez A, Jessop A, Santos E, Davies M, Dadu R. Anti-CTLA4-induced Graves disease: a rare cause of hyperthyroidism in 3 patients with metastatic melanoma. In: Proceedings of the 85th Annual Meeting of the American Thyroid Association; October 18–23, 2015; Buena Vista, FL.
14. Orlov S, Salari F, Kashat L, Walfish PG. Induction of painless thyroiditis in patients receiving programmed death 1 receptor immunotherapy for metastatic malignancies. *J Clin Endocrinol Metab.* 2015;**100**(5):1738–1741.
15. de Filette J, Jansen Y, Schreuer M, Everaert H, Velkeniers B, Neyns B, Bravenboer B. Incidence of thyroid-related adverse events in melanoma patients treated with pembrolizumab. *J Clin Endocrinol Metab.* 2016;**101**(11):4431–4439.
16. Lee H, Hodi FS, Giobbie-Hurder A, Ott PA, Buchbinder EI, Haq R, Tolaney S, Barroso-Sousa R, Zhang K, Donahue H, Davis M, Gargano ME, Kelley KM, Carroll RS, Kaiser UB, Min L. Characterization of thyroid disorders in patients receiving immune checkpoint inhibition therapy. *Cancer Immunol Res.* 2017;**5**(12):1133–1140.
17. Iyer P, Cabanillas ME, Waguespack SG, Busaidy NF, Hu MI, Dadu R. Immunotherapy mediated destructive thyroiditis: a cancer center's experience. Proceedings of the 86th Annual Meeting of the American Thyroid Association; September 21–25, 2016; Denver, CO.

NEUROENDOCRINOLOGY AND PITUITARY

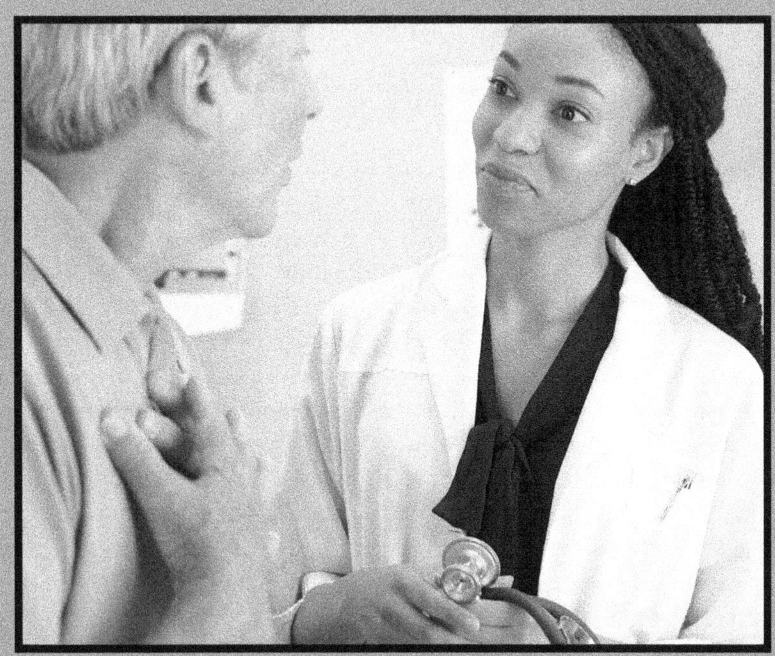

Pregnancy and Pituitary Tumors

M02

Presented, March 17–20, 2018

Mark E. Molitch, MD. Northwestern University Feinberg School of Medicine, Chicago, Illinois 60611, E-mail: molitch@northwestern.edu

CHANGES IN PITUITARY PHYSIOLOGY DURING PREGNANCY

The normal pituitary gland enlarges considerably during pregnancy, due to placental estrogen-stimulated lactotroph hyperplasia (1, 2). Concomitantly, prolactin (PRL) levels rise through gestation, preparing the breast for lactation (3). This lactotroph hyperplasia results in an increase in overall pituitary size as seen on magnetic resonance imaging (MRI) (2, 4, 5). After delivery, there is a rapid involution of the gland, so that normal pituitary size is found by 6 months postpartum (4, 5).

Circulating levels of a growth hormone (GH) variant made by the syncytiotrophoblastic epithelium of the placenta increase during the second half of pregnancy (6, 7). The GH variant is biologically active, stimulating the production of IGF-1, which causes a reduction in pituitary GH secretion via negative feedback (6, 7). In patients with acromegaly who have autonomous GH secretion and become pregnant, both forms of GH persist in the blood (8).

Over the course of gestation, cortisol levels rise progressively, due to an estrogen-induced increase in cortisol binding globulin levels and an increase in cortisol production, so that the bioactive "free" fraction, urinary free cortisol levels, and salivary cortisol levels are also increased (9, 10). Although there is placental production of adrenocorticotropic hormone (ACTH) and corticotropin-releasing hormone, they do not appear to be involved in the physiologic regulation of adrenal cortisol secretion during pregnancy (10). The elevated cortisol and ACTH levels may also be due to an antiglucocorticoid action of the elevated progesterone levels of pregnancy, with a resultant increase in the set-point for the negative feedback effects of cortisol (10).

Thyrotropin levels fall in the first trimester, in response to the rise in thyroid hormone levels, which are stimulated by placental chorionic gonadotropin, but return to the normal range by the third trimester (11). In response to placental sex steroid production, follicle-stimulating hormone and luteinizing hormone levels decline in the first trimester of pregnancy (12).

Pituitary adenomas cause problems because of hormone hypersecretion as well as by causing hypopituitarism because of mass effects. The pregnancy-induced alterations in hormone secretion complicate the evaluation of patients with pituitary adenomas. The influence of various types of therapy on the developing fetus also affects therapeutic decision making.

CASES

Case 1. Prolactinoma

This 42-year-old physician had initially presented with amenorrhea and galactorrhea and was found to have a 2-cm macroprolactinoma that extended inferiorly into the sphenoid sinus and had no suprasellar extension. With cabergoline 1 mg twice weekly, her PRL level normalized, her tumor reduced in size by ~50%, her menses regularized, and her galactorrhea resolved. She tried going off cabergoline a couple of times without maintaining normal PRL levels and also felt poorly off medication. Now she is 20 weeks pregnant and wonders if she should stop taking cabergoline. She feels so much better on compared with off cabergoline.

Case 1. Question

Which of the following should be the next step in management?

A. Switch cabergoline to bromocriptine and continue throughout pregnancy
B. Continue cabergoline throughout the pregnancy
C. Stop the cabergoline treatment now
D. Stop the cabergoline treatment now but restart if feeling badly

Case 1. Discussion

Answer: C. Stop the Cabergoline Treatment Now

Neither cabergoline nor bromocriptine should be continued once the pregnancy is diagnosed (answers A and B), so as to limit the exposure of the developing fetus to either drug (13). The chance of clinically significant tumor growth of a macroadenoma related to the pregnancy is ~16% (13), and this is not high enough to warrant continuing the drug. An exception might be made in a patient with a giant prolactinoma (>4 cm) in whom the risk of rapid tumor enlargement outweighs the risks of drug continuation. This is not the case in this patient with a 2-cm tumor. When either of these drugs is stopped within the first few weeks of pregnancy, the frequency of major malformations is not greater than would be expected in the general population (13). Because the risks are not increased for either drug, there is no justification for switching from cabergoline to bromocriptine (answer A), which is generally less effective. On the other hand, she has already been taking cabergoline for 20 weeks and is past the time of possible induction of malformations. Furthermore, we do occasionally reintroduce cabergoline when patients have tumor enlargement without adverse consequences. Interestingly, in a survey of Canadian endocrinologists, it was found that only 65% would discontinue dopamine agonists on confirmation of pregnancy in women with macroprolactinomas, and 82% stated they would continue the dopamine agonists in patients with large prolactinomas (14). In studies from Brazil and the Middle East/North Africa, only 58% and 38%, respectively, would withdraw dopamine agonists in women with macroadenomas (15, 16). Therefore, at 20 weeks of gestation, the best answer is not certain, but, in general, both drugs should be avoided during pregnancy.

Case 2. Acromegaly

This 28-year-old physician self-diagnosed acromegaly because of secondary amenorrhea, increasing foot size, change in facial appearance, increased sweating, and skin oiliness. On examination, she had mild facial features of acromegaly. Laboratory testing: GH 38.8 μg/L, IGF-1 518 ng/mL (117 to 329), PRL 115 μg/L [normal (nl) <26.3], AM cortisol 15.1, free T4 1.2 μg/dL (0.7 to 1.5), luteinizing hormone <1 IU/L, and follicle-stimulating hormone 2.8 IU/L. MRI showed a 2.7 × 1.6- × 2.1-cm tumor with right cavernous sinus invasion and was partially wrapped around the internal carotid. She recently married and wishes to get pregnant. She is concerned about her chances of remission and risks of hypopituitarism with surgery. She has also heard that medical treatments are only mediocre in their success rates.

Case 2. Question

Which of the following medical treatment options could be considered the safest to use during pregnancy?

A. Octreotide LAR
B. Pasireotide
C. Cabergoline
D. Pegvisomant
E. Lanreotide depot

Case 2. Discussion

Answer: C. Cabergoline

As discussed for case 1, cabergoline (answer C) has an established safety record during pregnancy (13). However, the efficacy of cabergoline in normalizing hormone levels is low, with only about one-third of individuals being controlled (17). Fewer than 50 pregnant patients treated with the somatostatin analogs octreotide and lanreotide have been reported; no malformations have been found in their children (18–21). However, a decrease in uterine artery blood flow has been reported with short-acting octreotide (21), and one fetus appeared to have intrauterine growth retardation that responded to a lowering of the dose of octreotide LAR (20). Octreotide binds to somatostatin receptors in the placenta (26) and crosses the placenta (21) and therefore can affect developing fetal tissues where somatostatin receptors are widespread, especially in the brain. Because of the limited data documenting safety, I recommend that octreotide and lanreotide analogs be discontinued if pregnancy is considered (answers A and E) and that contraception be used when these drugs are administered, and most (18–20) but not all (21) others concur. There are no safety data on using pasireotide (answer D) during pregnancy. Considering the prolonged nature of the course of most patients with acromegaly, interruption of somatostatin analogs for 9 to 12 months should not have a particularly adverse effect on the long-term outcome. On the other hand, these drugs can control tumor growth, and for enlarging tumors, their reintroduction during pregnancy may be warranted versus operating. Pegvisomant, a GH receptor antagonist, has been given to two patients with acromegaly during pregnancy without harm (19, 22), but the safety of this is certainly not established (answer D).

Case 3. Cushing Disease

This 30-year-old woman presented with 3 years of increasing facial hair, facial rounding, abdominal obesity, hypertension, diabetes, and oligomenorrhea. She had no muscle weakness or pigmented striae. She was taking a total of 140 U of insulin per day. Laboratory testing: 8:00 AM cortisol 30.2 μg/dL and ACTH 77 pg/mL (reference range, 5 to 27 pg/mL). With an overnight 1-mg dexamethasone suppression test, her 8:00 AM cortisol was 17.7 μg/dL. A 24-hour urine free cortisol was 305 μg (4.0 to 50). HbA_{1c} was 8.4%. An MRI showed a 5-mm pituitary tumor. Transsphenoidal surgery did not result in a cure. However, she now wishes to become pregnant.

Case 3. Question

Which of the following treatment options is absolutely contraindicated?

A. Ketoconazole
B. Repeat transsphenoidal surgery
C. Mifepristone
D. Pasireotide
E. Cabergoline

Case 3. Discussion

Answer: C. Mifepristone

Cushing syndrome is associated with a pregnancy loss rate of 25% due to spontaneous abortion, stillbirth, and early neonatal death because of extreme prematurity (23–25). The passage of cortisol across the placenta may rarely result in suppression of the fetal adrenals. Hypertension develops in most mothers with Cushing, and diabetes and myopathy are frequent (24, 25). Postoperative wound infection and dehiscence are common after cesarean section (24, 25). In a review of 136 pregnancies collected from the literature, Lindsay *et al.* (24) found that the frequency of live births increased from 76% to 89% when active treatment was instituted by a gestational age of 20 weeks. Therefore, treatment during pregnancy has been advocated (23–26).

All of the treatment modalities listed can improve Cushing disease (27), and treatment during pregnancy is advocated because it results in better fetal outcomes (23–26). Transsphenoidal surgery (answer B) has a cure rate of 80% to 90% in expert neurosurgical hands (28), with very low complication and fetal loss rates when done in the second trimester, but success of a second surgery is only ~50% (29). Experience with the various medical therapies is limited (26). Metyrapone has been used most often but can be associated with worsening hypertension and an increase in preeclampsia (26). Ketoconazole (answer A) now has a black box warning regarding liver function abnormalities; it has never been approved for use during pregnancy and is only modestly successful (26). Mifepristone (answer C) was originally developed as a progesterone receptor blocker and is a potent abortifacient (RU468) (30); therefore, its use in pregnancy is absolutely contraindicated. Pasireotide (answer D) is the only somatostatin analog with any success in patients with Cushing disease (31), but there is no experience with its use during pregnancy, and it would be expected to worsen glucose tolerance in this population susceptible to gestational diabetes. Although cabergoline (answer E) is safe when stopped after conception (see case 1 above), there is little experience when used throughout pregnancy, and its ability to normalize cortisol levels in Cushing disease is only modest (27). Neither pasireotide nor cabergoline is absolutely contraindicated during pregnancy.

REFERENCES

1. Scheithauer BW, Sano T, Kovacs KT, Young WF, Jr, Ryan N, Randall RV. The pituitary gland in pregnancy: a clinicopathologic and immunohistochemical study of 69 cases. *Mayo Clin Proc.* 1990;**65**(4): 461–474.
2. Elster AD, Sanders TG, Vines FS, Chen MY. Size and shape of the pituitary gland during pregnancy and post partum: measurement with MR imaging. *Radiology.* 1991;**181**(2):531–535.
3. Rigg LA, Lein A, Yen SSC. Pattern of increase in circulating prolactin levels during human gestation. *Am J Obstet Gynecol.* 1977;**129**(4): 454–456.
4. Gonzalez JG, Elizondo G, Saldivar D, Nanez H, Todd LE, Villarreal JZ. Pituitary gland growth during normal pregnancy: an in vivo study using magnetic rsonance imaging. *Am J Med.* 1988;**85**(8):217–220.
5. Dinç H, Esen F, Demirci A, Sari A, Resit Gümele H. Pituitary dimensions and volume measurements in pregnancy and *post partum.* MR assessment. *Acta Radiol.* 1998;**39**(1):64–69.
6. Frankenne F, Closset J, Gomez F, Scippo ML, Smal J, Hennen G. The physiology of growth hormones (GHs) in pregnant women and partial characterization of the placental GH variant. *J Clin Endocrinol Metab.* 1988;**66**(6):1171–1180.
7. Eriksson L, Frankenne F, Edèn S, Hennen G, Von Schoultz B. Growth hormone 24-h serum profiles during pregnancy: lack of pulsatility for the secretion of the placental variant. *Br J Obstet Gynaecol.* 1989; **96**(8):949–953.
8. Beckers A, Stevenaert A, Foidart J-M, Hennen G, Frankenne F. Placental and pituitary growth hormone secretion during pregnancy in acromegalic women. *J Clin Endocrinol Metab.* 1990;**71**(3): 725–731.
9. Nolten WE, Lindheimer MD, Rueckert PA, Oparil S, Ehrlich EN. Diurnal patterns and regulation of cortisol secretion in pregnancy. *J Clin Endocrinol Metab.* 1980;**51**(3):466–472.
10. Lindsay JR, Nieman LK. The hypothalamic-pituitary-adrenal axis in pregnancy: challenges in disease detection and treatment. *Endocr Rev.* 2005;**26**(6):775–799.
11. Glinoer D. The regulation of thyroid function in pregnancy: pathways of endocrine adaptation from physiology to pathology. *Endocr Rev.* 1997;**18**(3):404–433.
12. Jeppsson S, Rannevik G, Liedholm P, Thorell JI. Basal and LRH-stimulated secretion of FSH during early pregnancy. *Am J Obstet Gynecol.* 1977;**127**(1):32–36.
13. Molitch ME. Endocrinology in pregnancy: management of the pregnant patient with a prolactinoma. *Eur J Endocrinol.* 2015;**172**(5): R205–R213.
14. Almalki MH, Ur E, Johnson M, Clarke DB, Imran SA. Management of prolactinomas during pregnancy – a survey of four Canadian provinces. *Clin Invest Med.* 2012;**35**(2):E96–E104.
15. Vilar L, Naves LA, Casulari LA, Azevedo MF, Albuquerque JL, Serfaty FM, Pinho Barbosa FR, de Oliveira AR, Jr, Montenegro RM, Montenegro RM, Jr, Ramos AJ, Dos Santos Faria M, Musolino NR, Gadelha MR, Boguszewski CL, Bronstein MD. Management of prolactinomas in Brazil: an electronic survey. *Pituitary.* 2010;**13**(3):199–206.
16. Beshyah SA, Sherif IH, Chentli F, Hamrahian A, Khalil AB, Raef H, El-Fikki M, Jambart S. Management of prolactinomas: a survey of physicians from the Middle East and North Africa. *Pituitary.* 2017; **20**(2):231–240.
17. Sandret L, Maison P, Chanson P. Place of cabergoline in acromegaly: a meta-analysis. *J Clin Endocrinol Metab.* 2011;**96**(5):1327–1335.
18. Cheng V, Faiman C, Kennedy L, Khoury F, Hatipoglu B, Weil R, Hamrahian A. Pregnancy and acromegaly: a review. *Pituitary.* 2012; **15**(1):59–63.
19. Cheng S, Grasso L, Martinez-Orozco JA, Al-Agha R, Pivonello R, Colao A, Ezzat S. Pregnancy in acromegaly: experience from two referral centers and systematic review of the literature. *Clin Endocrinol (Oxf).* 2012;**76**(2):264–271.
20. Caron P, Broussaud S, Bertherat J, Borson-Chazot F, Brue T, Cortet-Rudelli C, Chanson P. Acromegaly and pregnancy: a retrospective multicenter study of 59 pregnancies in 46 women. *J Clin Endocrinol Metab.* 2010;**95**(10):4680–4687.
21. Maffei P, Tamagno G, Nardelli GB, Videau C, Menegazzo C, Milan G, Calcagno A, Martini C, Vettor R, Epelbaum J, Sicolo N. Effects of octreotide exposure during pregnancy in acromegaly. *Clin Endocrinol (Oxf).* 2010;**72**(5):668–677.
22. Brian SR, Bidlingmaier M, Wajnrajch MP, Weinzimer SA, Inzucchi SE. Treatment of acromegaly with pegvisomant during pregnancy: maternal and fetal effects. *J Clin Endocrinol Metab.* 2007;**92**(9): 3374–3377.
23. Bevan JS, Gough MH, Gillmer MD, Burke CW. Cushing's syndrome in pregnancy: the timing of definitive treatment. *Clin Endocrinol (Oxf).* 1987;**27**(2):225–233.
24. Lindsay JR, Jonklaas J, Oldfield EH, Nieman LK. Cushing's syndrome during pregnancy: personal experience and review of the literature. *J Clin Endocrinol Metab.* 2005;**90**(5):3077–3083.
25. Vilar L, Freitas MC, Lima LHC, Lyra R, Kater CE. Cushing's syndrome in pregnancy: an overview. *Arq Bras Endocrinol Metabol.* 2007;**51**(8): 1293–1302.
26. Bronstein MD, Machado MC, Fragoso MC. Management of endocrine disease: management of pregnant patients with Cushing's syndrome. *Eur J Endocrinol.* 2015;**173**:R85–R91.
27. Feelders RA, Hofland LJ. Medical treatment of Cushing's disease. *J Clin Endocrinol Metab.* 2013;**98**(2):425–438.
28. Petersenn S, Beckers A, Ferone D, van der Lely A, Bollerslev J, Boscaro M, Brue T, Bruzzi P, Casanueva FF, Chanson P, Colao A, Reincke M, Stalla G, Tsagarakis S. Therapy of endocrine disease: outcomes in patients with Cushing's disease undergoing transsphenoidal surgery: systematic review assessing criteria used to define remission and recurrence. *Eur J Endocrinol.* 2015;**172**(6):R227–R239.
29. Cohen-Kerem R, Railton C, Oren D, Lishner M, Koren G. Pregnancy outcome following non-obstetric surgical intervention. *Am J Surg.* 2005;**190**(3):467–473.
30. Marions L. Mifepristone dose in the regimen with misoprostol for medical abortion. *Contraception.* 2006;**74**(1):21–25.
31. Colao A, Petersenn S, Newell-Price J, Findling JW, Gu F, Maldonado M, Schoenherr U, Mills D, Salgado LR, Biller BM; Pasireotide B2305 Study Group. A 12-month phase 3 study of pasireotide in Cushing's disease. *N Engl J Med.* 2012;**366**(10):914–924.

Acromegaly: Diagnosis and Management

M04
Presented, March 17–20, 2018

Peter J. Trainer, MD. The Christie NHS Foundation Trust, University of Manchester, Manchester Academic Health Science Centre, Manchester M20 4BX, United Kingdom, E-mail: Peter.Trainer@manchester.ac.uk

SIGNIFICANCE OF THE CLINICAL PROBLEM

- Rare chronic disabling disease associated with premature death
- Incidence: five cases per million per year
- Prevalence: 60 cases per million
- Effective treatment relieves symptoms and restores life expectancy to near normal

Etiology

- 99% pituitary adenomas
  - >70% macroadenomas
- Rarely ectopic secretion of growth hormone (GH)–releasing hormone or somatotroph-cell hyperplasia
- Most cases sporadic
- Familial/genetic causes
  - Multiple endocrine neoplasia type 1
  - McCune-Albright syndrome
  - Familial acromegaly and Carney's syndrome
  - Aryl hydrocarbon receptor interacting protein gene mutations
  - X-LAG caused by microduplications on chromosome Xq26.3, encompassing the gene *GPR101*

BARRIERS TO OPTIMAL PRACTICE

- Delay in diagnosis
- Access to specialist pituitary surgeon
- Cost of medical therapy
- Biochemical definition of disease control; understanding the limitations of GH and insulin-like growth factor-1 (IGF-1) measurement

LEARNING OBJECTIVES

- Limitations of assays
- Importance of input of a multidisciplinary team including laboratory, pituitary surgeon, radiotherapist, and specialist nurse

STRATEGIES FOR DIAGNOSIS, THERAPY, AND MANAGEMENT

Diagnosis

- Varied presentation: soft tissue changes, headache, sleep apnea, carpal tunnel syndrome, visual field defect, hypertension, diabetes mellitus, sweating
- Typically, a decade lapses between development of symptoms and confirmation of diagnosis.
- Greatest challenge is for the diagnosis to be considered; thereafter, diagnosis is usually easily and rapidly confirmed.

Biochemical Confirmation

GH

- Undetectable (<0.3 μg/L) random GH measurement good evidence against acromegaly
- 75-g oral glucose tolerance test and serum IGF-1
  - Normal individuals, GH levels fall at least one value <0.3 μg/L
- Failure of suppression or a paradoxical rise in GH indicative of acromegaly
- Results usually unequivocal
- GH can fail to suppress in uncontrolled diabetes mellitus, liver or renal disease, patients receiving estrogen, during pregnancy and late adolescence, and malnutrition and anorexia (not difficult to distinguish anorexia from acromegaly), but in combination with IGF-1 measurement and examination, there is rarely a problem confirming the diagnosis.

IGF-1

- IGF-1 within the reference range in newly diagnosed acromegaly is rare.
- Utility of IGF-1 is hindered by concerns over the quality of some commercial assays and reference ranges.
- Levels may vary, typically being low in liver and renal dysfunction and uncontrolled diabetes mellitus.
- Nutrition, circadian rhythm, estrogen, insulin, glucocorticoid therapy, and thyroxine levels can affect IGF-1 levels

Imaging

Magnetic resonance imaging with gadolinium contrast

- >70% pituitary tumor >10 mm
- Hyperplastic gland in rare cases of ectopic GH-releasing hormone or somatotroph hyperplasia

Pituitary Function Testing

As per standard protocols

Therapy

Goals of Therapy/Criteria for Remission

- Nadir GH of <0.3 μg/L on oral glucose tolerance test and
- IGF-1 in the age-adjusted normal range

GH is not a measure of disease activity in patients receiving pegvisomant therapy; rely on IGF-1.

Surgery

- Choice of the surgeon is crucial.
- Transsphenoidal microsurgical approach is initial treatment in a majority of patients.
- In expert hands, approximately 80% and 50% of patients with micro- and macroadenomas, respectively, achieve normal IGF-1 levels.
- Morbidity and mortality lower in the hands of specialist pituitary surgeons.

Radiotherapy

- Effective at controlling tumor growth
- Slow to control GH secretion and normalize IGF-1

Conventional Multifractionated (three field, 4500 cGy)

- No longer routine because of the risk of cerebrovascular accidents but still has a place in the treatment of patients with large and growing residual tumor after surgery
- 50% reduction in GH levels in the first 2 years after radiotherapy, and a 75% fall by 5 years; the fall in circulating IGF-1 levels is more gradual
- Hypopituitarism: most common complication
- 10-year deficiencies: thyroid-stimulating hormone, 27%; follicle-stimulating hormone/luteinizing hormone, 18%; adrenocorticotropic hormone, 15%

Stereotactic High-Dose Irradiation

- In many centers supplanted conventional radiotherapy
- Most frequently being delivered by the stereotactic radiosurgery
- Requires precise delineation of the tumor to ensure minimal surrounding tissue exposure
- Suitable for smaller-volume residual tumor beyond reach of surgeon
- Tumor control attained in 97%
- Hormonal remission rates vary from 17% to 96%
- Hypopituitarism is the most common adverse effect.

Medical Treatment

Dopamine Receptor Agonists

- Act through D2 receptor
- Continue to have a place in treatment
- Often in combination with somatostatin analogs
- Twin virtues of relatively inexpensive and orally administered
- Cabergoline: long-acting ergot-derived dopamine agonist; superseded bromocriptine
  - More potent and better tolerated
  - Doses of up to 1 mg/d normalize IGF-1 in up to 30% of patients
  - Probably most effective in patients with prolactin cosecretion
  - May induce tumor shrinkage
  - Not licensed for the treatment of acromegaly
  - Large-scale prospective studies have not been undertaken

Adverse Effects

- Gastrointestinal discomfort, nausea, vomiting, dizziness, headache, and postural hypotension
- Manageable by slow-dose titration
- Depression or mania, often in patients with a history of such
- Rarely addictive behavior: gambling, alcohol, shopping, and sex
- Cardiac valve fibrosis
- Evidence in Parkinson's disease with ergot-derived dopamine agonists
- Lack of convincing evidence in pituitary disease
- Related to cumulative dose
- Doses in endocrine patients smaller than those for Parkinson's
- Annual echocardiograms recommended

Somatostatin Analogs

- Somatostatin peptide produced by neuroendocrine, inflammatory, and immune cells in response to specific stimuli
  - Actions mediated by five subtypes of receptors (SST1-5)
  - Somatostatin cannot be used for therapy of acromegaly: short plasma half-life (2 to 3 minutes), lack of specificity (binds all five receptor subtypes).
- Octreotide and lanreotide are somatostatin analogs with prolonged plasma half-lives and high affinity for the SST2 and SST5 receptors responsible for regulation of GH secretion from somatotrophs.
- Pasireotide: high affinity for SST1, 2, 3, and 5 (40-fold increased affinity to ST5 compared with other analogs)
- May be of value in patients with an inadequate response to octreotide
- Significantly higher rate of impaired glucose tolerance and diabetes
- Treatment of choice for most patients not cured by surgery
- Recent prospective clinical trial; biochemical disease control achieved by octreotide in 19%, pasireotide 31%
- Results better in patients with milder disease
- Addition of cabergoline may result in a further fall in GH and IGF-1 levels accompanied by relief of symptoms.
- Increasing interest in somatostatin analog therapy preoperatively, either as a short-term measure in the hope that surgical outcomes are improved or as a long-term alternative to surgery

- Impressive tumor shrinkage in patients as first-line therapy
- Few objective data showing preoperative somatostatin analog therapy improves the outcome of subsequent surgery

Adverse Effects

- Gastrointestinal symptoms
- Biliary tract abnormalities
- Hyperglycemia
- Asymptomatic sinus bradycardia

Pegvisomant

- Genetically engineered analog of human GH
- GH receptor antagonist
- IGF-1 main measure of disease activity (serum GH should not be measured)
- Normalized IGF-1 in 89% at dose of 20 mg/d, 97% using doses up to 40 mg/d
- Data from the postmarketing surveillance database: IGF-1 normalization rate is only ~70%, probably because of a failure of adequate dose titration
- Long half-life (>70 hours) of pegvisomant means probably a once weekly, rather than daily, medication.
- Place of pegvisomant in treatment algorithm: persisting symptoms and elevated IGF-1 despite surgery, possibly radiotherapy, and maximum doses of somatostatin analogs
- Monotherapy or combination with somatostatin analog both expensive but little to choose between the two in terms of cost
- Combination with cabergoline offers a more cost-effective option.

Adverse Effects

- Elevation of liver enzymes
- Magnetic resonance imaging initially every 6 months and ultimately annual
- Lipohypertrophy

GH and IGF-1 Measurement

- Serum GH and IGF-1 levels are closely correlated, but discordance can occur as a consequence of:
  - Biological factors
  - Artifact of the measurement
  - Definitions of normality
- Estrogens induce relative GH resistance such that for a given GH, IGF-1 is lower in women than men.
- After pituitary radiotherapy, GH declines faster than IGF-1. Pulsatility studies indicate that circulating IGF-1 values correlate most closely with trough, rather than mean or peak, GH values.
- Because >70% of circulating IGF-1 is hepatic in origin, liver disease can in impair IGF-1 generation.
- Vigilance is required when applying international criteria to local practice, because bias in assay performance can be significant, a problem compounded by quality assurance concerns with some commercial kits.
- The upper limit of normal of modern reference ranges for IGF-1 is significantly lower than historical limit, such that a patient regarded as controlled by IGF-1 criteria a decade ago may no longer be so.
- When GH and IGF-1 levels are grossly elevated, the factors described above are of little clinical relevance. The true challenge of discordant results is in the patient with nearly ideal control and who may benefit from additional treatment. In an era of ever-greater technology, seeking symptoms from patients remains critical to management and good outcomes.

CASES

Case 1

A 22-year-old woman presented to the neurosurgeons with grand mal seizures and a right temporal visual field defect. Laboratory values are as follows: fT4, 14.9 pmol/L (reference range, 10 to 22 pmol/L); thyroid stimulating hormone, 1.45 mU/L; random cortisol, 408 nmol/L (15 μg/dL); IGF-I, 363 ng/mL (reference range, 99 to 382 ng/mL); prolactin, 1580 mU/L (reference, <425 mU/L). The woman proceeded to transsphenoidal surgery. The tumor histology was positive staining for GH. Postoperative laboratory values were as follows: IGF-I, 538 ng/mL (reference range, 99 to 382 ng/mL; oral glucose tolerance test (OGTT) GH nadir, 30 ng/mL.

Question

What is the explanation of IGF-I being higher postoperatively?

Answer

The patient had acromegaly with a mild phenotype, although she was tall. At presentation, she was on an estrogen-containing oral contraceptive, which was discontinued at the time of surgery. Estrogen induces GH resistance, which resulted in a normal preoperative IGF-I and there was no preoperative assessment of GH status.

Learning Point

One should measure GH and IGF-I preoperatively.

Case 2

A 27-year-old man presented to the dentist with facial pain. Acromegaly was suspected and confirmed by elevated IGF-I and abnormal OGTT and a prolactin level of 1484 mU/L (reference, <400 mU/L). The patient was started on bromocriptine preoperatively. One year later, the patient had transsphenoidal hypophysectomy. At 2 years, the patient had the following treatment for persistent disease: transcranial surgery, postoperative multifractional radiotherapy, and ongoing bromocriptine and long-acting octreotide. At 4 years, the patient was jailed for defrauding family members of ~$200,000 to pay off gambling debts. At 6 years, the patient was released from prison; his IGF-I level was 678 ng/mL (reference range, 78 to 232 ng/mL).

Question

What therapeutic intervention was necessary?

Answer

Bromocriptine was discontinued as it is likely to have induced addictive behavior, namely compulsive gambling. Compulsive disorders, including pathological gambling, compulsive shopping, excessive alcohol consumption, and increased libido, have been suggested to be a class effect of dopamine agonists. Pegvisomant was added to ongoing octreotide therapy, and his most recent octreotide was 250 ng/mL (reference range, 78 to 219 ng/mL).

RECOMMENDED READING

Abs R, Verhelst J, Maiter D, Van Acker K, Nobels F, Coolens JL, Mahler C, Beckers A. Cabergoline in the treatment of acromegaly: a study in 64 patients. *J Clin Endocrinol Metab.* 1998;**83**(2):374–378.

Ahmed S, Elsheikh M, Stratton IM, Page RC, Adams CB, Wass JA. Outcome of transphenoidal surgery for acromegaly and its relationship to surgical experience. *Clin Endocrinol (Oxf).* 1999;**50**(5):561–567.

Bevan JS, Atkin SL, Atkinson AB, Bouloux PM, Hanna F, Harris PE, James RA, McConnell M, Roberts GA, Scanlon MF, Stewart PM, Teasdale E, Turner HE, Wass JA, Wardlaw JM. Primary medical therapy for acromegaly: an open, prospective, multicenter study of the effects of subcutaneous and intramuscular slow-release octreotide on growth hormone, insulin-like growth factor-I, and tumor size. J Clin *Endocrinol Metab.* 2002;**87**(10):4554–4563.

Brabant G, von zur Mühlen A, Wüster C, Ranke MB, Kratzsch J, Kiess W, Ketelslegers JM, Wilhelmsen L, Hulthén L, Saller B, Mattsson A, Wilde J, Schemer R, Kann P; German KIMS Board. Serum insulin-like growth factor I reference values for an automated chemiluminescence immunoassay system: results from a multicenter study. *Horm Res.* 2003; **60**(2):53–60.

Carlsen SM, Lund-Johansen M, Schreiner T, Aanderud S, Johannesen O, Svartberg J, Cooper JG, Hald JK, Fougner SL, Bollerslev J; Preoperative Octreotide Treatment of Acromegaly Study Group. Preoperative octreotide treatment in newly diagnosed acromegalic patients with macroadenomas increases cure short-term postoperative rates: a prospective, randomized trial. *J Clin Endocrinol Metab.* 2008;**93**(8):2984–2990.

Clayton RN, Stewart PM, Shalet SM, Wass JA. Pituitary surgery for acromegaly. Should be done by specialists. *BMJ.* 1999;**319**(7210): 588–589.

Colao A, Bronstein MD, Freda P, Gu F, Shen CC, Gadelha M, Fleseriu M, van der Lely AJ, Farrall AJ, Hermosillo Reséndiz K, Ruffin M, Chen Y, Sheppard M; Pasireotide C2305 Study Group. Pasireotide versus octreotide in acromegaly: a head-to-head superiority study. *J Clin Endocrinol Metab.* 2014;**99**(3):791–799.

Cozzi R, Attanasio R, Lodrini S, Lasio G. Cabergoline addition to depot somatostatin analogues in resistant acromegalic patients: efficacy and lack of predictive value of prolactin status. *Clin Endocrinol (Oxf).* 2004; **61**(2):209–215.

Giustina A, Chanson P, Kleinberg D, Bronstein MD, Clemmons DR, Klibanski A, van der Lely AJ, Strasburger CJ, Lamberts SW, Ho KK, Casanueva FF, Melmed S; Acromegaly Consensus Group. Expert consensus document: a consensus on the medical treatment of acromegaly. *Nat Rev Endocrinol.* 2014;**10**(4):243–248.

Jenkins PJ, Bates P, Carson MN, Stewart PM, Wass JA. Conventional pituitary irradiation is effective in lowering serum growth hormone and insulin-like growth factor-I in patients with acromegaly. *J Clin Endocrinol Metab.* 2006;**91**(4):1239–1245.

Melmed S. Medical progress: acromegaly. *N Engl J Med.* 2006;**355**(24): 2558–2574.

Melmed S, Colao A, Barkan A, Molitch M, Grossman AB, Kleinberg D, Clemmons D, Chanson P, Laws E, Schlechte J, Vance ML, Ho K, Giustina A; Acromegaly Consensus Group. Guidelines for acromegaly management: an update. *J Clin Endocrinol Metab.* 2009;**94**(5):1509–1517.

Sandret L, Maison P, Chanson P. Place of cabergoline in acromegaly: a meta-analysis. *J Clin Endocrinol Metab.* 2011;**96**(5):1327–1335.

Swearingen B, Barker FG 2nd, Katznelson L, Biller BM, Grinspoon S, Klibanski A, Moayeri N, Black PM, Zervas NT. Long-term mortality after transsphenoidal surgery and adjunctive therapy for acromegaly. *J Clin Endocrinol Metab.* 1998;**83**(10):3419–3426.

Trainer PJ, Drake WM, Katznelson L, Freda PU, Herman-Bonert V, van der Lely AJ, Dimaraki EV, Stewart PM, Friend KE, Vance ML, Besser GM, Scarlett JA, Thorner MO, Parkinson C, Klibanski A, Powell JS, Barkan AL, Sheppard MC, Malsonado M, Rose DR, Clemmons DR, Johannsson G, Bengtsson BA, Stavrou S, Kleinberg DL, Cook DM, Phillips LS, Bidlingmaier M, Strasburger CJ, Hackett S, Zib K, Bennett WF, Davis RJ. Treatment of acromegaly with the growth hormone-receptor antagonist pegvisomant. *N Engl J Med.* 2000;**342**(16):1171–1177.

van der Lely AJ, Biller BM, Brue T, Buchfelder M, Ghigo E, Gomez R, Hey-Hadavi J, Lundgren F, Rajicic N, Strasburger CJ, Webb SM, Koltowska-Häggström M. Long-term safety of pegvisomant in patients with acromegaly: comprehensive review of 1288 subjects in ACROSTUDY. *J Clin Endocrinol Metab.* 2012;**97**(5):1589–1597.

van der Lely AJ, Hutson RK, Trainer PJ, Besser GM, Barkan AL, Katznelson L, Klibanski A, Herman-Bonert V, Melmed S, Vance ML, Freda PU, Stewart PM, Friend KE, Clemmons DR, Johannsson G, Stavrou S, Cook DM, Phillips LS, Strasburger CJ, Hackett S, Zib KA, Davis RJ, Scarlett JA, Thorner MO. Long-term treatment of acromegaly with pegvisomant, a growth hormone receptor antagonist. *Lancet.* 2001;**358**(9295): 1754–1759.

Wang YY, Higham C, Kearney T, Davis JR, Trainer P, Gnanalingham KK. Acromegaly surgery in Manchester revisited—the impact of reducing surgeon numbers and the 2010 consensus guidelines for disease remission. *Clin Endocrinol (Oxf).* 2012;**76**(3):399–406.

Wieringa GE, Barth JH, Trainer PJ. Growth hormone assay standardization: a biased view? *Clin Endocrinol (Oxf).* 2004;**60**(5):538–539.

Diabetes Insipidus: Challenges in Diagnosis/Management

M07
Presented, March 17–20, 2018

Daniel G. Bichet, MD. University of Montreal, Montreal, Quebec H4J 1C5, Canada, E-mail: daniel.bichet@umontreal.ca

SIGNIFICANCE OF THE CLINICAL PROBLEM: HOW TO EVALUATE FLUID BALANCE

Simple Plasma and Urine Measurements to Differentiate Hypo-Osmotic Diuresis (Aquaresis) From Osmotic Diuresis: Measurements of Plasma Osmolality, Urine Osmolality, and Ratio of Urine $Na^+ + K^+$/Plasma $Na^+ + K^+$

Diabetes insipidus (DI) is characterized by the excretion of abnormally large volumes of hypo-osmotic urine (<250 mmol/kg).

This definition excludes osmotic diuresis, which occurs when excess solute is being excreted as with glucose in the polyuria of diabetes mellitus. In osmotic diuresis, the urine osmolality is >300 mmol/kg, and the total excretion of solutes per 24 hours is >900 mmol. The kidney neoglucogenesis is producing 15 to 55 g of glucose per day; 25 to 35 g are used for metabolic purposes, and 180 g of glucose are filtered and reabsorbed every day by the sodium-glucose cotransporter 2 expressed in proximal tubules. In nondiabetes mellitus subjects, the renal glucose reabsorption is around 180 g/d, and glycosuria is minimal. In patients taking sodium-glucose cotransporter 2 inhibitors, the additional osmotic diuresis is only 200 to 600 mL/d (1).

Other agents that produce osmotic diuresis are mannitol, urea, glycerol, contrast media, and loop diuretics. Total parenteral nutrition could induce an osmotic diuresis, because the catabolism of 100 g of proteins will produce 571 mmol of urea (2). Osmotic diuresis should be considered when solute excretion exceeds 60 mmol/h (3).

The urine excretion of electrolytes and not urine osmolality is a useful tool to predict the expected variations in plasma sodium. Urine osmolality includes $Na^+ + K^+$ + urea + glucose. A hypotonic urine is characterized by a concentration of $Na^+ + K^+$ less than the plasma $Na^+ + K^+$ concentration. In these calculations, urea, although the most abundant urine osmole, is not included, because it moves to achieve an equal concentration in the extracellular fluid and intracellular fluid compartments (4). As well, in the presence of insulin, the contribution of glucose to movements of water between extracellular fluid and intracellular fluid is minimal. The excretion of a hypotonic urine will increase plasma sodium and will result in compensatory thirst and vasopressin release. By contrast, the excretion of urine with a concentration of $Na^+ + K^+$ higher than the plasma $Na^+ + K^+$ concentration will decrease plasma sodium. Bockenhauer and Bichet (5) recently published an example of these tonicity calculations pertaining to the administration of fluid in a young patient with nephrogenic DI. A 10-kg congenital nephrogenic DI patient with an estimated 7 L of total body water and a hypotonic urine with an Na concentration of 10 mmol/L is receiving 1 L of 0.9% saline to replace a urine output of 1 L. This will not change the fluid balance, but it will lead to a net gain of 144 mmol of Na and would lead to a dangerous increase in the plasma Na concentration of ~144 mmol/7 L = 20 mmol/L.

Quantify the Severity of Polyuria and Do Short Dehydration Tests Not Reaching a Dehydration State Beyond a Plasma Sodium of 147 mEq/L

Polyuria has generally been defined as a urine output exceeding 3 L/d in adults and 2 L/m^2 in children. It must be differentiated from the more common complaints of frequency or nocturia, which are not associated with an increase in the total urine output. A precise quantification of 24-hour urine volume might be technically difficult in young patients and may necessitate >2 × 4-L urine collection containers in adults, but this measurement will determine the length of a dehydration test. Short dehydration tests with immediate results of plasma sodium, osmolality, urine osmolality, and $Na^+ + K^+$ concentrations will be done in severely polyuric patients, and dehydration will be stopped as soon as plasma sodium reaches 147 mEq/L. This plasma sodium concentration corresponds to a maximum stimulation of the antidiuretic hormone (ADH) arginine vasopressin (AVP). Thereafter, 2 μg of desamino-8D-arginine-vasopressin (dDAVP) is given subcutaneously, and urine osmolality measures are repeated every 30 minutes over the next 2 hours to differentiate central from nephrogenic DI.

Do Not Hesitate to Seek Genetic Testing in Patients With Congenital DI

Genetic testing will rapidly identify patients bearing *AVP* mutations (6) responsible for autosomal dominant central DI or arginine-vasopressin type 2 receptor (*AVPR2*) or aquaporin 2 (*AQP2*) mutations responsible for nephrogenic DI (7). The *AVP*, *AVPR2*, and *AQP2* genes are small genes easily sequenced. A rapid accurate diagnosis cuts the "diagnostic odyssey" that often involves many false leads and ineffective treatments, can reduce health costs, and can provide psychological benefit to patients and families (8).

BARRIERS TO OPTIMAL PRACTICE

Patients with DI are relatively rare, and their evaluation and treatment might not be as frequent as other common endocrine pathologies. I encourage endocrinologists to study these cases in collaboration with radiologists well versed in the interpretation of hypothalamic magnetic resonance imaging and with internists or nephrologists with a good grasp of electrolyte and tonicity evaluation and measurements. A clinical research unit used to do dehydration tests with online measures of sodium, osmolality, and electrolytes is a valuable resource in many academic centers. Finally, I recommend e-mail exchanges with individuals or centers used to do clinical and genetic tests for DI.

LEARNING OBJECTIVES

As a result of participating in this session, learners should be able to:

- Differentiate osmotic and nonosmotic polyuric states and memorize three examples of osmotic polyuria: glucose, mannitol, and urea
- Recognize three main entities in nonosmotic polyuric patients: central (neurohypophyseal) DI, nephrogenic DI, and psychogenic polydipsia
- Order a safe dehydration test with plasma and urine measurements pre- and post-dDAVP testing, never allowing a plasma sodium to be >147 mEq/L
- Seek genetic testing for the following genes responsible for congenital DI cases: *AVP*, *AVPR2*, and *AQP2*

STRATEGIES FOR DIAGNOSIS, THERAPY, AND/OR MANAGEMENT

- Primary polydipsia (sometimes called psychogenic polydipsia) is characterized by a primary increase in water intake. This disorder is most often seen in middle-aged women and patients with psychiatric illnesses, including those taking a phenothiazine, which can lead to the sensation of a dry mouth. Primary polydipsia can also be induced by hypothalamic lesions that directly affect the thirst center, such as may occur with an infiltrative disease, such as sarcoidosis.
- Central DI (also called neurohypophyseal or neurogenic DI) is associated with deficient secretion of ADH. This condition is most often idiopathic (possibly due to autoimmune injury to the ADH-producing cells) or can be induced by trauma, pituitary surgery, or hypoxic or ischemic encephalopathy. Rare familial cases have been described.
- Nephrogenic DI is characterized by normal ADH secretion but varying degrees of renal resistance to its water-retaining effect. This problem, in its mild form, is relatively common, because most patients who are elderly or who have underlying renal disease have a reduction in maximum concentrating ability. This defect, however, is not severe enough to produce a symptomatic increase in urine output.

Nephrogenic DI presenting in childhood is almost always caused by inherited defects. The most common are X-linked hereditary nephrogenic DI caused by mutations in the *AVPR2* gene encoding the ADH receptor V2 and autosomal recessive and dominant nephrogenic DI caused by mutations in the aquaporin-2 *AQP2* (water channel) gene.

Nephrogenic DI presenting in adults is almost always acquired, with chronic lithium use and hypercalcemia being the most common causes of a defect severe enough to produce polyuria.

Plasma Sodium and Urine Osmolality

Each of the three causes of polyuria—primary polydipsia, central DI, and nephrogenic DI—is associated with an increase in water output and the excretion of a relatively dilute urine. With primary polydipsia, the polyuria is an appropriate response to enhanced water intake; in comparison, the water loss is inappropriate with either form of DI. Measurement of the plasma sodium concentration and the urine osmolality response to dDAVP may be helpful in distinguishing between these disorders (9).

New Data Using Optogenetic Tools Allow the Identification and Functional Analysis of Thirst Neurons and Vasopressin-Producing Neurons

Two major advances provide a detailed anatomy of taste for water and the ADH AVP release. (1) Thirst and AVP release are regulated by not only the classical homeostatic, interosensory plasma osmolality negative feedback but also, novel exterosensory, anticipatory signals. These anticipatory signals for thirst and vasopressin release converge on the same homeostatic neurons circumventricular organs that monitor the composition of the blood (10). (2) Acid-sensing taste receptor cells (which express polycystic kidney disease 2–like 1 protein) on the tongue that were previously suggested as the sour taste sensors also mediate taste responses to water. The tongue has a taste for water (11).

Therapy and management of central and nephrogenic DI are discussed extensively in recent publications (7, 12).

CONCLUSIONS

The regulation of thirst and vasopressin release are now better characterized with modern genetic tools as well as the vasopressin action on principal cells of the collecting duct. The identification of osmotic diuresis vs aquaresis is simple, and the urine osmolality response to dDAVP differentiates central from nephrogenic DI. Congenital nephrogenic DI cases benefit from genetic testing.

CASES

Case 1: A Young Patient Thirsty Since Birth

E-mail was received March 3, 2010. "My son Ethan was born December ... 2005. Ever since that date, he has had a near-constant thirst. He would not take to breastfeeding, because the milk came out too slow. When he was of age to eat food, he would scream for drink instead.

By age 2, we were starting to get quite concerned with his size. He was only 21 lb at that point, but our family doctor shrugged it off. He was also still constantly thirsty and urinating frequently. He would often wake up at night screaming frantically for a drink. We could not wake him from these events. Once again, the family doctor was not concerned.

My son's pediatrician currently thinks that his excessive thirst is behavioral and has advised us to forcefully reduce his fluid intake. This is becoming very difficult, since Ethan is now finding more and more ways to sneak a drink secretly.

I am wondering if you might have any insight here ... we would certainly be willing to make the trip to Montreal."

Voting questions

1. The excessive thirst is likely behavioral and water should be restricted.
2. Excessive thirst and urination present since birth are likely secondary to congenital nephrogenic DI.

Answer

Mrs. ..., I do not think that the increased thirst and polyuria observed in your son Ethan are behavioral.

We would appreciate receiving blood from Ethan and from you.

E-mail April 19th: *AVPR2* mutation V88M; mother is a carrier.

Urine flow: 6 mL/min; UOsm: 55 pre-dDAVP and 57 post-dDAVP.

Case 2: Not Nephrogenic DI but Central DI Easily Treated With dDAVP

E-mail

"I was in contact with you about 2 mo ago about a patient with congenital nephrogenic DI. I sent you blood on the patient.

I am actually a hematologist who has seen the patient on two occasions with regard to his platelet function and how renal transplantation could most safely be performed. We did a dDAVP challenge test, and the platelet function reverted to normal post-dDAVP. We also measured a large increase in factor VIII and VWF, showing that his endothelial cells do respond to vasopressin.

This patient had been thoroughly evaluated at the Mayo Clinic when he was a child (probably close to 40 years ago). I do not have access to the exact results of urine studies and response to 'pitressin' (which apparently was used at that time).

My patient has a 13-year-old son who is affected, a 7-year-old son who is not affected, and a 9-year-old daughter who is not affected."

Question

X-linked nephrogenic DI with a father to son transmission?

Answer

Your patient has a central, autosomal dominant vasopressin-sensitive DI; my laboratory identified the G88V mutation in his *AVP* gene, the gene responsible for AVP coding in the hypothalamus. The G88V mutation is new, but G88S and G88R mutations have been identified previously.

This result is in line with your dDAVP test showing normal coagulation factor responses to dDAVP.

It is possible that the central DI was not recognized and that progressive dilatation of the urinary tract was the consequence with progressive renal failure. Progressive dilatation of urinary tract in untreated central DI and consequent renal failure are rare but already known.

The important lesson now is to make the appropriate diagnosis and prescribe treatment to the 13-year-old affected son. The best will be to send me blood (two 5-mL lavender stopper tubes from the two sons and the daughter) and do a 24-hour urine collection, a short dehydration test, and response to dDAVP for the 13-year-old son.

The affected brother of Mr. K should also be DNA tested (13).

REFERENCES

1. Ferrannini E, Solini A. SGLT2 inhibition in diabetes mellitus: rationale and clinical prospects. *Nat Rev Endocrinol.* 2012;**8**(8):495–502.
2. Lindner G, Schwarz C, Funk GC. Osmotic diuresis due to urea as the cause of hypernatraemia in critically ill patients. *Nephrol Dial Transplant.* 2012;**27**(3):962–967.
3. Bichet DG. Clinical manifestations and causes of central diabetes insipidus; clinical manifestations and causes of nephrogenic diabetes insipidus. In: *UptoDate.* Waltham, MA: Wolters Kluwer; 2017.
4. Carlotti AP, Bohn D, Mallie JP, Halperin ML. Tonicity balance, and not electrolyte-free water calculations, more accurately guides therapy for acute changes in natremia. *Intensive Care Med.* 2001;**27**(5):921–924.
5. Bockenhauer D, Bichet DG. Nephrogenic diabetes insipidus. *Curr Opin Pediatr.* 2017;**29**(2):199–205.
6. Bichet DG, Lussier Y. Mice deficient for ERAD machinery component Sel1L develop central diabetes insipidus. *J Clin Invest.* 2017;**127**(10): 3591–3593.
7. Bockenhauer D, Bichet DG. Pathophysiology, diagnosis and management of nephrogenic diabetes insipidus. *Nat Rev Nephrol.* 2015; **11**(10):576–588.
8. Green ED, Guyer MS; National Human Genome Research Institute. Charting a course for genomic medicine from base pairs to bedside. *Nature.* 2011;**470**(7333):204–213.
9. Bichet DG. Diagnosis of polyuria and diabetes insipidus. In: *UptoDate.* Waltham, MA: Wolters Kluwer; 2017.
10. Zimmerman CA, Leib DE, Knight ZA. Neural circuits underlying thirst and fluid homeostasis. *Nat Rev Neurosci.* 2017;**18**(8):459–469.
11. Zocchi D, Wennemuth G, Oka Y. The cellular mechanism for water detection in the mammalian taste system. *Nat Neurosci.* 2017;**20**(7): 927–933.
12. Bichet DG. Treatment of central diabetes insipidus. Treatment of nephrogenic diabetes insipidus. In: Rose BD, ed. *UptoDate.* Waltham, MA: Wolters Kluwer; 2017.
13. Bichet DG, Rice L, Levallois-Gignac J. A need for a systematic genetic evaluation of hereditary polyuric patients. *Clin Kidney J.* 2016;**9**(2): 177–179.

Diagnosis and Management of Hyponatremia in 2018

M16
Presented, March 17–20, 2018

Mark Sherlock, MB, BCh, BAO, MRCPI. Beaumont Hospital and Royal College of Surgeons in Ireland, Dublin 2, Ireland, E-mail: marksherlock@beaumont.ie

Joseph G. Verbalis, MD. Division of Endocrinology and Metabolism, Georgetown University, Washington, DC 20007, E-mail: verbalis@georgetown.edu

SIGNIFICANCE OF THE CLINICAL PROBLEM

Hyponatremia is the most common electrolyte abnormality and is encountered in all areas of clinical practice (1). Hyponatremia occurs in approximately 15% to 30% of hospitalized patients, with 1% to 2% of patients having a serum sodium level <125 mmol/L (2, 3). The risk of developing hyponatremia can be even higher in certain populations, including those in the critical care and neurosurgical environments (4–7). Similarly, there is an increased rate of hyponatremia with increasing age (8).

Hyponatremia is associated with increased morbidity and mortality (9). Acute severe symptomatic hyponatremia is a medical emergency that carries considerable morbidity and mortality if not addressed acutely. The related morbidity depends on the severity, acuity, and underlying etiology of hyponatremia. There is increasing evidence that patients with mild asymptomatic hyponatremia have increased risk of falls, osteoporosis, and fractures (10–13). In addition, inappropriate management of hyponatremia can lead to substantial morbidity because of the risk of osmotic demyelination syndrome (14). Mortality is also increased in patients with hyponatremia, and the risk of mortality is different depending on the etiology of hyponatremia (15).

Assessment and treatment of hyponatremia are often suboptimal. In recent years, expert guidance and recommendations have been published providing an evidence-based approach to diagnosis and treatment of hyponatremia (16, 17). There is still a paucity of data regarding a number of areas of hyponatremia management.

LEARNING OBJECTIVES

- Hyponatremia is common and is associated with increased morbidity and mortality
- How to differentiate between different etiologies of hyponatremia
- Management of severe symptomatic hyponatremia
- Management of chronic hyponatremia
- Approaches to decrease the risk of osmotic demyelination syndrome

PHYSIOLOGY OF WATER BALANCE

Plasma/serum sodium concentrations are maintained within a narrow range, despite wide variations in water and salt intake (18). Plasma sodium concentration rarely varies by more than 1% to 2% off baseline in normal physiological conditions if access to water is freely available. In health, plasma osmolality is closely regulated by the sophisticated interaction of the secretion and action of the antidiuretic hormone vasopressin (AVP) and the sensation of thirst, which promotes water intake. Changes in plasma osmolality are detected by specialized magnocellular neurones in the anterior hypothalamus, with resultant changes in AVP synthesis and secretion and thirst sensation.

ETIOLOGY AND CLASSIFICATION OF HYPONATREMIA

There are a number of etiologies of hypontremia, which can be divided into:

- Hypotonic hyponatremia (which is subdivided into hypovolemic, euvolemic, and hypervolemic causes)
- Less frequent causes of hyponatremia, including pseudohyponatremia and nonhypotonic hyponatremia

Other important subclassifications are based on whether the hyponatremia has developed acutely or chronically and is symptomatic or asymptomatic.

Hypotonic hyponatremia can be classified based on estimation of the extracellular volume status of the patient as hypovolemic, euvolemic, or hypervolemic hyponatremia (Table 1). In clinical practice, evaluation of volume status may be challenging.

Hypovolemic Hyponatremia

Hypovolemic hyponatremia occurs when there is depletion of both water and body sodium with a relative excess of sodium loss. Solute loss can be classified as renal and nonrenal. Thiazide diuretic–induced hyponatremia is the leading cause of drug-induced hyponatremia requiring hospital admission. Risk factors for the development of thiazide-induced hyponatremia include: increasing age, low body mass index, hypokalemia, and female sex. Other causes of hypovolemic hyponatremia include gastrointestinal losses, skin losses (burns and perspiration), and renal salt loss as a result of salt wasting nephropathy or mineralocorticoid deficiency (*e.g.*, Addison's disease/primary adrenal insufficiency).

Euvolemic Hyponatremia

Euvolemic hyponatremia is caused by a relative absolute increase in body water. It is the most heterogeneous and common cause of hyponatremia among hospitalized patients, and the syndrome of inappropriate antidiuresis (SIAD) is the most frequent underlying disorder. Patients with SIAD will be clinically

Table 1. Causes of Hyponatremia According to Volume Status and Urinary Sodium

	Urinary Sodium, mmol/L	
Clinical Signs	**≤30**	**≥40**
Hypovolemic		
Dry mucous membranes	GI losses	Diuretics
Decreased turgor	Mucosal losses	Addison's disease
Tachycardia	Pancreatitis	Cerebral salt wasting
Hypotension (orthostatic)	Sodium depletion post diuretics	Salt wasting nephropathy
Raised urea, renin		
Euvolemic		
Underlying illness	Hypothyroidism	SIAD
	SIAD with ongoing fluid restriction	ACTH deficiency
Hypervolemic		
Peripheral edema	Cirrhosis	Cardiac failure with diuretic therapy
Ascites	Cardiac failure	
Raised JVP	Nephrotic syndrome	
Pulmonary edema	Primary polydipsia	
Underlying illness		

Data adapted from Smith et al (19).
Abbreviations: ACTH, adrenocorticotrophic hormone; GI, gastrointestinal; JVP, jugular venous pressure; SIAD, syndrome of inappropriate antidiuresis;

euvolemic. Other causes of euvolemic hyponatremia include primary polydipsia, malnutrition, glucocorticoid deficiency (secondary adrenal insufficiency), and severe hypothyroidism.

SIAD

SIAD is the most common cause of euvolemic hyponatremia in hospitalized patients (20). The most common causes of SIAD are malignancy, pulmonary disorders, central nervous system disorders, and medications (21, 22). SIAD has been reported as an adverse effect of many drugs, including psychotropic medications (23) and chemotherapeutic drugs (24). The cardinal diagnostic criteria for SIAD are outlined in Table 2.

Glucocorticoid Deficiency

An important cause of euvolemic hyponatremia, which must be differentiated from SIAD, is adrenocorticotrophic hormone deficiency, which leads to isolated cortisol deficiency (which differs from Addison's disease patients who are also lacking mineralocorticoids and are as a result usually volume depleted).

Hypothyroidism

Determination of thyrotropin is important for evaluation of a patient with hyponatremia, because the exclusion of hypothyroidism is one of the prerequisites for the diagnosis of SIAD. However, recent data suggest that the hypothyroidism-induced hyponatremia is rare and probably occurs only in severe hypothyroidism and myxedema.

Hypervolemic Hyponatraemia

In hypervolemic hyponatremia, there is an increase in both total body water and total body sodium, with a relative excess of total

Table 2. Essential Diagnostic Criteria for SIAD

Criteria
Plasma hypoosmolality (<275 mOsm/kg)
Inappropriate urine concentration (urinary osmolality >100 mOsm/kg water)
Urinary sodium >30 mmol/L, with normal salt and water intake
Clinical euvolemia
Exclusion of hypothyroidism or glucocorticoid deficiency

Supplemental criteria are not included, because they are not used routinely in clinical practice.

body water, leading to dilutional hyponatremia. In both cardiac failure and cirrhosis, baroregulated vasopressin secretion and stimulation of the renin-angiotensin-aldosterone axis and increased sympathetic tone occur. Increased AVP leads to water retention, and the activation of the renin-angiotensin axis promotes sodium and water retention (25).

Pseudohyponatremia

Pseudohyponatremia is caused by a displacement of serum water by significantly elevated concentrations of serum lipids or proteins (26).

Nonhypotonic hyponatremia

Hyponatremia with normal or increased effective osmolality can occur when the serum contains additional osmoles that reduce serum sodium concentration by attracting water from the intracellular compartment. The most common cause of this is hyperglycemia.

CLINICAL APPROACH TO THE PATIENT WITH HYPONATREMIA

A majority of patients who have hyponatremia are asymptomatic. When present, the symptoms associated with hyponatremia are varied and are related to the severity and rapidity of the fall in plasma sodium concentration as well as the coexistence of neurologic disease or other electrolyte abnormalities. In acute hyponatremia, the main pathological consequence is the development of cerebral edema, which leads to raised intracranial pressure with the risk of cerebral herniation (27). In chronic hyponatremia, there is a lower risk of neurologic symptoms because of the presence of chronic cerebral adaptive mechanisms (28).

The initial diagnostic approach to the adult patient with hyponatremia consists of a directed history and physical examination, supported by laboratory tests. There should be a focus on assessment of the extracellular fluid volume status, symptoms and signs of hyponatremia, rate at which hyponatremia developed, and severity of hyponatremia.

Measurement of urinary sodium is crucial in the distinction of hyponatremia etiologies and can help guide optimal management (Table 1). However, low urinary sodium is also an early feature of the recovery phase from diuretic use or SIAD, highlighting the complexities in forming a diagnostic algorithm for hyponatremia. Recent studies have focused on the use of a novel parameter, copeptin, as a surrogate marker for vasopressin, and its potential role as a diagnostic parameter in the differential diagnosis of hyponatremia has been discussed (29).

Management of hyponatremia needs to be targeted at the underlying etiology. The urgency of intervention is determined by the severity of symptoms and the potential for an adverse outcome.

Management of Acute Symptomatic Hyponatremia

This is a medical emergency as there is considerable morbidity and mortality associated with symptomatic hyponatremia given the risk of cerebral edema and brain herniation, and as such, plasma sodium needs to be elevated acutely (the risk of not increasing plasma sodium needs to be weighed against the risk of osmotic demyelination syndrome) (30). The recent report by Verbalis *et al.* (16) recommends an initial rise in serum sodium of 4 to 6 mmol/L over 4 hours, using intravenous boluses of hypertonic (3%) sodium chloride in patients with severe symptomatic hyponatremia. This is based on published experience with hypertonic saline to treat cerebral edema in normotremic patients with neurosurgical conditions, where a 5-mmol/L rise in serum sodium reversed the clinical signs of herniation and reduced intracranial pressure by almost 50% within the first hour (31).

For severe symptoms, a 100-mL bolus of 3% saline infusion should be administered over 10 minutes and repeated up to three times if necessary depending on clinical and biochemical improvement. For mild to moderate symptoms with a low risk of cerebral herniation, 3% saline infusion is again recommended but at a slower rate of 0.5 to 2 mL/kg/h. In true acute hyponatremia (where the decrease in plasma sodium has been documented to have occurred in the prior 24 to 48 hours), the rate of correction need not be restricted as tightly as in chronic hyponatremia, because there is a lower risk of osmotic demyelination. However, if there is any uncertainty as to the rapidity of onset of hyponatremia (chronic versus acute), the target limits for correction of chronic hyponatremia should be respected (16).

Management of Chronic Hyponatremia

Patients with chronic asymptomatic hyponatremia are at a significantly lower risk of neurologic compromise and therefore do not require as aggressive sodium correction as those with acute or symptomatic hyponatremia. In patients with chronic asymptomatic hyponatremia, it is essential to avoid overly rapid rates of correction of hyponatremia, because this can lead to neurologic sequelae resulting from osmotic demyelination syndrome (ODS; previously known as pontine or extrapontine myelinolysis).

Current recommendations suggest a target rise in serum sodium concentration in patients with chronic hyponatremia stratified by the risk of developing ODS (Table 3). Factors that place patients at high risk of developing ODS with correction of chronic hyponatremia include: starting serum sodium concentration $\leq$105 mmol/L, hypokalemia, alcoholism, malnutrition, and advanced liver disease (16).

Management of Chronic Asymptomatic Hypovolemic Hyponatremia

In hypovolemic hyponatremia, the aim is to correct plasma sodium and also restore intravascular volume. Most patients will respond to intravenous infusion of physiological saline. Diuretic therapy should be discontinued where possible and any other underlying causes determined and treated. The

Table 3. Targets for Elevation in Plasma Sodium in Hyponatremic Patients

Patient Risk of ODS	Goal of Minimal Correction of Plasma Sodium in First 24 Hours, mmol/L	Limits Not To Exceed in Plasma Sodium per 24 hours, mmol/L
Normal	4–8	10–12[a]
High[b]	4–6	8

[a] Not >18 mmol/L in 48 hours in normal-risk patients.
[b] Patients with plasma sodium <105 mmol/L, hypokalemia, alcoholism, malnutrition, liver disease.

diagnosis of Addison's disease is suggested by history, examination, and presence of hyperkalemia.

Management of Chronic Asymptomatic SIAD

The first-line recommended treatment of chronic asymptomatic SIAD is fluid restriction. The current European guidelines and US consensus recommendations diverge in relation to the use of interventions after fluid restriction has failed. There are a number of options for second-line therapy, including demeclocycline, vaptan therapy, urea therapy, and frusemide with or without salt tablets.

Fluid Restriction

The first-line therapy for mild to moderate chronic asymptomatic hyponatremia secondary to SIAD is fluid restriction. Several factors may predict failure of fluid restriction, including high urine osmolality (>500 mOsm/kg water), low 24-hour urine volume (<1500 mL/d), and urinary sodium and potassium being greater than plasma sodium. In addition, failure of fluid restriction may prompt reconsideration for the presence of underlying causes such as malignancy or presence of clinically unapparent hypovolemia.

Fluid restriction of 800 to 1200 mL per day is generally advised, according to the severity of hyponatremia. As long as background water losses from the kidney, skin, and lungs exceed this amount, there is progressive depletion of total body water and a gradual rise in plasma sodium concentration. The principal drawback is that patients often find it extremely difficult to maintain fluid restriction. Hospitalized patients who can be supervised tend to do better with fluid restriction than outpatients, but even hospitalized patients who are receiving fluid with intravenous cytotoxic agents or antibiotics, for instance, find it hard to comply.

Demeclocycline

Demeclocycline is a tetracycline derivative, which is used in the treatment of SIAD because it causes nephrogenic diabetes insipidus in ~60% of patients. The degree and timing of vasopressin resistance are not predictable, and in a significant proportion of patients, it does not work. In some patients, polyuria can be profound, and patients can become markedly symptomatic, occasionally developing hypernatremia if access to water is compromised. Nephrotoxicity can arise, particularly in patients with cirrhosis, and although renal impairment is usually reversible with discontinuation, cases of permanent renal failure have been reported (16). It has also been associated with photosensitive skin rash, and appropriate ultraviolet protection is recommended.

Urea

A relatively small number of centers (predominantly in Europe) have experience in the use of urea, and it is recommended as a second-line therapy for use in the recent European hyponatremia guidelines. Human studies have shown that long-term (5-year) treatment of hyponatremia with urea is effective (24).

Frusemide

Frusemide was shown some years ago to be effective in the rapid correction of hyponatremia in SIAD (27), but it is of limited efficacy in long-term treatment, because the diuresis it induces includes natriuresis, which may occasionally worsen hyponatremia.

Vaptans

The vaptans are vasopressin receptor antagonists with V1a (relcovaptan) or V2 (tolvaptan, lixivaptan) selectivity or nonselective activity (conivaptan). The V2 receptors are located primarily in the collecting tubules and mediate free water absorption, whereas the V1b receptors are located in the anterior pituitary and mediate adrenocorticotropin hormone release (32).

The V1a/V2 nonselective vasopressin antagonist conivaptan was the first vaptan approved by the US Food and Drug Administration for the treatment of euvolemic and hypervolemic hyponatremia as an intravenous infusion. Its efficacy for the treatment of hyponatremia has been assessed in several double-blind, placebo-controlled clinical trials (33, 34). Like other vasopressin antagonists, its use is contraindicated in patients with hypovolemic hyponatremia.

Tolvaptan is an oral selective nonpeptide V2 receptor antagonist. The results of two large multicenter, randomized, placebo-controlled, double-blind trials of oral tolvaptan have been reported in patients with hyponatremia (resulting from chronic heart failure, cirrhosis, or SIAD) (35). Approximately 55% of patients in the tolvaptan group had normal serum sodium concentrations after 1 month of treatment (without the need for water restriction), compared with 25% in the placebo group. However, the benefit on serum sodium was more effective in patients with SIAD compared with those with heart failure or cirrhosis. Excessive correction of serum sodium concentrations was noted in this study (>12 mmol/L/d in 3% of patients). The SALTWATER (Safety and Sodium Assessment of Long-Term Tolvaptan With Hyponatremia To Gain Experience

Under Real-World Conditions) trial, an extension of the SALT (Study of Ascending Levels of Tolvaptan) study, showed that the effect of tolvaptan was sustained for the duration of the observation period, a maximum of 214 weeks (36).

The US consensus recommendations suggest certain precautions with use of vaptans to avoid overcorrection and subsequent ODS. Clinicians should monitor serum sodium levels frequently during the active phase of correction of the hyponatremia. In addition, fluid restriction should not be recommended, thereby allowing the patient's own thirst mechanism to compensate for the induced aquaresis. Goals and limits for safe correction are similar to those described for the treatment of chronic hyponatremia. Hepatotoxicity with tolvaptan is a concern based on the TEMPO (*Tolvaptan* Efficacy and Safety in Management of Autosomal Dominant Polycystic Kidney Disease and Its Outcomes) trial (this trial examined the effect of tolvaptan at a high dose on the progression of polycystic kidney disease) (37); it is therefore recommended that liver enzymes be checked in patients receiving tolvaptan.

Saline Infusion in SIAD

There are data to suggest that plasma sodium concentration will rise in some patients with SIAD who are treated with intravenous normal (0.9%) saline (28). However, treatment with normal saline is reserved for patients in whom the differentiation between hypovolemia and euvolemia is difficult. In this situation, intravenous saline is a safer first-line treatment than fluid restriction, but careful monitoring is required to ensure improvement in sodium concentrations while receiving saline.

Management of Hypervolemic Hyponatremia

In hypervolemic hyponatremia, therapy is aimed at treating the underlying cause. In congestive cardiac failure and cirrhosis, the mainstays of therapy are a combination of dietary sodium restriction, diuretics, and fluid restriction to restore total body water to normal, in combination with inhibition of the renin angiotensin aldosterone system using angiotensin-converting enzyme inhibitors, angiotensin receptor blockers, or mineralocorticoid receptor antagonists.

The use of vasopressin receptor antagonists in hypervolemic hyponatremia results in increased solute-free excretion without activation of the neurohumoral systems, as compared with loop diuretics. This provides a rationale for substitution in the management of heart failure. The efficacy of vaptans in hypervolemic hyponatremia and cirrhosis is limited (38), and given the potential hepatotoxicity seen with tolvaptan, it is recommended that tolvaptan not be administered to patients with chronic liver disease.

CONCLUSION

Hyponatremia is the most common electrolyte abnormality encountered in clinical practice and is a biochemical manifestation of a spectrum of illnesses. It is associated with considerable morbidity and mortality. The etiology of hyponatremia needs to be systematically determined; this is the critical step to ensure adequate treatment. SIAD is the most common cause of euvolemic hyponatremia in hospitalized patients. Clinical practice guidelines and consensus statements provide recommendations to help evidence-based practice. Acute hyponatremia should be promptly managed to protect from neurologic sequelae, whereas chronic hyponatremia should be investigated to establish etiology and cautiously treated to avoid overcorrection.

CLINICAL CASES FOR DISCUSSION

Case 1: Management of Severe Symptomatic Hyponatremia

A 42-year-old woman with a history of schizophrenia and substantial polydipsia presented in status epilepticus. Her serum sodium was 104 mmol/L, urea was low at 1.3 mmol/L (normal range, 2.0 to 7.0 mmol/L), and urine osmolality was 107 mOsm/kg.

The case discussion will include issues related to the use of hypertonic saline and prevention of rapid overcorrection and osmotic demyelination syndrome.

Case 2: Exercise-Associated Hyponatremia

A healthy 25-year-old woman just completed her first marathon race. She felt ill toward the end of the race but was able to walk back to her hotel unassisted. Six hours later, her roommate noticed that she was not making sense. She was taken to the nearby emergency room where she was found to be disoriented and confused but without focal neurologic deficits. Vital signs were stable except for an increased respiratory rate to 32 breaths/min, and the patient was euvolemic by clinical examination. Laboratory data from the ER were as follows:

- Sodium: 122 mEq/L
- Potassium: 3.5 mEq/L
- Plasma osmolality: 254 mOsm/kg water
- Blood urea nitrogen: 12 mg/dL
- Creatinine: 0.8 mg/dL
- Urine osmolality: 412 mOsm/kg water
- Urinary sodium: 50 mEq/L
- Urinary potassium: 40 mEq/L
- Glucose: 120 mg/dL

The case discussion will include issues related to treatment of an acute hyponatremia (*e.g.*, <48 hours in duration) to prevent fatal cerebral edema. Treatment strategies will be compared with those in Case 1, where risk of osmotic demyelination must be factored into the decision-making process.

Case 3: Treatment of Chronic SIAD When Fluid Restriction Fails

A 62-year-old man with small-cell lung cancer developed SIAD secondary to his malignancy. His serum sodium was

124 mmol/L, urinary sodium was 85 mmol/L, urinary potassium was 63 mmol/L, and urine osmolality was 636 mOsm/kg; his serum cortisol was normal at 440 nmol/L, and thyroid function tests were normal. He was treated with fluid restriction, but after 1 week, there was no improvement in his hyponatremia.

The case discussion will include issues related to predicting failure of fluid restriction and options for second-line therapy in SIAD.

Case 4: Adverse Events Associated With Asymptomatic Hyponatremia

An 80-year-old woman was seen as an outpatient for chronic hyponatremia with a serum sodium level that ranged from 125 to 129 mmol/L. Her main complaint was feeling unsteady on her feet, and she had a history of several falls in the past 2 years. Her only medication is hydrochlorothiazide 25 mg/d for systolic hypertension. A recent bone densitometry scan confirmed a diagnosis of osteoporosis in the LSS (T score, −3.3) and hip (T score, −2.7). Laboratory data were as follows:

- Sodium: 127 mEq/L
- Potassium: 3.9 mEq/L
- Plasma osmolality: 263 mOsm/kg water
- Blood urea nitrogen: 10 mg/dL
- Creatinine: 1.2 mg/dL
- Urine osmolality: 520 mOsm/kg water
- Urinary sodium: 75 mEq/L
- Urinary postassium: 52 mEq/L
- Thyrotropin: 2.9 μIU/L
- Plasma cortisol: 18 μg/dL

The case discussion will include issues related to long-term adverse effects of chronic hyponatremia, specifically falls, osteoporosis, and fractures, that may contribute to the long-standing association between hyponatremia and increased mortality, as well as treatment strategies for chronic hyponatremia.

REFERENCES

1. Upadhyay A, Jaber BL, Madias NE. Incidence and prevalence of hyponatremia. *Am J Med.* 2006;**119**(7, suppl 1)S30–S35.
2. Asadollahi K, Beeching N, Gill G. Hyponatraemia as a risk factor for hospital mortality. *QJM.* 2006;**99**(12):877–880.
3. Hoorn EJ, Lindemans J, Zietse R. Development of severe hyponatraemia in hospitalized patients: treatment-related risk factors and inadequate management. *Nephrol Dial Transplant.* 2006;**21**(1): 70–76.
4. DeVita MV, Gardenswartz MH, Konecky A, Zabetakis PM. Incidence and etiology of hyponatremia in an intensive care unit. *Clin Nephrol.* 1990;**34**(4):163–166.
5. Oude Lansink-Hartgring A, Hessels L, Weigel J, de Smet AMGA, Gommers D, Panday PVN, Hoorn EJ, Nijsten MW. Long-term changes in dysnatremia incidence in the ICU: a shift from hyponatremia to hypernatremia. *Ann Intensive Care.* 2016;**6**(1):22.
6. Sherlock M, O'Sullivan E, Agha A, Behan LA, Rawluk D, Brennan P, Tormey W, Thompson CJ. The incidence and pathophysiology of hyponatraemia after subarachnoid haemorrhage. *Clin Endocrinol (Oxf).* 2006;**64**(3): 250–254.
7. Hannon MJ, Finucane FM, Sherlock M, Agha A, Thompson CJ. Clinical review: disorders of water homeostasis in neurosurgical patients. *J Clin Endocrinol Metab.* 2012;**97**(5):1423–1433.
8. Miller M, Morley JE, Rubenstein LZ. Hyponatremia in a nursing home population. *J Am Geriatr Soc.* 1995;**43**(12):1410–1413.
9. Dineen R, Thompson CJ, Sherlock M. Hyponatraemia - presentations and management. *Clin Med (Lond).* 2017;**17**(3):263–269.
10. Renneboog B, Musch W, Vandemergel X, Manto MU, Decaux G. Mild chronic hyponatremia is associated with falls, unsteadiness, and attention deficits. *Am J Med.* 2006;**119**(1):71.e1–71.e8.
11. Hoorn EJ, Rivadeneira F, van Meurs JB, Ziere G, Stricker BH, Hofman A, Pols HA, Zietse R, Uitterlinden AG, Zillikens MC. Mild hyponatremia as a risk factor for fractures: the Rotterdam study. *J Bone Miner Res.* 2011;**26**(8):1822–1828.
12. Verbalis JG, Barsony J, Sugimura Y, Tian Y, Adams DJ, Carter EA, Resnick HE. Hyponatremia-induced osteoporosis. *J Bone Miner Res.* 2010;**25**(3):554–563.
13. Barsony J, Sugimura Y, Verbalis JG. Osteoclast response to low extracellular sodium and the mechanism of hyponatremia-induced bone loss. *J Biol Chem.* 2011;**286**(12):10864–10875.
14. Singh TD, Fugate JE, Rabinstein AA. Central pontine and extrapontine myelinolysis: a systematic review. *Eur J Neurol.* 2014;**21**(12): 1443–1450.
15. Cuesta M, Garrahy A, Slattery D, Gupta S, Hannon AM, McGurren K, Sherlock M, Tormey W, Thompson CJ. Mortality rates are lower in SIAD, than in hypervolaemic or hypovolaemic hyponatraemia: results of a prospective observational study. *Clin Endocrinol (Oxf).* 2017; **87**(4):400–406.
16. Verbalis JG, Goldsmith SR, Greenberg A, Korzelius C, Schrier RW, Sterns RH, Thompson CJ. Diagnosis, evaluation, and treatment of hyponatremia: expert panel recommendations. *Am J Med.* 2013;**126**(10, suppl 1) S1–S42.
17. Spasovski G, Vanholder R, Allolio B, Annane D, Ball S, Bichet D, Decaux G, Fenske W, Hoorn EJ, Ichai C, Joannidis M, Soupart A, Zietse R, Haller M, van der Veer S, Van Biesen W, Nagler E. Clinical practice guideline on diagnosis and treatment of hyponatraemia [published correction appears in Intensive Care Med. 2014;40(6):924]. *Intensive Care Med.* 2014;**40**(3):320–331.
18. Reynolds RM, Padfield PL, Seckl JR. Disorders of sodium balance. *BMJ.* 2006;**332**(7543):702–705.
19. Smith DM, McKenna K, Thompson CJ. Hyponatraemia. *Clin Endocrinol (Oxf).* 2000;**52**(6):667–678.
20. Baylis PH. The syndrome of inappropriate antidiuretic hormone secretion. *Int J Biochem Cell Biol.* 2003;**35**(11):1495–1499.
21. Verbalis JG, Greenberg A, Burst V, Haymann JP, Johannsson G, Peri A, Poch E, Chiodo JA III, Dave J. Diagnosing and treating the syndrome of inappropriate antidiuretic hormone secretion. *Am J Med.* 2016;**129**(5):537.e9–537.e23.
22. Shepshelovich D, Leibovitch C, Klein A, Zoldan S, Milo G, Shochat T, Rozen-zvi B, Gafter-Gvili A, Lahav M. The syndrome of inappropriate antidiuretic hormone secretion: distribution and characterization according to etiologies. *Eur J Intern Med.* 2015;**26**(10):819–824.
23. Lange-Asschenfeldt C, Kojda G, Cordes J, Hellen F, Gillmann A, Grohmann R, Supprian T. Epidemiology, symptoms, and treatment characteristics of hyponatremic psychiatric inpatients. *J Clin Psychopharmacol.* 2013;**33**(6):799–805.
24. Atas E, Kesik V, Karaoglu A, Kalkan G. Inappropriate antidiuretic syndrome hypersecretion after a single dose of cisplatin. *J Cancer Res Ther.* 2015;**11**(4):1032.
25. Oren RM. Hyponatremia in congestive heart failure. *Am J Cardiol.* 2005;**95**(9A)2B–7B.
26. Hussain I, Ahmad Z, Garg A. Extreme hypercholesterolemia presenting with pseudohyponatremia - a case report and review of the literature. *J Clin Lipidol.* 2015;**9**(2):260–264.
27. Ellis SJ. Severe hyponatraemia: complications and treatment. *QJM.* 1995;**88**(12):905–909.
28. Thompson CJ. Hyponatraemia: new associations and new treatments. *Eur J Endocrinol.* 2010;**162**(suppl 1):S1–S3.
29. Nigro N, Winzeler B, Suter-Widmer I, Schuetz P, Arici B, Bally M, Blum CA, Nickel CH, Bingisser R, Bock A, Huber A, Muller B, Christ-Crain M.

Evaluation of copeptin and commonly used laboratory parameters for the differential diagnosis of profound hyponatraemia in hospitalized patients: 'The Co-MED Study'. *Clin Endocrinol (Oxf)*. 2017;**86**(3): 456–462.
30. Sterns RH, Silver SM. Brain volume regulation in response to hypo-osmolality and its correction. *Am J Med*. 2006;**119**(7, suppl 1) S12–S16.
31. Koenig MA, Bryan M, Lewin JL III, Mirski MA, Geocadin RG, Stevens RD. Reversal of transtentorial herniation with hypertonic saline. *Neurology*. 2008;**70**(13):1023–1029.
32. Decaux G, Soupart A, Vassart G. Non-peptide arginine-vasopressin antagonists: the vaptans. *Lancet*. 2008;**371**(9624):1624–1632.
33. Zeltser D, Rosansky S, van Rensburg H, Verbalis JG, Smith N; Conivaptan Study Group. Assessment of the efficacy and safety of intravenous conivaptan in euvolemic and hypervolemic hyponatremia. *Am J Nephrol*. 2007;**27**(5):447–457.
34. Ghali JK, Koren MJ, Taylor JR, Brooks-Asplund E, Fan K, Long WA, Smith N. Efficacy and safety of oral conivaptan: a V1A/V2 vasopressin receptor antagonist, assessed in a randomized, placebo-controlled trial in patients with euvolemic or hypervolemic hyponatremia. *J Clin Endocrinol Metab*. 2006;**91**(6):2145–2152.
35. Schrier RW, Gross P, Gheorghiade M, Berl T, Verbalis JG, Czerwiec FS, Orlandi C; SALT Investigators. Tolvaptan, a selective oral vasopressin V2-receptor antagonist, for hyponatremia. *N Engl J Med*. 2006; **355**(20):2099–2112.
36. Berl T, Quittnat-Pelletier F, Verbalis JG, Schrier RW, Bichet DG, Ouyang J, Czerwiec FS; SALTWATER Investigators. Oral tolvaptan is safe and effective in chronic hyponatremia. *J Am Soc Nephrol*. 2010; **21**(4):705–712.
37. Torres VE, Higashihara E, Devuyst O, Chapman AB, Gansevoort RT, Grantham JJ, Perrone RD, Ouyang J, Blais JD, Czerwiec FS; TEMPO 3:4 Trial Investigators. Effect of tolvaptan in autosomal dominant polycystic kidney disease by CKD stage: results from the TEMPO 3:4 trial. *Clin J Am Soc Nephrol*. 2016;**11**(5):803–811.
38. Pose E, Solà E, Piano S, Gola E, Graupera I, Guevara M, Cárdenas A, Angeli P, Ginès P. Limited Efficacy of Tolvaptan in Patients with Cirrhosis and Severe Hyponatremia. Real Life Experience. *Am J Med*. 2016;**130**(3):372–375.

Neuroendocrine Tumors

M20
Presented, March 17–20, 2018

Ashley Grossman, BA, BSc, MD, FRCP, FMedSci. Royal Free Hospital, London, United Kingdom; University of Oxford, Oxford, United Kingdom; and Barts and the London School of Medicine, London NW3 2QG, United Kingdom, E-mail: ashley.grossman@ocdem.ox.ac.uk

SIGNIFICANCE OF THE CLINICAL PROBLEM

There seems to be little doubt that neuroendocrine tumors (NETs; now referred to generically as neuroendocrine neoplasms) are increasing in incidence and prevalence, at least in part because of better diagnostic techniques, but there does, in addition, seem to be a true increase in their occurrence (1). Such tumors are mainly those arising from the gastroenteropancreatic tract, so-called gastroenteropancreatic tract NETs, but they also include bronchopulmonary and thymic NETs, which are usually still referred to by their older names of bronchopulmonary and thymic carcinoids, respectively (2). Furthermore, such tumors are increasingly mandating the involvement of endocrinologists, because the value and indeed, necessity for a multidisciplinary team will generally require an endocrinologist to be present. Thus, many more patients with NETs are now being seen in endocrine services and demand expert care.

For bronchopulmonary carcinoids, the majority are identified when still small and often asymptomatic, and thus, surgical cure is a strong possibility, although much less so for thymic carcinoids. However, in the case of gastroenteropancreatic tract NETs, these are often slow growing and occult for many years, and they only become clinically evident when they cause secretory syndromes or local pressure effects. Pancreatic NETs or islet cell tumors are often nonfunctioning and present when large, whereas those arising from the midgut may only present with a carcinoid syndrome when metastases spread to the liver. Thus, many such patients, if not the majority, present with metastatic disease. The management and treatment of patients with NETs are often a considerable challenge, and they demand expertise from many specialties, which requires coordination by a knowledgeable endocrinologist.

BARRIERS TO OPTIMAL PRACTICE

Part of the problem in managing NET patients has been that, until very recently, all of the evidence for therapy has been based on small uncontrolled series, anecdotal reports, and poorly characterized heterogeneous patient groups. In addition, many of the therapeutic interventions were not widely available, required considerable local expertise, and have been very resource intensive, not to say highly expensive. What has compounded the problem has been the realization that the natural history of NETs is highly variable, quite unlike other more common tumors, such as adenocarcinomas; thus, prolonged survival may occur even in the absence of active therapy. Mandating onerous and expensive therapy has, therefore, sometimes been hard to justify when prolonged survival and a good (better?) quality of life may occur in its absence. Nevertheless, recent national and international trials, controlled and randomized in selected patient groups and using both "hard" end points and quality of life assessments, have led to the production of useful well-supported guidelines from national and international bodies, and therefore, some consensus on optimal therapy is taking place. Unfortunately, clinicians seeing patients with these conditions only occasionally may not be fully aware of such consensual statements, denying their patients the best possible management plans.

LEARNING OBJECTIVES

As a result of participating in this session, learners should be able to

- Identify NETs and optimize key diagnostic pathways in terms of pathology, biochemistry, and imaging
- Formulate a strategy for patient management involving expertise in surgery, oncology, interventional radiology, and nuclear medicine
- Use medical therapies and targeted agents in a considered and evidence-based manner, taking into account patient quality of life as well as overall survival

STRATEGIES FOR DIAGNOSIS

The critical first point is the accurate diagnosis of an NET; to this end, advances in pathological staging and the use of selected immunocytochemical stains have been vital. In almost every case, histopathological assessment is essential to both confirm the diagnosis and offer prognostic information. A specialist should assess tissue for chromogranin and synaptophysin immunostaining and calculate the proliferation index using the Ki-67 percentage; this will grade tumors into grade 1 (<2% of cells Ki-67 positive), grade 2 (2% to 20%), and grade 3 (>20%). In addition, grade 3 tumors should be defined in terms of small cell or large cell and well or poorly differentiated, because there is evidence that there are well-differentiated NETs, which respond differently to therapy than poorly differentiated neuroendocrine carcinomas. The tumor should then be assigned a tumor node metastasis classification (3).

Measurement of circulating chromogranin A is helpful in assessing progress or response to therapy, less so in confirming the diagnosis. Urinary 5-hydroxy-indoleacetic acid (5HIAA), either 24 hours or preferably, a random sample, is helpful in monitoring patients with a suspected carcinoid syndrome, generally, patients with midgut tumors and hepatic metastases, or occasionally, those with extensive peritoneal seeding or the rare ovarian carcinoid. Measurement of urinary 5HIAA will also alert the clinician to possible cardiac valvular involvement (4). For pancreatic NETs, measurement of circulating pancreatic hormones may be helpful in particular situations (insulin, gastrin, glucagon, *etc.*). There is also increasing evidence regarding the utility of the NETest, a measure of circulating RNA transcripts, but this remains a research procedure currently.

Radiological imaging is usually initially with computed tomography (CT) scanning, which will often show the "stellate" tethering of the fibrotic intestinal NET and incipient obstruction; magnetic resonance imaging is preferable for full assessment of possible liver metastases. It is then essential to consider radionuclide imaging for somatostatin receptors with either ^{111}in-octreotide single-photon emission computerized tomography imaging or ideally, ^{68}Ga-octreotate positron emission tomography/CT or magnetic resonance fusion images. This will tend to confirm the NET nature of lesions, identify those not previously apparent, and suggest therapeutic options (5). More specialized radiological techniques (endoscopic ultrasound, selected angiography, the use of alternative radionuclides, *etc.*) may also be considered.

MANAGEMENT AND THERAPY

The only curative option is surgery. However, there is evidence that removal of a midgut primary not only may reduce the possibility of intestinal obstruction but also, may itself prolong progression-free survival (PFS). Occasionally, removal of a primary tumor plus metastatectomy, as long as some 90% of the tumor burden is removed, may be appropriate (6). In general, it is generally accepted that gross removal of tumor and metastases is worthwhile, provided that the patient's performance status allows for it.

After surgery, the initial treatment of choice for residual disease is the use of a somatostatin analog, either octreotide LAR (Sandostatin) or lanreotide autogel (Somatuline). This is essential for all patients with a carcinoid syndrome. Furthermore, large-scale controlled trials have suggested that there is a class effect of somatostatin analogs in retarding tumor progression, including grade 1 and some grade 2 tumors (Ki-67 < 10%) (7, 8). This should probably be at least considered in all patients with residual tumor; we use a starting dose of octreotide LAR 30 mg or lanreotide autogel 120 mg given without "test dosing," with the first dose given in hospital and the patient observed for a period of hours.

Many patients can be treated by simple observation or with a somatostatin analog for long periods of time, with a good quality of life and few, if any, symptoms or adverse effects. Analog-induced diarrhea can be helped by use of pancreatic enzyme supplements. However, with tumor progression or a lack of symptomatic control, other options need to be considered. If disease is mainly locoregional to the liver, then radiofrequency or similar ablation of metastases is possible, but when more widespread, hepatic transarterial embolization can be performed in two stages for left and right hepatic arteries to improve symptoms, although its effect on overall survival is unclear. In my opinion, there is little evidence that embolization with chemotherapy or radionuclides offers important advantages over bland embolization. In general, the technique has risks attached to it and should only be performed in dedicated units.

For more widespread disease, the choices of systemic therapy include chemotherapy, radionuclide therapy, and targeted agents. Most would start with chemotherapy for pancreatic NETs, especially if grade 2, using either streptozotocin plus capecitabine or temozolomide and capecitabine. For patients with the majority of disease octreotide avid on scanning, recent data have indicated that therapeutic radionuclide treatment with ^{177}Lu-octreotate will markedly improve PFS in midgut NETs (9), and this may also apply to ^{90}Y-octreotide (although the latter agent has somewhat different radiobiological properties and may have higher renal toxicity). Most find that two to four courses of treatment in specialized centers involve no hospital or just overnight admission and few short- or medium-term toxicities; whether there will be long-term problems with myelodysplastic syndromes and other hematological disorders to any major extent remains unclear, but there may be a synergistic effect in such toxicities with the use of chemotherapy.

For patients with grade 3 tumors, the current approach is with chemotherapy, usually etoposide and a platinum; there is some evidence that radionuclide therapy can be beneficial with the better-differentiated grade 3 tumors with a Ki-67 between 20% and 55%.

Finally, large-scale trials have undoubtedly shown the value on PFS of both the mammalian target of rapamycin inhibitor everolimus (in a whole range of NETs) (10, 11) and the tyrosine kinase inhibitor sunitinib (for pancreatic NETs) (12); in both cases, the increase in PFS has been ~6 months, but these agents need to be monitored carefully for adverse events in a department, often oncological, familiar with these drugs.

MAIN CONCLUSIONS

NETs are being increasingly seen by endocrinologists as part of a large management team, with such tumors often metastatic at presentation. It is important to realize that even untreated metastatic tumors can be congruent with a prolonged survival and a good quality of life. Although only surgery can be truly curative, somatostatin analogs are very useful symptomatically and have been shown to retard tumor progression with minimal adverse effects; however, the initiation and sequencing of subsequent therapies (locoregional, chemotherapy, radionuclide, and/or targeted) require an individualized and customized approach. In such patients, the involvement of a specialist endocrine oncology nurse is of great value.

CASES

Case 1 (A)

A 52-year-old woman presents to your clinic with a 7-year history of "irritable bowel syndrome"; she has had gastroscopy and colonoscopy, which were normal, but her diarrhea has persisted with some response to codeine phosphate and is not especially troublesome. For the last 6 months, she has suffered infrequent episodes of flushing: these are "dry" in nature unassociated with sweating and can be particularly precipitated by alcohol. Her gastroenterologist ordered a CT scan of the abdomen and random urinary 5HIAA measurement; the CT revealed a spiculated mass in the right lower quadrant, with 11 to 12 liver lesions up to 6 cm in diameter. Urinary 5HIAA excretion was 23 mmol/mol creatinine (normal <5). A ^{68}Ga-DOTATATE scan confirmed markedly positive uptake in the abdominal mass and some of the hepatic lesions.

The most appropriate next step in management would be

A. Initiation of somatostatin analog therapy
B. Percutaneous liver biopsy
C. Radiolabeled octreotide therapy
D. Laparoscopy and biopsy
E. Targeted agent therapy

Discussion

The best answer is B.

The patient has a midgut "carcinoid" tumor or NET with a carcinoid syndrome associated with hepatic metastases and elevated urinary 5HIAA excretion. Although formerly this would have been sufficient diagnostically, we now know that prognosis is very dependent on confirmatory pathology. Urinary 5HIAA can be spuriously elevated because of various dietary constituents, and somatostatin receptors can be seen occasionally on other tumors and even inflammatory tissue. The hepatic lesions are large, such that liver biopsy is safest and most convenient, avoiding laparoscopy at this stage (D). It is essential to confirm the diagnosis before initiating treatment (C and E) unless symptoms are severe, which is not the case here (A). Histopathological conformation of an NET is combined with Ki-67 measurement and grading, which will also determine optimal therapy.

Case 1 (B)

Biopsy of the largest liver lesion proceeds uneventfully and shows a chromogranin-positive NET with a Ki-67 of 1%: hence, grade 1. The flushes continue occasionally, but the diarrhea becomes more resistant to simple measures.

The next step should be

A. Wait and see with regular follow-up
B. Resection of primary tumor with or without metastases
C. Resection of primary tumor and transarterial embolization
D. Initiation of somatostatin analog
E. Use of radiolabeled ^{177}Lu-octreotate

Discussion

Because of the fact that the patient has a carcinoid syndrome, albeit mild, and being aware of the tumoristatic effect of somatostatin analogs, the next step should be starting a depot somatostatin analog preparation (D).

Simple observation (A) would leave the patient with many symptoms, which can be alleviated in most cases. One could start with subcutaneous octreotide twice daily or thrice daily if the syndrome was more severe. This not only will relieve symptoms in the majority of cases but also, should render a carcinoid crisis less likely should surgery (B and C) or other therapies (E) be used. At this time, chromogranin A measurement will provide a useful baseline to gauge the effect of therapy, and many would assess right-sided cardiac function with an echocardiogram.

Case 1 (C)

The patient is symptomatically greatly improved, with some mild steatorrhea with her somatostatin analog and a normal echocardiogram. However, the tumor shows gradual growth over the next 6 months. Surgery is considered to remove the primary, but it is considered too complex. She has a good performance status and is keen on more definitive therapy if possible.

One would now consider the best next step to be

A. Radiolabeled radionuclide treatment
B. Chemotherapy with temozolomide and capecitabine
C. Orthotopic liver transplantation
D. Targeted therapy with everolimus
E. Wait and see

Discussion

The patient is keen on active therapy, and although there is some evidence that removal of the primary tumor can extend PFS, surgery is contraindicated. Most would consider (A) peptide radio-receptor therapy as an important therapeutic option, where available.

The patient is well, and one could make a case for a conservative observational approach (E). However, she is in good general health and enthusiastic for a more active approach, and the tumor is progressing. These tumors are poorly chemotherapy sensitive, especially when grade 1 (B), and molecular-targeted therapy should be reserved for progressive tumors unresponsive to simpler techniques (D). Liver transplantation should only be considered as a last resort in patients with an extensive hepatic load unresponsive to all other measures where there are no extrahepatic metastases (C).

Case 2

A 65-year-old man, previously well, with a long smoking history presents with weight loss and abdominal fullness. A CT scan of the abdomen shows widespread metastatic disease with liver involvement: an ^{111}In-octreotide single-photon emission computerized tomography scan shows marked uptake in all lesions; liver biopsy shows a poorly differentiated NET with positive chromogranin and synaptophysin staining, negative TTF-1 suggestive of a nonlung origin, and a Ki-67 of 80% to 90%. Your advice would be to

A. Arrange supportive and hospice care
B. Offer radiolabeled octreotide therapy
C. Chemotherapy with temozolomide and capecitabine
D. Chemotherapy with etoposide and a platinum
E. Arrange for a respiratory outpatient appointment

Discussion

The patient has a grade 3 tumor, which is probably of gut origin (negative TTF-1) and requires immediate treatment. Survival is poor but can be substantially extended with appropriate chemotherapy, which in this case, is with etoposide and a platinum (D).

Other types of chemotherapy are not indicated for this type of tumor (C), and although there have been some positive results with radiolabeled therapy in grade 3 tumors, this is principally in the well-differentiated grade 3 tumors with a Ki-67 < 55% to 60% (B). Supportive care alone is only indicated for patients with otherwise poor performance status (A), and chemotherapy should be initiated without delay (E). Other regimens are available for poor responders to etoposide and platinum, such as fluorouracil, folinic acid, and irinotecan.

REFERENCES

1. Huguet I, Grossman AB, O'Toole D. Changes in the epidemiology of neuroendocrine tumours. *Neuroendocrinology.* 2015;**104**(2):105–111.
2. Jia R, Sulentic P, Xu JM, Grossman AB. Thymic neuroendocrine neoplasms: biological behaviour and therapy. *Neuroendocrinology.* 2017;**105**(2):105–114.
3. Modlin IM, Oberg K, Chung DC, Jensen RT, de Herder WW, Thakker RV, Caplin M, Delle Fave G, Kaltsas GA, Krenning EP, Moss SF, Nilsson O, Rindi G, Salazar R, Ruszniewski P, Sundin A. Gastroeneteropancreatic neuroendocrine tumours. *Lancet Oncol.* 2008;**9**(1):61–72.
4. Grozinsky-Glasberg S, Grossman AB, Gross DJ. Carcinoid heart disease: from pathophysiology to treatment–';something in the way it moves.' *Neuroendocrinology.* 2015;**101**(4):263–273.
5. Sundin A. Radiological and nuclear medicine imaging of gastroenteropancreatic neuroendocrine tumours. *Best Pract Res Clin Gastroenterol.* 2012;**26**(6):803–818.
6. Ahmed A, Turner G, King B, Jones L, Culliford D, McCance D, Ardill J, Johnston BT, Poston G, Rees M, Buxton-Thomas M, Caplin M, Ramage JK. Midgut neuroendocrine tumours with liver metastases: results of the UKINETS study. *Endocr Relat Cancer.* 2009;**16**(3): 885–894.
7. Rinke A, Müller HH, Schade-Brittinger C, Klose KJ, Barth P, Wied M, Mayer C, Aminossadati B, Pape UF, Bläker M, Harder J, Arnold C, Gress T, Arnold R; PROMID Study Group. Placebo-controlled, double-blind, prospective, randomized study on the effect of octreotide LAR in the control of tumor growth in patients with metastatic neuroendocrine midgut tumors: a report from the PROMID Study Group. *J Clin Oncol.* 2009;**27**(28):4656–4663.
8. Caplin ME, Pavel M, Ćwikła JB, Phan AT, Raderer M, Sedláčková E, Cadiot G, Wolin EM, Capdevila J, Wall L, Rindi G, Langley A, Martinez S, Blumberg J, Ruszniewski P; CLARINET Investigators. Lanreotide in metastatic enteropancreatic neuroendocrine tumors. *N Engl J Med.* 2014;**371**(3):224–233.
9. Strosberg J, El-Haddad G, Wolin E, Hendifar A, Yao J, Chasen B, Mittra E, Kunz PL, Kulke MH, Jacene H, Bushnell D, O'Dorisio TM, Baum RP, Kulkarni HR, Caplin M, Lebtahi R, Hobday T, Delpassand E, Van Cutsem E, Benson A, Srirajaskanthan R, Pavel M, Mora J, Berlin J, Grande E, Reed N, Seregni E, Oberg K, Lopera Sierra M, Santoro P, Thevenet T, Erion JL, Ruszniewski P, Kwekkeboom D, Krenning E; NETTER-1 Trial Investigators. Phase 3 trial of 177-Lu-dotatate for midgut neuroendocrine tumors. *N Engl J Med.* 2017;**376**(2): 125–135.
10. Yao JC, Shah MH, Ito T, Bohas CL, Wolin EM, Van Cutsem E, Hobday TJ, Okusaka T, Capdevila J, de Vries EG, Tomassetti P, Pavel ME, Hoosen S, Haas T, Lincy J, Lebwohl D, Oberg K; RAD001 in Advanced Neuroendocrine Tumors, Third Trial (RADIANT-3) Study Group. Everolimus for advanced pancreatic neuroendocrine tumors. *N Engl J Med.* 2011;**364**(6):514–523.
11. Yao JC, Fazio N, Singh S, Buzzoni R, Carnaghi C, Wolin E, Tomasek J, Raderer M, Lahner H, Voi M, Pacaud LB, Rouyrre N, Sachs C, Valle JW, Fave GD, Van Cutsem E, Tesselaar M, Shimada Y, Oh DY, Strosberg J, Kulke MH, Pavel ME; RAD001 in Advanced Neuroendocrine Tumours, Fourth Trial (RADIANT-4) Study Group. Everolimus for the treatment of advanced, non-functional neuroendocrine tumours of the lung or gastrointestinal tract (RADIANT-4): a randomised, placebo-controlled, phase 3 study. *Lancet.* 2016;**387**(10022):968–977.
12. Raymond E, Dahan L, Raoul JL, Bang YJ, Borbath I, Lombard-Bohas C, Valle J, Metrakos P, Smith D, Vinik A, Chen JS, Hörsch D, Hammel P, Wiedenmann B, Van Cutsem E, Patyna S, Lu DR, Blanckmeister C, Chao R, Ruszniewski P. Sunitinib malate for the treatment of pancreatic neuroendocrine tumors. *N Engl J Med.* 2011;**364**(6):501–513.

Panhypopituitarism

M21
Presented, March 17–20, 2018

Laurence Katznelson, MD. Stanford School of Medicine, Stanford, California 94305, E-mail: lkatznelson@stanford.edu

SIGNIFICANCE OF THE CLINICAL PROBLEM

Hypopituitarism refers to a complete or partial deficiency in pituitary hormones. Anterior pituitary hormone deficiency includes adrenal insufficiency (AI) due to adrenocorticotropic hormone deficiency, hypogonadism due to luteinizing hormone (LH)/follicle-stimulating hormone (FSH) deficiency or hyperprolactinemia, hypothyroidism due to thyrotropin (TSH) deficiency, and growth hormone deficiency (GHD) due to hypothalamic GH-releasing hormone or pituitary gland GHD. Posterior gland deficiency primarily involves diabetes insipidus (DI), which is due to antidiuretic hormone (ADH) deficiency. Appropriate awareness of pituitary function testing as well as of therapeutic strategies is critical for accurate management of hypopituitarism. This review focuses on several clinical scenarios that offer effective lessons on the management of hypopituitarism, including perioperative management after pituitary surgery and traumatic brain injury (TBI). In both these settings, there is a range of approaches and, in the case of TBI, limited awareness of the impact on pituitary function. This Meet the Professor session focuses on the issues involved to facilitate a more-focused approach.

BARRIERS TO OPTIMAL PRACTICE

- Effective management of a patient who undergoes pituitary surgery: strategizing the appropriate tests
- Awareness of hypopituitarism following TBI and understanding an appropriate strategy for testing such patients

LEARNING OBJECTIVES

As a result of participating in this session, learners should be able to:

- Perform the appropriate pituitary function tests and endocrine management for a patient undergoing pituitary surgery
- Demonstrate the correct clinical approach to hypopituitarism in a patient with a history of TBI

STRATEGIES FOR DIAGNOSIS, THERAPY, AND/OR MANAGEMENT

Basic Pituitary Function Testing

Hypothyroidism is caused by insufficient TSH stimulation of thyroid gland function due to inadequate production of either TSH or thyrotropin-releasing hormone. The diagnosis is based on low free thyroxine (T4) in the setting of a low, normal, or mildly elevated TSH in pituitary disease.

AI is inadequate cortisol secretion due to inadequate adrenocorticotropic hormone and/or corticotropin-releasing hormone production. The diagnosis is based on low morning serum cortisol <3 μg/dL and inadequate serum cortisol response (<18 μg/dL) after 250 μg Cortrosyn (Amphastar Pharmaceuticals, Rancho Cucamonga, CA) intravenous/intramuscular injection at 30 or 60 minutes. The Cortrosyn stimulation test assesses the adrenal gland response to exogenous Cortrosyn and not to the hypothalamus or pituitary gland. A normal response assumes integrity of the entire axis, but this supposition may be incorrect, especially with acute trauma to the pituitary gland. The test should be performed at least 18 to 24 hours after the last hydrocortisone dose.

Central hypogonadism is caused by inadequate secretion of LH and FSH. In men, the diagnosis is based on low morning serum testosterone; in women, diagnosis is based on the presence of amenorrhea or oligomenorrhea with low estradiol in a premenopausal woman. In a postmenopausal woman, diagnosis is based on the absence of high FSH and LH.

GHD is caused by inadequate GH secretion due to pituitary dysfunction or GH-releasing hormone production by the hypothalamus. The diagnosis is based on low insulin-like growth factor 1 (IGF-1) in the setting of three other deficient anterior pituitary axes; otherwise, provocative testing with the use of glucagon, insulin, and/or other stimulation tests is necessary. Single, unstimulated GH levels are not useful for diagnosis.

Central DI is caused by inadequate secretion of ADH. The diagnosis is based on the determination of polyuria (>3.5 L/d in a 70-kg person); simultaneous measurement of serum and urine osmolarity, with high serum osmolarity (>295 mOsmol/L) and urine osmolarity (should be >600 mOsmol/L); and results of a dehydration test where urine osmolarity should be less than plasma osmolarity (ratio <0.5) and remain <600 mOsmol/L (1).

Approach to a Patient Undergoing Pituitary Surgery

Hypopituitarism may occur in the setting of a pituitary adenoma or result from the associated surgical and radiation treatments. Surgery may lead to pituitary axis recovery or dysfunction. Surgery for any form of sellar mass may lead to pituitary dysfunction. Transsphenoidal surgery traditionally has been performed by microscopic method but has been increasingly performed by using an endonasal endoscopic technique, often with both a neurosurgeon and otolaryngologist present. There are insufficient data on whether these techniques have a different impact on pituitary function. Either way, it is imperative that pituitary function be monitored and deficiency replaced appropriately both during and following pituitary surgery. The hormones monitored mostly closely during and immediately after surgery are cortisol and ADH because AI and DI need to be closely assessed peri- and postoperatively (2, 3). In general, thyroid, GH, and gonadal axes may be measured ≥6 weeks after surgery.

A thorough preoperative evaluation is necessary to determine whether hormone replacement should be administered before and during surgery. Baseline endocrine testing involves the assessment of hypercortisolism and acromegaly as well as of prolactin level to rule out prolactinoma.

In the case of hypofunction, if AI, glucocorticoids should be administered preoperatively and stress dose steroids given during surgery. DI usually is not present for most pituitary adenomas but may be present with cystic or other types of sellar mass. If present, DDAVP (Ferring Pharmaceuticals, Parsippany, NJ) may be started preoperatively.

In the case of hypothyroidism, if mild, replacement is not necessary, and surgery does not need to be postponed because there is no clear evidence for major associated adverse outcomes. For moderate hypothyroidism, surgery should be performed if there is urgency, such as in the setting of local mass effects. If elective, then thyroid hormone replacement should be initiated first and appropriate free T4 levels achieved. For severe hypothyroidism, levothyroxine therapy should be initiated before surgery, although this decision will be dictated by urgency for neurosurgical intervention. Gonadal insufficiency and GHD do not need replacement before surgery.

With regard to peri- and postoperative management, if the patient has AI preoperatively, then appropriate stress dose steroids should be administered during surgery, with postoperative taper and reassessment of adrenal function. If the patient has normal adrenal function preoperatively, an individualized approach can be taken. In some centers, steroids are administered to all patients to cover for possible AI. In other centers, including ours, steroids are withheld during surgery and postoperatively, and cortisol levels are measured postoperatively. With this protocol, we measure morning serum cortisol daily and initiate steroids if the serum cortisol is <5 μg/dL or if between 5 and 10 μg/dL and there are symptoms of AI. This method can reduce unnecessary steroid management in approximately one half of patients.

DDAVP is administered by using either subcutaneous aqueous or oral dosing as needed for DI, without prescheduled dosing given the risk of potentiation of hyponatremia and syndrome of inappropriate ADH secretion (SIADH) several days later (part of the triphasic response). After discharge, pituitary axes should be retested postoperatively starting at 6 weeks.

Management of Patients With TBI

Hypopituitarism occurs after both penetrating and blunt head trauma in ~25% of patients (range, 15% to 68%). The pathophysiology of hypopituitarism in patients with TBI includes direct injury to the gland; vasospasm of the hypothalamo-hypophyseal blood supply; and compression of the hypothalamus and pituitary gland by edema, hemorrhage, or elevated intracranial pressure (4). Genetic factors, including certain apolipoprotein E haplotypes, may affect this risk. In addition, studies have shown that antipituitary and antihypothalamic antibodies are found in patients with TBI, although the pathogenic role is unclear. Autopsy series have shown necrotic glands in up to 80% of fatal cases. GHD is the most common deficiency found, and this has critical implications because GHD may affect full convalescence.

All patients with moderate to severe TBI should be evaluated for hypopituitarism during the acute and chronic course of their recovery (5). Immediately following the TBI, emphasis on care during the first 2 weeks post-TBI should be on the adrenal axis and posterior pituitary function. In the subsequent months after injury, the entire anterior and posterior pituitary hormonal axes should be assessed. In addition, symptomatic patients with mild TBI (including those with repetitive mild TBI) and impaired quality of life are at risk for hypopituitarism and should be considered for neuroendocrine testing.

Testing for chronic hypopituitarism following TBI usually is performed at least 6 to 12 months after the event. Hormone replacement should be administered accordingly (6).

MAIN CONCLUSIONS

1. Evaluation of pituitary function following pituitary surgery should be performed by using a stepwise approach that incorporates preoperative function data with postoperative management. This approach involves temporal assessment of individual pituitary hormones following surgery.
2. TBI is associated with hypopituitarism, and assessment should be performed both immediately and at least 6 months after the event.

CASES

Case 1

A 34-year-old female has been diagnosed with a 2.5-cm clinically nonfunctioning pituitary macroadenoma that has caused chiasmal compression. She is being scheduled for surgery. Her history is notable for oligomenorrhea and bilateral galactorrhea but is otherwise adequate. Her test results are as follows: prolactin, 43 ng/mL (normal, <25 ng/mL); TSH, 2.1 U/mL; free T4 1.2 ng/mL; LH, 6 IU/L; FSH, 30 mIU/L; IGF-1, 87 ng/mL; and Cortrosyn stimulation test (250 μg) peak cortisol, 25 μg/dL. The patient undergoes surgery.

Question 1

Which of the following tests should be performed in the first 72 hours after surgery?

1. Cortrosyn stimulation test

2. IGF-1
3. Electrolytes
4. FSH

Answer: 3

Question 2

For the same patient, she is found on postoperative day 1 to have polyuria and polydipsia, nocturia 5 times a night, and a sodium level of 154 mEq/L. Which one of the following management options should be used for treating the DI?

1. DDAVP scheduled dosing 1 spray intranasally twice daily
2. Dehydration test
3. One-liter fluid restriction
4. DDAVP 0.1 to 0.2 mg by mouth as needed

Answer: 4

Case 2

A 28-year-old male presents with fatigue, an increase in abdominal girth, loss of strength, sexual dysfunction, and weight gain. Fourteen months earlier, he had a severe head trauma in a motor vehicle accident. There was cerebral edema and a small cerebral hemorrhage. The patient was in a coma for 10 days and then transferred to a rehabilitation facility. He has since undergone inpatient and outpatient rehabilitation. He denies polyuria and polydipsia. Because of fatigue, he was placed on Provigil (Cephalon, Frazer, PA). He is referred to an endocrinologist, and the following laboratory results are noted: TSH, 1.4 U/mL; free T4, 1.0 ng/mL; serum testosterone, 130 ng/dL; IGF-1, 65 ng/mL; and Cortrosyn stimulation test (250 μg) peak cortisol, 25 μg/dL.

Question 3

Which of the following tests should be performed next?

1. Morning plasma cortisol
2. Glucagon stimulation test
3. Reverse triiodothyronine
4. Plasma ADH

Answer: 2

DISCUSSION OF CASES AND ANSWERS

Question 1

After pituitary surgery, the two pituitary axes that need to be critically monitored are the pituitary-adrenal and ADH axes. Close monitoring for DI with appropriate DDAVP management is important, and electrolytes are necessary to assess the degree of hypernatremia. IGF-1 and FSH levels are not useful because the GH and gonadotropin axes should be assessed at least 6 weeks following surgery. A Cortrosyn stimulation test is not useful either to assess adrenal reserve at this time. Because it may take a number of weeks for the serum cortisol response to Cortrosyn to become blunted, this test should be performed well after surgery, such as at least 6 weeks later.

Question 2

If a patient has early postoperative central DI, then DDAVP should be administered as needed (either subcutaneously or as oral tablets). The concern is that DDAVP overdosing may exaggerate hyponatremia, particularly if SIADH begins a few days later as part of the triphasic response. Therefore, scheduled DDAVP dosing should not be administered at this time. A dehydration test is important for evaluating DI in a patient with polyuria but is not useful in a patient in this clinical setting where the risk of DI is relatively high. Fluid restriction is part of the management of SIADH, not DI.

Question 3

This patient has a history of TBI and is at risk for hypopituitarism. He has evidence of low serum testosterone as well as very low IGF-1. GHD is the most common deficient pituitary axis, and the low IGF-1 suggests this diagnosis. A provocative test, such as a glucagon stimulation test, should be performed as the next step to confirm this diagnosis. Cortrosyn stimulation test results were normal, so there is no need to obtain an additional cortisol level. The thyroid tests are sufficient, and there is no value here for a reverse triiodothyronine value. Plasma ADH is not useful. The patient has no clinical evidence to support DI, so this does not add to the diagnosis.

REFERENCES

1. Fleseriu M, Hashim IA, Karavitaki N, Melmed S, Murad MH, Salvatori R, Samuels MH. Hormonal replacement in hypopituitarism in adults: an Endocrine Society clinical practice guideline. *J Clin Endocrinol Metab.* 2016;**101**(11):3888–3921.
2. Jia X, Pendharkar AV, Loftus P, Dodd RL, Chu O, Fraenkel M, Katznelson L. Utility of a glucocorticoid sparing strategy in the management of patients following transsphenoidal surgery. *Endocr Pract.* 2016;**22**(9):1033–1039.
3. Woodmansee WW, Carmichael J, Kelly D, Katznelson L, Neuroendocrine A; AACE Neuroendocrine and Pituitary Scientific Committee. American Association of Clinical Endocrinologists and American College of Endocrinology disease state clinical review: postoperative management following pituitary surgery. *Endocr Pract.* 2015;**21**(7): 832–838.
4. Tritos NA, Yuen KC, Kelly DF, Neuroendocrine A; AACE Neuroendocrine and Pituitary Scientific Committee. American Association of Clinical Endocrinologists and American College of Endocrinology disease state clinical review: a neuroendocrine approach to patients with traumatic brain injury. *Endocr Pract.* 2015;**21**(7):823–831.
5. Klose M, Feldt-Rasmussen U. Chronic endocrine consequences of traumatic brain injury—what is the evidence? *Nat Rev Endocrinol.* 2018;**14**:57–62.
6. Giuliano S, Talarico S, Bruno L, Nicoletti FB, Ceccotti C, Belfiore A. Growth hormone deficiency and hypopituitarism in adults after complicated mild traumatic brain injury. *Endocrine.* 2017;**58**(1): 115–123.

Challenging Cushing Syndrome Cases

M23
Presented, March 17–20, 2018

John A. H. Wass, MD. Department of Endocrinology, Oxford Centre for Diabetes, Endocrinology and Metabolism, Oxford University, Oxford OX3 9DU, United Kingdom, E-mail: john.wass@nhs.net

SIGNIFICANCE OF THE CLINICAL PROBLEM

Cushing syndrome is one of the most difficult problems that an endocrinologist deals with. Untreated, it has a high mortality; thus, accurate diagnosis of the cause of Cushing syndrome is essential. Often, time lags between the diagnosis of possible Cushing syndrome and referral to an expert center and can lead to serious adverse consequences. Multidisciplinary involvement, including an endocrinologist, an endocrine surgeon, a neurosurgeon, an oncologist, a radiologist, and a pathologist, experienced in the diagnosis and management of Cushing syndrome is essential.

BARRIERS TO OPTIMAL PRACTICE

The barriers to accurate diagnosis can be considerable. Often these patients are unwell and for other reasons may lose their circadian rhythm of cortisol. Infection may be a problem, and patients may be elderly with other comorbidities.

LEARNING OBJECTIVES

As a result of participating in this session, learners should be able to:

- Understand the complicated nature of some patients with Cushing syndrome from the investigation and treatment point of view and understand the importance of rapid referral to clinicians with experience and expertise in diagnosing and managing this condition
- Understand the clinical and biochemical means of diagnosing Cushing syndrome and the potential pitfalls therein
- Understand the tests involved in making the differential diagnosis of Cushing syndrome together with the advantages, disadvantages, and reliability of these tests

STRATEGIES FOR THE MANAGEMENT OF CUSHING SYNDROME

In terms of the correct diagnosis of the cause of Cushing syndrome, a clear order is necessary. First is the establishment of cortisol hypersecretion. This is done through urinary cortisol and dexamethasone suppression tests as well as by midnight cortisol levels, and in cases that lack clarity, a dexamethasone-suppressed corticotropin-releasing hormone (CRH) test or an intravenous desmopressin test can be used.

A differential diagnosis is important, and tests include a corticotropin value (which if suppressed points to an adrenal cause), a serum potassium level (which if low points to an ectopic source), and suppression of cortisol in response to CRH (which suggests an ectopic source). Pituitary-dependent cases tend to suppress with exogenous dexamethasone and have an exaggerated response to CRH, whereas patients with ectopic corticotropin secretion have a flat CRH test. The differential diagnosis requires expert input, and this may include inferior petrosal sinus sampling.

The diagnosis may be complicated by the fact that a number of patients have cyclical Cushing syndrome. Most patients' Cushing disease is caused by a microadenoma. The pituitary surgeon must have experience in the treatment of not only macroadenomas but also microadenomas. Surgically, microadenomas are the most difficult to deal with and need the most surgical experience to optimize results.

The cases presented will highlight the difficulties in diagnosing Cushing syndrome as well as its causes.

In conclusion, Cushing syndrome is one of the most challenging conditions for an endocrinologist to diagnose and treat. Investigation and treatment in an experienced center is essential. Long-term follow-up is mandatory. Despite a cure, the current evidence is that mortality is increased significantly.

RECOMMENDED READING

Coelho MC, Santos CV, Vieira Neto L, Gadelha MR. Adverse effects of glucocorticoids: coagulopathy. *Eur J Endocrinol.* 2015;**173**(4):M11–M21.

Daniel E, Aylwin S, Mustafa O, Ball S, Munir A, Boelaert K, Chortis V, Cuthbertson DJ, Daousi C, Rajeev SP, Davis J, Cheer K, Drake W, Gunganah K, Grossman A, Gurnell M, Powlson AS, Karavitaki N, Huguet I, Kearney T, Mohit K, Meeran K, Hill N, Rees A, Lansdown AJ, Trainer PJ, Minder AE, Newell-Price J. Effectiveness of metyrapone in treating Cushing's syndrome: a retrospective multicenter study in 195 patients. *J Clin Endocrinol Metab.* 2015;**100**(11):4146–4154.

Ferriere A, Cortet C, Chanson P, Delemer B, Caron P, Chabre O, Reznik Y, Bertherat J, Rohmer V, Briet C, Raingeard I, Castinetti F, Beckers A, Vroonen L, Maiter D, Cephise-Velayoudom FL, Nunes ML, Haissaguerre M, Tabarin A. Cabergoline for Cushing's disease: a large retrospective multicenter study. *Eur J Endocrinol.* 2017;**176**(3):305–314.

Lacroix A, Feelders RA, Stratakis CA, Nieman LK. Cushing's syndrome. *Lancet.* 2015;**386**(9996):913–927.

Nieman LK, Biller BM, Findling JW, Murad MH, Newell-Price J, Savage MO, Tabarin A; Endocrine Society. Treatment of Cushing's syndrome: an Endocrine Society clinical practice guideline. *J Clin Endocrinol Metab.* 2015;**100**(8):2807–2831.

Ntali G, Asimakopoulou A, Siamatras T, Komninos J, Vassiliadi D, Tzanela M, Tsagarakis S, Grossman AB, Wass JA, Karavitaki N. Mortality in Cushing's syndrome: systematic analysis of a large series with prolonged follow-up. *Eur J Endocrinol.* 2013;**169**(5):715–723.

Pivonello R, De Leo M, Cozzolino A, Colao A. The treatment of Cushing's disease. *Endocr Rev.* 2015;**36**(4):385–486.

Pivonello R, Isidori AM, De Martino MC, Newell-Price J, Biller BM, Colao A. Complications of Cushing's syndrome: state of the art. *Lancet Diabetes Endocrinol.* 2016;**4**(7):611–629.

Storr HL, Savage MO. Management of endocrine disease: paediatric Cushing's disease. *Eur J Endocrinol.* 2015;**173**(1):R35–R45.

Tomlinson JW, Draper N, Mackie J, Johnson AP, Holder G, Wood P, Stewart PM. Absence of cushingoid phenotype in a patient with Cushing's disease due to defective cortisone to cortisol conversion. *J Clin Endocrinol Metab.* 2002;**87**(1):57–62.

Hypophysitis: New Understanding in Diagnosis and Management

M33
Presented, March 17–20, 2018

Paul V. Carroll, MD. Department of Endocrinology, Guy's and St Thomas' National Health Service Foundation Trust, London SE1 9RT, United Kingdom, and Faculty of Life Sciences and Medicine, King's College London, London WC2R 2LS, United Kingdom, E-mail: paul.carroll@gstt.nhs.uk

SIGNIFICANCE OF THE CLINICAL PROBLEM

Hypophysitis is the collective term for inflammation of the pituitary gland and infundibulum. Pituitary inflammation can occur as a primary condition or secondary to a predisposing systemic disorder. Hypophysitis is a rare condition; however, the recent recognition of immunoglobulin G4–related disease (IgG4-RD) and hypophysitis as adverse effects of immunotherapy in oncology has invigorated interest in inflammatory disorders affecting the pituitary gland. Understanding of pituitary inflammation has grown considerably in the last decade, with publications including large case series and comprehensive review articles (1). Compared with pituitary adenoma and other sellar mass lesions, relatively little is known about the optimal diagnostic approach and treatment of inflammatory pituitary disorders.

BARRIERS TO OPTIMAL PRACTICE

- Because hypophysitis is rare, a majority of endocrinologists have limited experience in diagnosing and managing pituitary inflammatory disorders.
- An evidence base and best practice guidance on the optimal management of hypophysitis are lacking.

LEARNING OBJECTIVES

As a result of participating in this session, learners should be able to:

- Recognize the clinical and radiological presentation of hypophysitis
- Better understand the classification of and conditions that result in pituitary inflammation
- Develop better knowledge of immunotherapy-related hypophysitis and IgG4-RD
- Consider the management strategy for the patient presenting with hypophysitis

STRATEGIES FOR DIAGNOSIS, THERAPY, AND/OR MANAGEMENT

Classification and Etiology of Hypophysitis/Inflammatory Pituitary Lesions

A number of classification systems are used to describe hypophysitis, because histology is not always available. Conventional classification is based on (presumed) etiology, with conditions described as either primary or secondary hypophysitis. The most common primary condition is lymphocytic hypophysitis, followed by granulomatous hypophysitis. Secondary causes include autoimmune conditions, infiltrative conditions [*e.g.*, Langerhans cell histiocytosis (LCH)], sarcoidosis, IgG4-RD, and immune therapy–induced hypophysitis. Historically, hypophysitis has also been classified based on the pattern of hypothalamic, pituitary, and pituitary stalk involvement. This approach is limited but does describe the associated pituitary hormone deficits. Patients with involvement of the neurohypophysis and those with panhypophysitis typically present with cranial diabetes insipidus (DI). Those with solely anterior pituitary involvement do not have DI but present with the consequences of anterior pituitary hormone deficiency. Hypophysitis can also be classified using histological appearance. Biopsy is most commonly performed to distinguish between neoplastic and inflammatory conditions and make a tissue diagnosis. Biopsy can result in hypopituitarism and DI and is indicated when there is mass effect or need to identify a neoplastic process. Successful biopsy can be useful in guiding management. There is overlap in the presentation of granulomatous, lymphocytic, and xanthomatous diseases, and making clear distinction among these can be difficult. It is important to acknowledge that although the term hypophysitis is used to refer to primary pituitary inflammation most commonly, it is also used to describe the consequences of other inflammatory and infiltrative conditions (*e.g.*, LCH). The classification of primary hypophysitis as well as secondary predisposing factors is summarized in Tables 1 and 2 (2, 3).

Clinical Presentation of Hypophysitis/Inflammatory Pituitary Disorders

Pituitary inflammation usually results in deficiency of pituitary hormones and increased size of the pituitary gland. This expansion may result in compression of the optic apparatus with resulting neuro-ophthalmic compromise. Involvement of the cavernous sinus with ophthalmoplegia is rare but described. Pituitary inflammation with enlargement commonly results in headache, which is a consistent feature in the patient with hypophysitis (4). Endocrine manifestations include anterior pituitary hormone deficiencies, DI, and abnormal serum prolactin. The pattern of endocrine dysfunction may be influenced by the etiology. Lymphocytic hypophysitis is considered to have a predilection to adrenocorticotropic hormone (ACTH), gonadotrophin, thyrotropin (TSH), and growth hormone (GH) deficiencies in that order, and although rare, isolated hormone deficiencies have been reported. When there is involvement of pituitary stalk and entire pituitary, DI is more likely. A relationship to pregnancy and the postpartum period

Table 1. Classification of Primary Hypophysitis

Classification
Based on anatomy
Lymphocytic adenohypophysitis
Lymphocytic infundibuloneurohypophysitis
Lymphocytic panhypophysitis
Based on histology
Lymphocytic hypophysitis
Xanthomatous hypophysitis
Granulomatous hypophysitis
Plasmacytic/IgG4-related hypophysitis
Necrotizing hypophysitis
Mixed forms (lymphogranulomatous, xanthogranulomatous)

supports the diagnosis of lymphocytic hypophysitis. Systemic conditions such as sarcoidosis or LCH may manifest with symptoms of respiratory or bone disease. Immune checkpoint inhibitors, most commonly ipilimumab, result in hypophysitis and thyroiditis as recognized consequences.

Investigation of the Patient With Hypophysitis

Biochemistry

A full early-morning pituitary hormone profile including cortisol, ACTH, insulin-like growth factor 1, GH, estradiol/testosterone, luteinizing hormone, follicle-stimulating hormone, free T4, TSH, prolactin, plasma/urine osmolality, and electrolytes should be performed. In patients with suspected DI, confirmatory tests are indicated. For potential systemic inflammatory conditions, other tests (*e.g.*, angiotensin-converting enzyme, antineutrophil cytoplasmic antibodies, human chorionic gonadotropin, double-stranded DNA) may be indicated.

Table 2. Conditions Predisposing Patients to Development of Hypophysitis

Condition
Autoimmune
Systemic lupus erythematosus
Systemic inflammatory disorders
Sarcoidosis
Granulomatosis with polyangitis (Wegener's granulomatosis)
IgG4-RD
Other granulomatous (Crohn's, Takayasu's, Castleman's disease)
Drug induced
Immune checkpoint therapy (CTLA-4 antibody, PD1 antibody)
Interferon α
Infiltrative lesions
LCH
Local tumor effect
Rupture of Rathke's cleft cyst
Germinoma
Infection
Tuberculosis
Syphilis
Fungal infections

Radiology

Gadolinium-enhanced pituitary magnetic resonance imaging (MRI) is the investigation of choice; radiological features suggestive of hypophysitis include a prompt, intense, and homogenously enhancing gland with no obvious stalk deviation. The posterior pituitary bright spot may be absent. The lesions are commonly associated with symmetrical suprasellar extension and enhancement of the dura, referred to as dural tail. Germ cell tumors and LCH have a predilection for involving the infundibulum and hypothalamus. IgG4 hypophysitis and immune checkpoint therapy–related hypophysitis have not been reported to have particular or unique characteristics that indicate etiology. Characterization of the unusual sellar mass is not straightforward and results in a wide differential. In patients with hypophysitis related to systemic pathology, additional imaging may identify other involved sites of disease. Computed tomography of the chest, abdomen, and pelvis is helpful in patients with potential sarcoidosis, tuberculosis, or connective tissue disorders or when malignancy is a potential differential diagnosis. Fluorodeoxyglucose (FDG) positron emission tomography (PET)/computed tomography has been shown to be helpful in confirming multisite disease (with FDG avidity demonstrated in sites other than the pituitary area, facilitating tissue diagnosis) and avoiding the need for pituitary biopsy in patients with IgG4-RD or LCH.

Immunology

A number of serological immune markers are under investigation but have yet to be established in clinical practice. Antipituitary antibodies have a low sensitivity and specificity. Coexisting autoimmune pathology in the patient with hypophysitis is uncommon, with autoimmune thyroid disease present in only 8% of patients with lymphocytic hypophysitis.

Histology

Histological assessment provides confirmation and classification of hypophysitis. Biopsy is associated with risk of morbidity, including DI and hypopituitarism. Histological stains to identify inflammatory cells and use of tissue [*e.g.*, CD45 (leukocyte common antigen), CD3 (T cells), CD20 (B cells), CD68 (macrophages), and CD138 (plasma cells)] and hormone-specific immune staining help to categorize different types of hypophysitis. Presence of histiocytes, granulomas, and xanthomas is essential to confirm specific subtypes of pituitary inflammatory lesions.

Treatment of Hypophysitis/Inflammatory Pituitary Disorders: General Principles

Hypophysitis has a variable natural history, and there is an absence of evidence-based treatment recommendations. Better understanding of the natural history and treatment responses of specific diagnoses (*e.g.*, IgG4-RD, immune checkpoint inhibitor treatment) will emerge with time. Hypopituitarism and DI should be treated according to current recommendations. Primary treatment of hypophysitis includes surgery, anti-inflammatory medical therapy, conservative management, and radiotherapy. An advantage of surgery is that it provides a histological diagnosis to guide future management. It also reliably and quickly treats mass effects and visual impairment resulting from the lesion. In a large German cohort, surgery for hypophysitis resulted in significant resolution of symptoms such as headaches and visual disturbances. The rate of recurrence is reported to be 11% to 25% (5). There are limited reports of spontaneous resolution of hypophysitis. In cases without pronounced mass effect or headache, surveillance of hypophysitis can be used in addition to replacement of endocrine insufficiencies.

Anti-inflammatory glucocorticoid therapy forms the cornerstone of medical management. Reports have confirmed initial good responses to steroid therapy, but the overall recurrence rate has been reported to be high and highlights the limitations of steroid treatment, with up to 38% of patients experiencing relapse (6). In cases of progressive or recurrent disease, steroid-sparing options such as alternative immune-suppressive agents or radiotherapy have been considered. Recent years have seen a rise in the use of immunosuppressive therapies for resistant lesions. Azathioprine is the most commonly used immune-suppressive agent at present, but in the future, we will see more focused monoclonal antibody–directed therapy such as rituximab. Treatment strategies and outcomes have been reported in a retrospective multicenter cohort from Germany (5).

Specific Conditions

Lymphocytic Hypophysitis

Lymphocytic hypophysitis is the most common primary hypophysitis. It occurs most frequently in women during reproductive years and has a strong association with pregnancy and the postpartum period. The condition may also occur in men, and there may be coexistent autoimmune conditions. Diagnosis is confirmed histologically, although clinical presentation may be classical, and therefore, biopsy may be avoided. Anti-inflammatory steroid therapy forms the cornerstone of management, but multimodal therapy may be required. There have been numerous comprehensive reviews of this condition (2).

Granulomatous Hypophysitis

Granulomatous hypophysitis is considered the second most common type of hypophysitis. Granulomatous disease can be seen as a primary entity (known as idiopathic primary granulomatous hypophysitis) or secondary to a systemic pathology such as sarcoidosis, tuberculosis, or granulomatosis with polyangitis (previously known as Wegener's granulomatosis). The histology is characterized by the presence of multinucleated giant cells, histiocytes, and lymphocyte infiltration along with plasma cells. It is still unclear if granulomatous changes represent a continuum of the lymphocytic inflammatory processes. Steroid treatment may be less effective than in lymphocytic hypophysitis, and surgery may be required for symptom control.

Xanthomatous Hypophysitis

Xanthomatous hypophysitis (XH) is considered to be the rarest of the histological subtypes, and it is unclear if XH constitutes a distinct entity or if it is a possible extension of the autoimmune or lymphocytic spectrum. As seen with xanthomatous lesions elsewhere in the body, it is postulated that xanthomatous infiltration results from macrophage activation secondary to chronic inflammation. It has been more commonly reported in women. Xanthomatous lesions present radiologically as cystic sellar masses on MRI and enhance on the postgadolinium contrast images. The gross lesion appears as a cyst filled with thick orange fluid with floating crystals. The diagnosis is only confirmed on tissue sections demonstrating xanthoma cells or lipid-laden macrophages in the pituitary tissue. It has been suggested that XH may be less responsive to steroid therapy as compared with lymphocytic hypophysitis, but because clinical experience is limited, this has yet to be established. Given the reported lack of effectiveness of medical management, most lesions are treated with surgery, if the patient has not already undergone surgery for diagnostic purposes. The response to treatment varies from complete to partial to no recovery from mass effect of symptoms, but endocrine deficiencies rarely recover (7).

IgG4-RD

IgG4-related hypophysitis was first reported in 2004 and is believed to be rare, but a recent retrospective histological review of cases previously thought to demonstrate lymphocytic hypophysitis showed that 41% were reclassified as IgG4-related hypophysitis (8). The previous lack of recognition of this etiology indicates that cases previously classified as hypophysitis or lymphocytic hypophysitis may in fact have been IgG4-RD. Additional retrospective and prospective studies will help us understand whether IgG4-RD represents a substantial cohort within the hypophysitis spectrum. The exact role of IgG4 in pathogenesis is uncertain, and it may well be considered a bystander in the inflammatory process. The condition commonly presents as pseudotumor lesions with IgG4-dominant plasmacytic infiltration of organs. The most common coexistent IgG4-related pathology associated with pituitary disease is retroperitoneal fibrosis. Leporati *et al.* (9)

suggested pituitary disease–specific diagnostic criteria for confirmation of the disease. Serum levels of IgG4 are not sensitive or specific for IgG4-RD, and elevated levels tend to normalize with steroid therapy, making them less useful as a diagnostic tool. FDG PET in IgG4-RD may be useful in characterizing systemic involvement of tissues. Steroids form the mainstay of treatment, with a beneficial early response, but recovery of endocrine function is rare.

Immune Checkpoint Therapy-Related Hypophysitis

Immunotherapy is associated with endocrine adverse effects including thyroiditis and hypophysitis. Ipilimumab (CTLA-4 antibody) was the first immune checkpoint inhibitor licensed for use in malignant melanoma, and nivolumab (PD1 antibody), pembrolizumab (PD1 antibody), and combination therapies are being used for a number of different metastatic malignancies. Pituitary inflammation is commonly noted before the third cycle of treatment and ranges from 5 to 36 weeks from the onset of therapy. The clinical presentation is similar to that of other forms of hypophysitis, and headache is a common feature (10). All patients receiving immune checkpoint therapy with new-onset headache or suspected cortisol deficiency should be evaluated for the likelihood of hypophysitis. Visual disturbance and DI are rare features. Endocrine deficiencies are noted in >70% patients. There are no obvious radiological features that can be used to differentiate primary from drug-induced hypophysitis, and as has been reported, the radiological findings can precede clinical diagnosis by several weeks. Numerous case reports have highlighted the incidental detection of hypophysitis, pancreatitis, adrenalitis, or thyroiditis when PET was used for surveillance purposes. Leporati *et al.* (9) described the biopsy results of CTLA-4–related hypophysitis, demonstrating pathological findings of complement fixation, macrophage infiltration, and lymphocyte activation and confirming that the mechanism of CTLA-4–related hypophysitis is largely a result of type II and type IV hypersensitivity reaction. The management of immune checkpoint therapy–related hypophysitis depends on the severity of the clinical presentation. For milder presentations, treatment involves replacing the hormone deficiency as standard. But in severe or life-threatening cases, the role of high-dose steroids and discontinuation of oncology therapy warrant consideration. Many centers have produced guidance on the recognition and management of adverse events related to immunotherapy.

MAIN CONCLUSIONS

Recognition of IgG4-RD has prompted reconsideration of the classification of hypophysitis, and clinicians are considering this diagnosis both in newly presenting cases and in ones previously labeled as lymphocytic hypophysitis. The advent of immune checkpoint inhibition has meant an increase in clinical experience with hypophysitis for endocrine physicians and provides insight into the pathophysiological mechanisms of disease. These increases in understanding will likely result in new diagnostic algorithms and more accurate classification of presentations. New serological markers are likely to emerge, and noninvasive diagnostics will improve. Future years will see more accurate diagnosis of inflammatory pituitary conditions and development of more consistent and specific treatments for these rare disorders.

CLINICAL CASES

Case 1

A 31-year-old woman presents at 38 weeks gestation. Clinical symptoms of persistent headache and nausea. Serum sodium low [125 mmol/L (normal range, 135 to 145 mmol/L)]. Cortisol low (25 nmol/L, 1.7 μg/dL) with undetectable ACTH. Low free T4. Visual function and fields normal.

- What is the likely diagnosis? Hypopituitarism, lymphocytic hypophysitis
- How should the case be managed? Assess visual function, imaging, birth plan, prednisolone
- What is the long-term outcome? Variable course, recurrence in subsequent pregnancy, permanent deficiency of ACTH and GH

Case 2

A 58-year-old woman with malignant melanoma, stage IIIA, midthoracic. Treated surgically and with chemotherapy: 12 months of vemurafenib; commenced ipilimumab 2 months before presentation with headache and fatigue. Elevated free thyroid hormones, TSH <0.01 mU/L. Cortisol 18 nmol/L (0.65 μg/dL).

- What is the diagnosis? Hypophysitis and thyroiditis related to ipilimumab
- Which investigations and management? Pituitary MRI, grade of adverse events, thyroid antibodies, replace hormones, manage thyrotoxicosis
- Should the drug be discontinued? Not necessarily; depends on clinical severity and mass effect

REFERENCES

1. Bellastella G, Maiorino MI, Bizzarro A, Giugliano D, Esposito K, Bellastella A, De Bellis A. Revisitation of autoimmune hypophysitis: knowledge and uncertainties on pathophysiological and clinical aspects. *Pituitary.* 2016;**19**(6):625–642.
2. Caturegli P, Newschaffer C, Olivi A, Pomper MG, Burger PC, Rose NR. Autoimmune hypophysitis. *Endocr Rev.* 2005;**26**(5):599–614.
3. Falorni A, Minarelli V, Bartoloni E, Alunno A, Gerli R. Diagnosis and classification of autoimmune hypophysitis. *Autoimmun Rev.* 2014; **13**(4-5):412–416.
4. Honegger J, Schlaffer S, Menzel C, Droste M, Werner S, Elbelt U, Strasburger C, Störmann S, Küppers A, Streetz-van der Werf C, Deutschbein T, Stieg M, Rotermund R, Milian M, Petersenn S; Pituitary Working Group of the German Society of Endocrinology. Diagnosis of primary hypophysitis in Germany. *J Clin Endocrinol Metab.* 2015; **100**(10):3841–3849.
5. Honegger J, Buchfelder M, Schlaffer S, Droste M, Werner S, Strasburger C, Störmann S, Schopohl J, Kacheva S, Deutschbein T, Stalla G, Flitsch J,

Milian M, Petersenn S, Elbelt U; Pituitary Working Group of the German Society of Endocrinology. Treatment of primary hypophysitis in Germany. *J Clin Endocrinol Metab.* 2015;**100**(9):3460–3469.

6. Khare S, Jagtap VS, Budyal SR, Kasaliwal R, Kakade HR, Bukan A, Sankhe S, Lila AR, Bandgar T, Menon PS, Shah NS. Primary (autoimmune) hypophysitis: a single centre experience. *Pituitary.* 2015; **18**(1):16–22.
7. Hanna B, Li YM, Beutler T, Goyal P, Hall WA. Xanthomatous hypophysitis. *J Clin Neurosci.* 2015;**22**(7):1091–1097.
8. Bernreuther C, Illies C, Flitsch J, Buchfelder M, Buslei R, Glatzel M, et al. IgG4-related hypophysitis is highly prevalent among cases of histologically confirmed hypophysitis. *Brain Pathol.* 2017;**27**(6):839–845.
9. Leporati P, Landek-Salgado MA, Lupi I, Chiovato L, Caturegli P. IgG4-related hypophysitis: a new addition to the hypophysitis spectrum. *J Clin Endocrinol Metab.* 2011;**96**(7):1971–1980.
10. Joshi MN, Whitelaw BC, Palomar MT, Wu Y, Carroll PV. Immune checkpoint inhibitor-related hypophysitis and endocrine dysfunction: clinical review. *Clin Endocrinol (Oxf).* 2016;**85**(3):331–339.

The Management of Nonfunctioning Pituitary Macroadenoma (NFPA)

M41
Presented, March 17–20, 2018

Frederic Castinetti, MD. Department of Endocrinology, Reference Center for Rare Pituitary Diseases, Aix-Marseille University, 13007 Marseille, France, E-mail: frederic.castinetti@ap-hm.fr

Henry Dufour, MD. Department of Neurosurgery, Reference Center for Rare Pituitary Diseases, Aix-Marseille University, 13007 Marseille, France, E-mail: henry.dufour@ap-hm.fr

SIGNIFICANCE OF THE CLINICAL PROBLEM

Nonfunctioning pituitary adenomas (NFPAs) are benign nonsecreting pituitary tumors, representing 15% to 30% of all pituitary adenomas. As they are frequently asymptomatic, their proper management is crucial to avoid the risk of visual disorders. The main issue is to determine the optimal timing for the surgical management of such tumors; a wait-and-see attitude is possible in some cases, provided a magnetic resonance imaging (MRI) follow-up is strictly performed. The problem is the same after surgery, as a proper follow-up is necessary to choose the best therapeutic strategy depending on the presence or absence of a remnant. We will not discuss in the following short text the case of silent pituitary adenomas or the initial workup necessary for proper evaluation of pituitary adenomas at initial diagnosis (shown in Table 1). We will mainly focus on the different steps in the management (mainly surgery or a wait-and-see attitude) and the follow-up of macro-NFPAs (1).

BARRIERS TO OPTIMAL PRACTICE

A barrier to optimal management is the fear of the clinicians to wait for too long before surgery, leading to nonreversible comorbidities due to the macroadenoma (visual field defects or pituitary deficiency). After surgery, the same applies for the fear of the growth of a pituitary remnant, which, in the majority of cases, will not happen rapidly.

LEARNING OBJECTIVES

As a result of participating in this session, learners should be able to:

- Determine the optimal therapeutic strategy at the time of diagnosis and the evidence for surgery or a wait-and-see approach
- Determine the optimal therapeutic strategy after surgery when a remnant is visualized on MRI

STRATEGIES FOR MANAGEMENT

At the Time of Diagnosis

Surgery and the Management of Symptomatic NFPAs

NFPAs With Visual Disorders. With surgery, improved vision is reported in ~80% to 90% of cases (including both partial and total recovery) (2–4). Recovery may be progressive, over a period of up to 1 year after surgery. Some studies highlighted a correlation between percentage recovery and duration and severity of visual field defect (acuity <1/10 or optic atrophy being of poor prognosis) (5, 6). In the case of demonstrable visual disorder, surgery should therefore not be delayed; the emergency depends on the severity of visual impact. There are no clear data for a threshold time beyond which visual recovery after chiasma decompression is no longer possible. Visual disorders are an indication for surgery, even though complete recovery cannot be guaranteed.

NFPAs With Pituitary Deficiency. The risk of onset of further pituitary deficiency associated with macroadenoma is estimated at 12% per year. Arafah *et al.* (7, 8) correlated preoperative deficiency, headaches, and hyperprolactinemia to the potential for postoperative recovery; when all the criteria were met, postoperative recovery of deficiency and improvement in headaches were more frequent, correlating with intrasellar pressure. Surgery provided recovery of normal anterior pituitary function in ~30% of cases, at a mean 1 year's follow-up (9); the rate was higher for earlier management. Some teams indeed recommend surgery at the asymptomatic stage of macroadenoma (9). The risk of postoperative deterioration in pituitary function is ~10% (5). Pituitary deficiency is thus probably not the main factor indicating surgery, postoperative recovery being uncertain.

NFPAs With Headaches. The involvement of pituitary adenoma in headaches can only be established after ruling out all other possible causes (possibly after referral to a neurologist) and determining time of onset in relation to the natural history of the adenoma. Disabling headache implicating adenoma could be an indication for nonemergency surgery, warning the patient that no direct causal relation can be proven and thus results cannot be guaranteed.

Wait-and-See Attitude or Surgery in the Management of Asymptomatic NFPAs

Surgical indications should be based on several factors.

Size of the Tumor. Progression is slow in microadenoma and surgery is not indicated. The natural progression of macroadenoma may indicate nonemergency surgery, depending

Table 1. Initial First-Line Evaluation of Nonfunctioning Pituitary Macroadenoma

Imaging	Dedicated Pituitary MRI
Biology	0800 h adrenocorticotropic hormone and cortisol
	24-h urinary free cortisol
	Thyrotropin, T4
	Luteinizing hormone, follicle-stimulating hormone, testosterone (estradiol depending on the menses)
	Prolactin
	IGF-1
	Clinical suspicion of hypersecretion should add:
	• 1 mg dexamethasone suppression test (Cushing)
	• Random growth hormone ± oral glucose tolerance test (acromegaly)
Ophthalmology	Visual field and acuity

on evolutive status, proximity to the optic pathways, and the patient's age. The spontaneous evolution of a nonsecreting macroadenoma has been evaluated at 17% increase and 12% decrease with a follow-up >4 years, and 30% to 40% increase with a longer follow-up (10).

Patient Age. Nonemergency surgery may be considered in young patients without awaiting progression, given the low risk of postoperative visual impairment, the almost inevitable progression of adenoma over the long-term, and the risk of definitive postoperative visual impairment if surgery is delayed awaiting onset of a campimetric visual-field effect. For young female patients, surgery should respond quickly to any impairment of visual field. Gonadotroph deficiency is also an indication for surgery, although postoperative recovery is unsure. Pregnancy is not theoretically a risk factor for increasing adenoma volume, but there is a risk of visual field defect if the adenoma is close to the optic pathways. In that case, surgery should be considered; if it is not implemented, close clinical surveillance and visual field testing should accompany the pregnancy. If no pregnancy is planned and the adenoma shows no impact, MRI surveillance should be proposed, or else surgical intervention without awaiting progression. Indications in 65- to 75-year-olds are the same as in young subjects, if comorbidity, anesthesia risk, and patient impact are well assessed. In the case of surgery, the approach should preferably be transsphenoidal, so as not to increase the risk of complications. In the absence of visual impact, simple annual MRI surveillance is sufficient. The lack of data for >75-year-olds is to be borne in mind.

Risk of Onset of Visual Field Defect, Pituitary Deficiency, and Apoplexy. The risk of onset of visual field defect correlates with the rate of tumor growth and proximity to the optic pathways. The risk of pituitary deficiency is 12% per year in macroadenoma. The risk of apoplexy is estimated at 1% per year in the absence of extra risk factors; the risk increases to 14% per year when the average growth of the adenoma is >3.5 mm per year (10).

Risks Inherent to Transsphenoidal Surgery. Mortality is <1%; the risk of severe adverse events (osteomeningeal breach, meningitis, or visual deterioration) is <5%; and the risk of diabetes insipidus may reach 10%.

In the absence of surgery, regular MRI follow-up should be performed for macro-NFPAs. This attitude does not sound necessary for micro-NFPAs. We usually perform a single MRI during the follow-up to confirm the lack of further growth and then stop the follow-up if the image remains stable.

After Surgery

The follow-up is based on regular pituitary MRI. The first MRI should be done 3 to 4 months after the surgery; the results of this MRI will determine the following therapeutic procedures (11, 12).

In the Absence of Visible Pituitary Adenoma Remnant

The risk of recurrence in the absence of pituitary adenoma remnant ranged from 0% to 24% in prospective and retrospective follow-up studies reported in the literature. Chen *et al.* (12) reported a 12% risk in their meta-analysis. Sheehan *et al.* (13) recently recommended (level II recommendation) to perform serial neuroimaging studies. Pituitary MRI might be performed every 1 to 2 years during at least 10 years. As recently stated by Ziu *et al.* (14), there is, however, insufficient evidence to make recommendations regarding the rhythm of MRI follow-up.

In the Presence of Visible Pituitary Adenoma Remnant

Further growth increase is observed in at least 20% of cases. Predictive factors of regrowth include pathological criteria of aggressiveness, such as Ki-67 >3%, genetic predisposition (AIP mutation for instance), and for some studies young age at diagnosis. Regular MRI might thus be performed on a lifelong basis, and at 1-year intervals during the first 5 years after surgery (15); again, no strong recommendation as recently stated (14). Two options can be discussed.

Surgical Revision. Second surgery is rarely curative; gross total resection is reported in 63% vs. 28% of cases in patients with primary vs. revision transsphenoidal resection (16). The benefits in terms of visual recovery are usually less important than for primary surgery (58% vs. 90% improvement). Surgical revision should be considered in cases for which complete resection is possible, when the remnant is symptomatic and close to the optic chiasm (in the aim of decreasing the volume to further treat by radiation techniques), or in rare cases of further regrowth after radiation techniques (15). Surgical side effects might include a higher risk of pituitary deficiency and diabetes insipidus than for primary surgery; however, a recent retrospective study comparing the side effects of primary vs. revision transsphenoidal resection only reported a higher risk of syndrome of inappropriate antidiuretic hormone secretion (SIADH; 17% vs. 4%), without increased risk of other surgical side effects such as hypopituitarism, diabetes insipidus, cerebrospinal fluid leak, or vascular injury (16).

Radiation Techniques. Several modalities are available with conformal or stereotactic radiation techniques depending on the size of the tumor, the proximity of the optic chiasm, *etc.* All these techniques are very effective in controlling tumor size even if they do not systematically lead to a decrease. Sheehan *et al.* (13) recently recommended the use of radiosurgery with a single session dose of at least 12 Gy or radiation therapy with a fractionated dose of 45 to 54 Gy. Usually, a stable or decreased tumor volume is observed in >90% of cases, provided the MRI definition of the target is optimal. The antitumor effect begins at the end of the first year after radiotherapy and is maintained on a long-term basis (17). Classical side effects include hypopituitarism (10% to 50%) and optic neuritis (for stereotactic radiosurgery when a sufficient distance between the target and the optic chiasm is not obtained). Research is still ongoing to determine the risk of extrapituitary side effects (stroke or brain tumors) for modern radiation techniques. Of note, Tampourlou *et al.* (18) recently reported that there was a 12.5% risk of further regrowth of NFPAs in patients treated by surgery and first radiotherapy. In these patients, no further regrowth was reported in patients treated with another radiation procedure.

The timing for performing surgical revision or radiation technique is also a matter of controversy. Although some teams recommend it to be performed on a systematic basis as soon as a remnant is visible, we recommend a wait-and-see attitude, provided the fact that the remnant is far from the optic chiasm, a regular MRI follow-up is performed, and the pathology is not in favor of an aggressive disease.

MAIN CONCLUSIONS

To conclude, the management of macro-NFPA requires a combined endocrinological, ophthalmological, and neurosurgical approach at first diagnosis. This will lead to a first decision of wait-and-see attitude or surgery. In both cases, regular MRI follow-up will be performed in the following years. In operated patients, the need for additional treatment (surgical revision or radiation technique) will be based on the presence of a postsurgical remnant, its growth through regular MRI, and pathological criteria of aggressiveness. Future studies are still needed to determine the optimal management of such patients.

DISCUSSION OF CASES AND ANSWERS

Case 1

Because he was complaining of occipital headaches, Mr. R (58 years old) had a brain MRI that showed a pituitary macroadenoma (largest size of 20 mm), close to the optic chiasm. Visual field is normal, and the patient is not complaining of any visual field defect. The evaluation of pituitary axes does not show any deficiency.

Question 1: How Would You Manage This Patient?

A. Immediate surgery
B. Fractionated radiotherapy
C. Pituitary MRI at 3 months without surgery
D. Pituitary MRI at 1 year without surgery

Explanation of Best Answer: C

The macroadenoma is close to the optic chiasm but the visual field is still normal. The headaches are posterior and are probably not due to the macroadenoma. Although surgery could be an option in this patient, we consider that a close follow-up would be enough. One year is too delayed due to the risk of tumor progression; scheduling pituitary MRI at 3 months sounds more reasonable. Obviously, this MRI should be performed earlier in the case of visual complaints.

Question 2: You Chose a Wait-and-See Attitude. Which Criteria Among the Following Could Have Been Additional Evidence in Favor of Surgery if Present in the Case?

A. Hypopituitarism
B. Bitemporal superior quadranopia
C. Anticlotting therapy
D. Older age (>75 years)

Explanation of Best Answers: A-B-C

These answers do not mean that surgery is mandatory in these situations except for the case of B, for which surgery should be performed rapidly to allow visual recovery. For answer A, there is a possibility of pituitary function recovery in ~30% of cases. For answer C, anticlotting therapy is a risk factor for pituitary apoplexy; given the fact that the macroadenoma is close to the optic chiasm, this is something to take into account when choosing the best therapeutic strategy. The patient should be warned of the clinical signs suggesting this diagnosis (strong headaches or visual nerve palsy) in the case of a wait-and-see attitude.

Case 2

Mr. B (48 years old) has been operated on for a pituitary macroadenoma with chiasm compression. The 3-month postoperative evaluation shows an 8-mm right cavernous sinus remnant. The patient has no pituitary deficiency and no clinical complaint.

Question 1: What Would You Recommend at This Stage?

A. Reoperation
B. Radiotherapy
C. Radiosurgery
D. 3- to 6-month pituitary MRI

Explanation for Best Answer: D

The laterosellar position of the remnant makes it difficult to be sure that a second surgery will be curative. The risk of further regrowth is estimated to be ~20% at 3 to 5 years follow-up. The remnant is far from the optic pathways. At this stage, MRI follow-up seems a reasonable option.

Question 2: The Ki-67 Was Actually 10% at the Pathology. Would This Change Your Management?

A. Yes, probably
B. No

Explanation for Best Answer: A

The high Ki-67 is in favor of an aggressive pituitary tumor. In this case, we usually recommend performing radiation techniques (radiosurgery in this instance, considering the small volume of the remnant and its location away from the optic chiasm) given the high efficacy in controlling tumor volume.

REFERENCES

1. Castinetti F, Dufour H, Gaillard S, Jouanneau E, Vasiljevic A, Villa C, Trouillas J. Non-functioning pituitary adenoma: when and how to operate? What pathologic criteria for typing? *Ann Endocrinol (Paris).* 2015;**76**(3):220–227.
2. Murad MH, Fernández-Balsells MM, Barwise A, Gallegos-Orozco JF, Paul A, Lane MA, Lampropulos JF, Natividad I, Perestelo-Pérez L, Ponce de León-Lovatón PG, Albuquerque FN, Carey J, Erwin PJ, Montori VM. Outcomes of surgical treatment for nonfunctioning pituitary adenomas: a systematic review and meta-analysis. *Clin Endocrinol (Oxf).* 2010;**73**(6):777–791.
3. Dehdashti AR, Ganna A, Karabatsou K, Gentili F. Pure endoscopic endonasal approach for pituitary adenomas: early surgical results in 200 patients and comparison with previous microsurgical series. *Neurosurgery.* 2008;**62**(5):1006–1015; discussion 1015–1017,
4. Tabaee A, Anand VK, Barrón Y, Hiltzik DH, Brown SM, Kacker A, Mazumdar M, Schwartz TH. Predictors of short-term outcomes following endoscopic pituitary surgery. *Clin Neurol Neurosurg.* 2009; **111**(2):119–122.
5. Dekkers OM, Pereira AM, Romijn JA. Treatment and follow-up of clinically nonfunctioning pituitary macroadenomas. *J Clin Endocrinol Metab.* 2008;**93**(10):3717–3726.
6. Gnanalingham KK, Bhattacharjee S, Pennington R, Ng J, Mendoza N. The time course of visual field recovery following transphenoidal surgery for pituitary adenomas: predictive factors for a good outcome. *J Neurol Neurosurg Psychiatry.* 2005;**76**(3):415–419.
7. Arafah BM, Kailani SH, Nekl KE, Gold RS, Selman WR. Immediate recovery of pituitary function after transsphenoidal resection of pituitary macroadenomas. *J Clin Endocrinol Metab.* 1994;**79**(2):348–354.
8. Arafah BM, Prunty D, Ybarra J, Hlavin ML, Selman WR. The dominant role of increased intrasellar pressure in the pathogenesis of hypopituitarism, hyperprolactinemia, and headaches in patients with pituitary adenomas. *J Clin Endocrinol Metab.* 2000;**85**(5):1789–1793.
9. Messerer M, Dubourg J, Raverot G, Bervini D, Berhouma M, George I, Chacko AG, Perrin G, Levivier M, Daniel RT, Trouillas J, Jouanneau E. Non-functioning pituitary macro-incidentalomas benefit from early surgery before becoming symptomatic. *Clin Neurol Neurosurg.* 2013; **115**(12):2514–2520.
10. Fernández-Balsells MM, Murad MH, Barwise A, Gallegos-Orozco JF, Paul A, Lane MA, Lampropulos JF, Natividad I, Perestelo-Pérez L, Ponce de León-Lovatón PG, Erwin PJ, Carey J, Montori VM. Natural history of nonfunctioning pituitary adenomas and incidentalomas: a systematic review and metaanalysis. *J Clin Endocrinol Metab.* 2011; **96**(4):905–912.
11. Chanson P, Raverot G, Castinetti F, Cortet-Rudelli C, Galland F, Salenave S; French Endocrinology Society Non-functioning Pituitary Adenoma Work-Group. Management of clinically non-functioning pituitary adenoma. *Ann Endocrinol (Paris).* 2015;**76**(3):239–247.
12. Chen Y, Wang CD, Su ZP, Chen YX, Cai L, Zhuge QC, Wu ZB. Natural history of postoperative nonfunctioning pituitary adenomas: a systematic review and meta-analysis. *Neuroendocrinology.* 2012;**96**(4): 333–342.
13. Sheehan J, Lee CC, Bodach ME, Tumialan LM, Oyesiku NM, Patil CG, Litvack Z, Zada G, Aghi MK. Congress of Neurological Surgeons systematic review and evidence-based guideline for the management of patients with residual or recurrent nonfunctioning pituitary adenomas. *Neurosurgery.* 2016;**79**(4):E539–E540.
14. Ziu M, Dunn IF, Hess C, Fleseriu M, Bodach ME, Tumialan LM, Oyesiku NM, Patel KS, Wang R, Carter BS, Chen JY, Chen CC, Patil CG, Litvack Z, Zada G, Aghi MK. Congress of Neurological Surgeons systematic review and evidence-based guideline on posttreatment follow-up evaluation of patients with nonfunctioning pituitary adenomas. *Neurosurgery.* 2016; **79**(4):E541–E543.
15. Cortet-Rudelli C, Bonneville JF, Borson-Chazot F, Clavier L, Coche Dequéant B, Desailloud R, Maiter D, Rohmer V, Sadoul JL, Sonnet E, Toussaint P, Chanson P. Post-surgical management of nonfunctioning pituitary adenoma. *Ann Endocrinol (Paris).* 2015;**76**(3): 228–238.
16. Przybylowski CJ, Dallapiazza RF, Williams BJ, Pomeraniec IJ, Xu Z, Payne SC, Laws ER, Jane JA, Jr. Primary versus revision transsphenoidal resection for nonfunctioning pituitary macroadenomas: matched cohort study. *J Neurosurg.* 2017;**126**(3):889–896.
17. Chen Y, Li ZF, Zhang FX, Li JX, Cai L, Zhuge QC, Wu ZB. Gamma Knife surgery for patients with volumetric classification of nonfunctioning pituitary adenomas: a systematic review and meta-analysis. *Eur J Endocrinol.* 2013;**169**(4):487–495.
18. Tampourlou M, Ntali G, Ahmed S, Arlt W, Ayuk J, Byrne JV, Chavda S, Cudlip S, Gittoes N, Grossman A, Mitchell R, O'Reilly MW, Paluzzi A, Toogood A, Wass JAH, Karavitaki N. Outcome of nonfunctioning pituitary adenomas that regrow after primary treatment: a study from two large UK centers. *J Clin Endocrinol Metab.* 2017;**102**(6): 1889–1897.

Hyperprolactinemia/Prolactinoma

M51
Presented, March 17–20, 2018

Vera Popovic, PhD, FRCP. Medical Faculty, University of Belgrade, 11000 Belgrade, Serbia, E-mail: popver@gmail.com

SIGNIFICANCE OF THE CLINICAL PROBLEM

Outside of gestation and lactation, the causes of persistent moderate hyperprolactinemia include drugs, hypothyroidism, and hypothalamic/pituitary disorders. A recent population-based study reported that the rising prevalence of hyperprolactinemia is probably due to an increased case ascertainment and increased incidence of psychoactive drug-related causes (1). Evaluation of the patient with drug-induced hyperprolactinemia may be challenging. If concomitant disease is present, management should be in conjunction with a psychiatrist. Prolactin-secreting pituitary adenomas are the most common type of pituitary tumors to cause pathological hyperprolactinemia.

BARRIERS TO OPTIMAL PRACTICE

The barriers to diagnosis are:

- The presence of macroprolactin may change the initial diagnosis in a large proportion of patients
- Misdiagnosis of patients with large tumors with moderate hyperprolactinemia (prolactin levels are falsely low due to the "hook effect") as clinically nonfunctioning tumor with stalk compression then followed by inappropriate management
- Overdiagnosing "microprolactinoma" in a patient with polycystic ovary syndrome (PCOS) and modest prolactin elevations who has a small tumor identified on magnetic resonance imaging (MRI); this may lead to unnecessary treatment with dopamine agonist

The barriers to treatment are:

- Failure to recognize the limitations of surgical treatment of microprolactinomas
- Uncertainty of how long to treat and when to withdraw treatment with dopamine agonists
- Unawareness of potential psychiatric adverse effects (impulse control disorder [ICD]) of dopamine agonists
- Limited experience in managing patients with macroprolactinoma in pregnancy
- Limited experience in the management of patients with aggressive prolactinomas resistant to conventional therapies

LEARNING OBJECTIVES

As a result of participating in this session, learners should be able to:

- Establish an accurate diagnosis before treatment of hyperprolactinemia
- Recognize the possibilities and limitations of surgical treatment options in microprolactinomas
- Recognize factors favorable to dopamine agonist withdrawal in responders and in special circumstances (pregnancy and menopause)
- Develop awareness of psychiatric adverse effects of dopamine agonists and reassure and explain to the patient the concern of valvular heart disease
- Understand the difficulties in the management of aggressive prolactinomas resistant to conventional therapies and plan a multidisciplinary approach

EPIDEMIOLOGY

Hyperprolactinemia may be physiological, pathological, or iatrogenic. The rising prevalence of hyperprolactinemia is due to increased ascertainment as well as the use of drugs that affect the hypothalamic dopamine system and/or pituitary dopamine receptors (most commonly antipsychotics). The occurrence of hyperprolactinemia depends on the study population. In a recent study of the overall prevalence of hyperprolactinemia over 20 years in Scotland, there was a fourfold increase in the number of prolactin assays performed and there was an increased rate of drug-induced hyperprolactinemia (tripled). The overall prevalence of ever-diagnosed hyperprolacinemia in Tayside, Scotland is 0.1% (1).

The prevalence of pituitary tumors is approximately one per 1,000 of the population. Prolactinomas account for ~44% of pituitary tumors. A population-based cohort study shows a prevalence of ever medically treated hyperprolactinemia to be ~0.2% (2).

STRATEGIES FOR DIAGNOSIS, THERAPY, AND MANAGEMENT

Clinical Cases

Although the diagnosis and treatment of hyperprolactinemia has been defined in guidelines, several challenging issues in the diagnosis and treatment remain (3).

Diagnostic Challenges

The association of certain drugs and hyperprolactinemia is well documented. Physicians should be aware that a large number of commonly prescribed medications are associated with hypeprolactinemia (antiemetics, prokinetics, antidepressants, antihypertensives, opiates, *etc.*), which suggests that it will occur frequently in the population. A Brazilian study reported a prevalence of 14.5% for drug-induced hyperprolactinemia, most commonly antipsychotics (4).

Macroprolactin results from the formation of big complexes between prolactin and immunoglobulins. Patients with hyperprolactinemia due to macroprolactin are usually asymptomatic. Detection of macroprolactin helps avoid miscategorization of patients with hyperprolactinemia. Macroprolactinemia may be associated with any cause of hyperprolactinemia and is reported in 5.8% of women with PCOS (5).

Prolactin levels >100 ng/mL are suggestive of microprolactinomas. However, as many as 25% of patients with microprolactinomas may present with prolactin levels <100 ng/mL. This is challenging in young women with moderate hyperprolactinemia (~50 to 75 ng/mL). The reason is that the peak incidence of idiopathic hyperprolactinemia and PCOS occurs most commonly in young women. The relationship between hyperprolactinemia and PCOS is considered a fortuitous association (6). In one-third of patients with idiopathic hyperprolactinemia, mildly elevated prolactin levels may resolve, and in others, it may remain stable. In some patients with mild/moderate hyperprolactinemia, MRI scan may detect pituitary hyperplasia or adenoma. Physicians should be aware that pituitary incidentalomas are frequent (10% of adult population) (7).

Large (macro) prolactinomas are diagnosed with prolactin levels >200 ng/mL. Potential pitfalls are falsely low prolactin levels in some patients with giant invasive skull base tumors ("hook effect"). This may lead to incorrect diagnosis and unnecessary surgery and/or radiotherapy. The solution is to repeat the assay after serum sample dilution. After dilution, the true magnitude of prolactin elevation confirms the diagnosis of macroprolactinoma. (8)

Treatment Challenges

The goals of treatment are (1) normalization of prolactin levels and pituitary function, (2) reduction of tumor size and prevention of recurrence, (3) relief of symptoms caused by excess prolactin, and (4) prevention of complications.

Medical treatment with dopamine agonists (cabergoline and bromocriptine) results in rapid and marked reduction in prolactin and tumor. High efficacy and good tolerability make these the first choice in the treatment of both micro- and macroadenomas (2). In partial responders, the dose of cabergoline may be increased stepwise to the maximal tolerable dose (up to 11 mg/wk) (9). It is not advised to start with a higher dose and/or to increase it more rapidly in patients with giant prolactinomas as some patients may normalize prolactin levels rapidly and show massive tumor size reduction, which may tend toward cerebrospinal fluid leakage or apoplexy. Ninety percent of prolactinomas are controlled by dopamine agonists, whereas 10% of macroprolactinomas remain uncontrolled and are truly resistant to cabergoline.

Can Prolactinomas Be Cured Medically?

There are several factors favorable to complete drug withdrawal: (1) treatment with cabergoline for >2 years (3–5 years), (2) maintenance of normoprolactinemia for at least 1 year after tapering to a dose of 0.5 mg/wk cabergoline, and (3) tumor no longer visible by MRI or a >50% reduction in the maximal tumor diameter (10).

What Are the Side Effects of Dopamine Agonists?

Dopamine agonists are generally safe. However patients on cabergoline may rarely exhibit psychiatric adverse effects, including ICD (gambling, compulsive shopping, and hypersexuality) and psychosis, which cause devastating effects on the patient's life (11). The symptoms of ICD are perhaps underreported because of a lack of awareness among patients and health care professionals. The condition is underreported due to the highly personal nature of the symptoms. If the patient has prolactinoma and psychosis, then the antipsychotic of choice could be aripiprazole. Aripiprazole is an atypical antipsychotic with partial dopamine agonist activity, which successfully suppresses prolactin levels in patients with microprolactinoma who develop psychosis while on cabergoline (12, 13). In the long-term, there might also be some risk of valvulopathy but only in patients treated with a high dose of cabergoline (>3 mg/wk) and long duration (cumulative dose effect). Cabergoline acts on the serotonin-5HT$_{2B}$R present in human cardiac valves with mitogenic activity. However at doses <2 mg/wk, the safety of cabergoline has been reported in a large UK follow-up study (14, 15).

Why Does Surgery Have Limited Use in Microprolactinomas?

Currently this is because the recurrence rate is high (20%) (long-term normalization of prolactin is achieved in 60% to 80%); relapse is very frequent if postoperative prolactin is >20 ng/mL. Low recurrence rates are seen only if postoperative prolactin is very low (5 ng/mL), *i.e.*, in the hypoprolactinemic range (16). Complications occur, such as diabetes insipidus and hypopituitarism, and the incidence depends on the experience of the surgeon and volume load of the respective center (17, 18). Surgical treatment is second-line therapy and has been reserved for patients with dopamine resistance or intolerance or poor compliance. The results of a primary surgical treatment approach for patients with microprolactinomas have been recently reported (19).

Tumor progression or regrowth despite treatment with dopamine agonists is a clear indication for surgery. Surgery could also be indicated as second-line therapy after medical treatment of macroprolactinomas, to reduce the duration of dopamine agonist therapy and thus avoid side effects (20). However during dopamine agonist treatment of macroprolactinomas and giant prolactinomas, the suprasellar and intrasellar parts of the tumor usually shrink first, and the residual tumor, which is located laterally in the cavernous sinus or posteriorly in the clivus, is often hardly resectable.

Aggressive Prolactinomas

Aggressive pituitary tumors are defined by clinical behavior. They invade surrounding tissues (invasion), have rapid growth potential (proliferation), are large in size, have a tendency to recur after initially successful treatment, are resistant to conventional therapies (medical and radiotherapy), and are potentially life threatening. Most dopamine agonist-resistant tumors have been recognized to have a particularly severe clinical course and are generally more frequent in men (21). Tumor size or the pretreatment serum prolactin levels are not predictive of the response to dopamine agonists. Such patients require a multidisciplinary approach. Radiotherapy comes only after failure of medical and/or surgical therapy to control tumor growth. This includes newer treatment modalities, such as stereotactic radiation therapy, stereotactic radiosurgery, and proton beam therapy (22). In a large meta-analysis of 923 patients in 32 studies, radiotherapy achieved partial endocrine response in 32.8% of patients and complete endocrine normalization in 28.8% of patients (23). Recent European Society of Endocrinology Guidelines recommend the use of temozolomide monotherapy as first-line chemotherapy for aggressive pituitary tumors and pituitary carcinomas after documented tumor growth and resistance to conventional treatment (24). The first evaluation of treatment response to temozolomide should take place after 3 months. In patients responding, treatment should be continued for at least 6 months. Despite a heterogeneous mix of patients, and differences in treatment schedules and imaging procedures, the response rate (defined as percentage of patients with a partial or complete tumor regression) has been broadly similar across the studies, with a reported volume reduction in 47% (95% CI 36 to 58). It should be noted that there are no head-to-head studies comparing temozolomide with other treatment options.

Special Circumstances: Management of Prolactinomas in Pregnancy and Menopause

In pregnancy, most women are treated for hyperprolactinemia to restore fertility. Withdrawal of dopamine agonists once pregnancy is confirmed is recommended (25). In case of pregnancy, the fetus will be exposed to dopamine agents, which cross the placenta. Bromocriptine taken in the first weeks of gestation is without adverse effects. Cabergoline is also withdrawn when pregnancy is established, but due to its long half-life, it can be detected in circulation until 30 days after its cessation. If, in the preconception period, a high dose of cabergoline (up to 9 mg/wk) has been used to normalize prolactin and shrink the tumor and spontaneous pregnancy occurs, then cabergoline can be slowly tapered until the fourth gestational week (26).

In Menopause

Women who pass through menopause have a substantial chance of normalizing prolactin levels, and usually treatment is withdrawn (24). The reasons for stopping treatment in menopause are as follows: no clinical evidence that normalization of prolactin levels in postmenopausal women improves bone mass density or reduces fracture risk, studies have not demonstrated an association of hyperprolactinemia with breast cancer, prolactin does not promote platelet aggregation, studies have not demonstrated that increased prolactin is associated with cardiovascular disease, and unclear and inconsistent results on the role of elevated prolactin in autoimmunity (27). In patients with macroprolactinomas, the cabergoline dose required to maintain a normal prolactin level during long-term follow-up is lower than the initial dosage. Withdrawal depends on whether there is invasion of the cavernous sinus. Prolactinomas are rarely diagnosed in postmenopausal women. Such women usually harbor large and invasive macroadenomas, secreting high prolactin levels, and usually respond well to dopamine agonist therapy (28).

CASE SUBJECTS

Case 1

A 28-year-old female 3 years prior to presentation had a serum prolactin concentration of 35 ng/mL, high androstenedione levels, mild hirsutism and acne, regular menstrual cycles, and polycystic ovary appearance of the ovaries. She was treated with oral contraceptive pills for 2 years and then stopped. Two years later on re-evaluation, serum prolactin concentrations rose to 65 to 75 ng/mL and cycles became irregular. MRI scan of the pituitary showed a macroadenoma 27 × 18 mm in size. She received cabergoline therapy. After 3 months of therapy, prolactin concentrations became extremely low (<5 ng/mL) and MRI scan showed a slight increase in tumor size.

Question: Should the Diagnosis and Treatment of This Patient Be Questioned?

ANSWER: Some patients may be miscategorized as having prolactinoma instead of nonfunctioning pituitary adenoma with a stalk effect and then treated long-term with dopamine agonists. Physicians should bear in mind that the diagnosis of prolactinoma is rarely confirmed by pathology because primary treatment is medical and surgery is not indicated. In a long-term follow-up study of patients who underwent transsphenoidal surgery for prolactin-secreting pituitary tumors, 78% were true prolactinomas by immunohistochemistry. Others were nonfunctioning pituitary adenomas or growth hormone– and prolactin-positive adenomas (common embryonic origin) and 20 were cysts and others (17). Because our patient had very low prolactin levels on cabergoline while the tumor slightly increased in size, the findings were not felt to be consistent with prolactinoma. Our patient underwent transsphenoidal surgery. The final diagnosis was silent adrenocorticotropic hormone adenoma.

Case 2

A 42-year-old female with a very large tumor of the skull base and unexplored primary amenorrhea had prolactin concentrations 120 ng/mL (normal <20 ng/mL).

Question: What Is the Diagnosis?

ANSWER: The diagnosis of giant prolactinomas may be delayed due to their atypical presentation (age and sex). Prolactin levels may be falsely low due to a prolactin assay problem, the high-dose "hook" effect. After dilution, the true magnitude of the prolactin elevation in our patient was 20,000 ng/mL, confirming the diagnosis of giant invasive prolactinoma. Cabergoline therapy restored menstrual cycles and caused a substantial reduction in tumor size.

Case 3

A 19-year-old female presented with amenorrhea, headache, 13-mm pituitary macroadenoma, and prolactin concentrations between 75 and 90 ng/mL. She was treated successfully with cabergoline 1 mg/wk and subsequently 0.5 mg/wk for 5 years. She resumed menstrual cycles, and prolactin quickly normalized, with a >50% reduction in the maximal tumor diameter (5 mm). After tapering the dose of cabergoline to 0.25 mg/wk and normal prolactin concentrations for 1 year, she withdrew from dopamine therapy. One year later, she was asymptomatic and prolactin concentrations measured were between 25 and 28 ng/mL, with slight tumor enlargement to 6 mm. Six months later, she suffered a severe headache, with prolactin concentration 26 ng/mL, and the tumor grew to a maximal tumor diameter of 11 mm.

Question: How Should This Case Further Be Managed?

ANSWER: This patient is clearly a responder to cabergoline and has fulfilled all the requirements necessary for withdrawal of dopamine therapy after 5 years of treatment. It was hoped that she would be in prolonged remission. We have informed her that when stopping treatment, long-term surveillance is necessary because according to meta-analysis performed by Dekkers *et al.*, including 19 studies and 743 patients, hyperprolactinemia recurred after drug withdrawal in 79% of patients previously treated with dopamine agonists (29). In that analysis, recurrence of hyperprolactinemia was not accompanied by an increase in tumor size but was associated with clinical symptoms of galactorrhea and hypogonadism. According to recent studies on long-term cabergoline treatment of macroprolactinomas, cabergoline can achieve remission maintenance in 73% of patients for at least 12 months after cessation of a 5-year course of therapy (28, 30). Our patient was in remission 1.5 years after cessation of a 5-year cabergoline course when headache and tumor regrowth occurred despite regular cycles and prolactin levels just slightly over the upper limit of normal. Treatment was reinstituted.

Case 4

A 14-year-old girl presented with secondary amenorrhea, galactorrhea, headache, and a 13 × 12 × 14 mm pituitary adenoma with slight suprasellar extension and invasion of the right cavernous sinus. Prolactin concentrations measured twice were 618 and 500 ng/mL. Macroprolactin was negative. Genetic testing for MEN1 and AIP mutations was negative. She was referred to us by a pediatric endocrinologist because 2 years of cabergoline 2 mg/wk did not normalize the prolactin level (~200 ng/mL). However, substantial tumor shrinkage occurred, loss of headache, and no galactorrhea was recorded. Amenorrhea persisted. We increased the cabergoline dose stepwise to 3.5 mg/wk, but the patient remained a partial responder with no further substantial reduction in prolactin concentrations.

Question: How Should This Patient Be Further Managed?

ANSWER: The challenge of this case is partial resistance to dopamine agonists (lack of prolactin normalization) in a young female patient with invasive macroadenoma in whom treatment caused tumor shrinkage despite the absence of hormonal normalization. Partial response is considered when the dose of cabergoline not normalizing prolactin is 3.5 mg/wk (18). Defining no response (true resistance) to cabergoline treatment is difficult because it has been shown that cabergoline may have its maximal antisecretory and/or antitumoral effects at very high doses (up to 11 mg/wk) (9). The question then is how long can the high doses be used safely? Our patient declined surgery, so we decided to continue with cabergoline 3.5 mg/wk and wait for the time effect (some prolactinomas are slow in responding). She has now received cabergoline for 7 years, and this has been effective in controlling the tumor volume. The tumor is now 4 mm maximal diameter and prolactin concentrations are reduced to 80 ng/mL. She continues with medical treatment with a yearly echocardiogram.

Case 5

A 14-year-old female with a 22-mm macroprolactinoma was treated with cabergoline 2× 0.5 mg/wk for 2 years. Tumor shrinkage occurred (tumor diameter 9 mm) and prolactin was rapidly normalized. At age 16 years on treatment, she developed promiscuous and hypersexual behavior that led to a volatile relationship with her parents and she became suicidal.

Question: How Should This Patient Be Further Managed?

ANSWER: This patient in her adolescent years developed ICD (hypersexuality). The condition is underreported, and in our case, the mother reported the symptoms. Impulse control disorders (ICDs) constitute socially disruptive behaviors such as pathological gambling, impulsive eating, compulsive shopping, and hypersexuality. These conditions are well recognized in patients on dopamine agonist therapy for Parkinson disease. Switching agents is not helpful because cabergoline, bromocriptine, and quinagolide are all implicated. Withdrawal of dopamine agonists should be considered, and pituitary surgery may be required. Dopamine agonist treatment was stopped. There was a period of 6 months with resolution of symptoms; however, during later follow-up, without treatment, a form of the disease recurred (ICD). Surgery was recommended but she declined. One year after stopping cabergoline, she has regular cycles and the prolactin concentration is in the upper limit of normal.

Case 6

A 29-year-old amenorrheic woman with a 12- × 11-mm invasive macroprolactinoma (left cavernous sinus) and prolactin 400 ng/mL requests pregnancy as soon as possible. She has been treated unsuccessfully with cabergoline 1 mg/wk in previous years. She did not tolerate bromocriptine. During a period of 1 year preconception, the cabergoline dose was gradually increased stepwise to a maximal tolerated dose of 7 mg/wk. Prolactin concentrations did not normalize and were 75 to 100 ng/mL. Conception (in vitro fertilization) was withheld until the MRI showed tumor reduction, and maximal tumor reduction was 6 mm.

Question: How Should This Case Be Managed?

ANSWER: The challenge was that our patient with an invasive macroprolactinoma failed to normalize prolactin, remained amenorrheic, and desired immediate pregnancy. She declined preconception surgery. After increasing the dose of cabergoline to 7 mg/wk, despite not normalizing prolactin levels, the tumor shrank to 6 mm (<1 cm) and she underwent in vitro fertilization. Twin pregnancy was established. We initiated stepwise cabergoline dose reduction during pregnancy, and cabergoline was withdrawn late in pregnancy (end of second trimester). The pregnancy was uneventful. She delivered two healthy babies via cesarean section and was allowed to breast feed.

Tumor enlargement in pregnancy is seen in 2.7% of patients with microprolactinomas and in 22.9% of patients with macroprolactinomas who did not receive previous therapy (25). It has been shown that cabergoline can control tumor growth and thereby achieve successful pregnancy in patients with macroprolactinomas (31). In a prospective Japanese study, 85 women with macroprolactinomas or microprolactinomas received prospective, high-dose cabergoline therapy for infertility (26). The dose of cabergoline was 2 to 9 mg/wk in the resistant patients. The authors concluded that cabergoline achieved a high pregnancy rate with uneventful outcomes in infertile women with prolactinoma, independent of tumor size and bromocriptine resistance or intolerance. Preconception surgery and/or radiotherapy was not necessary.

REFERENCES

1. Soto-Pedre E, Newey PJ, Bevan JS, Greig N, Leese GP. The epidemiology of hyperprolactinaemia over 20 years in the Tayside region of Scotland: the Prolactin Epidemiology, Audit and Research Study (PROLEARS). *Clin Endocrinol (Oxf)*. 2017;**86**(1):60–67.
2. Kars M, Souverein PC, Herings RM, Romijn JA, Vandenbroucke JP, de Boer A, Dekkers OM. Estimated age- and sex-specific incidence and prevalence of dopamine agonist-treated hyperprolactinemia. *J Clin Endocrinol Metab*. 2009;**94**(8):2729–2734.
3. Melmed S, Casanueva FF, Hoffman AR, Kleinberg DL, Montori VM, Schlechte JA, Wass JA; Endocrine Society. Diagnosis and treatment of hyperprolactinemia: an Endocrine Society clinical practice guideline. *J Clin Endocrinol Metab*. 2011;**96**(2):273–288.
4. Vilar L, Fleseriu M, Bronstein MD. Challenges and pitfalls in the diagnosis of hyperprolactinemia. *Arq Bras Endocrinol Metabol*. 2014; **58**(1):9–22.
5. Hayashida SA, Marcondes JA, Soares JM, Jr, Rocha MP, Barcellos CR, Kobayashi NK, Baracat EC, Maciel GA. Evaluation of macroprolactinemia in 259 women under investigation for polycystic ovary syndrome. *Clin Endocrinol (Oxf)*. 2014;**80**(4):616–618.
6. Robin G, Catteau-Jonard S, Young J, Dewailly D. Physiopathological link between polycystic ovary syndrome and hyperprolactinemia: myth or reality? [in French]. *Gynécol Obstét Fertil*. 2011;**39**(3): 141–145.
7. Galland F, Vantyghem MC, Cazabat L, Boulin A, Cotton F, Bonneville JF, Jouanneau E, Vidal-Trécan G, Chanson P. Management of nonfunctioning pituitary incidentaloma. *Ann Endocrinol (Paris)*. 2015; **76**(3):191–200.
8. Maiter D, Delgrange E. Therapy of endocrine disease: the challenges in managing giant prolactinomas. *Eur J Endocrinol*. 2014;**170**(6): R213–R227.
9. Ono M, Miki N, Kawamata T, Makino R, Amano K, Seki T, Kubo O, Hori T, Takano K. Prospective study of high-dose cabergoline treatment of prolactinomas in 150 patients. *J Clin Endocrinol Metab*. 2008;**93**(12): 4721–4727.
10. Molitch ME. Pituitary gland: can prolactinomas be cured medically? *Nat Rev Endocrinol*. 2010;**6**(4):186–188.
11. Noronha S, Stokes V, Karavitaki N, Grossman A. Treating prolactinomas with dopamine agonists: always worth the gamble? *Endocrine*. 2016;**51**(2):205–210.
12. Burback L. Management of a microprolactinoma with aripiprazole in a woman with cabergoline-induced mania. *Endocrinol Diabetes Metab Case Rep*. 2015;**2015**:150100.
13. Bakker IC, Schubart CD, Zelissen PM. Successful treatment of a prolactinoma with the antipsychotic drug aripiprazole. *Endocrinol Diabetes Metab Case Rep*. 2016;**2016**:160028.
14. Drake WM, Stiles CE, Howlett TA, Toogood AA, Bevan JS, Steeds RP; UK Dopamine Agonist Valvulopathy Group. A cross-sectional study of the prevalence of cardiac valvular abnormalities in hyperprolactinemic patients treated with ergot-derived dopamine agonists. *J Clin Endocrinol Metab*. 2014;**99**(1):90–96.
15. Drake WM, Stiles CE, Bevan JS, Karavitaki N, Trainer PJ, Rees DA, Richardson TI, Baldeweg SE, Stojanovic N, Murray RD, Toogood AA, Martin NM, Vaidya B, Han TS, Steeds RP, Baldeweg FC, Sheikh UE, Kyriakakis N, Parasuraman SK, Taylor L, Butt N, Anyiam S; UK Cabergoline valvulopathy study group. A follow-up study of the prevalence of valvular heart abnormalities in hyperprolactinemic patients treated with cabergoline. *J Clin Endocrinol Metab*. 2016; **101**(11):4189–4194.
16. Roelfsema F, Biermasz NR, Pereira AM. Clinical factors involved in the recurrence of pituitary adenomas after surgical remission: a structured review and meta-analysis. *Pituitary*. 2012;**15**(1): 71–83.
17. Feigenbaum SL, Downey DE, Wilson CB, Jaffe RB. Transsphenoidal pituitary resection for preoperative diagnosis of prolactin-secreting pituitary adenoma in women: long term follow-up. *J Clin Endocrinol Metab*. 1996;**81**(5):1711–1719.
18. Barker II FG, Klibanski A, Swearingen B. Transsphenoidal surgery for pituitary tumors in the United States, 1996-2000: mortality,

morbidity, and the effects of hospital and surgeon volume. *J Clin Endocrinol Metab.* 2003;**88**(10):4709–4719.

19. Babey M, Sahli R, Vajtai I, Andres RH, Seiler RW. Pituitary surgery for small prolactinomas as an alternative to treatment with dopamine agonists. *Pituitary.* 2011;**14**(3):222–230.
20. Képénékian L, Cebula H, Castinetti F, Graillon T, Brue T, Goichot B. Long-term outcome of macroprolactinomas. *Ann Endocrinol (Paris).* 2016;**77**(6):641–648.
21. Delgrange E, Daems T, Verhelst J, Abs R, Maiter D. Characterization of resistance to the prolactin-lowering effects of cabergoline in macroprolactinomas: a study in 122 patients. *Eur J Endocrinol.* 2009; **160**(5):747–752.
22. Sheplan Olsen LJ, Robles Irizarry L, Chao ST, Weil RJ, Hamrahian AH, Hatipoglu B, Suh JH. Radiotherapy for prolactin-secreting pituitary tumors. *Pituitary.* 2012;**15**(2):135–145.
23. Wattson DA, Tanguturi SK, Spiegel DY, Niemierko A, Biller BM, Nachtigall LB, Bussière MR, Swearingen B, Chapman PH, Loeffler JS, Shih HA. Outcomes of proton therapy for patients with functional pituitary adenomas. *Int J Radiat Oncol Biol Phys.* 2014;**90**(3):532–539.
24. Raverot G, Burman P, McCormack A, Heaney A, Petersenn S, Popovic V, Trouillas J, Deckkers OM; European Society of Endocrinology. Clinical practice guidelines for the management of aggressive pituitary tumours and carcinomas. *Euro J Endocrinol.* 2018;**178**(1):G1–G24.
25. Molitch ME. Endocrinology in pregnancy: management of the pregnant patient with a prolactinoma. *Eur J Endocrinol.* 2015;**172**(5): R205–R213.
26. Ono M, Miki N, Amano K, Kawamata T, Seki T, Makino R, Takano K, Izumi S, Okada Y, Hori T. Individualized high-dose cabergoline therapy for hyperprolactinemic infertility in women with micro- and macroprolactinomas. *J Clin Endocrinol Metab.* 2010;**95**(6): 2672–2679.
27. Karunakaran S, Page RC, Wass JA. The effect of the menopause on prolactin levels in patients with hyperprolactinaemia. *Clin Endocrinol (Oxf).* 2001;**54**(3):295–300.
28. Faje AT, Klibanski A. The treatment of hyperprolactinemia in postmenopausal women with prolactin-secreting microadenomas: cons. *Endocrine.* 2015;**48**(1):79–82.
29. Dekkers OM, Lagro J, Burman P, Jørgensen JO, Romijn JA, Pereira AM. Recurrence of hyperprolactinemia after withdrawal of dopamine agonists: systematic review and meta-analysis. *J Clin Endocrinol Metab.* 2010;**95**(1):43–51.
30. Shimon I, Bronstein MD, Shapiro J, Tsvetov G, Benbassat C, Barkan A. Women with prolactinomas presented at the postmenopausal period. *Endocrine.* 2014;**47**(3):889–894.
31. Liu C, Tyrell JB. Successful treatment of a large macroprolactinoma with cabergoline during pregnancy. *Pituitary.* 2001;**4**(3):179–185.

Unusual Sellar Masses

M62
Presented, March 17-20, 2018

Mark Gurnell, PhD, MA(MEd), FHEA, FAcadMEd, FRCP. Wellcome Trust-MRC Institute of Metabolic Science, Addenbrooke's Hospital, Cambridge CB2 0QQ, United Kingdom, E-mail: mg299@medschl.cam.ac.uk

> **Unusual:** ***adj:*** not habitually or commonly occurring or done; remarkable or interesting because different from or better than others...
> *Oxford English Dictionary*

SIGNIFICANCE OF THE CLINICAL PROBLEM

- Hormone-secreting (functioning) or nonsecreting (nonfunctioning) pituitary adenomas account for the majority of sella-based masses. However, in a substantial minority of cases (estimated at 5% to 10% in some surgical series) (1, 2), other etiologies are the cause of the sellar abnormality.
- Although some nonpituitary lesions have distinctive radiological appearances or are identified in a clinical context that lends itself to rapid diagnosis, others arise in isolation and/or are indistinguishable from a pituitary adenoma.
- Pituitary biopsy can help establish the diagnosis, but carries a small risk of damaging the remaining normal gland and may not be necessary in all cases.

Misdirected investigation may result in wasted resources and/or incorrect therapeutic intervention.

BARRIERS TO OPTIMAL PRACTICE

- Lack of familiarity with the rarer causes of a sellar mass may result in failure to distinguish it from a pituitary adenoma and result in either inappropriate observation or surgical intervention.
- Multidisciplinary expertise is required to ensure an appropriate management plan; decision making should reside within a team comprising neuroendocrinology, neurosurgery, neuroradiology, neuro-oncology, and neuro-ophthalmology (consistent with recent Pituitary Tumor Centers of Excellence guidance) (3).

LEARNING OBJECTIVES

As a result of participating in this session, learners should be able to:

- Readily identify the different (nonadenomatous) causes of a sellar mass (considering other benign neoplasia, malignancy, and inflammatory and cystic lesions)
- Instigate relevant investigations to allow distinction among different, rarer causes of a sellar mass and thus recommend appropriate management

CLINICAL CASES

Case 1

A 24-year-old woman was referred to the pituitary service with an 8-month history of secondary amenorrhea and bilateral galactorrhea. Her medical history was unremarkable, aside from Graves' disease, which was treated initially with medical therapy and then total thyroidectomy (at the age of 20 years). She was taking thyroxine 275 μg/d. Examination confirmed bilateral galactorrhea. She was clinically euthyroid with no palpable thyroid remnant. Visual acuity and visual field testing did not show any evidence of compression of the optic chiasm.

Endocrine testing confirmed hyperprolactinemia [1245 mU/L; reference range (RR) <620] and central hypogonadism. Serum cortisol at 9:00 AM was 450 nmol/L (RR 280 to 550). Free thyroxine was mildly raised [22.0 pmol/L (RR 9 to 20)], but thyrotropin (TSH) was significantly elevated [>100 mU/L (RR 0.4 to 4.0)]. IGF-1 was within the age- and sex-matched reference range. Pituitary magnetic resonance imaging (MRI) appearances are shown in Fig. 1.

Questions

1. What is the most probable cause of the sellar mass in this patient?
2. How would you further investigate and manage this case?

Answers

1. The presentation with secondary amenorrhea and galactorrhoea in a woman of this age is suggestive of a prolactinoma. However, because the prolactin level is only mildly raised, the differential diagnosis (prior to imaging) lies between a microprolactinoma and stalk disconnection syndrome due to local mass effect. The finding of a larger (>1 cm) lesion on MRI, with suprasellar extension, favors the latter. However, although nonfunctioning pituitary adenomas can occur in younger patients, they are less common than functioning tumors. In addition, in this case, thyroid function tests are clearly abnormal with a markedly elevated TSH despite mild hyperthyroxinemia. Although a TSH-secreting pituitary macroadenoma (with the added confounding effect of preceding thyroid surgery) should enter the differential diagnosis, another possibility must be considered—thyrotroph hyperplasia secondary to long-term intermittent/poor concordance with thyroxine therapy.

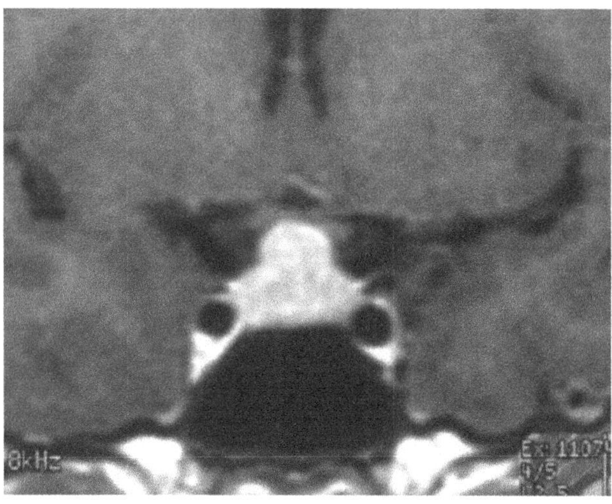

Figure 1. Coronal MRI with contrast.

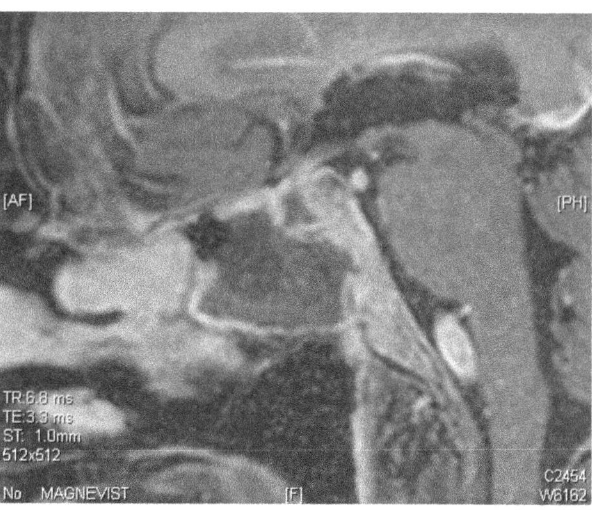

Figure 2. Sagittal MRI without contrast.

2. MRI appearances—symmetrical enlargement of the gland in the absence of expansion of the sella, with suprasellar extension that respects anatomical boundaries (including the diaphragma sellae)—are consistent with thyrotroph hyperplasia. Therefore, it is important to establish whether the patient is concordant with her thyroxine therapy. If doubt remains, then consideration should be given to a period of supervised thyroxine administration (after TSH assay interference has been excluded). If it is confirmed that the patient is taking her medication reliably, then further investigation will need to consider the possibility of a thyrotropinoma with tumor expansion following thyroidectomy. It is important to check whether the original pattern of thyroid function tests was consistent with primary thyrotoxicosis (*i.e.*, TSH fully suppressed). In such cases, it is generally advisable to seek expert advice (4).

Case 2

A 77-year-old man attended the emergency department with severe headache and blurred vision. He reported a 3-day history of nasal congestion and facial pain, which had worsened in the 12 hours prior to admission. He had no relevant medical history and was not taking any regular medications. Physical examination revealed mild pyrexia (37.9°C), pulse rate of 104 beats/min, and blood pressure of 120/70 mm Hg. Visual acuity was reduced in the left eye (6/60), with evidence of left cranial nerve III, IV, and VI palsies. There were no other focal neurologic signs nor clinical stigmata of hypercortisolism or acromegaly.

Endocrine assessment showed partial anterior hypopituitarism: random cortisol 468 nmol/L, free thyroxine 9.8 pmol/L (RR 10 to 20), TSH 0.25 mU/L (RR 0.35 to 5.5), testosterone 0.9 nmol/L (RR 8 to 29), luteinizing hormone 1.5 U/L (RR 1 to 6), prolactin 92 mU/L (RR 45 to 375), IGF-1 13.7 nmol/L (RR 10 to 25). MRI appearances are shown in Fig. 2.

Questions

1. What is the most probable cause of this patient's acute presentation?
2. How would you further investigate and manage this case?

Answers

1. Presentation with severe headache, reduced vision, and ophthalmoplegia raises the possibility of pituitary apoplexy with infarction/hemorrhage into a previously undiagnosed pituitary adenoma. Fever and meningitic features may also be present (secondary to an aseptic meningitis). However, this patient clearly described a prodromal period with nasal congestion and facial pain, which should raise concerns of a primary sinus infection (bacterial or fungal) with extension to involve the sella.
2. The patient is unwell with substantial cranial neuropathy and reduced vision. MRI findings are suggestive of a sphenoid sinus infection/mucopyocele with breech of the floor of the fossa and extension into the sella. After initial bedside investigations (including blood cultures) and in addition to supportive measures, the patient should be treated with broad-spectrum antibiotic and antifungal therapy and transferred for urgent transsphenoidal exploration. Although lumbar puncture may be considered, the need for an urgent tissue/microbiological diagnosis and decompression of the parasellar region renders this less relevant.

STRATEGIES FOR DIAGNOSIS AND MANAGEMENT

Etiopathogenesis

Sellar masses that are not primarily pituitary in origin can be considered under the following broad headings:

Cysts

- Rathke's cleft
- Arachnoid
- Epidermoid
- Other (*e.g.*, simple)

Benign Neoplasia

- Craniopharyngioma
- Meningioma
- Other (*e.g.*, ependymoma, hemangioma)

Malignancy

- Metastases (*e.g.*, breast, lung, prostate, renal)
- Chordoma
- Lymphoma
- Germinoma
- Other (*e.g.*, chondrosarcoma, hemangiopericytoma, sinonasal undifferentiated carcinoma, glioma)

Inflammatory/Infective

- Hypophysitis (lymphocytic/autoimmune/drug induced; granulomatous; IgG4-related disease)
- Sarcoidosis
- Bacterial/tuberculosis/fungal infection/abscess (with or without sinus origin)
- Other (*e.g.*, granulomatosis with polyangiitis)

Other

- Langerhans cell histiocytosis; Erdheim-Chester disease
- Aneurysm
- Mucocele
- Hyperplasia (*e.g.*, thyrotroph hyperplasia in severe/untreated primary hypothyroidism)
- Empty sella syndrome (cerebrospinal fluid–filled sella may occasionally be mistaken for a cystic lesion)

It is also important to note that rare tumors of pituitary (pituitary carcinoma) or stromal (pituicytoma) origin may also be encountered in the sella.

Clinical Presentation

Anterior pituitary dysfunction and typical features of local mass effect (hyperprolactinaemia, headache, reduced visual acuity with field defects, and/or ophthalmoplegia) may accompany any sella-based pathology.

Features that should raise concerns of an alternative (nonprimary pituitary) pathology include:

- Presence of diabetes insipidus prior to intervention
- Unusual pattern of anterior pituitary hormone loss
- Rapid speed of onset/progression (in the absence of apoplexy)
- Extensive cranial neuropathy
- Systemic upset
- History of previous/active malignancy or a systemic disorder with recognized propensity to involve the sellar/parasellar region

In a smaller number of patients, the presence of a sella mass will be an incidental finding on a scan performed for other purposes.

Investigation/Management

All cases of suspected atypical sellar/parasellar lesions should be referred for early discussion by a specialist pituitary multidisciplinary team (3). Clinical context is critical for guiding the tempo and nature of further investigations (compare and contrast cases 1 and 2).

In addition to assessment of anterior (and, when indicated, posterior) pituitary function and formal ophthalmic review, further investigations that may be indicated include the following.

Blood Profile

- Full blood count, erythrocyte sedimentation rate, C-reactive protein
- Blood cultures
- Serum angiotensin converting enzyme, IgG4, antineutrophil cytoplasmic antibody
- Tumor markers

Cerebrospinal Fluid

- Tumor markers (*e.g.*, human chorionic gonadotropin, α-fetoprotein), cytology

Radiology

Computed Tomography of the Sellar/Parasellar Region

- To provide better definition of bony landmarks

Computed Tomography of the Chest With or Without the Abdomen With or Without the Pelvis

- In cases of suspected malignancy or systemic disorders

^{18}F-Labeled Fluorodeoxyglucose Positron Emission Tomography

- In cases of suspected malignancy or systemic inflammatory disorders

Transsphenoidal Biopsy (With or Without Culture)

- Remains an important option when the primary diagnosis remains unclear and a period of observation is deemed inappropriate
- Can be combined with debulking/decompression in cases where there is substantial local mass effect

- May be complicated by worsening pituitary function

MAIN CONCLUSIONS

A. A substantial minority of sellar masses are not the result of primary pituitary pathology.

B. A high index of clinical suspicion is required, especially because many will present with symptoms, endocrine dysfunction, and radiological appearances that are typical of pituitary adenomas.

C. Careful clinical assessment and targeted investigation may facilitate early diagnosis and guide management.

D. However, many lesions will only be diagnosed at surgery.

REFERENCES

1. Freda PU, Wardlaw SL, Post KD. Unusual causes of sellar/parasellar masses in a large transsphenoidal surgical series. *J Clin Endocrinol Metab.* 1996;**81**(10):3455-3459.
2. Valassi E, Biller BM, Klibanski A, Swearingen B. Clinical features of nonpituitary sellar lesions in a large surgical series. *Clin Endocrinol (Oxf).* 2010;**73**(6):798-807.
3. Casanueva FF, Barkan AL, Buchfelder M, Klibanski A, Laws ER, Loeffler JS, Melmed S, Mortini P, Wass J, Giustina A; Pituitary Society, Expert Group on Pituitary Tumors. Criteria for the definition of Pituitary Tumor Centers of Excellence (PTCOE): A Pituitary Society Statement. *Pituitary.* 2017;**20**(5):489-498.
4. Koulouri O, Moran C, Halsall D, Chatterjee K, Gurnell M. Pitfalls in the measurement and interpretation of thyroid function tests. *Best Pract Res Clin Endocrinol Metab.* 2013;**27**(6):745-762.

PEDIATRIC ENDOCRINOLOGY

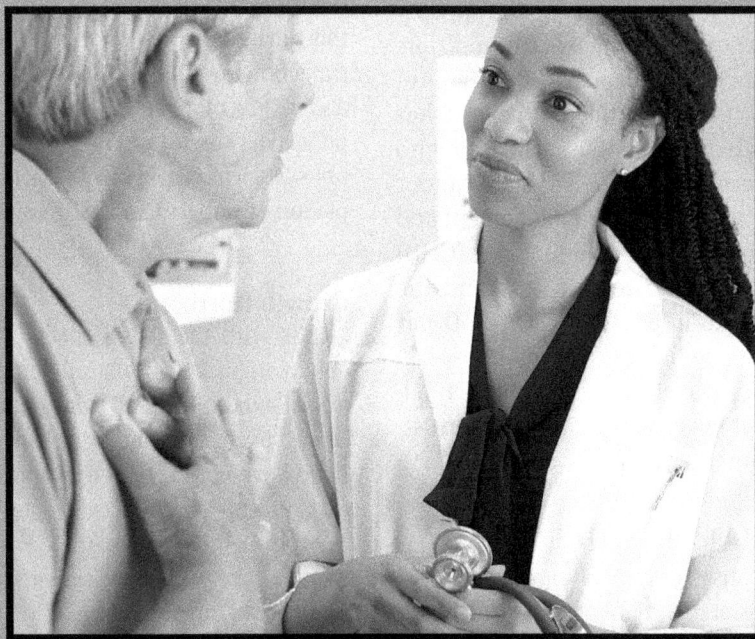

Transitioning Children With Panhypopituitarism to Adult Practice

M01
Presented, March 17–20, 2018

Sara DiVall, MD. Seattle Children's Hospital/University of Washington, Seattle, Washington 98105, E-mail: sara.divall@seattlechildrens.org

SIGNIFICANCE OF THE CLINICAL PROBLEM

Health care transition is the "purposeful, planned movement of adolescents and young adults (AYA) with chronic and physical medical conditions from child-centered care to the adult-oriented health care system" (1). Health care transition in patients with hypopituitarism involves transition of the following elements: (1) the endocrine medical "home"; (2) the burden of responsibility for daily disease management and coordination tasks from caregiver to patient; and (3) the disease treatment driven by physiological developmental changes. Hypopituitarism is an umbrella diagnosis that may involve a singular pituitary hormone deficiency or multiple pituitary hormone deficiencies. The causes of hypopituitarism are varied; many persons affected have other complex medical problems that also require transition into adult care and possibly neurocognitive defects that hinder the patient's ability to direct his/her daily management and care. The prevalence of growth hormone deficiency (GHD) in children is estimated at 1:4000 to 1:10,000 and the prevalence of hypopituitarism in adults at 30 to 50 per 100,000, with an estimated one-half of cases diagnosed in childhood. Thus, health care transition of AYA with hypopituitarism is a process that every pediatric and internist-endocrinologist will encounter.

BARRIERS TO OPTIMAL PRACTICE

Because there are diverse causes of hypopituitarism, the assessment of continuing medical treatment after linear growth is finished varies greatly by the underlying cause.

No studies exist that investigate a transition of care process that optimizes outcomes for patients with hypopituitarism; processes must be borrowed from other chronic disease models (*e.g.*, diabetes mellitus, cystic fibrosis).

Given the heterogeneity of patient readiness and cognitive abilities, effect and burden of coexisting diagnoses, and available expertise among internist endocrinologists, each transition process must be individualized, requiring substantial provider time and resources.

Competing academic, economic, and social priorities of AYA detract from their commitment to disease management and the transition process.

Learning Objectives

As a result of participating in this session, learners should be able to:

- Develop a strategy to re-evaluate the hypothalamic pituitary axes to optimize physiological outcomes in AYA
- Adapt transitions of care templates and checklists to clinical practice and individualize to patient needs
- Develop strategies for diagnosis, therapy, and/or management

MANAGEMENT OF PHYSIOLOGICAL TRANSITIONS

The greatest physiological change of adolescence is puberty with resultant development of secondary sex characteristics, pubertal growth spurt with subsequent fusion of the growth plates to achieve adult height, and maturation of the gonads for sperm or egg production. Depending upon extent of pituitary deficiency of the individual patient, the clinician must manage the replacement of one or multiple pituitary hormones during this time. At the age when most adolescents are considered for transition to adult care (≥16 years), the vast majority of women and many men have achieved adult height and completed puberty. Thus, the following discussion will center upon the physiological transitions of each pituitary hormone after completion of puberty and achievement of adult height.

Growth Hormone

Adults with childhood-onset GHD have alterations in body composition, bone mineral density, and lipid metabolism that are alleviated by GH treatment (2). Thirty percent to 50% of persons diagnosed with isolated, idiopathic GHD in childhood have normal somatotropic axis functioning in adulthood and do not experience the morbidities of adult GHD (3–5). Therefore, the clinician must develop a strategy to determine which adolescents need reassessment of the somatotropic axis after linear growth completion and thus potentially benefit from continued GH replacement. A strategy can be developed based upon the degree of pituitary hormone deficiency and underlying cause (Fig. 1). Individuals with multiple pituitary hormone deficiency of any cause, defined as three or more pituitary hormone deficiencies, develop bone and metabolic alterations associated with adult GHD and invariably meet criteria for adult GHD on provocative testing (6–8). Therefore, reassessment of the somatotropic axis is not needed in these persons, and a diagnosis of adult GHD can be made. Persons with two pituitary hormone deficiencies (or ectopic posterior pituitary) may or may not test as having persistent GHD; therefore, reassessment is advised (9). Reassessment should be done when the patient has not taken GH for 1 to 3 months. An insulin-like growth factor I (IGF-1) test may be performed

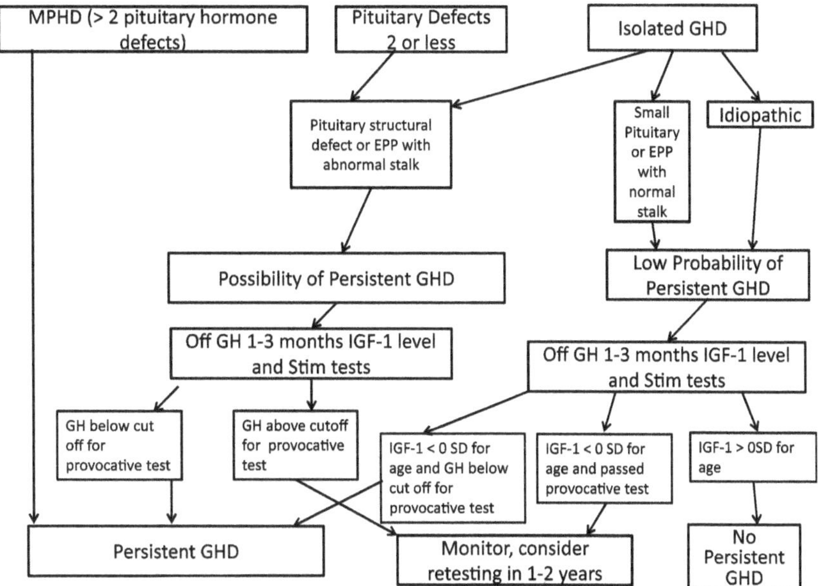

Figure 1. A diagnostic approach to evaluate the somatotropic axis after linear growth completion.

to serve as an off-treatment baseline; however, in persons with two or more pituitary hormone defects, diagnostic cut-offs for persistent GHD are unclear. Thus, provocative testing for GH should be done (agents discussed below) regardless of the IGF-1 level. In contrast, AYA with isolated, idiopathic GHD have a low probability of persistent GHD. Performing an IGF-1 test after the patient has not taken GH for 1 to 3 months is helpful, because persons with an IGF-1 level greater than zero standard deviation for age pass the GH stimulation testing in most series (9). If an IGF-1 level is less than zero standard deviation, then provocative testing is recommended. There is no IGF-1 level below which individuals invariably test as persistent GH on provocative testing.

The agent with the greatest sensitivity and specificity for determining persistent GHD in AYA is insulin. Growth hormone–releasing hormone (GHRH)-arginine has been tested in the transition period, but diagnostic cut-offs are different than when used to diagnose adult GHD (and GHRH is not available in the United States) (9). Glucagon is a promising alternative, but it has not been specifically tested in the transition period. In adults, the cut-off value is lower for those who are overweight/obese.

The optimal GH dose during the transition period is not clear. As in adults, IGF-1 levels are used with the goal to dose GH to normalize IGF-1 level for age and sex. Endocrine Society suggests starting at 400 to 500 μg daily, titrating dose to IGF-1 level. Persons taking oral estrogen may need higher doses (2).

Thyroid Hormone

Replacement of thyroid hormone in AYA is more straightforward. Endocrine Society Guidelines recommend monitoring with a free T4, aiming to keep free T4 in the mid-upper range of normal (10). No recommendations are given for frequency of free T4 determinations, except in the case of pregnancy, when free T4 should be checked monthly, when the rising estrogen thus hormone-binding globulins of pregnancy increases thyroid hormone–replacement needs. It makes sense to check free T4 at least yearly or as needed for symptoms or substantial changes in medication (*e.g.*, estrogen dose, introduction of anti-epileptic drugs).

Glucocorticoids

Treatment regimens for glucocorticoid replacement vary widely, from short-acting hydrocortisone one to three times daily to long-acting prednisone or dexamethasone. In general, pediatricians favor hydrocortisone two to three times daily to minimize the chances of glucocorticoid effect on linear growth, with doses calculated per body surface area. Endocrine Society guidelines suggest continuing hydrocortisone in adults to lower the possibility of overtreatment, which decreases quality of life (10). The recommended dose is 15 to 20 mg/d divided two to three times daily. The type of glucocorticoid used and frequency of dosing must adequately provide replacement and optimize quality of life, yet be a feasible regimen to encourage compliance. Instructions regarding possibility of adrenal crises and need for stress-dose steroids are lifelong. In multiple series examining causes of death in hypopituitarism, patients with adrenal insufficiency had the highest rates of death (11).

Sex Steroid Replacement

Sex steroid replacement after puberty is important for continued bone health, normal body composition, and libido. There are no studies comparing the efficacy of different replacement regimens on these outcomes. Therefore, replacement regimens are individualized to maximize compliance and quality of life. In men, testosterone levels are a reliable indicator of adequate dosing, but estrogen levels in women are not as reliable. Theoretically, estrogen doses sufficient to build a uterine lining should be sufficient for bone health, but studies have not been done.

If persons have pituitary dysfunction encompassing gonadotropins, fertility is typically compromised. There are different protocols of gonadotropin replacement to produce sperm or to induce ovulation (12) that have been effective in persons with hypogonadotropic hypogonadism. Reproductive endocrinology protocols and techniques are improving and providing the opportunity for some persons with hypogonadotropic hypogonadism to conceive biological children.

Diabetes Insipidus

Desmopressin treatment of diabetes insipidus allows patients with an intact thirst mechanism to obtain adequate rest at night and to function with adequate quality of life in society. Desmopressin is available orally, intranasally, and subcutaneously; dose is titrated to urine output. To avoid overdosing and inducing hyponatremia, polyuria should be experienced regularly. Patients with adipsia pose a therapeutic challenge, and doses of desmopressin must be matched to the amount and timing of fluid intake.

Transitioning Disease Management From Caregiver to Patient

The transition from pediatric to adult care is not unique to endocrinology. Much work has been done in other disciplines to detect gaps in process, develop and test tools and models of care, and identify best practices. Indeed, the provision of diabetes care from pediatric to adult care has been an area where transition concepts have been devised and models have been tested. Many resources are available that contain frameworks and tools to foster the transition process in clinical practice. Below are some reference Web sites; this is by no means an exhaustive list:

http://www.endocrinetransitions.org/
http://www.gottransition.org
http://depts.washington.edu/healthtr/
http://www.waisman.wisc.edu/wrc/pdf/pubs/THCL.pdf

The transition process can be conceptualized using a framework put forth by the Center for Health Care Transition Improvement. It can used by individual providers, practices, and systems to devise a transition process that optimizes outcomes. These elements are part of both pediatric and internal medicine practices and include the following: (1) transition policy; (2) transition tracking and monitoring; (3) transition readiness; (4) transition planning; (5) transfer of care; and (6) transfer completion (13). Although the framework can be implemented using a formal transition program or clinic with dedicated pediatric and adult providers, the relatively few patients with hypopituitarism in most practices make dedicated transition programs unfeasible for this population. Therefore, the framework can be distilled into distinct action items that can be implemented by the departing pediatric practice and the accepting internist-endocrinologist practice. Each party has its role and action items. The role of the AYA's pediatric practice is to (1) assess transition readiness of the youth, family, and provider; (2) plan a longitudinal process to outline goals (*e.g.*, skills, health outcomes) and a timeline for reaching goals; (3) implement the plan; and (4) document the progress of the plan. The role of the AYA and his/her family is to (1) partner with the providers on goal setting and follow through; (2) share information about the transition process with other medical care providers; and (3) engage in the process and gradually take on (or relinquish) health care responsibilities. The role of the AYA's internist practice is to (1) engage with the AYA's previous pediatric provider for continuity of care; (2) communicate to the AYA how the practice operates; (3) allow caregivers to be involved in the AYA's care as necessary, yet create clear boundaries of involvement; and (4) prepare to offer a higher level of education and support to the AYA population.

Purview of Pediatrics

Assess Transition Readiness

Assessment of transition readiness includes inquiries to the youth about knowledge of his/her illness, medications needed, self-management skills, when to seek care, when to seek emergency care, *etc.* It is assumed that the mastering of self-management skills will be a multiyear/multivisit process. The Web site http://www.endocrinetransitions.org/ has a checklist item for skills assessment tailored to persons with hypopituitarism. This can be done at each visit starting in the early teenage years.

Transition Plan

The timeline for each patient will be individualized. Content of the transition packet may vary from person to person; nonetheless, it will not only include mastery of the self-management skills, but also plans for emergency care, a summary of diagnoses, and treatment course (*e.g.*, transfer letter). Samples can also be found at http://www.endocrinetransitions.org/.

Documentation

Local electronic medical records may make documentation of the transition process seamless or cumbersome. Some may have to document the process within the body of the clinical visit note.

Purview of Adult Medicine

Engage With Pediatric Provider

The internist may provide information about the individual expertise of physicians in the practice to pediatric providers.

The internist may self-educate about endocrine diseases often diagnosed in pediatrics that will require adult care.

Communicate Practice Operations

The adult provider should explain consent and confidentiality policies of the practice to AYA and family. Practice operations (*e.g.*, procedures for medication refills, paperwork requests, and how to access after-hours care) should be communicated. Tools are available at http://www.gottransition.org.

Reimbursement (for the US Audience)

Reliable Current Procedural Terminology (CPT) reimbursement codes for outpatient transition work would be to bill for a prolonged encounter with an established patient (CPT code 99214 or 99215), stating the amount of time spent if necessary to meet the time requirements for each level. If a clinic visit is > 70 minutes (*e.g.*, 30 minutes beyond the 40 minutes required for CPT code 99215), then CPT code 99354 can be added. CPT code 99354 can only be used for provider time (not clinical staff time). CPT codes exist for Care Plan oversight (99339 and 99340), but many insurance companies and Medicaid will not reimburse for these codes or have byzantine rules regarding reimbursement.

CASES

Case 1

An 18.5-year-old man had a craniopharyngioma resection at the age of 11.5 years, with postoperative panhypopituitarism encompassing GHD, thyroid hormone deficiency, corticosteroid deficiency, gonadotropin deficiency, and diabetes insipidus. He is on full replacement therapy. His most recent growth rate is 2.1 cm/y while receiving a GH dose of 0.22 mg/kg/wk (approximately 30 μg/kg/d), with adherence on most days. His bone age is 17 years. His height is 163 cm (approximately 64 inches), and he receives testosterone (200 mg every 2 weeks) that maintains his mid-dose testosterone level at 360 ng/dL. He reports adherence to desmopressin (allowing a period of urination between doses), hydrocortisone, and levothyroxine regimens. His most recent free T4 level was 1.6 μg/dL (0.9 to 1.9 μg/dL), and his IGF-1 level on therapy was 362 ng/mL (153 to 542 ng/mL).

He reports that he is tired of receiving GH shots and wants to take a break. He does not feel different on days that he misses his GH shot. His provider has discussed with him the benefit of GH administration in adults, but he is doubtful that he will be able to be compliant. He is living with his parents while attending community college, but wants to transfer in 2 years to an art school that is out of the area. Now that their son is older than 18 years, his family wants to transfer care to a local internist-endocrinologist, because the 2.5- to 3.5-hour drive for the quarterly visits is taxing on the family. The patient manages his daily medication regimen and schedule, but relies on his parents to coordinate prescription refills and medical appointments. He has recently restarted wearing a medical alert bracelet, but reports that none of his friends know what to do in an emergency situation if he is injured. When questioned without his parents in the room, he asked about the safety of drinking alcohol and trying marijuana, given his medical conditions. He is not sexually active.

Discussion

This case demonstrates a number of issues that arise in caring for older AYA with panhypopituitarism. Given this patient's multiple pituitary hormone deficiencies, he will meet criteria for adult GHD and thus have persistent GHD; no further evaluation of the somatotropic axis is needed. He no longer requires childhood doses of GH, because his bone age is 17 years and his growth rate is < 2.0 to 2.5 cm/y. He does not want to continue receiving GH despite explanations of the benefits and risks. In these cases, a baseline and a repeat dual-energy x-ray absorptiometry scan every 1 to 2 years may be helpful to monitor bone mineral density in the face of untreated GHD.

Providing a plan consisting of discrete goals for the family to gradually relinquish prescription management and schedule coordination would be helpful (and is a process that should have started 1 or 2 years earlier). The skills inventory is helpful for tracking and reminds patients of the steps necessary to coordinate their care. A plan to transfer duties from parent to patient can be devised by the family upon minimal prodding from the provider. In this case, with little time to prepare, at a minimum the current endocrine provider should devise a short summary of the clinical history, either using tools at http://endocrinetransitions.org or data from the medical record to put in the current clinical note to share with the family/accepting provider.

In regard to the questions that the patient asked the provider in private, these are rarely asked by AYA; furthermore, many providers do not ask. Upon transfer to adult care and a new provider, the patient may not be forthcoming in inquiring about the health effects of these common risk-taking behaviors among AYA.

Case 2

A 14.5-year-old girl with ectopic posterior pituitary has GHD and thyroid hormone deficiency. She was diagnosed with GHD at the age of 2.5 years. Magnetic resonance imaging performed at that time showed ectopic posterior pituitary with small pituitary; the stalk was visualized and was normal. Six months after initiating GH therapy, she began levothyroxine replacement for a low free T4 level and has been receiving hormone replacement since that time; repeated testing of adrenal function has been normal. She spontaneously entered puberty at the age of 11.0 years and achieved menarche at the age of 13.5 years with regular menses. Her growth rate is currently 1.9 cm/y with reported adherence to hormone replacement therapy. Her bone age is 14 years. Her free T4 and IGF-1 levels are in goal range for age and pubertal stage.

Discussion

In this case, because fewer than three pituitary hormone defects are experienced and a pituitary anatomical defect is present, repeat GH provocative testing is necessary. The repeat testing should occur when the bone age is 14.0 years in girls with a growth rate of 2.0 to 2.5 cm/y, after not taking GH for 1 to 3 months. IGF-1 testing when the patient is not taking GH can be done to obtain an off-treatment baseline, but there is no IGF-1 level that is predictive of persistent GHD in this scenario. Repeat testing could be done with insulin, glucagon, or GHRH-arginine (if available). There are established cut-offs for defining persistent GHD in the transition population for insulin (5.6 μg/L) and GHRH-arginine (9 μg/L), but glucagon has not been specifically tested in this age group. GHRH-arginine should not be administered to patients with hypothalamic dysfunction, because it can give false normal results. In the absence of age-specific data for glucagon, cut-offs for defining GHD in adults (3 μg/L for normo–body mass index of 1 μg/L in overweight/obese persons) can be used. Secondary hypothyroidism is associated with GH treatment in both children and adults. If she does not test as having persistent GHD, then it may be reasonable to perform a trial when she is not taking levothyroxine to test if it is still necessary.

Given her age, steps must also be taken to assess her knowledge regarding her condition, skills in managing her condition, and skills in navigating the health care system.

REFERENCES

1. Blum RW, Garell D, Hodgman CH, Jorissen TW, Okinow NA, Orr DP, Slap GB. Transition from child-centered to adult health-care systems for adolescents with chronic conditions. A position paper of the Society for Adolescent Medicine. *J Adolesc Health.* 1993;**14**(7): 570–576.
2. Molitch ME, Clemmons DR, Malozowski S, Merriam GR, Vance ML; Endocrine Society. Evaluation and treatment of adult growth hormone deficiency: An Endocrine Society clinical practice guideline. *J Clin Endocrinol Metab.* 2011;**96**(6):1587–1609.
3. Tauber M, Moulin P, Pienkowski C, Jouret B, Rochiccioli P. Growth hormone (GH) retesting and auxological data in 131 GH-deficient patients after completion of treatment. *J Clin Endocrinol Metab.* 1997; **82**(2):352–356.
4. Juul A, Kastrup KW, Pedersen SA, Skakkebaek NE. Growth hormone (GH) provocative retesting of 108 young adults with childhood-onset GH deficiency and the diagnostic value of insulin-like growth factor I (IGF-I) and IGF-binding protein-3. *J Clin Endocrinol Metab.* 1997; **82**(4):1195–1201.
5. Quigley CA, Zagar AJ, Liu CC, Brown DM, Huseman C, Levitsky L, Repaske DR, Tsalikian E, Chipman JJ. United States multicenter study of factors predicting the persistence of GH deficiency during the transition period between childhood and adulthood. *Int J Pediatr Endocrinol.* 2013;**2013**(1):6.
6. Maghnie M, Strigazzi C, Tinelli C, Autelli M, Cisternino M, Loche S, Severi F. Growth hormone (GH) deficiency (GHD) of childhood onset: Reassessment of GH status and evaluation of the predictive criteria for permanent GHD in young adults. *J Clin Endocrinol Metab.* 1999; **84**(4):1324–1328.
7. Donaubauer J, Kiess W, Kratzsch J, Nowak T, Steinkamp H, Willgerodt H, Keller E. Re-assessment of growth hormone secretion in young adult patients with childhood-onset growth hormone deficiency. *Clin Endocrinol (Oxf).* 2003;**58**(4):456–463.
8. Nicolson A, Toogood AA, Rahim A, Shalet SM. The prevalence of severe growth hormone deficiency in adults who received growth hormone replacement in childhood [see comment]. *Clin Endocrinol (Oxf).* 1996;**44**(3):311–316.
9. Grimberg A, DiVall SA, Polychronakos C, Allen DB, Cohen LE, Quintos JB, Rossi WC, Feudtner C, Murad MH; Drug and Therapeutics Committee and Ethics Committee of the Pediatric Endocrine Society. Guidelines for growth hormone and insulin-like growth factor-I treatment in children and adolescents: Growth hormone deficiency, idiopathic short stature, and primary insulin-like growth factor-I deficiency. *Horm Res Paediatr.* 2016;**86**(6): 361–397.
10. Fleseriu M, Hashim IA, Karavitaki N, Melmed S, Murad MH, Salvatori R, Samuels MH. Hormonal replacement in hypopituitarism in adults: An Endocrine Society clinical practice guideline. *J Clin Endocrinol Metab.* 2016;**101**(11):3888–3921.
11. Johannsson G, Falorni A, Skrtic S, Lennernäs H, Quinkler M, Monson JP, Stewart PM. Adrenal insufficiency: Review of clinical outcomes with current glucocorticoid replacement therapy. *Clin Endocrinol (Oxf).* 2015;**82**(1):2–11.
12. Boehm U, Bouloux PM, Dattani MT, de Roux N, Dodé C, Dunkel L, Dwyer AA, Giacobini P, Hardelin JP, Juul A, Maghnie M, Pitteloud N, Prevot V, Raivio T, Tena-Sempere M, Quinton R, Young J. Expert consensus document: European Consensus Statement on congenital hypogonadotropic hypogonadism—pathogenesis, diagnosis and treatment. *Nat Rev Endocrinol.* 2015;**11**(9):547–564.
13. American Academy of Pediatrics; American Academy of Family Physicians; American College of Physicians; Transitions Clinical Report Authoring Group, Cooley WC, Sagerman PJ. Supporting the health care transition from adolescence to adulthood in the medical home. *Pediatrics.* 2011;**128**(1):182–200.

Transitioning Childhood Cancer Survivorship

M01
Presented, March 17-20, 2018

Laurie E. Cohen, MD. Division of Endocrinology, Boston Children's Hospital, Boston, Massachusetts 02115, E-mail: laurie.cohen@childrens.harvard.edu

SIGNIFICANCE OF THE CLINICAL PROBLEM

Both the incidence and survival rates of childhood cancer have been increasing over time. Since 1975, the incidence rate of cancer in children aged 0 to 14 years has increased by 0.6% per year (1). In the United States in 2017, the estimate is that 15,270 children and adolescents aged 0 to 19 years will be diagnosed with cancer. At the same time, their survival rate has increased due to improvements in cure, from an overall 5-year survival rate of 50% in 1975, to 83% in 2007 to 2013 (2). There has also been a decrease in late mortality due to the lowering of treatment exposures (3). As of 1 January, 2014, there were approximately 419,000 childhood cancer survivors (CCS) in the United States (2).

Adult CCS have a high incidence of chronic health conditions that increase over time. In a study of 10,397 CCS at a median age of 26.6 years (range, 18.0 to 48.0 years), 62.3% had at least one chronic disorder; in particular, secondary malignancies, cardiovascular disease, renal dysfunction, severe musculoskeletal problems, and endocrine disorders (4). Endocrine disorders are the most common late effect in multiple studies (5). Radiation therapy and alkylating agent chemotherapy are the most highly associated treatment risk factors for the development of endocrinopathies (6).

Prevalence and incidence rates of endocrinopathies may vary depending on the population studied (*e.g.*, different diagnoses, treatment exposures, or sample sizes), length of follow-up, screening methods, lack of standardization of laboratory assays, diagnostic thresholds, and other factors such as genetics. In a study of 310 Italian adult CCS, Brignardello *et al.* (5) determined that 57% had developed an endocrine disorder at a median age of 25.31 years (median of 16.38 years after cancer diagnosis): growth hormone deficiency (GHD) in 16.13%, all diagnosed prior to transition; spermatogenesis damage in 42.22% of males (confirmed by semen analysis in about 40% of the cases); primary hypogonadism in 13.33% of males and primary hypogonadism in 21.54% of females; and primary hypothyroidism in 17.74%. Other endocrinopathies were less common: low bone mineral density with z score <-2.0 in 7.74%, papillary thyroid cancer in 5.81%, thyrotropin deficiency in 2.26%, hyperprolactinemia in 1.94%, adrenocorticotropin deficiency in 1.29%, and type 2 diabetes mellitus in 1.29%. Overweight/obesity and dyslipidemia were not assessed (5). In the St. Jude Lifetime Cohort Study (SJLIFE), of 748 adult CCS at a mean age of 34.2 years who had been treated with cranial irradiation and observed for a mean of 27.3 years, 46.5% had GHD, 10.8% had central hypogonadism, 7.5% had thyrotropin deficiency, and 4% had adrenocorticotropin deficiency (7); these are likely underestimates because they were based on criteria that increased sensitivity but lowered specificity. Because the risk for late effects does not appear to plateau, lifelong follow-up is necessary.

The transition from pediatric to adult care is recommended to occur between the ages of 18 and 21 years (8). However, that timing may not be appropriate for many CCS who may have multiple chronic health conditions, cognitive late effects, problems with psychosocial functioning, and delayed physical development (9), as well as dependence on their parent(s)/caregiver(s). Thus, the transition process may need to be individualized for each patient. There are no studies that have assessed the transition of care process from pediatric to adult endocrine care in CCS, although a transition tool has been developed with content validation (10).

BARRIERS TO OPTIMAL PRACTICE

Barriers to Patient Independence

- Cognitive late effects
- Psychosocial dysfunction
- Physical limitations
- Delayed physical development (9)

In addition, it is difficult to translate population-based relative risk to the individual and communicate it effectively, especially to adolescents who have not yet fully developed abstract thinking.

Barriers to Transfer of Care From the Pediatric to Adult Physician

- Patients not wanting to leave their pediatric physician and not ready to manage their own medical care
- Parents not trusting the new physician
- Pediatric physicians thinking adult physicians do not spend enough time with their patients or do not understand the complexities of the conditions
- Adult physicians thinking pediatric physicians are overprotective (11)

In addition, about one-half of hematology-oncology programs continue to follow their patients as adults (10), which may make it difficult to convince patients, parents, and oncology providers of the need to transition from pediatric to adult endocrine care.

LEARNING OBJECTIVES

As a result of participating in this session, learners should be able to:

- Recognize the challenges of transitioning CCS from pediatric to adult care
- Recognize the risk of GHD in CCS and the outcomes of its therapy
- Recognize the risk factors for male infertility in CCS and describe the diagnostic challenges
- Recognize the risk factors for female infertility in CCS and describe the diagnostic challenges

STRATEGIES FOR DIAGNOSIS, THERAPY, AND/OR MANAGEMENT

Managing the Transition of CCS From Pediatric to Adult Care

The pediatric endocrinologist, patient, and family all need to be ready to transition care, and there must be an adult endocrinologist who will assume care. The needs for the transition of endocrinology care for CCS may be extrapolated from studies of transition of oncology care. In a study by DiNofia *et al.* (12), 100% of parent respondents believed that it was important to support CCS independence. Although the traditional models of transition aim for adult independence, CCS want some continued parental involvement in their care (13); however, only 43% of CCS reported parental inclusion as "very important" compared with 83% of parents (9). CCS would like to see providers by themselves and gradually assume responsibility for their health care, but they also want ongoing support from their parents in scheduling appointments, medical decision making, and dealing with new clinical symptoms. Young adult CCS feel the transition process should start in early adolescence (13). The ability to be self-sufficient may be delayed or may not occur, however, because some CCS have physical limitations that require help in activities of daily living or have cognitive conditions that require help in decision making (9). Some CCS have an unnecessary and unhealthy reliance on their parents/caregivers and may not know about their cancer history, its significance, their current medical conditions, or their need for long-term assessment (12). The adult provider who may be used to dealing with just the patient may need to learn how to navigate between patient and parent.

CCS who had recently completed cancer therapy or who perceived a higher risk of late effects were more likely to indicate a preference to never transition to adult care or to transition at an older age (14). A survey of Children's Oncology Group medical providers found that the most frequent barriers to transition of care were perceived attachment to provider (91%), lack of adult providers with cancer survivor expertise (86%), patient's cognitive/emotional delay (81%), unstable social situation (80%), patient noncompliance (68%), instability of survivors' medical condition (63%), and health insurance issues (55%) (15). If oncology providers are not comfortable with transition, it may hinder the process for other subspecialists.

Preparation for transition requires developmentally appropriate one-on-one education (13) from the pediatric endocrinologist, with reinforcement from the patient's oncologist. The oncologist can help educate the patient that they will likely have side effects from the underlying malignancy and/or its treatments and thus will need lifelong monitoring, as well as educate on such matters as healthy weight, proper nutrition, and fertility (11). Written documents, online documents, peer support groups, and Web-based resources need to be developed (13).

Regardless of variable practices concerning transition for oncology care and other chronic health conditions, an expert panel of European pediatric and adult endocrinologists all concurred that CCS should have long-term follow-up with adult endocrinologists, although there was not agreement on the frequency of visits. Many of the outcomes of endocrine late effects are conditions more commonly seen in adults than in children and include high risk of developing metabolic syndrome and fertility issues (11). In addition, many pediatric endocrinologists are not comfortable with taking care of older adults. Age at transition, however, should not be an absolute, because each patient may have his or her unique needs.

Adult GHD in CCS

GHD is the most common anterior pituitary hormone deficiency in CCS and occurs as a result of hypothalamic-pituitary tumors or from radiation therapy to the hypothalamic-pituitary axis. It is directly related to radiation dose and inversely related to the number of radiation fractions and can occur after ≥18 Gy. It can also occur after a single total body irradiation (TBI) dose of 10 Gy or fractionated doses of 12 Gy (6); however, there can be recovery over time (16). The cumulative incidence of GHD after ≥18 Gy was 17.3% within 15 years in the Childhood Cancer Survivor Study, although cases may have been missed because of lack of systematic evaluation (17).

Adult CCS with untreated GHD are more likely to have increased weight-to-height-ratio, decreased lean muscle mass, low energy expenditure, muscle weakness, and poor exercise tolerance compared with those without GHD (7). Outcome data of growth hormone (GH) replacement in adult CCS are limited, but some studies suggest improvement in metabolic parameters and quality of life. As in non-CCS, adult CCS who had childhood GHD should be retested with provocative testing unless they have three or more anterior pituitary hormone deficits (18). GH-releasing hormone alone, or in combination with arginine, should not be used because the damage is primarily hypothalamic, and testing may give a false-negative result (6). Similar to non-CCS, insulin-induced hypoglycemia is considered the most reliable test (19).

GH and insulinlike growth factor-I have mitogenic properties, stimulate cellular proliferation, and inhibit apoptosis in *in vitro* assays, so concern has been raised that GH therapy might result in primary tumor recurrence or secondary neoplasms (SNs) (20). SNs are most common after radiation therapy, and CCS who have received cranial irradiation are, in particular, at increased risk for the development of meningiomas and gliomas. Initial data suggested that the relative risk of SNs in CCS treated with GH compared with CCS not treated with GH was 3.21 [95% confidence interval (CI), 1.88 to 5.46], with meningioma the most common SN (21), but decreased to 2.15 (95% CI, 1.3 to 3.5) with longer follow-up (22). However, more recent data from the same Childhood Cancer Survivor Study cohort have shown no significant association between GH therapy and the development of a central nervous system SN (23); similar results have been seen in other studies (24). Likewise, these studies have shown no significant increase in risk of tumor recurrence in GH-treated CCS. There are fewer data for adult GH replacement. In a study by Mackenzie *et al.* (24) of 220 patients who had received cranial irradiation, 110 GH-treated patients (median of 8 years of treatment; range, 4 to 10 years; 69 adult-onset tumors) and 110 control patients (68 adult-onset tumors) at a median follow-up of 14.5 years, there was no statistical difference in the incidence rate of SN in GH-treated *vs* non-GH-treated patients. A postmarket surveillance study of 280 CCS, including 252 patients on adult GH replacement and 28 non-GH-treated control patients, had a duration of follow-up of only 2.9 years (95% CI, 1.5 to 5.1) and 2.6 years (95% CI, 1.8 to 3.7), respectively. Twenty-three of the GH-treated patients and four of the non-GH-treated control patients developed SNs. Ten developed SNs prior to enrollment, with four naïve to GH therapy and six previously treated. The SN proportion during the study was 6.0% (95% CI, 3.4 to 9.6) based on 15 cases in the 252 GH-treated patients and 7.1% (95% CI, 0.9 to 23.5) based on 2 cases in the 28 non-GH-treated patients (20).

Testicular Hypofunction in CCS

Impaired spermatogenesis is the most common endocrinopathy in male CCS (5). Risk factors include the following:

- Cyclophosphamide (highest risk of azoospermia at doses >19 g/m^2, abnormal semen parameters at doses >5 to 7.5 g/m^2 or lower)
- Chlormethine
- Procarbazine (highest risk of azoospermia at doses >4 g/m^2)
- Ifosfamide (highest risk of azoospermia at doses >60 g/m^2)
- Busulfan/cyclophosphamide
- Fludarabine/melphalan
- Hematopoietic stem cell transplantation (HSCT) conditioning
- Radiotherapy potentially exposing the testes (highest risk at doses >2 to 3 Gy; may be reversible at lower doses) (25, 26)

There is not a cumulative alkylating agent exposure dose-below which azoospermia is always absent, nor one above which azoospermia is always present, although a cyclophosphamide equivalent dose (CED) of ≥4000 mg/m^2 is high risk, where CED (based on hematotoxicity) (27) is equal to

$$
\begin{aligned}
&1.0 \times [\text{cumulative cyclophosphamide dose}(\text{mg/m}^2)]\\
&\quad + 0.244 \times [\text{cumulative ifosfamide dose}(\text{mg/m}^2)]\\
&\quad + 0.857 \times [\text{cumulative procarbazine dose}(\text{mg/m}^2)]\\
&\quad + 14.286 \times [\text{cumulative chlorambucil dose}(\text{mg/m}^2)]\\
&\quad + 15.0 \times [\text{cumulative carmustine(BCNU)dose}(\text{mg/m}^2)]\\
&\quad + 16.0 \times [\text{cumulative lomustine(CCNU)dose}(\text{mg/m}^2)]\\
&\quad + 40.0 \times [\text{cumulative melphalan dose}(\text{mg/m}^2)]\\
&\quad + 50.0 \times [\text{cumulative thiotepa dose}(\text{mg/m}^2)]\\
&\quad + 100.0 \times [\text{cumulative chlormethine dose}(\text{mg/m}^2)]\\
&\quad + 8.823 \times [\text{cumulative busulfan dose}(\text{mg/m}^2)]
\end{aligned}
$$

Nonalkylating chemotherapeutic agents appear to be associated with only transient impairment in spermatogenesis (28). There are no studies of the probability, rate, or timing of impaired spermatogenesis, nor whether there is deterioration or improvement of spermatogenesis over time (26). In addition, some patients with normospermia have impaired sperm motility and morphology (28).

Evaluation should include Tanner staging and testicular size (26). Those patients with spermatozoa on semen analysis tend to have larger testicular volumes and lower follicle-stimulating hormone (FSH) levels. Using a cutoff of 15 mL [the lower two standard deviations (SDs) of adult volume], 80% of non-azoospermic survivors were identified with 91% specificity (29). If a patient has risk factors for impaired spermatogenesis, fertility surveillance should be performed when the patient requests it (after receiving in-depth education from the provider) or if fatherhood is desired in the near future. Screening investigations may include serum FSH and inhibin B, but they are limited in their specificity and positive predictive value. In the SJLIFE cohort, azoospermia correlated with levels of FSH >11.5 mIU/mL and inhibin B ≤31 ng/mL; however, that FSH level had only a specificity of 74.1% and a positive predictive value of 65.1%, and that inhibin B level had only a specificity of 45% and a positive predictive value of 52.1% (30). A semen analysis is the gold standard (26) but should be reserved for the determination of potential for paternity or when conception has been difficult (30). With advances in reproductive technology, patients with low sperm counts may achieve paternity, and those with ejaculatory azoospermia may still have sperm present in the testis that can be retrieved by testicular microdissection with sperm extraction (25).

Radiation treatment is also a risk factor for hypoandrogenism, with increased risk after testicular irradiation of 12 Gy or TBI of 7.5 to 15 Gy. Gonadotoxic chemotherapy alone is less likely to be a risk factor (26); the prevalence rate of Leydig cell failure is 10% to 57%, but it is generally subclinical (6).

Premature Ovarian Insufficiency in CCS

Premature ovarian insufficiency (POI) is the most common endocrinopathy in female CCS. CCS have an absolute risk of premature menopause of 8% and a 13-fold increased risk compared with siblings (31). Up to 25.8% of medulloblastoma survivors and 84% of HSCT survivors have POI (6). Gonadotoxic agents accelerate the natural age-related decline of the primordial follicle pool. Using the criteria of FSH >30 IU/L before age 40 years, 921 patients in the SJLIFE cohort at a median age of 31.7 years who were evaluated at a median of 24.0 years after diagnosis had a prevalence of POI of 10.9%. Risk factors were older age at therapy (due to the natural decrease in follicular reserve as a female ages), ovarian radiation treatment of any dose, and a CED ≥8000 mg/m^2 (32). Of HSCT survivors who have received TBI as a conditioning regimen for their HSCT, up to 50% of those treated before age 10 years have spontaneous pubertal onset, although the arrest of puberty and premature menopause can still occur. Those treated after age 10 years almost all have POI. Whether heavy metals are gonadotoxic is still debatable (6).

Anti-Müllerian hormone (AMH) is fairly constant across the menstrual cycle and becomes abnormal before the onset of irregular menses or a rise in FSH and is thus thought to be a good marker for the decline in oocyte reserve. AMH levels rise until around 9 years of age, slightly decline during pubertal age (9 to 15 years), rise again and peak at about age 25 years, and then decline until they are undetectable at menopause (33). Thus, an increase in AMH levels in late adolescence and young adulthood is typical and does not indicate improving ovarian function. In a study of 66 women at a median age of 23.3 years (range, 18.2 to 34.2 years) who had received alkylating-agent chemotherapy, 34.8% had a low AMH level (34). In a study of 49 girls at a mean age of 14.9 years (SD, 3.3 years) with a mean time off therapy of 7.5 years (SD, 3.6 years), 28.6% had diminished ovarian reserve with AMH below the fifth percentile for age and 35.7% had menopausal FSH levels. Twenty percent of patients with normal menstrual cycles had diminished ovarian reserve. In a multivariate analysis, older age at diagnosis and bilateral ovarian irradiation were associated with a low AMH level, and increased CED showed a trend (35). Diagnostic cutoffs are dependent on the assay used because there is substantial variability in AMH levels between assays and, at higher AMH levels, the differences are larger (36). At the present time, the predictive value of a low AMH level in adolescent patients on their future ability to conceive a pregnancy or their age at menopause is not known. AMH levels are associated with oocyte yield for assisted reproductive techniques (37). If a patient is thought to be at risk for POI and did not have fertility preservation prior to treatment, pubertal CCS can be offered oocyte cryopreservation (6), although insurance may not cover it. In a study of adults, those postchemotherapy had higher cycle cancellation rates than those prechemotherapy, but those who were able to have oocyte retrieval had similar oocyte yield to patients undergoing this procedure prechemotherapy (37). Of note, patients with elevated gonadotropin levels may still intermittently ovulate and, therefore, should be counseled about the risk for pregnancy (35).

MAIN CONCLUSIONS

Endocrinopathies are common late effects of the treatment of childhood cancer. During the adolescent period, the goals of therapy may change, such as from a focus on height attainment to metabolic and quality-of-life outcomes in GHD. As they become more independent, adolescent patients should be apprised of their risk for infertility. A patient's transition away from health care dependence on the parent/caregiver and from pediatric to adult providers may be more challenging in this population due to other, concomitant chronic health conditions and developmental and cognitive delays.

CASES

Case 1

A 15-year-old girl presented with a standard-risk medulloblastoma at age 7.5 years. Treatment included tumor resection, craniospinal proton radiation therapy at a dose of 23.4 Gy with a boost to the posterior fossa to 54 Gy, and chemotherapy with vincristine, lomustine, and cisplatin. She was diagnosed with GHD at age 11 years and has been treated with recombinant human GH. Her growth velocity has slowed to <2 cm/y, and her bone age is concordant with her chronologic age. She has no other anterior pituitary hormone deficiencies but was diagnosed with primary hypothyroidism at age 11 years and has been treated with levothyroxine, with normal thyroid function tests. You discuss the potential for GH treatment of adult GHD with her and her father. She is otherwise healthy and is working at grade level in school. Of the following, the MOST correct statement is:

A. The diagnosis of GH deficiency does not need to be reassessed.
B. Further GH therapy should not be considered, because of its high risk of inducing SNs.
C. Her medical care should be transitioned to an adult endocrinologist because she is done growing.
D. She should have a discussion about her medical condition without her parents present.

Answer: D

Discussion

This child is 15 years old, and transition of care from a pediatric to adult physician generally should occur between age 18 and 21 years (it may need to occur later in patients with chronic health conditions). However, the transition process includes making sure patients have personal knowledge about their illness and its treatment, and it is necessary for the provider and patient to meet one-on-one to ensure the patient's transition to independence. Given that she does not appear to have substantial cognitive delays, it is appropriate for the physician to meet with her independently from her parent, as well as meet with them together. Because she has an isolated pituitary hormone deficiency, reassessment is recommended to confirm the diagnosis before suggesting adult GH. Although long-term risks of GH therapy remain unclear, to date, studies suggest that there is not an increased risk of SNs over the increased risk expected after radiation therapy.

Case 2

A 15-year-old boy was treated for an osteosarcoma of the left distal femur at age 11 years. He received 10 weeks of chemotherapy with methotrexate, doxorubicin, and cisplatin, followed by surgery to remove the tumor, and then methotrexate, doxorubicin, cisplatin, ifosfamide, and etoposide for 29 weeks. No chemotherapy doses were noted on his treatment summary. On examination, he has Tanner stage V pubic hair, an adult size phallus, and 10-mL testes. When told his testes are small for his stage of development, his mother asks if his fertility can be assessed. He says he is not interested and does not even think he wants to be a father. Of the following, the BEST next step is:

A. Do no testing.
B. Obtain an FSH level.
C. Obtain an inhibin B level.
D. Perform a semen analysis.
Answer: A

Discussion

This patient received the alkylating agent ifosfamide, which can cause Sertoli cell and germ cell damage. Although a CED of ≥4000 mg/m^2 is high risk for infertility, there is not a cumulative alkylating-agent exposure dose below which azoospermia is always absent, nor one above which azoospermia is always present, so he is at risk for infertility. However, fertility surveillance should be performed only when the patient requests it or if paternity is desired in the near future. A semen analysis is the gold standard, although patients with low sperm counts may achieve paternity, and those with ejaculatory azoospermia may still have sperm present in the testis that can be retrieved surgically. FSH and inhibin B levels may be used for screening but have poor specificity and positive predictive value.

Case 3

A 14-year-old girl was treated for relapsed acute lymphoblastic leukemia with HSCT after conditioning with a cumulative dose of 3.6 g/m^2 of cyclophosphamide and 14 Gy of TBI at age 8 years. She progressed through puberty and is having monthly menses. You are considering whether to do a laboratory evaluation to assess ovarian function. Of the following statements, the MOST correct is:

A. An AMH level can be used to predict her age at menopause.
B. An FSH level that is elevated rules out the ability for her to get pregnant.
C. Her normal puberty suggests she does not have ovarian damage.
D. She may be a candidate for oocyte cryopreservation.
Answer: D

Discussion

Up to 50% of girls treated with HSCT before age 10 years have spontaneous pubertal entry, although pubertal arrest and premature menopause can still occur. Because she is at risk for POI, she can be evaluated to see whether she is a candidate for oocyte cryopreservation, although this may not be covered by insurance. Although a low AMH level is associated with a decreased oocyte yield after oocyte stimulation, its predictive value in adolescent patients on their future ability to conceive a pregnancy or their age at menopause is not known. Patients with elevated gonadotropin levels may still intermittently ovulate and, therefore, there is a risk of pregnancy if she is sexually active.

REFERENCES

1. Cancer Facts & Figures 2017. American Cancer Society 2017, https://www.cancer.org/content/dam/cancer-org/research/cancer-facts-and-statistics/annual-cancer-facts-and-figures/2017/cancer-facts-and-figures-2017.pdf. Accessed 24 November 2017.
2. Cancer in Children and Adolescents. National Cancer Institute fact sheet 2017; https://www.cancer.gov/types/childhood-cancers/child-adolescent-cancers-fact-sheet. Accessed 24 November 2017.
3. Armstrong GT, Conklin HM, Huang S, Srivastava D, Sanford R, Ellison DW, Merchant TE, Hudson MM, Hoehn ME, Robison LL, Gajjar A, Morris EB. Survival and long-term health and cognitive outcomes after low-grade glioma. *Neuro-oncol.* 2011;**13**(2):223–234.
4. Oeffinger KC, Mertens AC, Sklar CA, Kawashima T, Hudson MM, Meadows AT, Friedman DL, Marina N, Hobbie W, Kadan-Lottick NS, Schwartz CL, Leisenring W, Robison LL; Childhood Cancer Survivor Study. Chronic health conditions in adult survivors of childhood cancer. *N Engl J Med.* 2006;**355**(15):1572–1582.
5. Brignardello E, Felicetti F, Castiglione A, Chiabotto P, Corrias A, Fagioli F, Ciccone G, Boccuzzi G. Endocrine health conditions in adult survivors of childhood cancer: the need for specialized adult-focused follow-up clinics. *Eur J Endocrinol.* 2013;**168**(3):465–472.
6. Chemaitilly W, Cohen LE. Diagnosis of endocrine disease: endocrine late-effects of childhood cancer and its treatments. *Eur J Endocrinol.* 2017;**176**(4):R183–R203.
7. Chemaitilly W, Li Z, Huang S, Ness KK, Clark KL, Green DM, Barnes N, Armstrong GT, Krasin MJ, Srivastava DK, Pui CH, Merchant TE, Kun LE, Gajjar A, Hudson MM, Robison LL, Sklar CA. Anterior hypopituitarism in adult survivors of childhood cancers treated with cranial radiotherapy: a report from the St Jude Lifetime Cohort study. *J Clin Oncol.* 2015; **33**(5):492–500.
8. American Academy of Pediatrics, American Academy of Family Physicians, American College of Physicians, Transitions Clinical Report Authoring Group. Supporting the health care transition from adolescence to adulthood in the medical home. *Pediatrics.* 2011; **128**(1):182–200.
9. Barakat LP, Hobbie W, Minturn J, Deatrick J. Survivors of childhood brain tumors and their caregivers: transition to adulthood. *Dev Med Child Neurol.* 2017;**59**(8):779–780.
10. Schwartz LA, Hamilton JL, Brumley LD, Barakat LP, Deatrick JA, Szalda DE, Bevans KB, Tucker CA, Daniel LC, Butler E, Kazak AE, Hobbie WL, Ginsberg JP, Psihogios AM, Ver Hoeve E, Tuchman LK. Development and content validation of the Transition Readiness Inventory item pool for adolescent and young adult survivors of childhood cancer. *J Pediatr Psychol.* 2017;**42**(9):983–994.

11. Hokken-Koelega A, van der Lely AJ, Hauffa B, Häusler G, Johannsson G, Maghnie M, Argente J, DeSchepper J, Gleeson H, Gregory JW, Höybye C, Keleştimur F, Luger A, Müller HL, Neggers S, Popovic-Brkic V, Porcu E, Sävendahl L, Shalet S, Spiliotis B, Tauber M. Bridging the gap: metabolic and endocrine care of patients during transition. *Endocr Connect.* 2016;**5**(6):R44–R54.
12. DiNofia A, Shafer K, Steacy K, Sadak KT. Parent-perceived facilitators in the transition of care for young adult survivors of childhood cancer. *J Pediatr Hematol Oncol.* 2017;**39**(7):e377–e380.
13. Frederick NN, Bober SL, Berwick L, Tower M, Kenney LB. Preparing childhood cancer survivors for transition to adult care: the young adult perspective. *Pediatr Blood Cancer.* 2017;**64**(10):e265444.
14. Fardell JE, Wakefield CE, Signorelli C, Hill R, Skeen J, Maguire AM, McLoone JK, Cohn RJ; ANZCHOG Survivorship Study Group. Transition of childhood cancer survivors to adult care: The survivor perspective. *Pediatr Blood Cancer.* 2017;**64(6)**:e26354.
15. Kenney LB, Melvin P, Fishman LN, O'Sullivan-Oliveira J, Sawicki GS, Ziniel S, Diller L, Fernandes SM. Transition and transfer of childhood cancer survivors to adult care: a national survey of pediatric oncologists. *Pediatr Blood Cancer.* 2017;**64**(2):346–352.
16. Brennan BM, Shalet SM. Endocrine late effects after bone marrow transplant. *Br J Haematol.* 2002;**118**(1):58–66.
17. Mostoufi-Moab S, Seidel K, Leisenring WM, Armstrong GT, Oeffinger KC, Stovall M, Meacham LR, Green DM, Weathers R, Ginsberg JP, Robison LL, Sklar CA. Endocrine abnormalities in aging survivors of childhood cancer: a report from the Childhood Cancer Survivor Study. *J Clin Oncol.* 2016;**34**(27):3240–3247.
18. Grimberg A, DiVall SA, Polychronakos C, Allen DB, Cohen LE, Quintos JB, Rossi WC, Feudtner C, Murad MH; Drug and Therapeutics Committee and Ethics Committee of the Pediatric Endocrine Society. Guidelines for growth hormone and insulin-like growth factor-I treatment in children and adolescents: growth hormone deficiency, idiopathic short stature, and primary insulin-like growth factor-I deficiency. *Horm Res Paediatr.* 2016;**86**(6):361–397.
19. Lissett CA, Saleem S, Rahim A, Brennan BM, Shalet SM. The impact of irradiation on growth hormone responsiveness to provocative agents is stimulus dependent: results in 161 individuals with radiation damage to the somatotropic axis. *J Clin Endocrinol Metab.* 2001;**86**(2):663–668.
20. Woodmansee WW, Zimmermann AG, Child CJ, Rong Q, Erfurth EM, Beck-Peccoz P, Blum WF, Robison LL; GeNeSIS and International Advisory Boards. Incidence of second neoplasm in childhood cancer survivors treated with GH: an analysis of GeNeSIS and HypoCCS. *Eur J Endocrinol.* 2013;**168**(4):565–573.
21. Sklar CA, Mertens AC, Mitby P, Occhiogrosso G, Qin J, Heller G, Yasui Y, Robison LL. Risk of disease recurrence and second neoplasms in survivors of childhood cancer treated with growth hormone: a report from the Childhood Cancer Survivor Study. *J Clin Endocrinol Metab.* 2002;**87**(7):3136–3141.
22. Ergun-Longmire B, Mertens AC, Mitby P, Qin J, Heller G, Shi W, Yasui Y, Robison LL, Sklar CA. Growth hormone treatment and risk of second neoplasms in the childhood cancer survivor. *J Clin Endocrinol Metab.* 2006;**91**(9):3494–3498.
23. Patterson BC, Chen Y, Sklar CA, Neglia J, Yasui Y, Mertens A, Armstrong GT, Meadows A, Stovall M, Robison LL, Meacham LR. Growth hormone exposure as a risk factor for the development of subsequent neoplasms of the central nervous system: a report from the childhood cancer survivor study. *J Clin Endocrinol Metab.* 2014;**99**(6):2030–2037.
24. Mackenzie S, Craven T, Gattamaneni HR, Swindell R, Shalet SM, Brabant G. Long-term safety of growth hormone replacement after CNS irradiation. *J Clin Endocrinol Metab.* 2011;**96**(9):2756–2761.
25. Kenney LB, Cohen LE, Shnorhavorian M, Metzger ML, Lockart B, Hijiya N, Duffey-Lind E, Constine L, Green D, Meacham L. Male reproductive health after childhood, adolescent, and young adult cancers: a report from the Children's Oncology Group. *J Clin Oncol.* 2012;**30**(27):3408–3416.
26. Skinner R, Mulder RL, Kremer LC, Hudson MM, Constine LS, Bardi E, Boekhout A, Borgmann-Staudt A, Brown MC, Cohn R, Dirksen U, Giwercman A, Ishiguro H, Jahnukainen K, Kenney LB, Loonen JJ, Meacham L, Neggers S, Nussey S, Petersen C, Shnorhavorian M, van den Heuvel-Eibrink MM, van Santen HM, Wallace WH, Green DM. Recommendations for gonadotoxicity surveillance in male childhood, adolescent, and young adult cancer survivors: a report from the International Late Effects of Childhood Cancer Guideline Harmonization Group in collaboration with the PanCareSurFup Consortium. *Lancet Oncol.* 2017;**18**(2):e75–e90.
27. Green DM, Nolan VG, Goodman PJ, Whitton JA, Srivastava D, Leisenring WM, Neglia JP, Sklar CA, Kaste SC, Hudson MM, Diller LR, Stovall M, Donaldson SS, Robison LL. The cyclophosphamide equivalent dose as an approach for quantifying alkylating agent exposure: a report from the Childhood Cancer Survivor Study. *Pediatr Blood Cancer.* 2014;**61**(1):53–67.
28. Green DM, Liu W, Kutteh WH, Ke RW, Shelton KC, Sklar CA, Chemaitilly W, Pui CH, Klosky JL, Spunt SL, Metzger ML, Srivastava D, Ness KK, Robison LL, Hudson MM. Cumulative alkylating agent exposure and semen parameters in adult survivors of childhood cancer: a report from the St Jude Lifetime Cohort Study. *Lancet Oncol.* 2014;**15**(11):1215–1223.
29. Wilhelmsson M, Vatanen A, Borgström B, Gustafsson B, Taskinen M, Saarinen-Pihkala UM, Winiarski J, Jahnukainen K. Adult testicular volume predicts spermatogenetic recovery after allogeneic HSCT in childhood and adolescence. *Pediatr Blood Cancer.* 2014;**61**(6):1094–1100.
30. Green DM, Zhu L, Zhang N, Sklar CA, Ke RW, Kutteh WH, Klosky JL, Spunt SL, Metzger ML, Navid F, Srivastava D, Robison LL, Hudson MM. Lack of specificity of plasma concentrations of inhibin B and follicle-stimulating hormone for identification of azoospermic survivors of childhood cancer: a report from the St Jude lifetime cohort study. *J Clin Oncol.* 2013;**31**(10):1324–1328.
31. Green DM, Kawashima T, Stovall M, Leisenring W, Sklar CA, Mertens AC, Donaldson SS, Byrne J, Robison LL. Fertility of female survivors of childhood cancer: a report from the childhood cancer survivor study. *J Clin Oncol.* 2009;**27**(16):2677–2685.
32. Chemaitilly W, Li Z, Krasin MJ, Brooke RJ, Wilson CL, Green DM, Klosky JL, Barnes N, Clark KL, Farr JB, Fernandez-Pineda I, Bishop MW, Metzger M, Pui CH, Kaste SC, Ness KK, Srivastava DK, Robison LL, Hudson MM, Yasui Y, Sklar CA. Premature ovarian insufficiency in childhood cancer survivors: a report from the St. Jude Lifetime Cohort. *J Clin Endocrinol Metab.* 2017;**102**(7):2242–2250.
33. Dewailly D, Andersen CY, Balen A, Broekmans F, Dilaver N, Fanchin R, Griesinger G, Kelsey TW, La Marca A, Lambalk C, Mason H, Nelson SM, Visser JA, Wallace WH, Anderson RA. The physiology and clinical utility of anti-Mullerian hormone in women. *Hum Reprod Update.* 2014;**20**(3):370–385.
34. Charpentier AM, Chong AL, Gingras-Hill G, Ahmed S, Cigsar C, Gupta AA, Greenblatt E, Hodgson DC. Anti-Müllerian hormone screening to assess ovarian reserve among female survivors of childhood cancer. *J Cancer Surviv.* 2014;**8**(4):548–554.
35. Elchuri SV, Patterson BC, Brown M, Bedient C, Record E, Wasilewski-Masker K, Mertens AC, Meacham LR. Low anti-Müllerian hormone in pediatric cancer survivors in the early years after gonadotoxic therapy. *J Pediatr Adolesc Gynecol.* 2016;**29**(4):393–399.
36. Su HI, Sammel MD, Homer MV, Bui K, Haunschild C, Stanczyk FZ. Comparability of antimullerian hormone levels among commercially available immunoassays. *Fertil Steril.* 2014;**101**(6):1766–1772.e1.
37. Chan JL, Johnson LN, Efymow BL, Sammel MD, Gracia CR. Outcomes of ovarian stimulation after treatment with chemotherapy. *J Assist Reprod Genet.* 2015;**32**(10):1537–1545.

Childhood Obesity

M06
Presented, March 17–20, 2018

Ellen Lancon Connor, MD. University of Wisconsin–Madison, Madison, Wisconsin 53706, E-mail: elconnor@wisc.edu

SIGNIFICANCE OF THE CLINICAL PROBLEM

Obesity in children and adolescents portends a risk for adult obesity and associated cardiovascular and other comorbidities. In the United States, approximately one third of children are overweight or obese. Six percent have extreme obesity, with a body mass index (BMI) >120th percentile for age and sex. Increasing BMI in US youth 6 to 19 years of age leads to costs of $1.4 billion more for health care than in youth with a normal BMI. If all 12.7 million US children with obesity <18 years of age become adults with obesity, lifetime societal costs would be >$1.1 trillion.

Worldwide, childhood obesity is now emerging in developing nations as a major concern, particularly in those with lower socioeconomic status. Globally, 41 million children <5 years of age are obese or overweight. If trends continue, by 2025, expected numbers would rise to 70 million children. In Africa, between 1990 and 2014, the incidence of overweight and obesity doubled. Almost one half the world's children who are obese or overweight live in Asia. The rate of obesity incidence increase is 30% greater in developing nations.

BARRIERS TO OPTIMAL PRACTICE

Multiple barriers affect the endocrinologist's optimal delivery of care to a child with obesity or an overweight condition. These barriers include familial beliefs, customs, and financial constraints; lack of infrastructure to support an environment in which children can increase activity; lack of infrastructure to give families access to healthier food options; media bombardment with food and drink advertised to children; consumption of sugar-sweetened beverages and foods with added sugar; lack of nutritional knowledge by caregivers; lack of provider access to psychologists and nutritionists who can work with families to affect BMI; and health care providers' limitations of office time for working with patients with obesity.

LEARNING OBJECTIVES

As a result of participating in this session, learners should be able to:

- Diagnose obesity-related comorbidities by using evidence-based guidelines for laboratory evaluation of children and adolescents
- Identify patients with obesity who should have genetic evaluations
- Select patients who have failed lifestyle intervention and may be candidates for psychological, pharmaceutical, and/or surgical intervention for obesity

STRATEGIES FOR DIAGNOSIS, THERAPIES, AND MANAGEMENT

Diagnosis of Comorbidities and Syndromes

Comorbidities

Comorbidities associated with obesity include impaired glucose tolerance/diabetes mellitus, hyperlipidemia, hepatic steatosis, hypertension, polycystic ovary syndrome (PCOS), renal insufficiency, and psychiatric disease. Screening should include hemoglobin A_{1c} (HbA_{1c}), fasting plasma glucose and/or oral glucose tolerance test fasting lipid profile, alanine aminotransferase (ALT), blood pressure measurements, free and total testosterone, sex hormone–binding globulin for PCOS, polysomnography, and psychiatric history.

Syndromes

Who needs evaluation for genetic syndromes that cause obesity (Fig. 1)?

- The child with developmental delays
- The child with rapid weight gain before age 5 years
- The child with congenital anomalies or early-onset visual or auditory loss
- The child with short stature/attenuated height velocity and obesity

Therapy for the Child/Adolescent With Obesity and Obesity Comorbidities

Therapy for pediatric obesity and related comorbidities includes lifestyle changes that are family centered, culturally appropriate, and age appropriate, including increased exercise duration and intensity (daily and weekly goals) and dietary modifications; psychological counseling; and medications. Pharmaceutical options for children and adolescents can be considered. Bariatric surgery in a pediatric bariatric surgery center of excellence should only be offered after an adequate trial of intensive lifestyle measures in physically mature and psychologically stable adolescents with a BMI $\geq$40 kg/m^2 or $\geq$35 kg/m^2 with extreme comorbidities.

Management of Obesity Comorbidities

Management of obesity comorbidities is needed in cases of impaired glucose tolerance/diabetes mellitus, hyperlipidemia, hypertension, hepatic steatosis, PCOS, renal insufficiency, and psychiatric disease.

CASES WITH QUESTIONS

Case 1

A 13-year-old boy is referred to endocrinology because he has acanthosis nigricans, hypertension, fatigue, and BMI at the

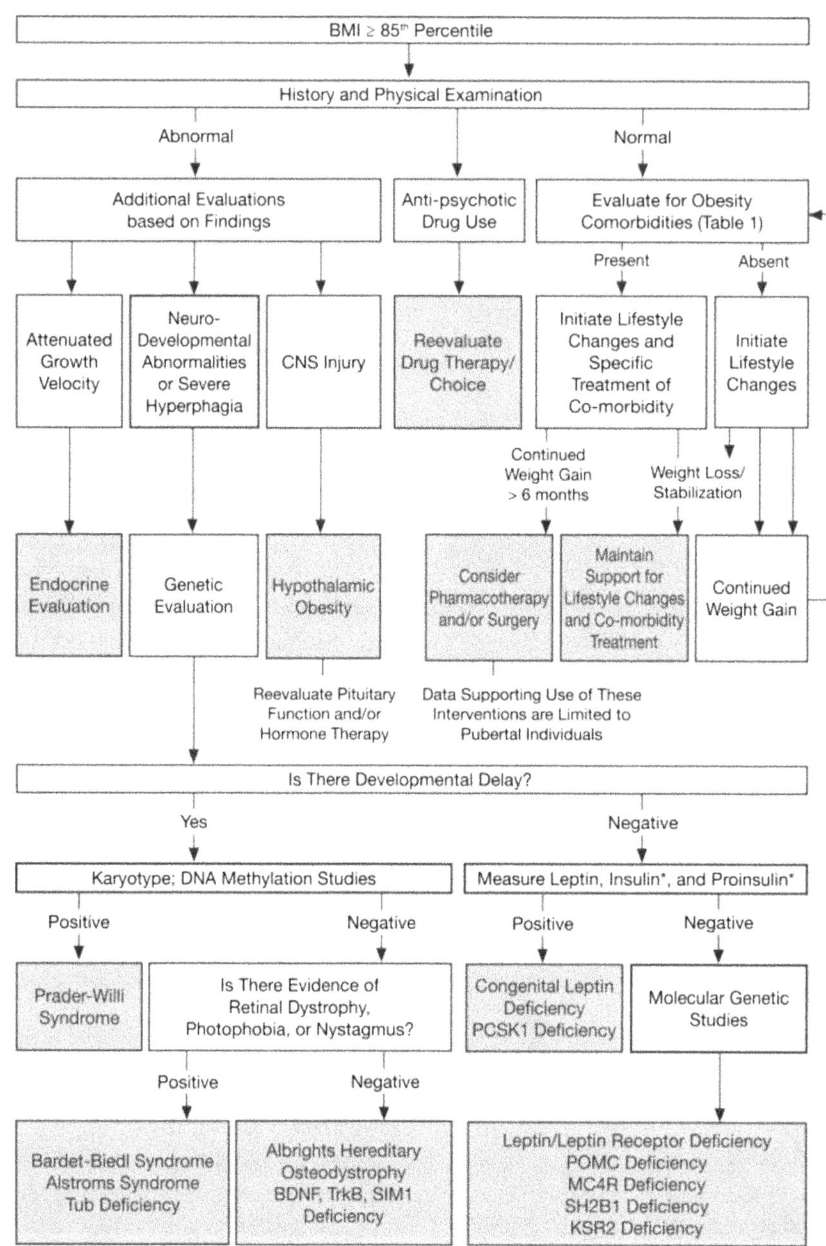

Figure 1. Diagnosis and management flowchart. Reprinted with permission from the Endocrine Society: Styne DM, Arslanian SA, Connor EL, et al. Pediatric obesity-assessment, treatment, and prevention: an Endocrine society clinical practice guideline. *J Clin Endocrinol Metab.* 2017;102(3):709–757.

98th percentile for age and sex. Weight is >95th percentile, and height is 70th percentile. He has had a 10-kg weight gain in 3 months. He denies polyuria or polydipsia but endorses occasional nocturia, falling asleep after school, and wheezing with exercise, so he has stopped participating in gym class. His mother has borderline diabetes, and both paternal grandparents have hyperlipidemia and type 2 diabetes. The child had a previous hospitalization for tonsillectomy and adenoidectomy at age 9 years. Review of the growth chart shows a BMI >95th percentile since age 8 years and a growth velocity >6 cm/y since he was in kindergarten. The primary care provider would like to know what laboratory tests should be obtained before you see the child in the clinic.

What laboratory studies should be assessed?

A. Free thyroxine, thyrotropin, alkaline phosphatase
B. Reverse triiodothyronine and thyrotropin, fasting lipids
C. Fasting lipids, fasting glucose, ALT
D. 8:00 AM cortisol, aspartate aminotransferase, fasting insulin

The correct answer is C.

Case 2

A 6-year-old girl is seen for impaired glucose tolerance with scant past medical records available. Her BMI is 98th percentile for age and sex and height at the 7th percentile. Midparental height is at the 80th percentile. She is repeating kindergarten and struggling with reading concepts. She had a birth weight of 3.1 kg at term and was noted by her mother to have rapid weight gain between 2 and 4 years of age. The child has been referred to ophthalmology after failing school vision screening. In infancy, the patient had surgery to remove extra sixth digits on her hands. Family history is positive for a grandfather receiving dialysis because of diabetes and parents with hypertension and BMIs in the 85th to 95th percentiles. The child is noted to have generalized obesity, blood pressure in the 91st percentile for age and sex, acanthosis nigricans, and fatty breast tissue bilaterally.

Which statement is true about this child?

A. She has familial obesity and her weight gain is not unexpected.
B. Fasting insulin and glucose levels should be obtained.
C. Because she is <9 years old, she does not need lipid screening.
D. Genetic consultation should be sought.

The correct answer is D.

Case 3

A 17-year-old boy is seen by the endocrinologist for concerns of increased HbA_{1c} not responding to insulin, BMI >140th percentile for age, refractory hypertension, and nocturia. Two years ago, his primary care provider prescribed lifestyle changes, and he was subsequently prescribed caloric restriction, psychological counseling for low self-esteem, and metformin XR 2000 mg/d for high insulin requirements. The patient has a full moustache and some beard hair. He is 170 cm tall and has generalized obesity with acanthosis nigricans of the posterior neck, axillae, and inner thighs. Laboratory evaluation reveals an HbA_{1c} of 9.4%; fasting glucose of 236 mg/dL; urinalysis positive for protein on random and timed samples; ALT of 145 U/L; and total cholesterol of 245 mg/dL, with triglycerides of 382 mg/dL, low-density lipoprotein of 198 mg/dL, and high-density lipoprotein of 28 mg/dL. He describes fatigue, exercise intolerance, and symptoms of obstructive sleep apnea. He is interested in a pill or surgery for weight loss.

How should this patient be counseled?

A. Basal insulin should be increased by 20%, and he should return to the clinic in 3 months for scheduling of bariatric surgery.
B. He might benefit from medication or bariatric surgery after a demonstrated trial of supervised dietary and activity changes and psychological evaluation and counseling.
C. Metformin dosing should increase because metformin can lead to considerable weight loss.
D. He is too young for weight loss medications and should continue his current insulin plan.

The correct answer is B.

CONCLUSIONS

Untreated pediatric obesity will become adult obesity with comorbidities that threaten both lifespan and global economic health. From preconception planning and counseling to successful lobbying for infrastructure changes that increase physical activity, nutrition knowledge, and access to healthy but economical food choices, many opportunities exist for governments to prevent childhood obesity. Although it is difficult to achieve and maintain weight loss through lifestyle changes, such changes result in measurable differences in cardiovascular parameters. Future research efforts locally and globally should seek to improve lifestyle interventions. For those in whom lifestyle interventions are not adequate, pharmaceutical interventions or bariatric surgery may ameliorate severe comorbidities of obesity.

RECOMMENDED READING

Afshin A, Forouzanfar MH, Reitsma MB, Sur P, Estep K, Lee A, Marczak L, Mokdad AH, Moradi-Lakeh M, Naghavi M, Salama JS, Vos T, Abate KH, Abbafati C, Ahmed MB, Al-Aly Z, Alkerwi A, Al-Raddadi R, Amare AT, Amberbir A, Amegah AK, Amini E, Amrock SM, Anjana RM, Arnlöv J, Asayesh H, Banerjee A, Barac A, Baye E, Bennett DA, Beyene AS, Biadgilign S, Biryukov S, Bjertness E, Boneya DJ, Campos-Nonato I, Carrero JJ, Cecilio P, Cercy K, Ciobanu LG, Cornaby L, Damtew SA, Dandona L, Dandona R, Dharmaratne SD, Duncan BB, Eshrati B, Esteghamati A, Feigin VL, Fernandes JC, Fürst T, Gebrehiwot TT, Gold A, Gona PN, Goto A, Habtewold TD, Hadush KT, Hafezi-Nejad N, Hay SI, Horino M, Islami F, Kamal R, Kasaeian A, Katikireddi SV, Kengne AP, Kesavachandran CN, Khader YS, Khang YH, Khubchandani J, Kim D, Kim YJ, Kinfu Y, Kosen S, Ku T, Defo BK, Kumar GA, Larson HJ, Leinsalu M, Liang X, Lim SS, Liu P, Lopez AD, Lozano R, Majeed A, Malekzadeh R, Malta DC, Mazidi M, McAlinden C, McGarvey ST, Mengistu DT, Mensah GA, Mensink GBM, Mezgebe HB, Mirrakhimov EM, Mueller UO, Noubiap JJ, Obermeyer CM, Ogbo FA, Owolabi MO, Patton GC, Pourmalek F, Qorbani M, Rafay A, Rai RK, Ranabhat CL, Reinig N, Safiri S, Salomon JA, Sanabria JR, Santos IS, Sartorius B, Sawhney M, Schmidhuber J, Schutte AE, Schmidt MI, Sepanlou SG, Shamsizadeh M, Sheikhbahaei S, Shin MJ, Shiri R, Shiue I, Roba HS, Silva DAS, Silverberg JI, Singh JA, Stranges S, Swaminathan S, Tabarés-Seisdedos R, Tadese F, Tedla BA, Tegegne BS, Terkawi AS, Thakur JS, Tonelli M, Topor-Madry R, Tyrovolas S, Ukwaja KN, Uthman OA, Vaezghasemi M, Vasankari T, Vlassov VV, Vollset SE, Weiderpass E, Werdecker A, Wesana J, Westerman R, Yano Y, Yonemoto N, Yonga G, Zaidi Z, Zenebe ZM, Zipkin B, Murray CJL; GBD 2015 Obesity Collaborators. Health effects of overweight and obesity in 195 countries over 25 years. *N Engl J Med.* 2017;**377**(1):13–27.

Centers for Disease Control and Prevention. Overweight & obesity, 2017. Available at: http://www.cdc.gov/obesity. Accessed 25 October 2017.

Grossman DC, Bibbins-Domingo K, Curry SJ, Barry MJ, Davidson KW, Doubeni CA, Epling JW Jr, Kemper AR, Krist AH, Kurth AE, Landefeld CS, Mangione CM, Phipps MG, Silverstein M, Simon MA, Tseng CW; US Preventive Services Task Force. Screening for obesity in children and adolescents: US Preventive Services Task Force recommendations statement. *JAMA.* 2017;**317**(23):2417–2426.

Styne DM, Arslanian SA, Connor EL, Farooqi IS, Murad MH, Silverstein JH, Yanovski JA. Pediatric obesity-assessment, treatment, and prevention: an Endocrine Society clinical practice guideline. *J Clin Endocrinol Metab.* 2017;**102**(3):709–757.

World Health Organization. 2016 Report of the Commission on Ending Childhood Obesity. Available at: http://apps.who.int/iris/bitstream/10665/204176/1/9789241510066_eng.pdf?ua=1. Accessed 19 January 2018.

Perinatal Thyroid Function: Truth and Controversies

M11
Presented, March 17–20, 2018

Scott A. Rivkees, MD. Department of Pediatrics, University of Florida, Gainesville, Florida 32601, E-mail: srivkees@ufl.edu

SIGNIFICANCE OF THE CLINICAL PROBLEM

Proper circulating levels of thyroid hormone are essential for normal embryonic and fetal development. The fetal thyroid gland does not begin to produce substantial amounts of thyroid hormone until after midgestation. Because the fetus is totally dependent on maternal sources for thyroid hormone during early gestation, maternal hypothyroidism can have adverse impacts on the fetus. Maternal Graves disease and its treatment can also adversely influence the fetus. As such, understanding fetal thyroid physiology and the impact of maternal thyroid disease is important for guiding therapy in the perinatal period (1–4).

LEARNING OBJECTIVES

- Discuss the ontogeny of the fetal thyroid axis
- Discuss the consequences of maternal hypothyroidism
- Discuss the consequences of fetal hyperthyroidism and Graves disease therapy during pregnancy
- Discuss controversies in the management of thyroid abnormalities during pregnancy

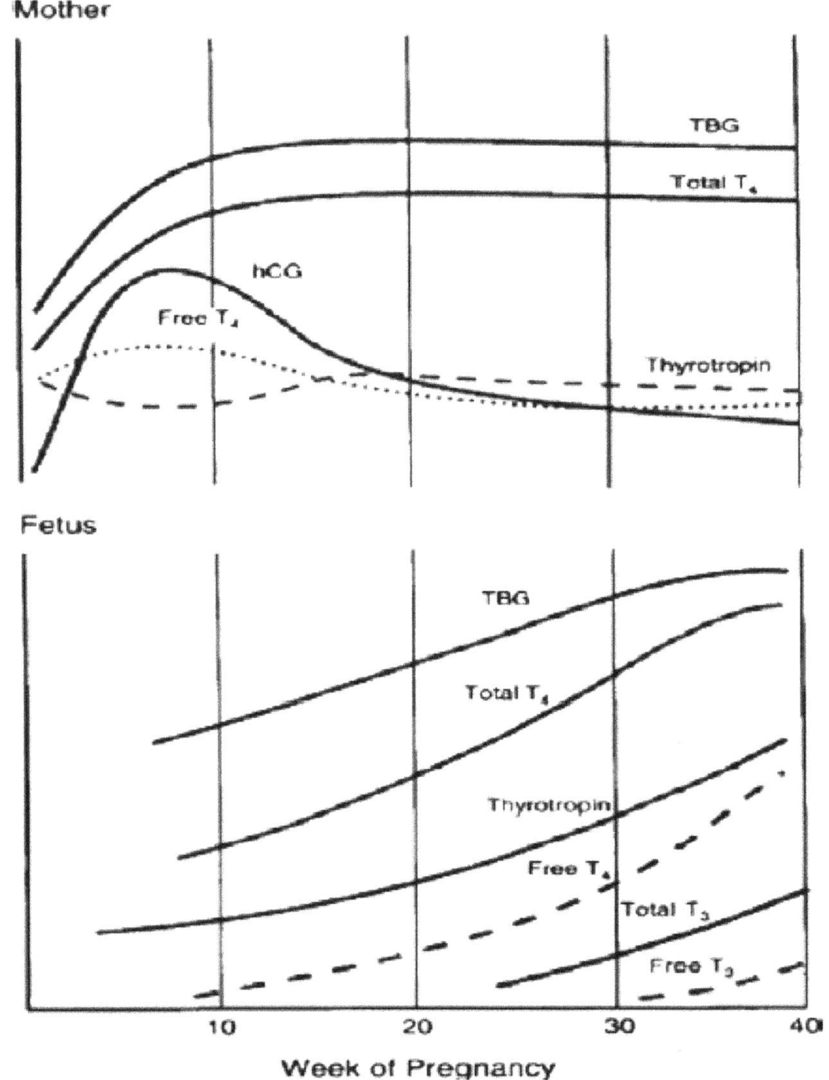

Figure 1. Thyroid hormone profile in the mother and fetus during pregnancy. From Ramprasad *et al.* (3). hCG, human chorionic gonadotropin; T_3, triiodothyronine; TBG, thyroid-binding globulin.

STRATEGIES FOR DIAGNOSIS, THERAPY, AND/OR MANAGEMENT

Fetal Thyroid Development

In humans, the thyroid gland originates from epithelial cells in the foramen cecum and migrates to the pretracheal region about 10 weeks after conception (4–7). Follicular thyroid cells are present at about 11 weeks after conception, and the fetal thyroid can produce thyroid hormones, albeit at very low levels, at approximately 12 weeks after conception. During the first half of pregnancy, the fetus is dependent on maternal thyroid hormone, with thyroxine (T_4) crossing the placenta to reach the fetus. The fetal hypothalamic-pituitary axis begins producing thyrotropin (TSH) at about 20 weeks' gestation, and the fetus accounts for *in utero* thyroid hormone production during the second half of pregnancy. After midgestation, fetal T_4 and triiodothyronine levels rise steadily (Fig. 1) (3).

In about 1 in 2500 infants, the thyroid gland does not develop or function normally at birth. Congenital hypothyroidism is the most common preventable form of mental retardation (5); therefore, beginning about four decades ago, newborn screening was introduced for the detection of congenital hypothyroidisms.

Maternal Hypothyroidism

Thyroid hormone is essential for normal fetal brain development, and during the first half of gestation, the fetus is dependent on maternal thyroid hormone for its supply. It is recognized that maternal hypothyroidism during pregnancy is associated with reduced neurocognitive outcomes in offspring (8, 9). As such, there has been considerable discussion related to the potential merits of universal screening for hypothyroidism during pregnancy (1, 2, 10).

Recent clinical trials, though, have not reported beneficial outcomes in the offspring of mothers who were identified as having hypothyroidism and treated (10, 11). However, supplementation in these studies was initiated close to halfway through gestation, past the critical periods of early brain development. Studies evaluating the potential effects of earlier interventions are not available at the present time.

Although debate continues on the potential merit of universal screening for maternal hypothyroidism during pregnancy, recent guidelines of the American Thyroid Association are prudent to follow at present (Table 1) (2, 10). First, screening pregnant women at risk for hypothyroidism and those with a history of infertility or pregnancy loss should be performed. When TSH elevation is detected, replacement therapy should be initiated because this treatment is of low cost and low risk.

Maternal Hypothyroidism and Graves Disease

The treatment of Graves disease during pregnancy has undergone considerable review after observing the risks of liver failure associated with propylthiouracil (PTU), coupled with concerns about the potential teratogenic risks of methimazole (MMI) (12, 13). As such, recent guideline recommendations suggest that PTU be used within the first trimester, followed by MMI for the remainder of the pregnancy (14). Recent clinical and animal data, however, cast doubt on the notion that MMI is significantly more teratogenic than PTU (15–18).

Other concerns related to Graves disease during pregnancy relate to the transplacental passage of thyroid-stimulating immunoglobulins (TSIs) (4, 7, 15, 19). If the levels of TSIs are elevated after 20 weeks' gestation, they can stimulate the fetal thyroid to elaborate excess amounts of thyroid, resulting in fetal hyperthyroidism that can exert severe adverse effects on the fetus. Thus, women with active Graves disease or a history of the disease need to be closely monitored throughout pregnancy, via monitoring of TSI levels, fetal heart rate, and

Table 1. American Thyroid Association Recommendations for the Management of Subclinical Hypothyroidism and Hypothyroxinemia in Pregnancy

Laboratory Data	Levothyroxine Therapy	Recommendation Strength	Evidence Quality
Anti-TPO–positive and thyrotropin level > pregnancy-specific reference range	Yes	Strong	Moderate
Anti-TPO–negative and thyrotropin level >10 mU/liter	Yes	Strong	Low
Anti-TPO–positive and thyrotropin level >2.5 mU/liter and < upper limit of the reference range	Consider	Weak	Moderate
Anti-TPO–negative and thyrotropin level > upper limit of the reference range and <10 mU/liter	Consider	Weak	Low
Isolated maternal hypothyroxinemia[a]	No	Weak	Low

From Cooper and Pearce (10), which was adapted from Alexander *et al.* (2).
Abbreviations: Anti-TPO, anti-thyroperoxidase antibody.
[a] Isolated maternal hypothyroxinemia is defined as an FT_4 level that is less than the 2.5th or 5th percentile and a normal TSH level.

fetal growth. When fetal thyrotoxicosis is observed, the fetus can be treated indirectly via the administration of antithyroid medications to the mother. The importance of preventing fetal hyperthyroidism is highlighted by recent basic studies showing long-term anatomical problems after fetal hyperthyroidism (19).

Most important, the controversies related to maternal thyroid disease management can be avoided by prepregnancy recognition of thyroid disease in women of childbearing age. With proper prepregnancy treatment of either hypo- or hyperthyroidism, the risks to the fetus can be greatly reduced (20).

REFERENCES

1. Committee on Practice Bulletins–Obstetrics, American College of Obstetricians and Gynecologists. Practice Bulletin No. 148: Thyroid disease in pregnancy. *Obstet Gynecol.* 2015;**125**(4): 996–1005.
2. Alexander EK, Pearce EN, Brent GA, Brown RS, Chen H, Dosiou C, Grobman WA, Laurberg P, Lazarus JH, Mandel SJ, Peeters RP, Sullivan S. 2017 Guidelines of the American Thyroid Association for the diagnosis and management of thyroid disease during pregnancy and the postpartum. *Thyroid.* 2017;**27**(3):315–389.
3. Ramprasad M, Bhattacharyya SS, Bhattacharyya A. Thyroid disorders in pregnancy. *Indian J Endocrinol Metab.* 2012;**16**(Suppl 2):S167–S170.
4. Rivkees SA, Mandel SJ. Thyroid disease in pregnancy. *Horm Res Paediatr.* 2011;**76**(Suppl 1):91–96.
5. Grüters A, Biebermann H, Krude H. Neonatal thyroid disorders. *Horm Res.* 2003;**59**(Suppl 1):24–29.
6. Lazarus JH. Thyroid function in pregnancy. *Br Med Bull.* 2011;**97**(1): 137–148.
7. Polak M. Human fetal thyroid function. *Endocr Dev.* 2014;**26**: 17–25.
8. Haddow JE, Palomaki GE, Allan WC, Williams JR, Knight GJ, Gagnon J, O'Heir CE, Mitchell ML, Hermos RJ, Waisbren SE, Faix JD, Klein RZ. Maternal thyroid deficiency during pregnancy and subsequent neuropsychological development of the child. *N Engl J Med.* 1999;**341**(8): 549–555.
9. Gronowski AM, Haddow J, Kilpatrick S, Lazarus JH, Negro R. Thyroid function during pregnancy: who and how should we screen? *Clin Chem.* 2012;**58**(10):1397–1401.
10. Cooper DS, Pearce EN. Subclinical hypothyroidism and hypothyroxinemia in pregnancy—still no answers. *N Engl J Med.* 2017;**376**(9):876–877.
11. Casey BM, Thom EA, Peaceman AM, Varner MW, Sorokin Y, Hirtz DG, Reddy UM, Wapner RJ, Thorp JM Jr, Saade G, Tita AT, Rouse DJ, Sibai B, Iams JD, Mercer BM, Tolosa J, Caritis SN, VanDorsten JP; Eunice Kennedy Shriver National Institute of Child Health and Human Development Maternal-Fetal Medicine Units Network. Treatment of subclinical hypothyroidism or hypothyroxinemia in pregnancy. *N Engl J Med.* 2017;**376**(9):815–825.
12. Bahn RS, Burch HS, Cooper DS, Garber JR, Greenlee CM, Klein IL, Laurberg P, McDougall IR, Rivkees SA, Ross D, Sosa JA, Stan MN. The role of propylthiouracil in the management of Graves' disease in adults: report of a meeting jointly sponsored by the American Thyroid Association and the Food and Drug Administration. *Thyroid.* 2009;**19**(7):673–674.
13. Cooper DS, Rivkees SA. Putting propylthiouracil in perspective. *J Clin Endocrinol Metab.* 2009;**94**(6):1881–1882.
14. Ross DS, Burch HB, Cooper DS, Greenlee MC, Laurberg P, Maia AL, Rivkees SA, Samuels M, Sosa JA, Stan MN, Walter MA. 2016 American Thyroid Association guidelines for diagnosis and management of hyperthyroidism and other causes of thyrotoxicosis. *Thyroid.* 2016; **26**(10):1343–1421.
15. Schurmann L, Hansen AV, Garne E. Pregnancy outcomes after fetal exposure to antithyroid medications or levothyroxine. *Early Hum Dev.* 2016;**101**:73–77.
16. Mallela MK, Strobl M, Poulsen RR, Wendler CC, Booth CJ, Rivkees SA. Evaluation of developmental toxicity of propylthiouracil and methimazole. *Birth Defects Res B Dev Reprod Toxicol.* 2014;**101**(4):300–307.
17. Laurberg P, Andersen SL. Antithyroid drug use in pregnancy and birth defects: why some studies find clear associations, and some studies report none. *Thyroid.* 2015;**25**(11):1185–1190.
18. Andersen SL, Olsen J, Wu CS, Laurberg P. Birth defects after early pregnancy use of antithyroid drugs: a Danish nationwide study. *J Clin Endocrinol Metab.* 2013;**98**(11):4373–4381.
19. Strobl MJ, Freeman D, Patel J, Poulsen R, Wendler CC, Rivkees SA, Coleman JE. Opposing effects of maternal hypo- and hyperthyroidism on the stability of thalamocortical synapses in the visual cortex of adult offspring. *Cereb Cortex.* 2017;**27**(5):3015–3027.
20. Rivkees SA. Propylthiouracil versus methimazole during pregnancy: an evolving tale of difficult choices. *J Clin Endocrinol Metab.* 2013; **98**(11):4332–4335.

Differentiated Thyroid Carcinoma in Children

M26
Presented, March 17–20, 2018

Steven G. Waguespack, MD. Department of Endocrine Neoplasia and Hormonal Disorders and the Children's Cancer Hospital, The University of Texas MD Anderson Cancer Center, Houston, Texas 77030, E-mail: swagues@mdanderson.org

SIGNIFICANCE OF THE CLINICAL PROBLEM

Differentiated thyroid cancer (DTC) is uncommon in the pediatric population but its incidence is increasing. Compared with adults, children present with larger tumors and a higher prevalence of regional lymph node (LN) disease and pulmonary metastases. Despite this, pediatric DTC patients paradoxically have a very low disease-specific mortality. DTC can be an incurable yet indolent disease, and the main challenge for clinicians is to appropriately treat and monitor the child with persistent disease while not overzealously pursuing a cure and thereby increasing the risks for lifelong complications and late effects. Unfortunately, there remain very few centers with large multidisciplinary teams who specialize in pediatric thyroid cancer, and many children cannot access such centers due to logistical and financial reasons. Guidelines from the American Thyroid Association (ATA) (1) and elsewhere have been developed for the management of pediatric DTC. However, the care of children with DTC continues to evolve, and more research is required to better understand the genomics of pediatric thyroid cancer and to improve risk-stratification systems to determine who may or may not benefit from more aggressive treatment and surveillance during childhood.

BARRIERS TO OPTIMAL PRACTICE

- The low incidence and indolent course of pediatric DTC make large-scale prospective studies difficult. Thus, there are substantial barriers to incorporating evidence-based decisions in patient care. The main challenge is balancing the risks of overtreatment during childhood with the risks of the underlying disease itself.
- The care of pediatric DTC remains poorly centralized. Few centers have multidisciplinary teams that see high volumes of children with DTC, which increases the risks of treatment, may lead to inappropriate treatment due to the lack of familiarity with the natural history of the disease, and may worsen oncologic outcomes.

LEARNING OBJECTIVES

As a result of participating in this session, learners should be able to:

- Describe the types of childhood DTC and their clinical presentation
- Identify genetic and environmental risk factors for pediatric DTC
- Discuss the evaluation and treatment of DTC when diagnosed during childhood
- Apply contemporary guidelines to the care of children with DTC and recognize the areas of uncertainty that require further research

STRATEGIES FOR DIAGNOSIS, THERAPY, AND/OR MANAGEMENT

Introduction

Pediatric DTC comprises two major histopathologic variants, papillary thyroid carcinoma (PTC; >90%) and follicular thyroid carcinoma (FTC; <10%). Children with PTC commonly present with a palpable thyroid nodule and/or malignant lymphadenopathy or their cancer may be identified incidentally in the context of imaging studies done for another reason. Pediatric PTC can also present as a diffusely infiltrative carcinoma without a discrete nodule, which can sometimes coexist with thyroid autoimmunity and be misdiagnosed as goiter due to autoimmune thyroid disease; in these cases, thyroid asymmetry and/or palpable cervical LN disease can be clues to a malignant diagnosis. In PTC, children with substantial cervical LN disease are at the highest risk for hematogenously spread lung metastases. The diagnosis of FTC is almost always made in children after the histopathologic identification of capsular and/or vascular invasion in a nodule surgically removed after an indeterminate fine-needle aspiration biopsy (FNAB). In contrast with PTC, FTC is usually a unifocal neoplasm that is not associated with locoregional LN metastases, but patients with FTC are at risk for distant metastases with any degree of angioinvasion (2). Given the rarity of FTC in the pediatric population, it remains poorly studied in this age-group.

Epidemiology and Prognosis

Individuals <20 years of age represent ~1.4% of thyroid cancers, and the incidence of DTC has been rising over the decades. Adolescents (ages 15 to 19 years) are the most commonly affected pediatric age-group (29 cases/million/y) and the female-to-male ratio is 5.4:1 in this subgroup (3). Children with DTC have an excellent prognosis, and survival over decades is the norm, even in patients with distant metastases (4, 5). However, a subset of patients diagnosed during childhood will ultimately succumb to their DTC or die of treatment-related complications.

Risk Factors

Thyroid exposure to ionizing radiation (primarily in the context of cancer therapy) is the major established DTC risk factor, especially in children who are exposed at a very young age. DTC is one of the most frequently diagnosed subsequent primary malignancies in childhood cancer survivors, and the latency period between radiation exposure and diagnosis is typically long in this setting (~20 years). Exposure to ionizing radiation can also occur via the ingestion of radionuclides, epitomized by the large environmental exposure to radioactive materials as a result of the Chernobyl nuclear accident and possibly the more recent Fukushima incident. Radiation-induced tumors do not appear to be inherently more aggressive compared with sporadic, non–radiation-induced disease. Other risk factors for DTC include living in a volcanic region, iodine deficiency, and possibly obesity. Whether there is a strong association between autoimmune thyroid disease and DTC in children remains largely unknown. Finally, although accounting for <5% of pediatric DTC, germ line variants in several genes have been associated with syndromic and nonsyndromic hereditary DTC (see below).

Molecular Mechanisms of Disease

In pediatric PTC, somatic gene rearrangements are the most common molecular event, especially fusions involving the rearranged during transfection (*RET*) proto-oncogene and the neurotropic tyrosine receptor kinase (*NTRK*) gene (6–8). In FTC, gene rearrangements of peroxisome proliferator–activated receptor gamma (*PPARG*) and paired box gene 8 (*PAX8*) are more common. $BRAF^{V600E}$ point mutations in pediatric PTC are also prevalent, although not as common as in adults. Accumulating data suggest that *BRAF* mutations are more common in older pediatric patients and may not be associated with more aggressive disease. Rat sarcoma (*RAS*) mutations are also rarely identified in pediatric PTC and FTC.

Germ line mutations that predispose children to DTC are quite rare. Multiple genes and heritable tumor syndromes have been associated with both benign and malignant thyroid neoplasia: *APC*-associated polyposis (*APC* gene; Online Mendelian Inheritance in Man® [OMIM] no. 175100), Birt-Hogg-Dubé syndrome (*FLCN* gene; OMIM no. 135150), the Carney complex (*PRKAR1A* gene; OMIM no. 160980), CHEK2-related cancer (*CHEK2* gene; OMIM no. 604373), DICER1-pleuropulmonary blastoma familial tumor predisposition syndrome (*DICER1* gene; OMIM no. 606241), familial nonmedullary thyroid carcinoma (multiple genes; OMIM no. 188550), Li-Fraumeni syndrome (*TP53* gene; OMIM no. 151623), *PTEN* (phosphatase and tensin homolog) hamartoma tumor syndrome (*PTEN* gene; OMIM no. 601728), Pendred syndrome (*SLC26A4* gene; OMIM no. 274600), and Werner syndrome (*WRN* gene; OMIM no. 277700). It should be emphasized that the association of DTC with a tumor predisposition syndrome does not necessarily indicate causality. Other than the child's personal and family history, a clue to the diagnosis of syndromic DTC can be macrocephaly, which is nearly universal in the *PTEN* hamartoma tumor syndrome and common in *DICER1* mutation carriers.

Evaluation, Treatment, and Follow-Up

The evaluation and treatment of pediatric DTC has evolved over the years, which in part is due to better preoperative staging/imaging, more appropriate initial surgical therapy, and the ever-changing perspective on the role of radioactive iodine (RAI) in the pediatric population.

Initial Workup and Staging

Figure 1 outlines an approach to the evaluation and treatment of pediatric PTC once the diagnosis is confirmed. Universally recommended is a high-resolution cervical ultrasound (US) performed by an experienced ultrasonographer to interrogate the thyroid and lateral neck LNs (1, 9). US-guided FNAB should be used to confirm a malignant diagnosis and the extent of regional metastases. Children with bulky cervical disease, a primary tumor that appears fixed to underlying aerodigestive structures, or vocal cord paralysis should have a contrast-enhanced computed tomography (CT) (preferred) or magnetic resonance imaging of the neck to help inform surgical decisions (1, 9). Because only a minority of children will have pulmonary metastases and because the detection of pulmonary metastatic disease does not change the initial therapeutic approach, guidelines do not suggest routine chest imaging in all pediatric DTC patients, although some centers do obtain preoperative chest imaging either via chest x-ray or chest CT (especially in high-risk children in whom a neck CT scan is also planned). Although not recommended by all, some experts obtain baseline thyroglobulin (Tg) and Tg antibody (TgAb) after confirmation of PTC (9).

Surgery

The surgical treatment of pediatric DTC is the single most important factor for improving long-term disease-free survival. For most children, especially given the high rate of clinical LN and pulmonary metastases in PTC, total thyroidectomy is typically needed (1). However, in low-risk children with small, incidentally discovered tumors, no previous radiation exposure, and no evidence of contralateral disease or cervical LN disease, thyroid lobectomy ± ipsilateral central neck dissection may result in similar long-term outcomes (5, 10). Compartment-oriented neck dissection is recommended for biopsy-proven LN disease, and central neck dissection, in the absence of documented LN metastases, can be selectively considered in children and guided by intraoperative findings (1). Recognizing that complication rates are higher in children, especially in those requiring neck dissection, it is imperative that surgery be performed by a high-volume thyroid cancer surgeon.

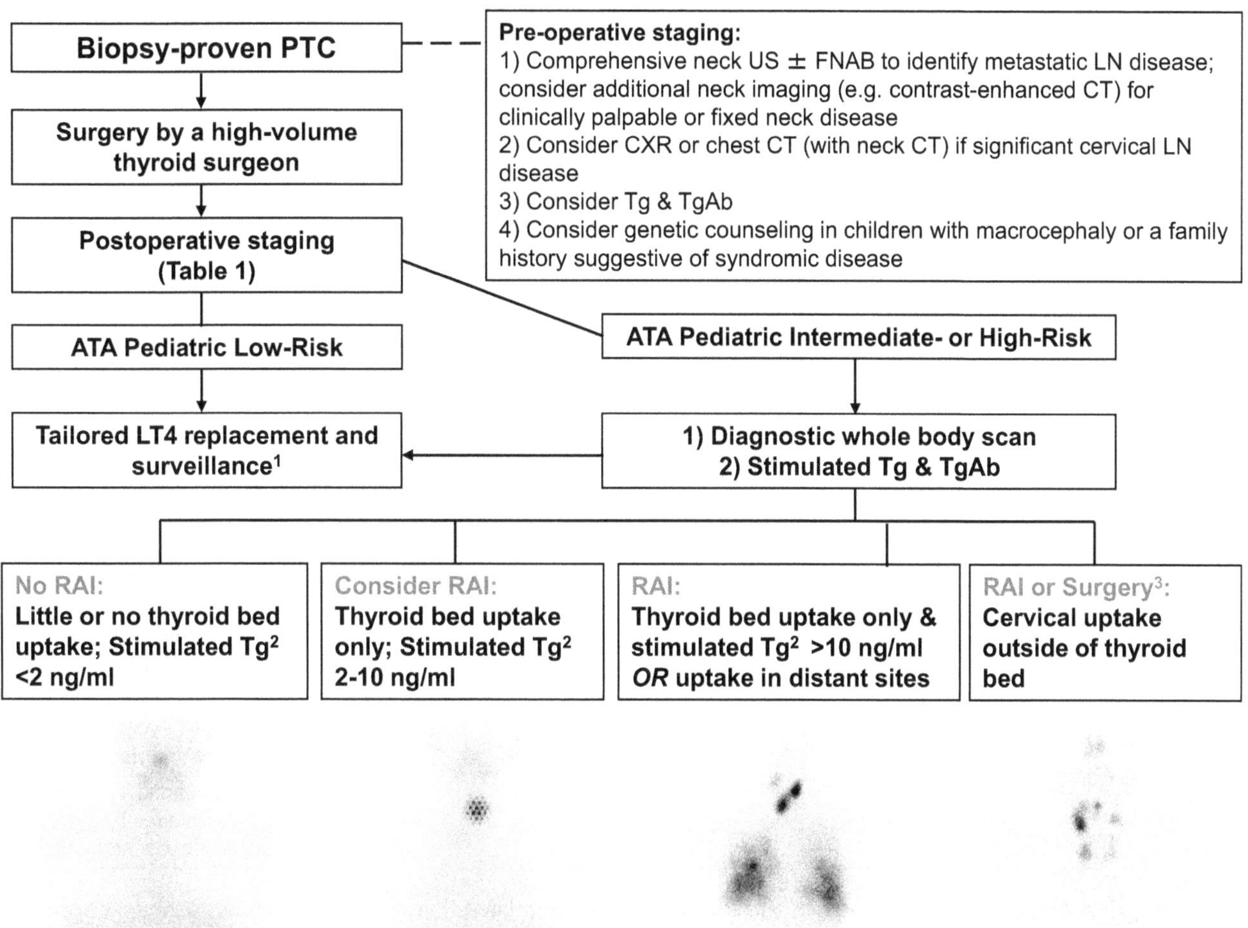

Figure 1. Initial evaluation and treatment of biopsy-proven pediatric PTC. [1]If residual/recurrent PTC is suspected during long-term follow-up of low-risk patients, and assuming neck US is negative, further evaluation and treatment with RAI is recommended. [2]Assumes negative TgAb; if TgAb is positive and there is no evidence of iodine-avid disease on the diagnostic scan, consideration can be given to deferring RAI treatment, especially in intermediate-risk patients. [3]RAI only if surgery deemed unsafe or not feasible. Reprinted with permission from Waguespack and Wasserman. Differentiated thyroid cancer in children. In: *Practical Management of Thyroid Cancer: A Multidisciplinary Approach.* 2nd ed. Springer International Publishing, In Press (18).

Postoperative Staging

The pathological tumor node metastasis (TNM) classification developed by the American Joint Committee on Cancer (AJCC) and the Union for International Cancer Control is the international reference staging system for thyroid cancer. This has recently been updated to the 8th edition, which was implemented in January 2018 (11). Utilizing AJCC 7th edition TNM staging, a novel risk categorization for PTC (ATA pediatric low, intermediate, and high risk) was introduced in the ATA pediatric guidelines (1) (Table 1).

This risk stratification was intended to be used in PTC patients to identify those at risk for persistent cervical disease and distant metastases to determine which patients would benefit from more intensive postoperative staging, thyrotropin (TSH) suppression, and surveillance. As increasingly used in adults (12), dynamic risk stratification based on the response to initial therapy may also predict outcomes in pediatric DTC.

RAI Therapy

Almost universally administered in the past, ^{131}I therapy is currently used more selectively in children and only after incorporating new data obtained from initial postoperative staging (1, 9) (Fig. 1). Two of the greatest remaining challenges surrounding the use of RAI in pediatric DTC are dose selection and how to determine when additional ^{131}I therapy is warranted. Recognizing that 50% of children with pulmonary metastases have chronic persistent disease (13), understanding that the Tg decline after ^{131}I treatment may continue for years (14), and asserting that an undetectable serum Tg level should no longer be the sole goal of therapy,

Table 1. ATA Pediatric Risk Categories and Recommendations for Postoperative Staging and Clinical Follow-up[a]

ATA Risk Level	Definition[b]	Postoperative Staging[c]	TSH Target[d]	Surveillance of Patients With No Evidence of Disease[e]
ATA pediatric low risk	Disease grossly confined to the thyroid (T1–T3) with N0/Nx disease or patients with incidental N1a disease (metastasis <0.2 cm to ≤5 central neck LNs)	Nonstimulated Tg[f] on LT4 therapy	0.5–1.0 mIU/L	US at 6 months postoperatively and then annually for 5 years
				Tg[f] on LT4 every 6 months for 2 years and then annually
ATA pediatric intermediate risk	Extensive N1a (>5 central neck LNs or LNs >0.2 cm) or minimal N1b disease (≤5 lateral neck LNs)	TSH-stimulated Tg[f] and diagnostic ^{123}I scan in most patients (see Fig. 1)	0.1–0.5 mIU/L	US at 6 months postoperatively, every 6–12 months for 5 years, and then every 2–3 years
				Tg[f] on LT4 every 6 months for 3 years and then annually
				Consider TSH-stimulated Tg[6] ± diagnostic ^{123}I scan after 1–2 years (or longer) in patients treated with ^{131}I
ATA pediatric high risk	Regionally extensive disease (extensive N1b; >5 lateral neck LNs) or locally invasive disease (T4 tumors); known distant metastasis	TSH-stimulated Tg[f] and diagnostic ^{123}I scan in all patients (see Fig. 1)	<0.1 mIU/L	US at 6 months postoperatively, every 6–12 months for 5 years, and then every 2–3 years
				Tg[f] on LT4 every 6 months for 3 years and then annually
				TSH-stimulated Tg[f] ± diagnostic ^{123}I scan after 1–2 years (or longer) in patients treated with ^{131}I

Reprinted with permission from Waguespack and Wasserman. Differentiated thyroid cancer in children. In: *Practical Management of Thyroid Cancer: A Multidisciplinary Approach.* 2nd ed. Springer International Publishing, In Press (18).

[a] Adapted from the ATA pediatric thyroid nodule and DTC guidelines. These recommendations apply to pediatric PTC and not to FTC or other rare pathologic variants.

[b] Utilizing TNM staging from the AJCC, 7th edition, *Cancer Staging Manual* (11).

[c] Postoperative staging that is done within 12 weeks after initial definitive thyroid surgery.

[d] Initial targets for TSH suppression. These are subsequently adapted to the patient's disease status on long-term follow-up. In higher-risk patients who have no evidence of disease after 3 to 5 years, the TSH can be allowed to rise to the low normal range.

[e] Surveillance after surgery ± RAI therapy in patients who are believed to be disease free; these recommendations do not apply to patients with known or suspected residual disease who require additional imaging and possibly treatment (see Fig. 2).

[f] Assumes negative TgAb. In patients with elevated TgAb titers, serial monitoring of the antibody level (using the same assay at the same laboratory) may be used as a surrogate for disease trajectory, although elevated titers alone do not imply residual or recurrent disease.

the ATA guidelines have recommended longer intervals between ^{131}I courses, suggesting that treatment be given no sooner than 12 months after the last dose (1). In all cases, the decision to prescribe ^{131}I should be individualized and incorporate knowledge regarding prognosis, tumor avidity for RAI, and the previous response to therapy (Fig. 2).

Different opinions remain as to how to best prepare the child for RAI (withdrawal vs. recombinant human TSH stimulation), how to determine the optimal ^{131}I-administered activity, and whether a diagnostic thyroid scan is needed in all cases (1, 15). What is not controversial is the importance of obtaining a posttreatment scan in all children 4 to 7 days after therapy. The incorporation of single-photon emission computed tomography/CT with nuclear scintigraphy has markedly improved our ability to localize disease and distinguish benign from malignant sites of RAI uptake.

TSH Suppression and Follow-Up

TSH suppression is universally used in the management of pediatric DTC, and the degree of initial TSH suppression depends on the child's ATA risk category (Table 1). In general, the TSH goal can be loosened in patients who have no evidence of disease after a 1- to 3-year period of follow-up.

In addition to tailored TSH suppression, the long-term surveillance of pediatric DTC includes the periodic assessment of Tg and TgAb levels, routine neck US, and the selective use of diagnostic thyroid scans and other cross-sectional imaging of the neck ± chest (Fig. 2). The intensity and type

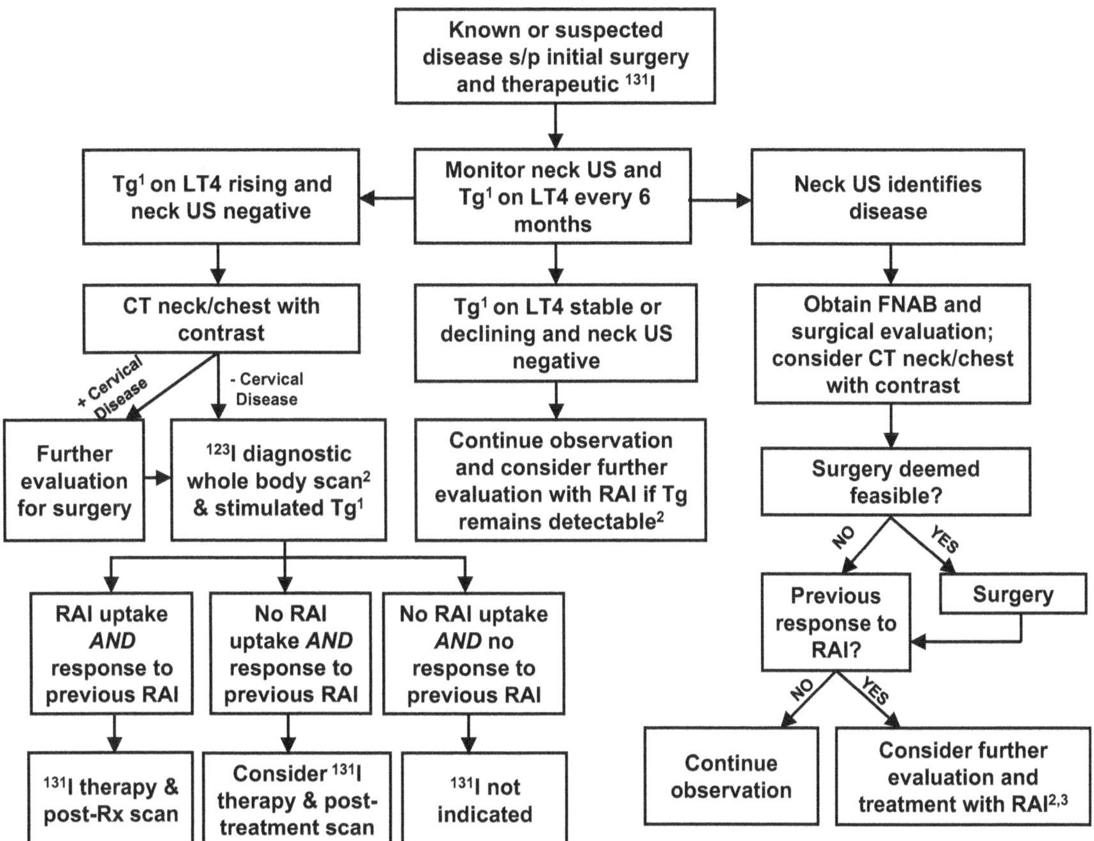

Figure 2. Follow-up of the pediatric patient with known or suspected residual/recurrent PTC after initial surgery and RAI. [1]Assumes a negative TgAb; in TgAb-positive patients, the singular presence of TgAb cannot be interpreted as a sign of disease unless the titer is clearly rising over time; a declining TgAb titer would suggest ongoing response to treatment. [2]Further evaluation and treatment with RAI should only be considered after a reasonable period of time (1–2 years) has elapsed in order not to overtreat a patient who may have a delayed clinical response to prior RAI. [3]Repeated courses of ^{131}I should be considered only if iodine-avid disease is proven/suspected and there was a previous clinical response to ^{131}I therapy. Reprinted with permission from Waguespack and Wasserman. Differentiated thyroid cancer in children. In: *Practical Management of Thyroid Cancer: A Multidisciplinary Approach.* 2nd ed. Springer International Publishing, In Press (18).

of follow-up is primarily based on the postoperative ATA pediatric risk categorization and dynamic risk restratification, modifying the surveillance plan as new clinical data become available (1, 12). Follow-up of children with DTC should be lifelong, given that the probability of recurrence continues to increase over time and because clinical disease may not be identified until decades after initial treatment (5). Clinical recurrences primarily occur in cervical LNs, underscoring the critical importance of neck US during long-term surveillance.

Around 40% of children with DTC have measurable TgAb (16), which renders the Tg uninterpretable. In such cases, the antibody titer itself can be followed, and it is the trend of this analyte over time (using the same assay and laboratory) that is more important than its absolute value. In children with evaluable Tg levels, an undetectable stimulated Tg correlates with a very low risk of recurrence. However, the exact Tg values that indicate residual, clinically relevant disease in children that would warrant more intensive surveillance or treatment remain largely unstudied; although a stimulated Tg >10 ng/mL may represent an actionable threshold (1, 17). Even if ^{131}I therapy is not used or a total thyroidectomy not done, Tg levels and their trend over time serve as a useful indicator of disease status.

Systemic Therapy for Advanced Disease

The development of progressive pediatric DTC that warrants systemic treatment outside of repeated courses of ^{131}I is very rare. The definition of RAI-refractory disease remains poorly defined in children, but if present, contemporary guidelines state that repeated courses of RAI should not be administered when there was no documented response to previous ^{131}I therapy (1). In such cases, the disease may remain quite indolent for years while continuing TSH suppression alone. In the rare event of a child with progressive DTC needing alternative approaches to care, consultation with providers who are experienced in the use of the available oral multikinase inhibitors is recommended.

MAIN CONCLUSIONS

- Greater than 90% of children with DTC have PTC; FTC occurs in <10%.
- Easily diagnosed with FNAB, PTC is frequently a multifocal tumor associated with a high rate of LN metastases and an increased rate of distant metastases (usually to the lungs), especially in the presence of bulky cervical disease. In contrast, FTC is a unifocal tumor not associated with LN disease and usually diagnosed after definitive surgery; distant metastases to lung and bone can occur in angioinvasive FTC.
- The major risk factor for the development of DTC is exposure to ionizing radiation.
- The molecular signature of pediatric PTC is different from adults. Gene rearrangements (*RET/PTC* and *NTRK* fusions) are most common, followed by the V600E *BRAF* mutation. These molecular differences may, in part, explain the excellent long-term outcome of children with DTC.
- The care of children with DTC is ideally done at specialized centers with multidisciplinary expertise.
- Surgery is the mainstay of management, especially for PTC, and surgery by a high-volume surgeon is associated with better outcomes.
- The role of RAI therapy is evolving, and more children are not being given routine treatment if postoperative staging does not document residual disease. Uncertainty remains as to how to optimally determine the ^{131}I-administered activity and how often to use ^{131}I in children with RAI-avid disease.
- For children with persistent disease despite appropriate initial therapy, early recognition that thyroid cancer may become a chronic disease, albeit one with low morbidity and mortality, may justify a more restrained approach to treatment.
- Further research geared toward postoperative risk stratification, better understanding the optimal use of RAI, and predicting long-term outcomes based on clinical presentation and tumor mutational status is needed.

CASES/DISCUSSION OF CASES AND ANSWERS

CASE 1

An asymptomatic 13-year-old female with a strong family history of PTC (mother and older sister) had a US at Mom's request that identified a 1.5-cm thyroid nodule. On exam, the thyroid gland has slight asymmetry and fullness in the right thyroid lobe. There is no macrocephaly, and no enlarged, firm, or asymmetric cervical LNs are appreciated.

Question: What is the next best step?

A. Refer to surgery for a diagnostic lobectomy
B. Review the US images and pursue FNAB
C. Order genetic testing for germ line mutations in the known DTC susceptibility genes
D. Order a thyroid uptake and scan

Answer: B. Although it was once common practice to treat pediatric thyroid nodules with surgery, due to the higher risk of malignancy (~25%), the recognition that FNAB is a safe and reliable test has led to the recommendation that FNAB should be the initial diagnostic procedure in most children presenting with a thyroid nodule. Therefore, going directly to surgery without biopsy is currently not advocated because a malignant diagnosis might change the plan for surgery (total thyroidectomy ± LN dissection vs. lobectomy) and because surgery may ultimately not be indicated, *e.g.*, in the event of a purely cystic nodule or a nodule <4 cm with benign cytopathology. Ultrasonographic features help to determine the risk of cancer in a given nodule, and FNAB is recommended in all solid or mostly solid nodules to determine the diagnosis. Although the patient may have a hereditary component to her thyroid nodule, immediately pursuing genetic testing would not be appropriate, especially in the absence of other features or family history suggestive of syndromic DTC. Finally, ordering a thyroid scan and uptake is a valuable test in patients with a suppressed TSH, but it would not be the ideal test before a TSH level has been checked.

CASE 2

A 6-year-old male was found to have a pea-sized swelling in the right lower neck. Observation was recommended by his provider, but it continued to grow. No pertinent family history or other risk factors. On examination, the thyroid is diffusely enlarged and firm. There is subtle asymmetry (right > left) and several firm, palpable LNs are palpated in the lateral neck bilaterally.

Question 1: Suspecting PTC, which of the following would be most appropriate to secure the diagnosis and plan treatment?

A. Contrast-enhanced CT neck and chest
B. ^{18}F-FDG positron emission tomography/CT scan
C. ^{123}I thyroid scan and uptake
D. Neck US with FNAB of the thyroid and testing for known PTC driver mutations
E. Neck US with FNAB of lateral neck LNs

Answer: E. The patient presents with an abnormal thyroid exam and bilateral palpable lymphadenopathy, which is highly suspicious for a diagnosis of locally metastatic PTC. FNAB is necessary to make the diagnosis. In this case, biopsy of a lateral neck LN with immediate cytologic assessment would be the best way to make the diagnosis and plan treatment. A finding of PTC in a lateral neck LN would indicate the need for a comprehensive lateral neck dissection, in addition to a total thyroidectomy and central neck dissection. In contrast, a biopsy of the thyroid would secure the diagnosis, but further tissue confirmation of lateral neck disease would still be required for definitive surgical planning, especially for subclinical LN disease. Although molecular testing may identify the driver mutation, and in the case of indeterminate cytology may help to secure a malignant diagnosis, it is not currently indicated at this stage. A contrast-enhanced CT of the neck will be important for surgery, but imaging alone cannot make a definitive diagnosis. In turn, this patient is at high risk for pulmonary metastases, but knowledge regarding distant metastases will not change the initial cancer management. ^{18}F-FDG positron emission tomography/CT scans are not indicated or useful in the diagnosis of pediatric thyroid cancer. Finally, a thyroid scan will not secure a diagnosis and is also a poor tool to assess for PTC metastases because the bulk of the iodine uptake will be in the normal thyroid gland.

Question 2: The patient is confirmed to have PTC. Chest imaging reveals evidence for pulmonary metastases. He has surgery and his cancer is staged as pmT3N1bcM1 (ATA high risk). Which of the following would you recommend to his parents now?

A. Start TSH suppressive therapy to keep his TSH 0.1 mIU/L or less and check a neck US in 6 months
B. Start an oral multikinase inhibitor for distant metastases
C. Proceed to a diagnostic thyroid scan and check a stimulated Tg to determine whether RAI is needed
D. Proceed directly to RAI therapy and obtain a posttreatment scan

Answer: C. The patient has a stage 2 PTC with locoregional and distant metastases. Although TSH suppression and monitoring of neck US are critical in the long-term treatment and follow-up of pediatric PTC, it would not be the next step in this case due to the patient being ATA high risk with known pulmonary metastases. Starting an oral multikinase inhibitor for distant metastases would be inappropriate in a child who has never received therapeutic RAI and who does not have progressive disease. In addition, it is anticipated that such treatment will not be required over the ensuing years because children at this age are likely to have iodine-avid and nonprogressive metastases. Many experts do proceed directly to treatment with RAI, whereas the ATA guidelines suggest getting a diagnostic thyroid scan and a stimulated Tg to better inform treatment decisions. Obtaining these data can identify those children with no evidence of disease (defined as those with an undetectable serum Tg and the absence of structurally apparent disease) who can avoid unnecessary RAI exposure, children with extensive RAI-avid cervical disease who may benefit from reoperation, and those with RAI-avid distant metastases who may need to have their planned administered ^{131}I activity adjusted because of either the extent of disease or the intensity of the pulmonary uptake. What remains difficult to know is what activity of therapeutic ^{131}I to administer to a given patient and how frequently to use RAI, recognizing that many patients develop incurable disease that ultimately will not be cured by RAI.

Other questions for discussion will be covered during the session.

REFERENCES

1. Francis GL, Waguespack SG, Bauer AJ, Angelos P, Benvenga S, Cerutti JM, Dinauer CA, Hamilton J, Hay ID, Luster M, Parisi MT, Rachmiel M, Thompson GB, Yamashita S; American Thyroid Association Guidelines Task Force. Management guidelines for children with thyroid nodules and differentiated thyroid cancer. *Thyroid.* 2015;**25**(7):716–759.
2. Enomoto K, Enomoto Y, Uchino S, Yamashita H, Noguchi S. Follicular thyroid cancer in children and adolescents: clinicopathologic features, long-term survival, and risk factors for recurrence. *Endocr J.* 2013; **60**(5):629–635.
3. Howlader N, Noone AM, Krapcho M, Miller D, Bishop K, Kosary CL, Yu M, Ruhl J, Tatalovich Z, Mariotto A, Lewis DR, Chen HS, Feuer EJ, Cronin KA. SEER cancer statistics review, 1975-2014. 2017. Accessed 18 July 2017. https://seer.cancer.gov/csr/1975_2014/.
4. Golpanian S, Tashiro J, Sola JE, Allen C, Lew JI, Hogan AR, Neville HL, Perez EA. Surgically treated pediatric nonpapillary thyroid carcinoma. *Eur J Pediatr Surg.* 2016;**26**(6):524–532.
5. Sugino K, Nagahama M, Kitagawa W, Shibuya H, Ohkuwa K, Uruno T, Suzuki A, Akaishi J, Masaki C, Matsuzu K, Ito K. Papillary thyroid carcinoma in children and adolescents: long-term follow-up and clinical characteristics. *World J Surg.* 2015;**39**(9):2259–2265.
6. Bauer AJ. Molecular genetics of thyroid cancer in children and adolescents. *Endocrinol Metab Clin North Am.* 2017;**46**(2):389–403.
7. Cordioli MI, Moraes L, Cury AN, Cerutti JM. Are we really at the dawn of understanding sporadic pediatric thyroid carcinoma? *Endocr Relat Cancer.* 2015;**22**(6):R311–R324.
8. Picarsic JL, Buryk MA, Ozolek J, Ranganathan S, Monaco SE, Simons JP, Witchel SF, Gurtunca N, Joyce J, Zhong S, Nikiforova MN, Nikiforov YE. Molecular characterization of sporadic pediatric thyroid carcinoma with the DNA/RNA ThyroSeq v2 next-generation sequencing assay. *Pediatr Dev Pathol.* 2016;**19**(2):115–122.
9. Waguespack SG, Francis G. Initial management and follow-up of differentiated thyroid cancer in children. *J Natl Compr Canc Netw.* 2010;**8**(11):1289–1300.
10. Golpanian S, Perez EA, Tashiro J, Lew JI, Sola JE, Hogan AR. Pediatric papillary thyroid carcinoma: outcomes and survival predictors in 2504 surgical patients. *Pediatr Surg Int.* 2016;**32**(3):201–208.
11. Amin MB, Edge S, Greene F, Byrd DR, Brookland RK, Washington MK, Gershenwald JE, Compton CC, Hess KR, Sullivan DC, Jessup JM, Brierley JD, Gaspar LE, Schilsky RL, Balch CM, Winchester DP, Asare EA, Madera M, Gress DM, Meyer LR, eds. *AJCC Cancer Staging Manual.* 8th ed. New York, NY: Springer International Publishing.
12. Haugen BR, Alexander EK, Bible KC, Doherty GM, Mandel SJ, Nikiforov YE, Pacini F, Randolph GW, Sawka AM, Schlumberger M, Schuff KG, Sherman SI, Sosa JA, Steward DL, Tuttle RM, Wartofsky L. 2015 American Thyroid Association management guidelines for adult patients with thyroid nodules and differentiated thyroid cancer: the American Thyroid Association Guidelines Task Force on Thyroid Nodules and Differentiated Thyroid Cancer. *Thyroid.* 2016;**26**(1):1–133.
13. Pawelczak M, David R, Franklin B, Kessler M, Lam L, Shah B. Outcomes of children and adolescents with well-differentiated thyroid carcinoma and pulmonary metastases following ^{131}I treatment: a systematic review. *Thyroid.* 2010;**20**(10):1095–1101.
14. Biko J, Reiners C, Kreissl MC, Verburg FA, Demidchik Y, Drozd V. Favourable course of disease after incomplete remission on (131)I therapy in children with pulmonary metastases of papillary thyroid carcinoma: 10 years follow-up. *Eur J Nucl Med Mol Imaging.* 2011; **38**(4):651–655.
15. Verburg FA, Hänscheid H, Luster M. Radioactive iodine (RAI) therapy for metastatic differentiated thyroid cancer. *Best Pract Res Clin Endocrinol Metab.* 2017;**31**(3):279–290.
16. Wassner AJ, Della Vecchia M, Jarolim P, Feldman HA, Huang SA. Prevalence and significance of thyroglobulin antibodies in pediatric thyroid cancer. *J Clin Endocrinol Metab.* 2017;**102**(9):3146–3153.
17. Vali R, Rachmiel M, Hamilton J, El Zein M, Wasserman J, Costantini DL, Charron M, Daneman A. The role of ultrasound in the follow-up of children with differentiated thyroid cancer. *Pediatr Radiol.* 2015;**45**(7):1039–1045.
18. Waguespack SG, Wasserman JD. Differentiated thyroid cancer in children. In: Mallick U, Harmer C, eds. *Practical Management of Thyroid Cancer: A Multidisciplinary Approach.* 2nd ed. New York, NY: Springer International Publishing, In Press.

Managing the Patient With Precocious Puberty: A Case-Based Discussion

M40
Presented, March 17–20, 2018

Karen Oerter Klein, MD. University of California, San Diego, La Jolla, California 92093; and Rady Children's Hospital, Sand Diego, California 92123, E-mail: kklein@ucsd.edu

SIGNIFICANCE OF THE CLINICAL PROBLEM

Diagnosing true precocious puberty continues to pose many challenges. This presentation will help the clinician think through the differential diagnosis of precocious puberty and distinguish true puberty from benign variants of puberty, as well as central vs peripheral puberty. The treatment options for central precocious puberty have expanded over the last several years, so considerations for choosing whom to treat and how to treat will also be discussed. Once a patient is receiving treatment, the next challenges are how to monitor treatment and optimize outcomes. Growth response, rate of bone maturation, hormonal suppression, and individualizing patient care will be considered. Deciding when to stop treatment and what to expect after discontinuation of treatment will be reviewed. We will explore how to answer patient and family questions about menarche, fertility, bone health, weight gain, and other long-term health considerations. Cases will be presented to address each of these issues. We will also discuss tools for evaluating the timing of puberty in children, essentials of physical pubertal examination, growth rate evaluation, and laboratory and radiographic studies.

BARRIERS TO OPTIMAL PRACTICE

- Clinicians face the challenge of the borderline patient who may or may not have pathology. This can be compounded by parents who insist on treatment.
- Lack of data on optimal suppression of hormones during Gonadotropin-releasing hormone (GnRH) analog treatment may appear as a barrier; however, we will review data available that help overcome this barrier.
- Another challenge clinicians face is when to stop treatment.

LEARNING OBJECTIVES

As a result of participating in this session, learners should be able to:

- Diagnose true central precocious puberty as distinguishable from other causes of pubertal change
- Normal range of pubertal onset and variables influencing onset
- Physical examination, growth patterns, laboratory testing, and imaging nuances
- Differential diagnosis
- Know the various treatment option pros and cons, and understand how to monitor treatment and evaluate growth during treatment
- Deciding whom to treat; age, bone age (BA), and growth variables
- Treatment options
- Laboratory and BA evaluation during treatment
- Know the variables involved in the decision of when to stop treatment and how to inform families what to expect long term after treatment is discontinued
- Factors involved in the decision of when to stop treatment
- Treatment outcomes: height, weight gain, menarche, fertility, bone health

STRATEGIES FOR DIAGNOSIS, THERAPY, AND/OR MANAGEMENT

1. Normal pubertal onset and progression based on National Health and Nutrition Examination Survey and Pediatric Research in Office Settings data (1–6)
   a. Average ages (AAs) in girls

	Breasts	Pubic Hair	Menses
AA	8.87 ± 1.93 y	8.78 ± 2.00 y	12.16 ± 1.21 y
White	9.96 ± 1.82 y	10.51 ± 1.67 y	12.88 ± 1.20 y

   b. AAs in boys

	Genital Stage 2	Pubic Hair	Testes ≥ 4 mL
White	10.14 y	11.47 y	11.46 y
AA	9.14 y	10.25 y	11.75 y
Hispanic	10.04 y	11.43 y	11.29 y

   c. Influences on onset
      i. Genetics, family history
      ii. Rate of weight gain
      iii. Geography
      iv. Ethnicity
2. The hypothalamic-pituitary-gonadal axis is inhibited before pubertal onset and activated by stimulatory neurotransmitters at the onset of puberty. This careful balance partially explains precocious puberty etiology.
   a. Negative feedback loops: between sex steroids, inhibin, anti-Müllerian hormone, and the pituitary and hypothalamus
   b. GnRH secretion pattern changes over lifetime and is pulsatile in nature.

3. Precocious puberty is defined as the onset of clinical signs of puberty before the age of 8 years in girls or 9 years in boys. The onset of puberty is influenced by genetics, ethnicity, weight gain, and environment (7).
   a. Precocious puberty can be central or peripheral and usually needs treatment when it is rapidly progressive, when compromises potential adult height, and/or for various psychosocial reasons.
   b. The diagnosis of precocious puberty is made by physical examination, BA radiographs, laboratory testing, and other imaging studies based on whether it is central or peripheral. Laboratory testing includes random estradiol or testosterone levels and luteinizing hormone (LH) and follicle-stimulating hormone (FSH) as well as stimulated LH and FSH levels.
4. Central pathology
   a. Idiopathic
   b. CNS lesions: hypothalamic hamartomas, tumors
   c. Genetic/familial: *MKRN3* inactivation mutations, *KISS1* and *KISS1R* activating mutations, and more (8–10)
5. Peripheral etiologies
   a. McCune-Albright syndrome: activating mutation of G protein
      i. Precocious puberty
      ii. Café au lait pigmentation
      iii. Polyostotic fibrous dysplasia of bones
      iv. Associated problems
         (1) Gigantism
         (2) Hyperthyroidism
         (3) Ovarian cysts
         (4) Cushing's syndrome
      v. Treatment
         (1) Block estrogen action: tamoxifen
         (2) Block estrogen production: aromatase inhibitors
   b. Familial male precocious puberty (testotoxicosis)
      i. Autosomal dominant/sex limited
      ii. Activation of G protein
      iii. Treatment
         (1) Antiandrogen plus aromatase inhibition
   c. Congenital adrenal hyperplasia
   d. Adrenal tumors
   e. Ovarian or testicular tumors (Leydig cell)
   f. Ectopic gonadotropins: teratomas, hepatoblastomas, choriocarcinomas, pineal tumors
6. Variations on puberty
   a. Premature thelarche
   b. Premature adrenarche
   c. Exogenous exposures: phytoestrogens (*i.e.*, lavender and tea tree oil)
   d. Obesity: drives earlier puberty
7. Diagnosis
   a. Thorough physical and pubertal examination
   b. Family history
   c. Growth assessment
   d. LH, FSH, sex steroid measures: baseline and GnRH stimulated
   e. BA radiograph
   f. Possible gonad, adrenal, or brain imaging
8. Whom to treat (11)?
   a. Early onset (age <8 years in girls, <9 years in boys)
   b. Rapid progression > 1 stage/yr
   c. Advanced BA: BA/chronologic age (CA) >1; BA >2 standard deviations
   d. Psychosocial issues
   e. Short predicted adult height for family
   f. Anyone with growth potential remaining (BA <13 years)
9. When to treat? Age and BA limit discussion
   a. As soon as rapid progression confirmed; better outcome with earlier treatment
   b. As long as growth potential exists
10. How to treat? Options (12–14)
   a. Monthly leuprolide depot: 7.5, 11.25, 15 mg
   b. Leuprolide depot every 3 months: 11.25 or 30 mg
   c. Histrelin implant yearly: 65 μg/d
   d. Triptorelin 22.5 mg every 6 months
   e. Safety and efficacy of all look good; no comparison studies done; individualize per family and patient preferences
11. How to monitor?
   a. Pubertal advance by physical examination
   b. Bone maturation: goal to slow BA/CA ≤1
   c. Growth: normal prepubertal rates
   d. Estimates of predicted adult height; should steadily improve on treatment
   e. Hormonal suppression: no definitive threshold levels; peak LH ≤4 to 5 IU/L; random LH levels ≤0.3 to 0.6 IU/L
   f. Important to consider all factors together; no one variable determines suppression
12. When to stop treatment (15, 16)?
   a. Age-appropriate development for peers
   b. Improved height predictions; almost always decrease once treatment stopped
   c. Concerns about decreased height potential if treatment stopped too soon
13. Outcomes (17–20)
   a. Height reaches midparental height if treated early and long enough
   b. Bone density: normal for pubertal stage
   c. Fertility: long-term data with fertility rates similar to general population
   d. Body mass: normal
   e. Menarche: occurs 3 months to 3 years after discontinuation of treatment; irregular cycles similar to general population
   f. Psychological: still being studied

MAIN CONCLUSIONS

- True central precocious puberty must have early onset of pubertal changes and rapid progression. This is usually before age 8 years in girls and 9 years in boys. Rapid progression includes physical changes, accelerated growth rate, and rapid maturation of BA.
- Age of onset of puberty is influenced by family background, ethnicity, weight gain, and exogenous exposures.
- Precocious puberty may be central or peripheral and may be idiopathic or caused by pathology requiring treatment.
- There are three main GnRH analogs available in the United States for treatment, and all show good safety and efficacy. Some have longer-term use than others. Patient and parent preferences can be considered.
- Treatment is monitored by physical examination, growth assessment, BA, and hormonal laboratory measures. GnRH-stimulated LH levels are still the most helpful.
- Treatment should be discontinued when child has age-appropriate development for peers, improvement in predicted adult height, and CA close to BA. Caution that predicted adult height decreases after treatment stopped.
- Outcome of treatment is good in all categories, with normal height, weight gain, menarche, fertility, bone health, and psychosocial health reported.

CASES

Case 1

- African American girl age 6 years 4 months
- Breast onset at age 6 years
- Height always 95%
- BA 7 years 6 months
- Predicted adult height = midparental height
- By age 7 years, breasts still stage 2 and BA 8 years
- Question: What is your diagnosis?

Case 2

- 4-year-old white girl with onset of breasts
- Growth acceleration
- BA 7 years 10 months
- Pubertal LH after GnRH stimulation
- Leuprolide treatment (every 3 months) started
- Peak LH of 3.2 IU/L after second injection
- Breasts softer and flatter
- Growth rate slightly slower
- BA advanced 1 year in 6 months
- Question: Is she adequately suppressed?

Case 3

- True central precocious puberty: when to stop treatment?
- 5-year-old with breasts since age 3 years, now pubic hair
- BA 9 years
- Growth rapid
- Hypothalamic hamartoma on central nervous system magnetic resonance imaging
- Predicted adult height 4 feet 8 inches
- GnRH analog treatment started
- By age 10 years, she is complaining that she wants to stop treatment; she is tired of shots, and some of her friends have bought bras.
- BA now 12 years; predicted height 5 feet 1 inch
- Question: What is your advice to the family about whether to stop treatment now?

DISCUSSION OF CASES AND ANSWERS

Case 1

Question: What Is Your Diagnosis?

Answer: Normal early puberty consistent with ethnic background. Key factors are: height consistent with no growth rate, height predicted similar to that of family, onset of breasts within expected time for ethnic background, and no rapid progression of physical findings or bone maturation.

Case 2

Question: Is She Adequately Suppressed?

Answer: Yes; BA maturation does not slow in first 6 months, so not concerning that it is advancing. With further follow-up, bone maturation starts to slow. If it did not, that would then be a concern. Clinical examination shows softer breasts and growth rate slowing down some. Again, it is early in treatment, so evaluation in 6 more months will be more helpful, but softer breasts reassures clinician he or she can keep watching. Reasonable hormone levels are reassuring. LH peak is <4 IU/L. This alone does not prove suppression, but with other findings, it is consistent with suppression. With time, bone maturation rate slowed further and LH decreased more.

Case 3

Question: What Is Your Advice to the Family About Whether to Stop Treatment Now?

Answer: Predicted height will decrease after treatment is stopped, and she does not yet have CA close to BA. Although some girls her age are now starting breast development, your daughter is already in midpuberty, and that will resume when treatment stopped. Strongly recommend continuing treatment longer to stop when age-appropriate development for peers, improved adult predicted height, and CA close to BA are achieved, as long as growth rate continues to be reasonable. If growth rate slows below normal prepubertal rates, then consider stopping treatment.

REFERENCES

1. Herman-Giddens ME, Slora EJ, Wasserman RC, Bourdony CJ, Bhapkar MV, Koch GG, Hasemeier CM. Secondary sexual characteristics and menses in young girls seen in office practice: a study from the Pediatric Research in Office Settings network. *Pediatrics*. 1997;**99**(4):505–512.
2. Herman-Giddens ME, Steffes J, Harris D, Slora E, Hussey M, Dowshen SA, Wasserman R, Serwint JR, Smitherman L, Reiter EO. Secondary

sexual characteristics in boys: data from the Pediatric Research in Office Settings Network. *Pediatrics.* 2012;**130**(5):e1058–e1068.

3. Kaplowitz PB, Oberfield SE. Reexamination of the age limit for defining when puberty is precocious in girls in the United States: implications for evaluation and treatment. Drug Therapeutics and Executive Committees of the Lawson Wilkins Pediatric Endocrine Society. *Pediatrics.* 1999;**104**(4 Pt 1):936–941.
4. Parent AS, Teilmann G, Juul A, Skakkebaek NE, Toppari J, Bourguignon JP. The timing of normal puberty and the age limits of sexual precocity: variations around the world, secular trends, and changes after migration. *Endocr Rev.* 2003;**24**(5):668–693.
5. Sørensen K, Mouritsen A, Aksglaede L, Hagen CP, Mogensen SS, Juul A. Recent secular trends in pubertal timing: implications for evaluation and diagnosis of precocious puberty. *Horm Res Paediatr.* 2012; **77**(3):137–145.
6. Tanner JM. *Growth at Adolescence*, 2nd ed. Oxford, United Kingdom: Blackwell Scientific Publications; 1962.
7. Kaplowitz P, Bloch C; Section on Endocrinology, American Academy of Pediatrics. Evaluation and referral of children with signs of early puberty [published online ahead of print December 14, 2015]. *Pediatrics.* doi: 10.1542/peds.2015-3732.
8. Abreu AP, Dauber A, Macedo DB, Noel SD, Brito VN, Gill JC, Cukier P, Thompson IR, Navarro VM, Gagliardi PC, Rodrigues T, Kochi C, Longui CA, Beckers D, de Zegher F, Montenegro LR, Mendonca BB, Carroll RS, Hirschhorn JN, Latronico AC, Kaiser UB. Central precocious puberty caused by mutations in the imprinted gene MKRN3. *N Engl J Med.* 2013;**368**(26):2467–2475.
9. Teles MG, Bianco SD, Brito VN, Trarbach EB, Kuohung W, Xu S, Seminara SB, Mendonca BB, Kaiser UB, Latronico ACA. A GPR54-activating mutation in a patient with central precocious puberty. *N Engl J Med.* 2008;**358**(7):709–715.
10. Bulcao Macedo D, Nahime Brito V, Latronico AC. New causes of central precocious puberty: the role of genetic factors. *Neuroendocrinology.* 2014;**100**(1):1–8.
11. Carel JC, Léger J. Clinical practice. Precocious puberty. *N Engl J Med.* 2008;**358**(22):2366–2377.
12. Lee PA, Klein K, Mauras N, Neely EK, Bloch CA, Larsen L, Mattia-Goldberg C, Chwalisz K. Efficacy and safety of leuprolide acetate 3-month depot 11.25 milligrams or 30 milligrams for the treatment of central precocious puberty. *J Clin Endocrinol Metab.* 2012;**97**(5): 1572–1580.
13. Silverman LA, Neely EK, Kletter GB, Lewis K, Chitra S, Terleckyj O, Eugster EA. Long-term continuous suppression with once-yearly histrelin subcutaneous implants for the treatment of central precocious puberty: a final report of a phase 3 multicenter trial. *J Clin Endocrinol Metab.* 2015;**100**(6):2354–2363.
14. Klein K, Yang J, Aisenberg J, Wright N, Kaplowitz P, Lahlou N, Linares J, Lundström E, Purcea D, Cassorla F. Efficacy and safety of triptorelin 6-month formulation in patients with central precocious puberty. *J Pediatr Endocrinol Metab.* 2016;**29**(11):1241–1248.
15. Carel JC, Lahlou N, Roger M, Chaussain JL. Precocious puberty and statural growth. *Hum Reprod Update.* 2004;**10**(2):135–147.
16. Carel JC, Eugster EA, Rogol A, Ghizzoni L, Palmert MR, Antoniazzi F, Berenbaum S, Bourguignon JP, Chrousos GP, Coste J, Deal S, de Vries L, Foster C, Heger S, Holland J, Jahnukainen K, Juul A, Kaplowitz P, Lahlou N, Lee MM, Lee P, Merke DP, Neely EK, Oostdijk W, Phillip M, Rosenfield RL, Shulman D, Styne D, Tauber M, Wit JM; ESPE-LWPES GnRH Analogs Consensus Conference Group. Consensus statement on the use of gonadotropin-releasing hormone analogs in children. *Pediatrics.* 2009;**123**(4):e752–e762.
17. Klein KO, Barnes KM, Jones JV, Feuillan PP, Cutler GB, Jr. Increased final height in precocious puberty after long-term treatment with LHRH agonists: the National Institutes of Health experience. *J Clin Endocrinol Metab.* 2001;**86**(10):4711–4716.
18. Fuqua JS. Treatment and outcomes of precocious puberty: an update. *J Clin Endocrinol Metab.* 2013;**98**(6):2198–2207.
19. Thornton P, Silverman LA, Geffner ME, Neely EK, Gould E, Danoff TM. Review of outcomes after cessation of gonadotropin-releasing hormone agonist treatment of girls with precocious puberty. *Pediatr Endocrinol Rev.* 2014;**11**(3):306–317.
20. Lazar L, Lebenthal Y, Yackobovitch-Gavan M, Shalitin S, de Vries L, Phillip M, Meyerovitch J. Treated and untreated women with idiopathic precocious puberty: BMI evolution, metabolic outcome, and general health between third and fifth decades. *J Clin Endocrinol Metab.* 2015;**100**(4):1445–1451.

Hypophosphatemic Rickets: Modern Molecules and Medical Management

M52
Presented, March 17–20, 2018

Michael A. Levine, MD, MACE, FAAP, FACP. Division of Endocrinology and Diabetes, The Children's Hospital of Philadelphia and Department of Pediatrics, University of Pennsylvania Perelman School of Medicine, Philadelphia, Pennsylvania 19104, E-mail: levinem@chop.edu

SIGNIFICANCE OF THE CLINICAL PROBLEM

The term rickets describes a childhood condition of defective skeletal mineralization and abnormal development of the growth plate. Rickets is a clinical and radiological diagnosis, and biochemical and genetic testing is used to identify or confirm the underlying cause. Rickets concerns the disruption of the growth plate architecture, whereas the term osteomalacia refers to impaired mineralization of the bone matrix. Rickets and osteomalacia occur together in children, whereas in adults, the equivalent defects in mineral metabolism result only in osteomalacia. In rickets, the chondrocytes in the growth plate become disorganized, and the normal columnar orientation is replaced with an expanded and irregular hypertrophic zone. In the bone tissue below the growth plate (metaphysis), the mineralization defect leads to the accumulation of osteoid. These abnormalities reduce bone strength and lead to compensatory widening of the growth plate and the associated metaphysis. The long bones are nevertheless weak, and skeletal deformities ensue.

Although nutritional vitamin D deficiency is the most common cause of rickets and osteomalacia (1), these conditions can also result from genetic defects that impair activation of vitamin D, reduce target tissue responsiveness to $1,25(OH)_2D$, or impair phosphorus reabsorption in the kidney. The most common form of genetic rickets is X-linked hypophosphatemic rickets (XLH), in which a defect in the *PHEX* gene results in increased circulating levels of the phosphatonin FGF23. Other genetic defects can also cause hypophosphatemic rickets through either excess FGF23 or impaired expression of the renal sodium phosphate cotransporters NPT2a and NPT2c that are FGF23 targets. Hypophosphatemic rickets can also result from certain tumors that produce excess FGF23, defects of the proximal renal tubule, or inadequate dietary supply or absorption of phosphorus.

It is important to distinguish vitamin D–deficient rickets from hypophosphatemic rickets, because the treatments for these two conditions are very different, and delay in prescribing the proper therapy for hypophosphatemic rickets can result in needless suffering, skeletal deformities, and impaired growth. Early recognition of hypophosphatemic rickets is particularly important, because more innovative and effective treatments for hypophosphatemic rickets will soon be available.

BARRIERS TO OPTIMAL PRACTICE

- The omission of a serum phosphorus test from most standard commercial "comprehensive metabolic panels" can delay recognition of hypophosphatemic rickets.
- Widespread deficiency or insufficiency of vitamin D can complicate the laboratory diagnosis of hypophosphatemic rickets.
- Restricted access to or lack of experience with genetic testing can delay or impede proper diagnosis of different forms of genetic rickets.

LEARNING OBJECTIVES

- As a result of participating in this session, learners should be able to recognize hypophosphatemic rickets and distinguish this form of rickets from nutritional rickets using specific biochemical and endocrine tests.
- Participants will be able to apply genetic testing to distinguish among the various forms of inherited hypophosphatemic rickets.
- Participants will be able explain the risks and benefits of conventional therapy for hypophosphatemic rickets and will be familiar with emerging treatments.

STRATEGIES FOR DIAGNOSIS, THERAPY, AND/OR MANAGEMENT

Etiology and Genetics

Hypophosphatemia is a general characteristic of rickets (2). In cases of rickets caused by deficiency or impaired action of vitamin D or calcium deficiency, hypophosphatemia is a consequence of secondary hyperparathyroidism, such that elevated serum levels of parathyroid hormone (PTH) reduce the renal tubular reabsorption of phosphate (TRP). Hypophosphatemic rickets also occurs in the absence of elevated serum levels of PTH in patients with genetic forms of hypophosphatemic rickets, tumor-induced osteomalacia, nutritional phosphorus deficiency, and primary renal tubular disorders (3). In all cases, the extracellular phosphate concentration is lower than that needed for optimal skeletal mineralization and proper maturation of the growth plate (4).

Genetic defects that affect phosphate homeostasis are important causes of hypophosphatemic rickets (4–6), and XLH [formerly termed hypophosphatemic vitamin D–resistant rickets; Mendelian Inheritance in Man (MIM) 307800] is the most common form of genetic rickets overall, with a prevalence of about 1 in 20,000. Serum levels of phosphate are reduced, and serum 1,25(OH)$_2$D levels are reduced or inappropriately normal; serum levels of total and/or bone-specific alkaline phosphatase are elevated, and serum calcium and PTH levels are normal. Hypophosphatemia results from decreased renal tubular reabsorption of phosphorus, but in children with active rickets, there is also a variable degree of reduced intestinal absorption of both phosphate and calcium. XLH is a dominant condition, and there is little if any difference in the severity or extent of the disorder in affected males and females. XLH is associated with defective bone mineralization, lower-extremity deformities, short stature, bone pain, enthesopathy, and dental abscesses.

XLH is caused by mutations in the *PHEX* gene (phosphate-regulating gene with homologies to endopeptidases on the X chromosome) that lead to a loss of enzymatic function. *PHEX* defects have been identified throughout the gene in patients with XLH and invariably lead to a loss of function (http://data.mch.mcgill.ca/phexdb for Phexdatabase). Although the genetic defect is highly penetrant, the severity of disease and specific clinical manifestations are variable, even among members of the same family. Commercial laboratories now provide clinical testing for mutations in the *PHEX* gene, and defects can be identified in 80% of patients with suspected XLH. However, the presence of the trait may be readily ascertained in most patients by 6 months of age by documentation of a reduced age-corrected concentration of plasma phosphate.

Patients with XLH have elevated plasma levels of FGF23, a phosphate-regulating hormone that is the principal circulating "phosphatonin" (4, 6). Osteocytes are the predominant FGF23 secretion site, and kidneys are its main targets. FGF23 acts directly on the kidney to alter phosphate transport and renal parameters of vitamin D metabolism. FGF23 reduces expression of the renal tubular sodium phosphate cotransporters Npt2a and Npt2c, thereby reducing the TRP or the maximum renal tubular phosphate reabsorption in mass per unit volume of glomerular filtrate (TmP/GFR). The loss of renal phosphate and to a lesser extent, decreased intestinal phosphate absorption lead to hypophosphatemia. In addition, FGF23 suppresses activity of the renal CYP27B1 (1α-hydroxylase), while inducing activity of the renal CYP24A1 (24-hydroxylase), which may, in part, explain the inappropriately normal (or low) circulating concentrations of 1,25(OH)$_2$D, despite hypophosphatemia.

In addition to XLH, at least four additional forms of inherited hypophosphatemic rickets have now been identified. Autosomal dominant hypophosphatemic rickets (MIM 193100) is caused by mutations in the *FGF23* gene encoding the phosphatonin FGF23 that prevents degradation of the protein. In addition, two forms of autosomal recessive hypophosphatemic rickets have been described that are caused by loss-of-function mutations in genes that encode proteins that are involved in FGF23 expression: (1) ARHR1 [Online Mendelian Inheritance in Man (OMIM) 241520] caused by the *DMP1* gene encoding dentin matrix protein 1, a noncollagenous bone matrix protein expressed in osteoblasts and osteocytes; and (2) ARHR2 (OMIM 613312) caused by the *ENPP1* gene encoding a phosphodiesterase that hydrolyzes adenosine triphosphate. Finally, it is worth noting that biallelic mutations in *FAM20C* have been identified in patients with elevated serum levels of FGF23, hypophosphatemia, hyperphosphaturia, dental anomalies, intracerebral calcifications, and osteosclerosis of the long bones in the absence of rickets. Hypophosphatemic rickets also occurs in patients with hereditary hypophosphatemic rickets with hypercalciuria (HHRH; OMIM 241530), which is caused by homozygous mutations in the *SLC34A3* gene encoding the renal Npt2c sodium phosphate cotransporter.

Circulating levels of FGF23 are usually elevated (or inappropriately normal) when measured with immunoassays that detect either intact or C-terminal FGF23 proteins in subjects with XLH, autosomal dominant hypophosphatemic rickets (ADHR), and autosomal recessive hypophosphatemic rickets (ARHR). By contrast, FGF23 is low or suppressed in patients with HHRH. Synthesis and processing of FGF23 are affected by iron (7), and iron deficiency leads to increased serum levels of C-terminal fragments of FGF23; levels of intact FGF23 remain normal in normal subjects and patients with XLH and ARHR, but they are elevated in patients with ADHR.

In addition to these hereditary conditions, hypophosphatemia, rickets, and/or osteomalacia can also occur because of excessive production of FGF23 by rare paraneoplastic and other disorders, including tumor-induced osteomalacia, fibrous dysplasia, neurofibromatosis, linear nevus sebaceous syndrome, and osteoglophonic dysplasia (8–10).

Pathophysiology

Hypophosphatemia usually appears in the first year of life. The biochemical findings are dominated by hypophosphatemia, with normal serum levels of calcium, PTH, and 25(OH)D. The ratio of TmP/GFR is subnormal in hypophosphatemic rickets, but age-dependent reference ranges must be used. The normal 1,25(OH)$_2$D concentration in the context of hypophosphatemia, which generally stimulates formation of 1,25(OH)$_2$D, reflects the elevated circulating concentrations of FGF23 in these disorders. HHRH can be distinguished from other forms of genetic hypophosphatemic rickets by the presence of low circulating levels of FGF23 and elevated levels of 1,25(OH)$_2$D that lead to hypercalciuria. Hypophosphatemic rickets can also develop in babies who are premature and/or receiving elemental formulas, in which case urinary phosphorus will be low and the TmP/GFR will be normal or elevated (11).

Diagnostic Findings

The primary clinical manifestations of hypophosphatemic rickets are skeletal pain and deformity, bone fractures, slipped epiphyses, and poor statural growth. Classic skeletal features of rickets, such as frontal bossing, may appear as early as 6 months of age in untreated infants. Early severe deformities (*viz.*, short stature and skeletal disproportion) become apparent during childhood, with the lower extremities short relative to the trunk. Notable deformities include coxa vara, anterior and lateral femoral bowing, genu valgum or varum, and medial deviation and torsion of the lower third of the tibia. A waddling gait is common. Unlike the findings in infants with vitamin D deficiency rickets, craniotabes and rachitic rosary are not present. In addition to the mineralization defect induced by hypophosphatemia, an intrinsic osteoblast defect also contributes to the bone disease and does not seem to respond to conventional treatment (see below). Proximal myopathy is absent in contrast to the findings in hypophosphatemia that occur later in life in patients with tumor-induced osteomalacia or antacid-induced hypophosphatemia. Poor dental development and spontaneous tooth abscesses may occur. Children with ARHR caused by *ENPP1* mutations often develop hearing loss (12).

In middle age, other clinical problems begin to appear, with mineralization of the spinal ligaments and thickening of the neural arches. There is loss of mobility of the spine, shoulders, elbows, and hips. The lumbar spine is flat and rigid, and reduction in the diameter of the spinal canal can lead to cord compression at more than one level. Painful secondary osteoarthritis in the hips and knees is common, as is a unique disorder of the entheses (tendons, ligaments, and joint capsules), with calcification of tendon and ligament insertions and joint capsules, particularly in the hand and sacroiliac joints.

Radiologic manifestations are evident by 1 to 2 years of age and include widening, splaying, and cupping of the metaphyses and coarse trabeculation of the whole skeleton. These findings are most pronounced in the lower extremities. The characteristic wedge-shaped defect of the medial surface of the proximal tibia in patients with genu varum deformity is probably the result of the increased weight on the medial side of the knee. Areal bone density as determined by dual energy x-ray absorptiometry is usually increased, but volumetric bone density may be reduced (13, 14). In rare cases, radiographs may not show growth plate changes that are diagnostic of rickets. In these patients, magnetic resonance imaging, particularly with diffusion tensor imaging, may disclose growth plate defects (15–17).

In contrast to XLH and ARHR, there seems to be greater variability in the age of onset and expression of the biochemical and clinical features of ADHR. Those with childhood onset look phenotypically like those with XLH, but some patients present with an apparent adult-onset form of the disorder, with reduced bone density (osteomalacia?), bone pain, weakness, and fractures but no skeletal deformity. Thus, ADHR is a phenotypically variable disorder with incomplete penetrance, delayed onset, and in several kindred, post-pubertal spontaneous resolution of the biochemical defect. A late-onset, milder form of HHRH has been described in adults who are carriers of only one defective SLC34A3 allele, which is characterized by hypophosphatemia, reduced bone mass, and renal stones (18).

Conventional Therapy

A combination of activated vitamin D (*e.g.*, calcitriol or 1α-cholecalciferol) and oral phosphorus constitutes conventional therapy and is currently the most effective treatment of genetic and acquired forms of hypophosphatemic rickets (19, 20). The main role of activated vitamin D is to counter the tendency of phosphate therapy to induce hypocalcemia and secondary hyperparathyroidism. Current practice is to use calcitriol (25 to 50 ng/kg/d) together with a neutral phosphate preparation (25 to 50 mg/kg phosphorus/d). Calcitriol can be given once or twice per day, whereas phosphate supplements should be given in four to five divided doses over the day. The dosage of calcitriol is adjusted to maintain the PTH in the midnormal range without inducing hypercalciuria or hypercalcemia. Patients with HHRH will require only phosphate salts, because they have elevated serum levels of 1,25$(OH)_2$D. The goal of therapy is to heal rickets and is not to normalize the serum phosphate level; hence, a normal age-adjusted serum alkaline phosphatase level and height velocity are appropriate indicators of therapeutic efficacy. The kidneys should be monitored by regular renal sonography; medullary nephrocalcinosis is common and usually caused by excessive urinary phosphate excretion, but it can be associated with nephrolithiasis when hypercalciuria occurs as well. Tertiary hyperparathyroidism can occur in patients who do not receive sufficient calcitriol to prevent secondary hyperparathyroidism. Although conventional therapy can improve bone mineralization, heal rickets, and in many cases, reduce dental abscesses (21, 22), it does not reverse the elevated serum level of FGF23 and does not seem to reduce the progression of other associated clinical features, such as enthesopathy. Moreover, statural deficits remain despite adequate treatment, and adult height is compromised (23). Small clinical trials of recombinant growth hormone have shown some improvement in growth (24, 25). Patients who have tumor-induced osteomalacia will receive the greatest benefit from surgical removal of the tumor that is producing FGF23, but these lesions are often quite small and difficult to locate.

Emerging Therapies

Antagonizing FGF23-mediated signaling seems to be a very promising approach to treatment of the hypophosphatemic disorders associated with FGF23 excess (26). Clinical trials of an investigational recombinant fully human monoclonal immunoglobulin G1 monoclonal antibody against FGF23 (KRN23, burosumab) have shown substantial efficacy and an acceptable safety profile in children and adults with XLH (27, 28). This antibody substantially increased the TmP/GFR, serum phosphorus concentration, and 1,25$(OH)_2$D without inducing secondary hyperparathyroidism and resulted in improvement in the rickets severity score in children and quality of life in adults (29). An alternative approach may be to reduce activity of CYP24, because genetic or pharmacological interventions that reduce CYP24 activity in murine models of hypophosphatemic rickets have been shown to result in near-complete recovery of rachitic/osteomalacic bony abnormalities in the absence of any improvement in the serum biochemical profile (30).

MAIN CONCLUSIONS

The diagnosis of hypophosphatemic rickets requires a high degree of suspicion, and standard biochemical testing should enable the physician to differentiate between nutritional vitamin D deficiency rickets and hypophosphatemic rickets. The family history and/or genetic testing provide important diagnostic insights and enable distinction among the various genetic forms of hypophosphatemic rickets. Although current therapy with conventional treatment can heal or improve rickets in XLH patients, this requires substantial effort and diligence. Treatment failure is common in many patients largely because of poor or inadequate compliance.

DISCUSSION OF CASES AND ANSWERS

Case 1

A 3-year, 2-month-old white male was referred to The Children's Hospital of Philadelphia for consultation regarding possible rickets. He was born to a G8P6A1 (ectopic) 33-year-old mother; there were no complications with pregnancy. The mother took prenatal vitamins from 6 months but cannot recall whether she took a multivitamin before that time. Pregnancy was to term, and the delivery was spontaneous vaginal delivery with no complications. Birth weight was 10 lb, 1 oz, and length was 22.5 in.

The child was breastfed for about a year and also received some infant formula (~4 to 8 oz/d almost every day). Solid foods were introduced at age 5 to 6 months old. He did not receive vitamin supplements. Growth and development were appropriate, except for large motor ability; weight has been consistently at 70% to 80%, but his height has been dropping consistently to the current 5%. Head circumference has been in 75th to 90th percentile.

Eruption of his first tooth was late, possibly at 12 months. He has not lost any teeth. He began to walk late at 20 months, and the parents noted abnormal gait at that time. Up until that time, he had no noticeable skeletal deformities and no fractures. At 26 months old, the mother took him to an orthopedist who diagnosed bilateral internal tibial torsion. No laboratory tests or radiographs were obtained. The parents were told that he needed physical therapy and would outgrow the problem.

About 10 weeks before our consultation, he was seen by another orthopedic surgeon who performed radiographs of the pelvis and lower extremities that showed rounding or cupping of the metaphysis. The distal femoral metaphyses were irregular. The hips were well seated and developing well. Morning laboratory tests showed serum phosphorus of 2.2 mg/dL, calcium of 8.7 mg/dL, creatinine of 0.2 mg/dL, 25(OH)D of 11 ng/mL, and PTH of 90 pg/mL. He was referred to a pediatric endocrinologist who repeated laboratory testing.

Urine phosphorus: 129 mg/dL
Urine creatinine: 47.90 mg/dL
Urine calcium: 2 mg/dL
25(OH)D: 10 ng/mL
Phosphorus: 2.5 mg/dL
Magnesium: 2.2 mg/dL
Calcium: 9.2 mg/dL
PTH: 95 pg/mL
Creatinine: 0.3 mg/dL
Alkaline phosphatase: 418 (40 to 290)

A diagnosis of healing nutritional rickets was made.

There is no family history of consanguinity, bone dysplasia, metabolic bone disease, renal stones, or fragility fractures.

Two weeks later at The Children's Hospital of Philadelphia, physical examination indicated the 4th percentile for height, with midparental height prediction of 69 in or nearly the 50th percentile. There was notable bowing of lower extremities, tibial torsion, and a stiff, waddling gait.

Questions

(1) What is the child's diagnosis?
(2) How would you treat this condition?
(3) What additional laboratory testing would you order?

Assessment

The history, physical examination, and laboratory studies suggested that this child had both nutritional vitamin D deficiency and hypophosphatemic rickets. Our plan was to treat first with vitamin D plus calcium: a loading dose of 50,000 IU of cholecalciferol followed by 2000 U of cholecalciferol per day plus 200 mg of elemental calcium three times daily for 1 month. At the conclusion of this treatment, we repeated laboratory tests: serum calcium was 9.5 mg/dL, creatinine was 0.3 mg/dL, alkaline phosphatase was 325, phosphorus was 2.6 mg/dL, magnesium was 2.2, 25(OH)D was 54 ng/dL, 1,25(OH)$_2$D was 67 pg/mL, and intact PTH was 60 pg/mL. The urine calcium/creatinine ratio was now 0.3 mg/mg, and the TRP was 75%. The patient was then started on conventional therapy for hypophosphatemic rickets with calcitriol and phosphate, and genetic studies were ordered.

Case 2

This 11-year, 11-month-old female was referred for consultation regarding hypophosphatemic rickets. She had originally presented to her endocrinologist for treatment of newly diagnosed hypophosphatemic rickets at age 8 years, 5 months old. There was a longstanding history of lower extremity stiffness and pain. Her older sister had been under treatment of years for hypophosphatemic rickets, and our patient was incidentally diagnosed with rickets when she accompanied her sister to a clinic visit. Laboratory testing revealed a low phosphorous of 2.6 mg/dL, with a low TRP of 70%. Her father is also very short and has a coincidental history of recurrent renal stones. The patient's older brother, now in his 20s, has recurrent knee pain and is same height as father. The paternal grandmother is short with bowed legs. The patient also has two other brothers who are taller than their father. The mother is very short and has no history of metabolic bone disease or renal stones.

The patient had been receiving calcitriol and phosphate treatment for years. In the past, laboratory studies had shown normal serum levels of 25(OH)D. Serum FGF23 was 20 (normal <230); PTH levels were low, and $1,25(OH)_2D$ levels were increased, even preceding treatment with calcitriol. There was no history of consanguinity. There were no dental problems. There was a history of hypercalciuria and bilateral renal stones. She has had one fracture (right forearm) after a fall. Radiographs commented on osteopenia. She had not had a dual energy x-ray absorptiometry scan.

She had been treated with recombinant growth hormone at age 5 years old for short stature when she fell off the growth curve, and since that time, she has been growing steadily at 1%. Recent radiographs of the lower extremities showed reduced mineralization, with down sloping of the distal femoral articular surfaces, and bilateral genu valgum widened growth plates.

Questions

(1) What is the child's diagnosis?

(2) What is the significance of the hypercalciuria and renal stones?

(3) How do you interpret the various biochemical tests?

(4) Based on the pedigree, what genetic tests would you order?

Assessment

The history and laboratory tests reveal an elevated serum $1,25(OH)_2D$ with a low PTH and hypercalciuria before beginning treatment with calcitriol and phosphate salts. In addition, serum levels of FGF23 are low. These are not typical features of hypophosphatemic rickets. In addition, the inheritance pattern is not consistent with X linkage or autosomal recessive forms of hypophosphatemic rickets. Dominantly inherited hypophosphatemic rickets is usually caused by mutations in the *FGF23* gene, which causes ADHR. Although the clinical and biochemical features in this case are most consistent with HHRH, the pattern of inheritance seems more dominant than recessive. Genetic testing revealed a unique pattern of digenic inheritance, in which the affected children carry heterozygous loss-of-function mutations in two different genes, *SLC34A1* and *SLC34A3*, encoding the two sodium phosphate cotransporters NPT2a and NPT2c, respectively. The proper treatment is to administer phosphate salts only.

REFERENCES

1. Uday S, Högler W. Nutritional rickets and osteomalacia in the twenty-first century: revised concepts, public health, and prevention strategies [published correction appears in *Curr Osteoporos Rep.* 2017; 15(5):507]. *Curr Osteoporos Rep.* 2017;**15**(4):293–302.
2. White KE, Hum JM, Econs MJ. Hypophosphatemic rickets: revealing novel control points for phosphate homeostasis. *Curr Osteoporos Rep.* 2014;**12**(3):252–3262.
3. Penido MG, Alon US. Hypophosphatemic rickets due to perturbations in renal tubular function. *Pediatr Nephrol.* 2014;**29**(3):361–373.
4. Goldsweig BK, Carpenter TO. Hypophosphatemic rickets: lessons from disrupted FGF23 control of phosphorus homeostasis. *Curr Osteoporos Rep.* 2015;**13**(2):88–97.
5. Razali NN, Hwu TT, Thilakavathy K. Phosphate homeostasis and genetic mutations of familial hypophosphatemic rickets. *J Pediatr Endocrinol Metab.* 2015;**28**(9-10):1009–1017.
6. Kinoshita S, Kawai M. The FGF23/KLOTHO regulatory network and its roles in human disorders. *Vitam Horm.* 2016;**101**:151–174.
7. Imel EA, Gray AK, Padgett LR, Econs MJ. Iron and fibroblast growth factor 23 in X-linked hypophosphatemia. *Bone.* 2014;**60**:87–92.
8. De Beur SM, Finnegan RB, Vassiliadis J, Cook B, Barberio D, Estes S, Manavalan P, Petroziello J, Madden SL, Cho JY, Kumar R, Levine MA, Schiavi SC. Tumors associated with oncogenic osteomalacia express genes important in bone and mineral metabolism. *J Bone Miner Res.* 2002;**17**(6):1102–1110.
9. Burckhardt MA, Schifferli A, Krieg AH, Baumhoer D, Szinnai G, Rudin C. Tumor-associated FGF-23-induced hypophosphatemic rickets in children: a case report and review of the literature. *Pediatr Nephrol.* 2015;**30**(1):179–182.
10. Ovejero D, Lim YH, Boyce AM, Gafni RI, McCarthy E, Nguyen TA, Eichenfield LF, DeKlotz CM, Guthrie LC, Tosi LL, Thornton PS, Choate KA, Collins MT. Cutaneous skeletal hypophosphatemia syndrome: clinical spectrum, natural history, and treatment. *Osteoporos Int.* 2016; **27**(12):3615–3626.
11. Gonzalez Ballesteros LF, Ma NS, Gordon RJ, Ward L, Backeljauw P, Wasserman H, Weber DR, DiMeglio LA, Gagne J, Stein R, Cody D, Simmons K, Zimakas P, Topor LS, Agrawal S, Calabria A, Tebben P, Faircloth R, Imel EA, Casey L, Carpenter TO. Unexpected widespread hypophosphatemia and bone disease associated with elemental formula use in infants and children. *Bone.* 2017;**97**:287–292.
12. Brachet C, Mansbach AL, Clerckx A, Deltenre P, Heinrichs C. Hearing loss is part of the clinical picture of ENPP1 loss of function mutation. *Horm Res Paediatr.* 2014;**81**(1):63–66.
13. Shanbhogue VV, Hansen S, Folkestad L, Brixen K, Beck-Nielsen SS. Bone geometry, volumetric density, microarchitecture, and estimated bone strength assessed by HR-pQCT in adult patients with hypophosphatemic rickets. *J Bone Miner Res.* 2015;**30**(1):176–183.
14. Colares Neto GP, Pereira RM, Alvarenga JC, Takayama L, Funari MF, Martin RM. Evaluation of bone mineral density and microarchitectural parameters by DXA and HR-pQCT in 37 children and adults with X-linked hypophosphatemic rickets. *Osteoporos Int.* 2017;**28**(5):1685–1692.
15. Tencza AL, Ichikawa S, Dang A, Kenagy D, McCarthy E, Econs MJ, Levine MA. Hypophosphatemic rickets with hypercalciuria due to mutation in SLC34A3/type IIc sodium-phosphate cotransporter: presentation as hypercalciuria and nephrolithiasis. *J Clin Endocrinol Metab.* 2009; **94**(11):4433–4438.
16. Lempicki M, Rothenbuhler A, Merzoug V, Franchi-Abella S, Chaussain C, Adamsbaum C, Linglart A. Magnetic resonance imaging features as surrogate markers of X-linked hypophosphatemic rickets activity. *Horm Res Paediatr.* 2017;**87**(4):244–253.
17. Ecklund K, Doria AS, Jaramillo D. Rickets on MR images. *Pediatr Radiol.* 1999;**29**(9):673–675.
18. Dhir G, Li D, Hakonarson H, Levine MA. Late-onset hereditary hypophosphatemic rickets with hypercalciuria (HHRH) due to mutation of SLC34A3/NPT2c. *Bone.* 2017;**97**:15–19.
19. Linglart A, Biosse-Duplan M, Briot K, Chaussain C, Esterle L, Guillaume-Czitrom S, Kamenicky P, Nevoux J, Prié D, Rothenbuhler A, Wicart P, Harvengt P. Therapeutic management of hypophosphatemic rickets from infancy to adulthood. *Endocr Connect.* 2014;**3**(1):R13–R30.

20. Sharkey MS, Grunseich K, Carpenter TO. Contemporary medical and surgical management of X-linked hypophosphatemic rickets. *J Am Acad Orthop Surg.* 2015;**23**(7):433–442.
21. Connor J, Olear EA, Insogna KL, Katz L, Baker S, Kaur R, Simpson CA, Sterpka J, Dubrow R, Zhang JH, Carpenter TO. Conventional therapy in adults with X-linked hypophosphatemia: effects on enthesopathy and dental disease. *J Clin Endocrinol Metab.* 2015;**100**(10): 3625–3632.
22. Biosse Duplan M, Coyac BR, Bardet C, Zadikian C, Rothenbuhler A, Kamenicky P, Briot K, Linglart A, Chaussain C. Phosphate and vitamin d prevent periodontitis in X-linked hypophosphatemia. *J Dent Res.* 2017;**96**(4):388–395.
23. Fuente R, Gil-Peña H, Claramunt-Taberner D, Hernández O, Fernández-Iglesias A, Alonso-Durán L, Rodríguez-Rubio E, Santos F. X-linked hypophosphatemia and growth. *Rev Endocr Metab Disord.* 2017; **18**(1):107–115.
24. Rothenbuhler A, Esterle L, Gueorguieva I, Salles JP, Mignot B, Colle M, Linglart A. Two-year recombinant human growth hormone (rhGH) treatment is more effective in pre-pubertal compared to pubertal short children with X-linked hypophosphatemic rickets (XLHR). *Growth Horm IGF Res.* 2017;**36**:11–15.
25. Meyerhoff N, Haffner D, Staude H, Wühl E, Marx M, Beetz R, Querfeld U, Holder M, Billing H, Rabl W, Schröder C, Hiort O, Brämswig JH, Richter-Unruh A, Schnabel D, Živičnjak M; Hypophosphatemic Rickets Study Group of the "Deutsche Gesellschaft für Kinderendokrinologie und -diabetologie" and "Gesellschaft für Pädiatrische Nephrologie". Effects of growth hormone treatment on adult height in severely short children with X-linked hypophosphatemic rickets [published online ahead of print October 20, 2017]. *Pediatr Nephrol.*.
26. Katoh M. Therapeutics targeting FGF signaling network in human diseases. *Trends Pharmacol Sci.* 2016;**37**(12):1081–1096.
27. Carpenter TO, Imel EA, Ruppe MD, Weber TJ, Klausner MA, Wooddell MM, Kawakami T, Ito T, Zhang X, Humphrey J, Insogna KL, Peacock M. Randomized trial of the anti-FGF23 antibody KRN23 in X-linked hypophosphatemia. *J Clin Invest.* 2014;**124**(4):1587–1597.
28. Imel EA, Zhang X, Ruppe MD, Weber TJ, Klausner MA, Ito T, Vergeire M, Humphrey JS, Glorieux FH, Portale AA, Insogna K, Peacock M, Carpenter TO. Prolonged correction of serum phosphorus in adults with X-linked hypophosphatemia using monthly doses of KRN23. *J Clin Endocrinol Metab.* 2015;**100**(7):2565–2573.
29. Ruppe MD, Zhang X, Imel EA, Weber TJ, Klausner MA, Ito T, Vergeire M, Humphrey JS, Glorieux FH, Portale AA, Insogna K, Peacock M, Carpenter TO. Effect of four monthly doses of a human monoclonal anti-FGF23 antibody (KRN23) on quality of life in X-linked hypophosphatemia. *Bone Rep.* 2016;**5**:158–162.
30. Bai X, Miao D, Xiao S, Qiu D, St-Arnaud R, Petkovich M, Gupta A, Goltzman D, Karaplis AC. CYP24 inhibition as a therapeutic target in FGF23-mediated renal phosphate wasting disorders. *J Clin Invest.* 2016;**126**(2):667–680.

Neonatal Hypoglycemia

M57
Presented, March 17–20, 2018

Mark A. Sperling, MD. Department of Pediatric Endocrinology and Diabetes, Icahn School of Medicine, Mount Sinai Hospital, New York, New York 10029, E-mail: masp@pitt.edu

SIGNIFICANCE OF THE CLINICAL PROBLEM

During pregnancy, human fetal glucose requirements are met entirely by placental transfer from mother to fetus, without any endogenous fetal glucose production (1, 2). At birth, clamping of the umbilical cord interrupts this glucose supply and imposes an immediate need to mobilize endogenous sources by breaking down glycogen and fat stores, deposited largely in the third trimester, to meet nutritional requirements. This is accomplished by hormonal changes characterized by a surge in glucagon and epinephrine with a simultaneous transient decline in insulin (3, 4); growth hormone [GH (20 to 40 ng/mL)] and cortisol are high at birth (5, 6). Until these counterregulatory hormones take effect, glucose may fall to a nadir of ~40 mg/dL, or occasionally less, which generally recovers after ~6 to 24 hours and is followed over the next 24 to 48 hours by the establishment of glucose values ≥60 mg/dL (7). In addition, the hormonal changes, accompanied by maturation of enzyme systems and hormone-receptor coupling, permit the induction of gluconeogenesis and ketogenesis by 24 to 48 hours of life to sustain energy needs between feedings (2, 7). Insulin values are lower in the newborn, but insulin action is facilitated by insulin receptors in liver and other tissues that are several times higher in number and affinity than in an adult so that the fetus and newborn are exquisitely sensitive to insulin action (8). Variable insulin extraction by the liver means that C-peptide is a better marker of endogenous secretion than a peripheral insulin level (9). In a healthy, full-term, vaginally delivered infant, these transitional adaptations generally are completed by 72 hours so that glucose metabolism and values are highly similar to that of adults with normal glucose concentrations of ≥70 mg/dL. The rate of glucose turnover in a normal infant is 4 to 6 mg/kg/min or about two- to threefold higher than in adults; most of the glucose is used by the brain, an obligatory glucose utilizer (7, 10). Counterregulation of impending hypoglycemia occurs at higher glucose levels in newborns than in adults, possibly as a neuroprotective safeguard. Thus, any deviation of these normal adaptive events predisposes to hypoglycemia, which recently has been defined as <55 mg/dL in an infant at 24 to 48 hours and <60 mg/dL in an infant at ≥72 hours (7, 11). In premature newborns or newborns with intrauterine growth restriction, the lack of tissue stores of glycogen, fat, and protein and delayed enzyme maturation may prolong the period of adaptation, but generally speaking, a blood glucose <55 mg/dL at or beyond day 3 of life requires confirmation and evaluation and should be considered as possible persistent hypoglycemia (7, 11). The major symptoms and signs of hypoglycemia are nonspecific but are focused on disturbed brain functions (Table 1). There are four major causes of persistent hypoglycemia. Persistent hyperinsulinism (HI) is the most common and most serious cause because the metabolic profile of low glucose, low ketones, and low fatty acids caused by excess insulin action leave the brain with no alternate fuel, so permanent neurologic sequelae may be severe. Neurologic sequelae are more likely when clinical manifestations appear in the neonatal period rather than in infancy and when there is no or poor response to medical therapy, implying a more severe defect in dysregulated insulin secretion. Counterregulatory hormone deficiency, usually cortisol or GH, is the next major cause. Clues such as midline facial cleft features, nystagmus, microphallus, and hyperpigmentation may point to pituitary-adrenal axis defects or primary adrenal insufficiency syndromes (Table 2). Glycogen storage diseases (GSDs) do not usually manifest in a neonate because the three to four hourly feedings mask the appearance. Hepatomegaly and a distinct metabolic profile point to these entities. Finally, fatty acid oxidation (FAO) defects, included in current neonatal screening programs, have distinct metabolic profiles and generally do not present in the newborn period when the baby receives frequent feedings but, rather, during an intercurrent illness with fasting that provokes a hypoglycemic response.

We will discuss several cases of persistent HI and counterregulatory hormone deficiency, omitting GSDs and FAO defects because these are rare and less likely to manifest in the neonatal period. The metabolic profile (Fig. 1) is the most useful aid in focusing the investigation of hypoglycemia. Note that in the immediate newborn period, hypopituitarism may mimic HI, which is the most severe problem because of neurologic sequelae; the earlier the manifestations occur, the more severe the hypoglycemia, the least responsive the newborn is to medical therapy, and the more likely the prediction for permanent neurologic sequelae.

BARRRIERS TO OPTIMAL PRACTICE

The major barrier to optimal practice is the nonspecific nature of the symptoms (Table 2). When severe, neurologic pathology is considered, but hypoglycemia may not be rapidly excluded as the cause because of a lack of awareness of the entity. A second major barrier is the practice of discharging newborns as early as day 2 of life without confirming that

Table 1 Signs of Hypoglycemia in the Neonate

Lethargy/somnolence
Irritability/fussiness
Feeding difficulty
Jitteriness/myoclonic jerks
Hypotonia/wilting spells
Temperature instability (subnormal temperature)
High-pitched cry
Sweating
Apnea
Seizures
Coma

glucose levels remain >55 mg/dL before a scheduled feed or after missing a feed (6- to 8-hour fast) or on day 3 if glucose is not maintained >60 mg/dL.

LEARNING OBJECTIVES

As a result of participating in this session, participants should be able to:

- Be familiar with the major causes of persistent hypoglycemia in the newborn and distinguish the etiology on the basis of the hormonal and metabolic profile
- Be aware of and diagnose the common genetic causes as well as more recently described entities of HI that cause hypoglycemia
- Describe the dangers and consequences of severe hypoglycemia in the newborn and formulate management strategies by using available technology

STRATEGIES FOR DIAGNOSIS, THERAPY, AND/OR MANAGEMENT

There has been much controversy about what constitutes hypoglycemia in the newborn. In the past, values of ≤45 or ≤40 mg/dL have been used. On the basis of an abundance of caution and review of normal physiology, any value <60 mg/dL (at which point counterregulation has been shown to occur in newborns) on day 3 of life should be evaluated and a value of <55 mg/dL (3 mmol/L) should be treated and investigated, according to recently proposed guidelines from the Pediatric Endocrine Society (7, 11). Whether such values are associated with neurologic deficits has not been determined, however. Although no specific single glucose concentration defines hypoglycemia, which will cause neurologic deficits, glucose values <40 mg/dL are more likely to do so, and severity of deficits may be determined by additional coexisting factors, such as duration of hypoglycemia, hypoxia, or sepsis (12, 13). Insulin secretion ceases at glucose concentrations <50 mg/dL, so any measurable insulin value at the time of hypoglycemia is possibly abnormal. Because of variable glucose extraction by the liver, a C-peptide value is a better reflection of insulin secretion. A C-peptide value of ≥0.5 ng/mL has been reported to strongly predict HI with a sensitivity of 85%; a coexisting β-hydroxybutyrate (β-OHB) concentration of ≤1.8 mmol/L was 100% sensitive (9). At the time of hypoglycemia, an injection of 1 mg of glucagon intramuscularly or intravenously (IV), which raises glucose concentrations by ≥30 mg/dL 30 minutes after injection, also strongly predicts HI because it indicates that endogenous glycogen breakdown had been inhibited by insulin but that glycogen reserves are adequate and glycogen breakdown mechanisms are intact. Although bedside measurements through point-of-care meters for glucose and ketones are useful, a definitive diagnosis must rely on formal laboratory measurements (7, 11). Thus, the criteria for establishing the diagnosis of HI are as follows:

- A high index of suspicion exists on the basis of clinical signs and history (*e.g.*, family history of a similar problem in a first-degree relative), as outlined in Table 1.
- Coexisting features are present on clinical examination of the patient (Table 2).
- Laboratory-based low glucose concentration values confirm a point-of-care value together with other laboratory features of HI, such as low β-OHB, inappropriate insulin/C-peptide for a newborn (reference range should be for newborns and infants not for adults, where insulin values of 5 to 20 μU/mL are considered normal), absence of acidosis, and a low free fatty acid (FFA) concentration (Fig. 1). These are the essential elements of the critical sample taken at the time of hypoglycemia. Missing the opportunity to take the sample at the time of hypoglycemia requires provoking hypoglycemia through a short fast, which may provoke hypoglycemia in as little

Table 2 Diagnostic Clues for Hypoglycemia

Cause of Hypoglycemia	Diagnostic Clues
HI	Born large for gestational age
	Requirement for glucose infusion rate >10 mg/kg/min; positive family history for prior case
Hypopituitarism (ACTH and/or GH deficiencies)	Midface hypoplasia
	Cleft lip/palate
	Nystagmus
	Microphallus, cryptorchidism
	Prolonged jaundice
Adrenal insufficiency	Ambiguous genitalia
	Hyperpigmentation
	Hyponatremia/hyperkalemia
Gluconeogenic defect	Hepatomegaly
Beckwith-Wiedemann syndrome	Macroglossia
	Earlobe fissures
	Hemihypertrophy
	Umbilical hernia/omphalocele

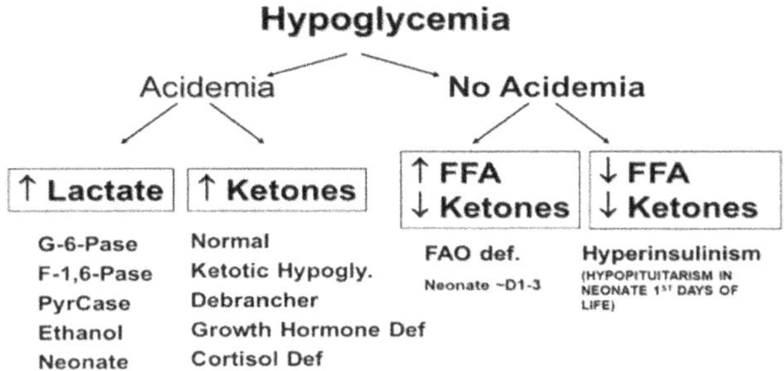

Figure 1. Metabolic profiles of the major categories of hypoglycemia. Concurrent acidemia implies a defect in gluconeogenesis or glycogen storage/release. In the absence of acidemia, a defect in FAO or HI are the likely causes. However, with FAO, FFA levels are increased, whereas in HI, all nutrients are depressed, the only entity in which this occurs and the reason for neurologic deficits that occur with HI. Note that in the first days of life, these changes may exist in infants with FAO or hypopituitarism because of a delay in maturation of enzyme systems.

as 6 hours in a newborn (*i.e.*, missing one feeding) or longer in older infants. At the time of the critical sample, following up with a glucagon challenge may provide further indirect evidence for HI. If the infant is on IV glucose infusion, a requirement of ≥10 mg/kg/min to maintain glucose concentrations >60 mg/dL is also indirect evidence for HI because the normal glucose requirement would be 4 to 6 mg/kg/min (10).

- Critical sample assessment for a diagnosis of HI when glucose is ≤50 mg/dL shows insulin ≥2.5 μU/mL or C-peptide ≥0.5 ng/mL (C-peptide likely offers best discrimination), β-OHB ≤2.0 mmol/L, and FFA ≤1.7 mmol/L.
- Indirect evidence would be an increase in glucose by ≥30 mg/dL 30 min after a 1 mg IV glucagon challenge and a glucose infusion rate necessary to maintain a glucose concentration of ≥10 mg/kg/min.

Therapy and Management

Once established as the diagnosis, treatment of HI should be initiated through supplemented caloric intake or IV glucose infusion to maintain glucose concentrations ≥60 mg/dL (≥3.5 mmol) as well as testing whether the entity is sensitive to diazoxide. This drug acts on the adenosine triphosphate (ATP)–regulated potassium channel (K_{ATP}) to inhibit closure and, hence, insulin secretion and is effective in some patients. A starting daily dose of 5 to 10 mg/kg/d (depending on severity) given orally in three divided doses is recommended. Although serious side effects may occur, they are reduced by concomitant use of hydrochlorothiazide 10 mg/kg/d to minimize fluid retention, and a recent analysis from a single institution revealed a good safety and effectiveness profile (14). Changes in dosage should only be made every 3 days to allow for the pharmacokinetics to reveal the desired effect. Although other experimental therapies have been proposed [*e.g.*, the use of sirolimus (15) and others (16)], none are approved for use in HI. Although these measures are ongoing, consideration must be given to the underlying cause, especially whether the genetic basis indicates a diffuse or focal lesion in the pancreas. The causes of HI include hypoxia (*e.g.*, as occurs with difficult delivery and preeclampsia) by mechanisms that are not understood but which usually respond to supplemental nutrition and may require the use of diazoxide. Genetic disturbances in the regulation of insulin secretion, especially those involving the K_{ATP} channel and including defects in imprinted genes associated with methylation defects, are the most common causes of persistent HI (11, 16, 17). Table 3 lists a classification of hypoglycemia in the newborn, and Fig. 2 illustrates the nine currently identified genetic defects regulating insulin secretion and causing hypoglycemia. The most common defects affect the sulfonylurea subunit of K_{ATP} defined by inactivating mutations in the *ABCC8* gene; inactivating mutations in the inwardly rectifying potassium channel itself, specified by the gene *KCNJ11*, also occur but are less common. Mutations occurring within families as autosomal dominant tend to have a milder course and to be sensitive to treatment with diazoxide. In the absence of a family history (*e.g.*, MEN1 with pancreatic insulinomas), mutational analysis for common mutations may be obtained commercially or possibly in centers with a research interest in these entities. A mutation in the patient together with the same mutation in both parents suggest an autosomal-recessive condition associated with diffuse pancreatic involvement and distinct histologic features that may require subtotal pancreatectomy; residual hypoglycemia and/or insulin-requiring diabetes frequently occur after this procedure. However, absence of the mutation in the mother but presence of a paternal mutation suggest a focal lesion that could be surgically resected and result in a cure. The focal lesion may be localized through 18F-fluoro-L-DOPA positron emission tomography (PET) scanning (18), which only is available in some institutions; studies suggest that ~50% of patients with K_{ATP} mutations have the focal form (11, 19). Mutations in *GLUD* (glutamate dehydrogenase) give rise to another common genetic form of HI previously known as leucine-sensitive hypoglycemia, but these may present later, have a milder course, are characterized by a modest increase in plasma ammonia levels, and respond to diazoxide (11, 19). Abnormal methylation patterns are found in Beckwith-Wiedemann syndrome [BWS (16, 20)]; Kabuki syndrome (16, 21); and, occasionally, the 6q24 chromosome region, which is more commonly associated with neonatal diabetes mellitus rather than with hypoglycemia (22).

Table 3 Hypoglycemia in Neonates and Infants: Working Classification

Classification	Description
Postprandial	Galactosemia
Postabsorptive	
HI	Infant of a diabetic mother
	Neonatal asphyxia
	Erythroblastosis fetalis
	Maternal tocolytics (β-sympathomimetic terbutaline)
	Genetic causes: insulin secretion, action, methylation
Non-HI	Hormone deficiency: cortisol/GH
	Systemic: sepsis, prematurity, liver disease
	GSD (I, III, IV): uncommon in the newborn
	Fatty acid metabolism defects: uncommon in the newborn

Table 3 displays a working classification of hypoglycemia in the neonate and infant beyond the first 3 days of life in a full-term baby. GSD rarely presents in the newborn because the frequent feedings every 3 to 4 hours mask the existence of hypoglycemia in most cases so that later manifestations of poor growth, hepatomegaly, and lordosis with ketosis predominate (23). Similarly, FAO defects rarely become apparent unless unmasked by very poor feeding during an intercurrent illness usually beyond 3 months of life; neonatal screening programs do test for FAO defects. HI and hormone deficiencies are the most common causes of persistent hypoglycemia in the newborn (11).

Methylation Disorders

Disorders such as BWS are frequently associated with hypoglycemia and HI because of differential methylation of imprinted maternal and paternal genes in a region of chromosome 11. Uniparental disomy of the paternal gene allows for expression of IGF2, which promotes growth without the restraining effects of maternal genes such as *H19* (Kip57); such changes also may occur randomly, affecting the maternal or paternal region (16, 20). Kabuki syndrome also results from defects in methylation or demethylation and, hence, may have HI among other endocrine manifestations (16, 21).

SUMMARY

HI is the most common cause of persistent hypoglycemia in the newborn that continues into infancy, resulting in a high risk of seizures and mental retardation unless recognized and treated promptly. Inheritance is heterogeneous, and many have spontaneous mutations most commonly in the K_{ATP} genes *ABCC8* (SUR1) and *KCNJ11* (Kir6.2), which may yield a diffuse lesion as a result of autosomal-recessive or -dominant mutations or focal lesions as a result of inheritance of a paternal mutation together with a maternal allele mutation early in embryogenesis that lead to loss of the normal maternal gene in a discrete region of the pancreas. Focal lesions can be identified by 18F-fluoro-L-DOPA PET scanning and can be surgically resected, resulting in a cure, whereas diffuse lesions, if unresponsive to medical management, may require subtotal pancreatectomy with a high risk for subsequent diabetes. Medical management through increasing caloric intake, with diazoxide, and/or with long-acting somatostatin analogs is effective in controlling hypoglycemia in some patients; side effects of somatostatin analogs include tachyphylaxis and necrotizing enterocolitis, particularly in premature babies in whom this drug is best avoided. Novel therapies are being attempted through such agents as sirolimus but are not approved for routine clinical use. Methylation defects are responsible for the HI seen in BWS and Kabuki syndrome. In ~30% to 50% of HI, the genetic basis remains to be discovered. Congenital defects in pituitary development resulting in adrenocorticotropic hormone (ACTH)-cortisol and/or GH deficiency as well as primary defects in adrenal development also result in neonatal hypoglycemia and must be excluded and treated.

CASES WITH DISCUSSION AND ANSWERS

Case 1

A baby boy was born at term to African parents who immigrated from a village in Conakry, Guinea, with a normal birth weight (3195 g) and length (50 cm), normal male genitalia, and no recognizable anomalies apart from darkly melanotic skin (Fig. 3). He developed hypoglycemia of 18 mg/dL at 4 hours, which persisted and was treated in the neonatal intensive care unit with glucose infusion of 5 mg/kg/min and by supplementing normal feedings. Critical samples drawn at the time of severe hypoglycemia (on more than one occasion) showed an undetectable cortisol level (<1 μg/dL) that failed to increase with exogenous ACTH along with a basal GH level of 7.5 ng/mL that failed to increase with glucagon stimulation. Thyroid function and prolactin levels were normal for his age. Insulin and β-OHB were both low. While awaiting results from laboratory testing, he developed cholestatic jaundice. Sodium was 130 to 134 mmol/L, and potassium was 4.7 to 5.0 mmol/L. All the results of newborn screening were normal.

What is your presumptive diagnosis? What other information and tests would you require to define the problem? Magnetic resonance imaging of the brain/pituitary gland was considered normal; ACTH levels ranged from 3885 to 4868 pg/mL. Treatment with high-dose cortisol (50 mg/m^2/d) resulted in alleviation of hypoglycemia, lightening of the skin, resolution of cholestasis, and restoration of normal GH associated with normal growth.

In what organ is the primary problem, the adrenal or pituitary gland? If the adrenal gland (because ACTH is markedly elevated) why is there GH deficiency? If the pituitary gland is

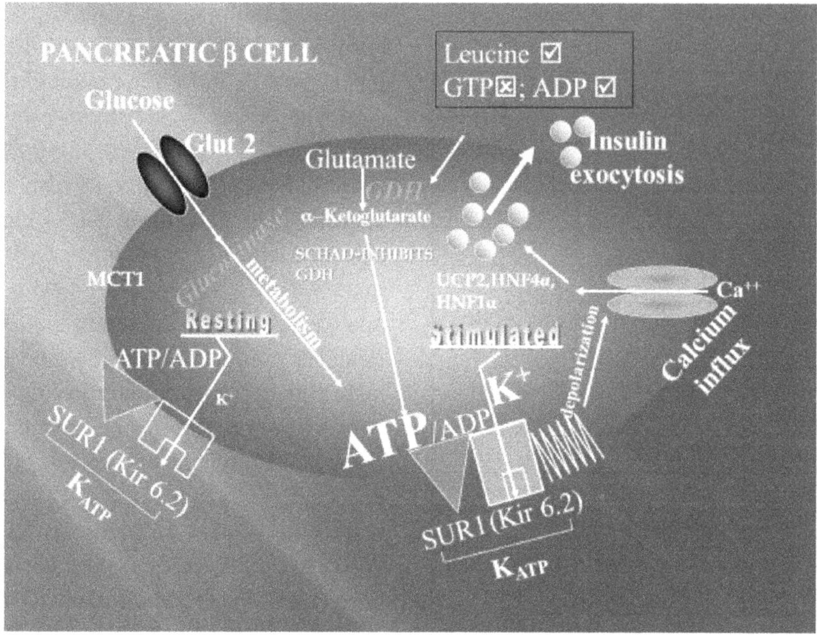

Figure 2. Genetic forms of congenital HI. Glucose triggers insulin release through its metabolism to produce ATP; the rise in ATP/adenosine diphosphate (ADP) ratio causes closure of the K_{ATP} channel, depolarization of the plasma membrane; activation of voltage-dependent calcium channels; and a rise in cytosolic calcium, which results in the release of insulin from stored granules. Note that diazoxide suppresses insulin release by opening K_{ATP} channels, whereas sulfonylureas promote insulin release by closing the channels. Leucine is an allosteric stimulus for glutamate dehydrogenase (GDH), the cause of leucine-sensitive hypoglycemia. A check mark indicates a positive stimulating signal; an *x*, a negative inhibitory signal. The nine currently identified genetic product defects regulating insulin secretion and causing hypoglycemia are glucokinase (GK); GDH; sulfonylurea receptor (SUR1); potassium ion pore (Kir6.2); pyruvate transporter (MCT1); short-chain 3-OH-acyl-CoA dehydrogenase (SCHAD), which normally inhibits GDH; hepatocyte nuclear factors 4α and 1α (HNF4α and HNF1α), which are most commonly associated with maturity onset diabetes of the young 1 and 3, respectively, but early in life, may have HI; and uncoupling protein 2 (UCP2), a mitochondrial gene (11, 19). An activating mutation in hexokinase, a homolog of GK, has been reported (27), as has an activating mutation in a calcium channel, but their roles in HI are not yet fully established (28).

the site of GH deficiency, why is ACTH elevated? Molecular testing of the ACTH resistance custom gene panel (*NNT, MC2R, MRAP*) revealed a known inactivating homozygous mutation in the *MC2R* gene, the ACTH receptor (c.634del, p.Arg212Fs*). Additional questioning of the parents suggested that they are likely distant cousins. A similar constellation of congenital cortisol deficiency with transient GH deficiency was reported in a patient with ACTH receptor deficiency (high ACTH) as well as in another with ACTH deficiency; therefore, the authors postulated that physiologic glucocorticoid levels are required for the development and function of somatotrophic cells during fetal life and infancy (24).

Case 2

A baby girl was born at term to unrelated young healthy parents, with a birth weight of 4840 g. At 2 hours of life, she was noted to be jittery, and plasma glucose was reported as 9 mg/dL. Physical examination revealed no abnormalities, in particular absence of macroglossia, umbilical hernia, and hemihypertrophy; family history was negative for any disorders associated with hypoglycemia. Her urine tested negative for ketones. A critical blood sample during a hypoglycemic episode of 29 mg/dL showed an insulin level of 36 μU/mL, GH of 30 ng/mL, and cortisol of 35 μg/dL. Glucose-infused IV at a rate of 15 mg/kg/min stabilized blood glucose, and she experienced treatment failure of a trial of diazoxide at 10 mg/kg/d. Genetic analysis revealed a heterozygous mutation in the *ABCC8* gene c.3989 G>A, which is known to be associated with HI. What should be the next steps in managing this patient?

The father had the same heterozygous mutation but was asymptomatic; the mother did not have any mutation. Could this be an autosomal-dominant form of HI? What are the next steps? An 18F-fluoro-L-DOPA PET scan showed a solitary lesion in the head of the pancreas, and this was surgically resected with resultant cure of hypoglycemia and no disturbances in glucose homeostasis. How did this solitary

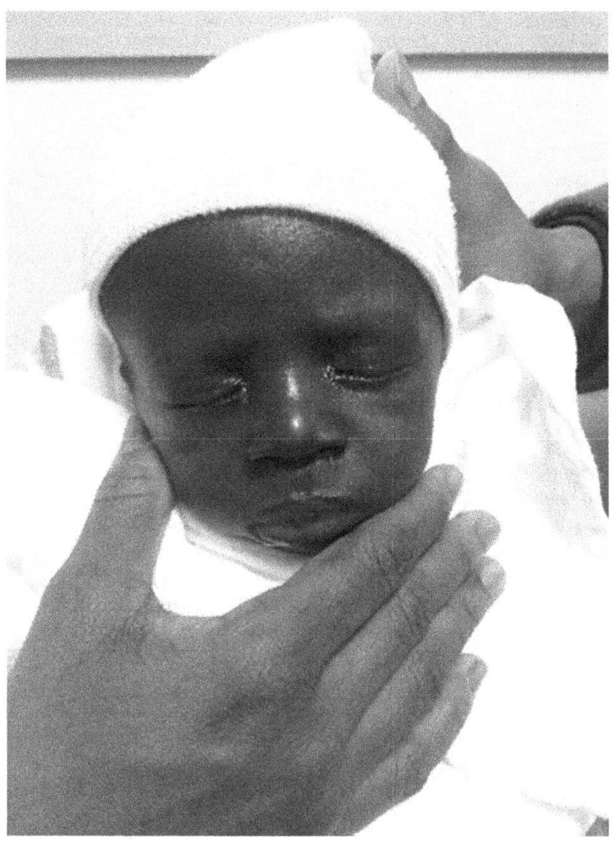

Figure 3. A newborn boy with normal birth weight and length, normal male genitalia, and hyperpigmentation who developed hypoglycemia at 4 hours of age. The hand is that of the biologic father. For details, please see text for case 1.

lesion arise? What is the significance of this particular mutation (25)?

Case 3

An infant male with vague symptoms and nonspecific dysmorphic features was found to have a glucose level of 28.8 mg/dL; concomitant β-OHB was 1.04 mmol/L, and FFA was 9.6 mg/dL (normal up to 20 mg/dL). After glucagon challenge, his blood glucose increased from a baseline of 23 mg/dL to 113 mg/dL at 30 minutes postchallenge. The hypoglycemia can be overcome by a glucose infusion of 4 mg/kg/min.

The degree of hypoglycemia together with low ketones, fairly low FFAs, and glycemic response to glucagon all suggest hyperinsulinism, but insulin was <0.4 μU/mL, and C-peptide was <0.02 ng/mL. How can these features be reconciled (26)?

Case 4

A newborn male large for gestational age has macroglossia, umbilical hernia, earlobe fissures, and hypoglycemia with HI. Testing for BWS reveals paternal uniparental isodisomy of chromosome 11p, a situation that alters the normal expression of maternal and paternal imprinted genes.

Comment

Hypoglycemia as a result of HI occurs in ~50% of BWS cases; in the majority of cases, the HI is mild and transient, but in ~5% of case, HI can be severe and persistent. In one half of BWS cases, the cause is isolated hypomethylation of imprinting control region 2, leading to loss of expression of CDKN1C and the adjacent voltage-gated potassium channel KCNQ1; in another 5% to 10% of cases, the cause is isolated hypermethylation of imprinting control region 1, leading to loss of expression of H19 and biallelic expression of IGF2; the remaining 20% of cases are caused by chromosome 11p paternal uniparental isodisomy, leading to loss of expression of CDKN1C and KCNQ1 and to overexpression of IGF2.

Kabuki syndrome is another entity that may be associated with HI; autosomal-recessive mutations in lysine-specific methyltransferase 2D are responsible for ~75% of cases, and X-linked mutations in lysine-specific demethylase 6A account for ~10%. HI in Kabuki syndrome usually is responsive to diazoxide.

REFERENCES

1. Kalhan SC, D'Angelo LJ, Savin SM, Adam PA. Glucose production in pregnant women at term gestation. Sources of glucose for human fetus. *J Clin Invest.* 1979;**63**(3):388–394.
2. Menon RK, Sperling MA. Carbohydrate metabolism. *Semin Perinatol.* 1988;**12**(2):157–162.
3. Sperling MA, DeLamater PV, Phelps D, Fiser RH, Oh W, Fisher DA. Spontaneous and amino acid-stimulated glucagon secretion in the immediate postnatal period. Relation to glucose and insulin. *J Clin Invest.* 1974;**53**(4):1159–1166.
4. Sperling MA, Ganguli S, Leslie N, Landt K. Fetal-perinatal catecholamine secretion: role in perinatal glucose homeostasis. *Am J Physiol.* 1984;**247**(1 Pt 1):E69–E74.
5. Kaplan SL, Grumbach MM, Shepard TH. The ontogenesis of human fetal hormones. I. Growth hormone and insulin. *J Clin Invest.* 1972; **51**(12):3080–3093.
6. Iwata O, Okamura H, Saitsu H, Saikusa M, Kanda H, Eshima N, Iwata S, Maeno Y, Matsuishi T. Diurnal cortisol changes in newborn infants suggesting entrainment of peripheral circadian clock in utero and at birth. *J Clin Endocrinol Metab.* 2013;**98**(1):E25–E32.
7. Stanley CA, Rozance PJ, Thornton PS, De Leon DD, Harris D, Haymond MW, Hussain K, Levitsky LL, Murad MH, Simmons RA, Sperling MA, Weinstein DA, White NH, Wolfsdorf JI. Re-evaluating "transitional neonatal hypoglycemia": mechanism and implications for management. *J Pediatr.* 2015;**166**(6):1520–1525.
8. Chernausek SD, Beach DC, Banach W, Sperling MA. Characteristics of hepatic receptors for somatomedin-C/insulin-like growth factor I and insulin in the developing human. *J Clin Endocrinol Metab.* 1987; **64**(4):737–743.
9. Ferrara C, Patel P, Becker S, Stanley CA, Kelly A. Biomarkers of insulin for the diagnosis of hyperinsulinemic hypoglycemia in infants and children. *J Pediatr.* 2016;**168**:212–219.
10. Bier DM, Leake RD, Haymond MW, Arnold KJ, Gruenke LD, Sperling MA, Kipnis DM. Measurement of "true" glucose production rates in infancy and childhood with 6,6-dideuteroglucose. *Diabetes.* 1977; **26**(11):1016–1023.
11. Thornton PS, Stanley CA, De Leon DD, Harris D, Haymond MW, Hussain K, Levitsky LL, Murad MH, Rozance PJ, Simmons RA, Sperling MA, Weinstein DA, White NH, Wolfsdorf JI; Pediatric Endocrine Society. Recommendations from the Pediatric Endocrine Society for evaluation and management of persistent hypoglycemia in neonates, infants, and children. *J Pediatr.* 2015;**167**(2):238–245.

12. Menni F, de Lonlay P, Sevin C, Touati G, Peigné C, Barbier V, Nihoul-Fékété C, Saudubray JM, Robert JJ. Neurologic outcomes of 90 neonates and infants with persistent hyperinsulinemic hypoglycemia. *Pediatrics.* 2001;**107**:476–479.
13. Meissner T, Wendel U, Burgard P, Schaetzle S, Mayatepek E. Long-term follow-up of 114 patients with congenital hyperinsulinism. *Eur J Endocrinol.* 2003;**149**(1):43–51.
14. Truong N, Reynolds C, Rodriguez L, Thornton P. Diazoxide side effects in the treatment of children with congenital hyperinsulinism In: 10th Joint Meeting of Paediatric Endocrinology, September 14–17, 2017; Washington, DC. Poster presentation.
15. Senniappan S, Alexandrescu S, Tatevian N, Shah P, Arya V, Flanagan S, Ellard S, Rampling D, Ashworth M, Brown RE, Hussain K. Sirolimus therapy in infants with severe hyperinsulinemic hypoglycemia. *N Engl J Med.* 2014;**370**(12):1131–1137.
16. De Leon DD, Stanley CA. Congenital hypoglycemia disorders: new aspects of etiology, diagnosis, treatment and outcomes: highlights of the Proceedings of the Congenital Hypoglycemia Disorders Symposium, Philadelphia April 2016. *Pediatr Diabetes.* 2017;**18**(1): 3–9.
17. Sperling MA. New insights and new conundrums in neonatal hypoglycemia: enigmas wrapped in mystery. *Diabetes.* 2013;**62**(5): 1373–1375.
18. Arnoux JB, Verkarre V, Saint-Martin C, Montravers F, Brassier A, Valayannopoulos V, Brunelle F, Fournet JC, Robert JJ, Aigrain Y, Bellanné-Chantelot C, de Lonlay P. Congenital hyperinsulinism: current trends in diagnosis and therapy. *Orphanet J Rare Dis.* 2011; **6**(1):63.
19. Güemes M, Hussain K. Hyperinsulinemic hypoglycemia. *Pediatr Clin North Am.* 2015;**62**(4):1017–1036.
20. Kalish JM, Boodhansingh KE, Bhatti TR, Ganguly A, Conlin LK, Becker SA, Givler S, Mighion L, Palladino AA, Adzick NS, De León DD, Stanley CA, Deardorff MA. Congenital hyperinsulinism in children with paternal 11p uniparental isodisomy and Beckwith-Wiedemann syndrome. *J Med Genet.* 2016;**53**(1):53–61.
21. Subbarayan A, Hussain K. Hypoglycemia in Kabuki syndrome. *Am J Med Genet A.* 2014;**164**(2):467–471.
22. Flanagan SE, Mackay DJ, Greeley SA, McDonald TJ, Mericq V, Hassing J, Richmond EJ, Martin WR, Acerini C, Kaulfers AM, Flynn DP, Popovic J, Sperling MA, Hussain K, Ellard S, Hattersley AT. Hypoglycemia following diabetes in patients with 6q24 methylation defects. Expanding the clinical phenotype. *Diabetologia.* 2013;**56**(1):218–221.
23. Dambska M, Labrador EB, Kuo CL, Weinstein DA. Prevention of complications in glycogen storage disease type Ia with optimization of metabolic control. *Pediatr Diabetes.* 2017;**18**(5):327–331.
24. McEachern R, Drouin J, Metherell L, Huot C, Van Vliet G, Deal C. Severe cortisol deficiency associated with reversible growth hormone deficiency in two infants: what is the link? *J Clin Endocrinol Metab.* 2011; **96**(9):2670–2674.
25. Glaser B, Blech I, Krakinovsky Y, Ekstein J, Gillis D, Mazor-Aronovitch K, Landau H, Abeliovich D. ABCC8 mutation allele frequency in the Ashkenazi Jewish population and risk of focal hyperinsulinemic hypoglycemia. *Genet Med.* 2011;**13**(10):891–194.
26. Hussain K, Challis B, Rocha N, Payne F, Minic M, Thompson A, Daly A, Scott C, Harris J, Smillie BJ, Savage DB, Ramaswami U, De Lonlay P, O'Rahilly S, Barroso I, Semple RK. An activating mutation of AKT2 and human hypoglycemia. *Science.* 2011;**334**(6055):474.
27. Pinney SE, Ganapathy K, Bradfield J, Stokes D, Sasson A, Mackiewicz K, Boodhansingh K, Hughes N, Becker S, Givler S, Macmullen C, Monos D, Ganguly A, Hakonarson H, Stanley CA. Dominant form of congenital hyperinsulinism maps to HK1 region on 10q. *Horm Res Paediatr.* 2013;**80**(1):18–27.
28. Flanagan SE, Vairo F, Johnson MB, Caswell R, Laver TW, Lango Allen H, Hussain K, Ellard S. A CACNA1D mutation in a patient with persistent hyperinsulinaemic hypoglycaemia, heart defects, and severe hypotonia. *Pediatr Diabetes.* 2017;**18**(4):320–323.

The Initial Approach to Evaluating Atypical Genitalia

M60
Presented, March 17–20, 2018

S. Faisal Ahmed, MD, FRCPCH. Developmental Endocrinology Research Group, University of Glasgow, Royal Hospital for Children, Glasgow G51 4TF, Scotland, United Kingdom, E-mail: faisal.ahmed@glasgow.ac.uk

SIGNIFICANCE OF THE CLINICAL PROBLEM

In many languages and cultures, the first question that is usually posed by new parents is, "Is it a boy or a girl?" Without this information, the parents cannot even formulate the second question, which is usually, "Is he/she all right?" The parents do not generally expect that the health care professional will have any difficulty in answering this most basic of questions. It is no wonder that the birth of a child with genitalia that are so atypical that the sex of rearing is uncertain can be a difficult neonatal scenario. However, the extent of genital ambiguity may depend on the expertise of the observer; although the birth prevalence of atypical genitalia may be even higher than one in 300 births, the birth prevalence of cases where there is true genital ambiguity on expert examination may be lower than one in 4000 births. Rather than treating every child with atypical genitalia as a medical emergency, it is paramount that such a child is first assessed by clinicians with adequate knowledge about the extent of variation in the physical appearance of genitalia, the underlying pathophysiology that may give rise to a disorder of sex development (DSD), and the strengths and weaknesses of the tests that can be performed in early infancy. Unlike 46,XX DSD, where the cause is usually clear, identification of a cause of an XY DSD is often unclear and may be attributed to a disorder of gonadal development, androgen synthesis, or androgen action. Furthermore, many genetic conditions that give rise to XY DSDs are associated with a wide range of manifestations, from mild atypicalities to quite severe phenotypes that could be associated with sex reversal. Reaching a firm underlying diagnosis in such cases is challenging and requires expertise within a framework that abides by the highest standards of clinical care. Although conditions associated with altered sex development have improved our fundamental understanding of sex and gonadal development, it is debatable whether this improvement in our understanding has improved the long-term as well as immediate care of people with DSDs. Thus, there is a need for more emphasis on showing that a firm diagnosis for conditions associated with DSDs is associated with a change in clinical practice that benefits the patient. With the rapid advances in diagnostic technology, there is also a need for clearer guidance on the relative merits of biochemical vs genetic evaluation. An expert should be able to ensure that parents' need for information and support is comprehensively addressed while appropriate investigations are performed in a timely fashion. This expert also needs to have immediate access to a clinical team with multidisciplinary skills. In the field of rare conditions, it is imperative that this clinician share experience and knowledge with others through platforms and forums that facilitate national and international clinical and research collaboration.

BARRIERS TO OPTIMAL PRACTICE

- The lack of experience of health care professionals in the front line who are involved at the time of initial presentation; first impression is often the last impression
- Lack of care pathways that allow seamless care of a person with a rare condition
- Provision of unbiased education, counseling, and support for parents
- Availability of specialist investigations
- Understanding of specialist investigations by those who use them
- The ethical challenges of making decisions for minors, especially when it relates to irreversible interventions
- Lack of unbiased evidence on long-term outcome
- The binary view of sex and the perceived stigma of DSDs in many societies
- Blurring of the margins between a difference and a DSD

LEARNING OBJECTIVES

The session will focus primarily on the evaluation of the affected infant with a suspected DSD. As a result of participating in this session, attendees should become familiar with:

- Clinical evaluation of the new infant with suspected DSD
- Strengths and weaknesses of biochemical and genetic tests, especially in context of XY DSD
- Use of networks for effective service and research

COMMUNICATION

Optimal communication with the parents is a critical part of the initial evaluation and management. Usually, by the time a specialist becomes involved in the case, the parents may have already spoken to three health care professionals, including a midwife, junior doctor, and possibly a neonatologist. The initial contact with the parents of a child with a suspected DSD is important because first impressions from these encounters often persist. A key point to emphasize is that the child has the potential to become a well-adjusted, functional member of society. The use of the phrase "differences or variations in sex development" may be useful in introducing the concept of the extent of variation in sex development. The analogy between a common condition such as variation in stature and associated functional disability may be easy to explain and understand, both for the parent as well as the health professional. Most differences in stature do not have any consequences, but marked tall or short stature can affect function. In addition, in many cases, although the abnormality in stature itself may not be profound and may not have a functional consequence, it may be a pointer toward coexisting health issues and thus require thorough clinical evaluation. Although it is likely a DSD may be a more complex and challenging group of conditions, discussions that use the above approach as the first step may reduce the stigma that is often experienced by families. The term DSD itself is not a diagnosis but simply a general description that will allow the expert to embark on a diagnostic pathway based on the DSD nomenclature described in Chicago in 2005. To the parent, it may be simpler to describe the differences in genitalia that have prompted a need for further investigation. In those cases where there is no doubt on expert examination about sex assignment, it should not be assumed that the parents' need for information and psychological help is any less, because the parents' perception of their own child's condition may be quite different from the clinician's perception of the severity of illness. In those cases where there is true genital ambiguity, it should be explained to the parents that the best course of action may not initially be clear, but the health care team will work with the family to reach the best possible set of decisions in the circumstances. The health care team should discuss with the parents the information to be shared in the early stages with family members and friends.

ASSESSMENT OF THE NEWBORN

It is important that a detailed family history and birth history are obtained from the parents of the affected infant before the infant undergoes a full systematic examination. It is also useful to clearly understand the parents' own understanding of their child's condition. Assessment of blood glucose and urinalysis for proteinuria should be routine. For the infant with atypical genitalia, the following details need to be recorded: size of the phallus, presence of chordee, site of urethral opening, single or dual openings on the perineum, development of labioscrotal folds or a bifid scrotum, whether gonads are palpable and their site, and scrotal rugosity and development. Although anogenital distance and anoscrotal index have often been used in clinical and epidemiological studies, their place in clinical practice is unclear. Although scoring systems such as the Prader scoring system for XX DSDs and modifications of this system for XY DSDs may provide an integrated summary description of the genitalia, these scoring systems are not sufficiently discriminating to portray the full spectrum of the variation encountered in the external genitalia. The external masculinisation score, which individually scores external genitalia for scrotal fusion, microphallus, location of urethral meatus, and location of each gonad, may be a more discriminatory and objective method of describing the external appearance. Reference ranges for dimensions of genitalia such as the phallus exist but are rarely necessary.

INVESTIGATIONS IN THE NEWBORN

Infants with suspected DSDs who require further clinical evaluation and need to be considered for investigation by a specialist should include those with isolated proximal hypospadias, isolated micropenis, isolated clitoromegaly, any form of familial hypospadias, or a combination of genital anomalies with an external masculinisation score of <11. This will avoid unnecessary detailed investigations of boys with isolated glandular or midshaft hypospadias and boys with a unilateral inguinal testis. In approximately 25% of affected patients, the DSD is part of a complex condition, and the coexistence of a systemic metabolic disorder, other malformations, or dysmorphic features would lower the threshold for investigation, as would a family history of consanguinity, stillbirths, multiple miscarriages, fertility problems, genital abnormalities, hernias, delayed puberty, genital surgery, unexplained deaths, or the need for steroid replacement. In addition, maternal health and pregnancy history themselves may hold key information. In those with ambiguous genitalia and/or bilateral impalpable gonads, a first tier of investigations should be undertaken to define the sex chromosomes and delineate, by pelvic ultrasound, the internal genitalia and exclude congenital adrenal hyperplasia (CAH). This first tier should therefore also include plasma glucose, serum 17OH-progesterone (17OHP), and serum electrolytes. Serum 17OHP is usually unreliable before the age of 36 hours, and in the salt-losing form of CAH, serum electrolytes usually do not become abnormal before day 4 of life. The results of polymerase chain reaction or fluorescence *in situ* hybridization analysis using Y- and X-specific markers should be available within 2 working days, and laboratories should attempt to report 17OHP results in such a circumstance within 2 working days. In situations where the level of suspicion of CAH is high, and the infant needs immediate steroid replacement therapy, additional serum samples should be collected and stored before starting therapy. These should be of a sufficient volume to assess 17OHP, testosterone, androstenedione, and possibly renin activity or concentration, in that order of priority. At the author's center, at least one spot urine sample for a urine steroid profile is also collected before starting therapy. The results of these initial investigations often dictate the second tier of investigations. In an infant with impalpable gonads, a karyotype of 46,XX, a significantly elevated serum 17OHP, and the presence of a uterus, CAH resulting from 21-hydroxylase deficiency is likely. A urine steroid profile can confirm this diagnosis and can also identify other rare forms of CAH, which may also be associated with a raised 17OHP level in the newborn, such as 11β-hydroxylase deficiency or 3β-hydroxysteroid dehydrogenase deficiency. For the XY or X/XY infant with a DSD, anti-Müllerian hormone (AMH) and testosterone measurement will provide information about the presence of functioning testes. Depending on the age of the child, a human chorionic gonadotropin (hCG) stimulation test may be required. Confirmation of a specific diagnosis will often require further biochemical identification of a defect in the androgen biosynthesis pathway and detailed genetic analysis. Imaging studies (ultrasonography and magnetic resonance imaging) may locate the site of gonads, but often laparoscopy is the only reliable method to identify gonads. This also provides the opportunity to obtain biopsies for histology, the only way to establish a diagnosis of ovotesticular DSD with certainty.

STRENGTHS AND WEAKNESSES OF DIAGNOSTIC TESTS, ESPECIALLY IN XY DSD

In an infant with a karyotype other than 46,XX, there is a need to understand whether the child has any testicular tissue, whether this tissue is functional, whether it has the capacity to produce testosterone in the future, whether the testosterone it produces can be converted into dihydrotestosterone (DHT), and whether the child has any evidence of androgen resistance. In addition, there is a need for careful assessment of the internal as well as the external anatomy of the reproductive organs, and there is a need to assess the possibility of coexisting conditions, including adrenal insufficiency. An assessment of functional testicular tissue is usually performed by a combination of examination, imaging, and biochemical investigations, including measurement of AMH and the synthesis of testosterone after stimulation with hCG. Testes that are descended are more likely to produce testosterone on hCG stimulation and are more likely to be associated with normal AMH. Many diagnostic algorithms exist in the literature to guide the clinician in this diagnostic journey.

Although a single assessment of AMH, especially in combination with an assessment of androgen synthesis, can be informative, a low AMH level does not necessarily predict suboptimal testicular function. A low AMH level in a boy with functional testes may be recorded during the newborn period, in the presence of hypogonadotrophic hypogonadism, or in the case of persistent Müllerian duct syndrome with an AMH gene mutation. Identification of the gonads by ultrasound examination is an established cornerstone of first-line assessment but is clearly associated with pitfalls and relies on expertise of the examiner as well as an optimal state of the child. More detailed and direct imaging by laparoscopy is increasingly advocated, but this procedure is not without its own risk. Although the biochemical investigations mentioned above can provide an assessment of testicular function at the point of assessment, their value in predicting long-term function has not been clearly studied. However, it is clear that in some conditions presenting as XY DSD with normal testosterone synthesis, such as those associated with a mutation in *NR5a1*, a deterioration of testis function may only occur over time. Disorders of testosterone biosynthesis, such as 17-β-hydroxysteroid dehydrogenase type 3 deficiency or 5α-reductase 2 (5ARD2) deficiency, are typically associated with a reduction in conversion of androstenedione to testosterone (T) or T to DHT, respectively. However, a low T-to-androstenedione ratio may not be sensitive or specific for 17-β-hydroxysteroid dehydrogenase type 3 deficiency, and the high T-to-DHT ratio may not be sufficiently sensitive for identifying cases of 5ARD2 deficiency. Although in the past, assessment of serum androgens was performed by immunoassays, which were difficult to interpret in the newborn period because of cross-reaction with other conjugated steroids, the introduction of liquid chromatography–mass spectrometry has improved the accuracy of androgen measurements. However, the specificity and sensitivity of using ratios to identify abnormalities of androgen synthesis by these specialist techniques remain unclear, because a clear overlap exists between those with true pathology and those without pathology. Although mass spectrometry–based methods are powerful tools for assessing disorders of androgen synthesis, the reliability of these techniques is dependent on the age-dependent variation in steroid synthesis and metabolism such that urine steroid analysis by gas chromatography–mass spectrometry is generally not recommended for assessment of 5ARD2 deficiency within the first 3 months of life. Androgen insensitivity has often been considered a diagnosis of exclusion in those cases of XY DSD where androgen production is deemed to be normal. However, in many cases of confirmed androgen insensitivity, androgen synthesis is not normal. Clinicians often use the effect of short-term exogenous testosterone on penile growth as a diagnostic test of androgen insensitivity. Some experts have suggested that clinical androgen insensitivity may be objectively assessed by a dynamic test of measurement of androgen-responsive proteins, such as sex hormone binding globulin, after androgen exposure. However, given the wide range of normal variation in SHBG, the diagnostic reliability of these clinical and functional tests of androgen sensitivity is unclear. It is possible that other androgen-responsive proteins or circulating noncoding RNAs may be more reliable measures of androgen sensitivity, and this requires further exploration in sufficiently large cohorts.

STRENGTHS AND WEAKNESSES OF GENETIC TETS, ESPECIALLY IN XY DSD

Strengths:

- Confirms the clinical suspicion
- Allows counseling
- No age-related reference ranges
- Increasing availability
- May predict long-term outcome
- In some situations, may influence sex of rearing
- May identify multiple genetic variations

Weaknesses:

- Poor correlation between genotype and phenotype

- Needs expert input and interpretation
- Functional studies may be required in some cases
- Unclear whether laboratory-based functional studies necessarily predict long-term clinical outcome
- Turnaround time needs to be faster
- Quality control: research vs clinical laboratory

The suggested pathway for investigating cases of 46,XY DSD is shown in Figure 1.

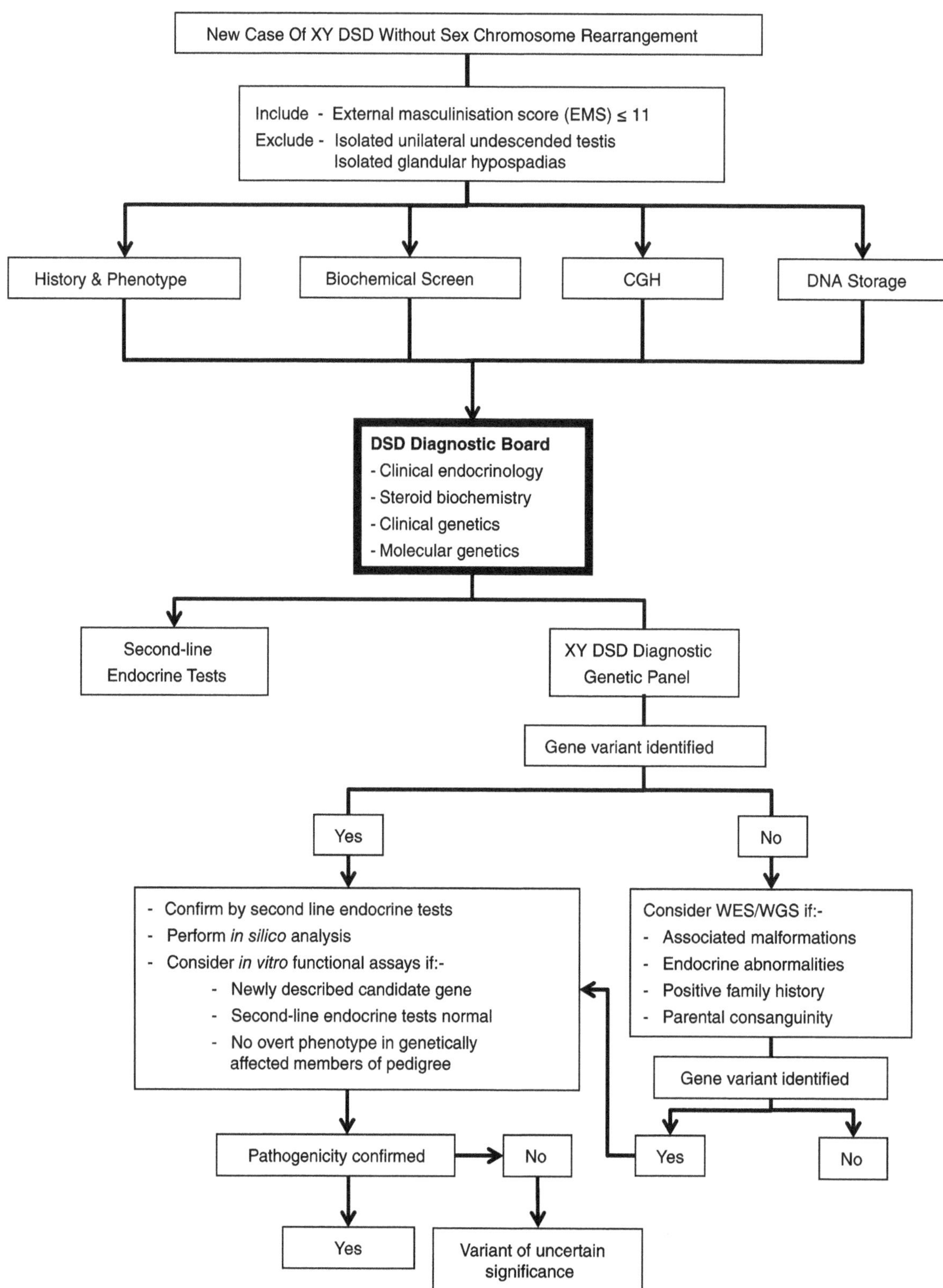

Figure 1. Suggested pathway for investigating cases of 46,XY DSD through an integrated endocrine and genetic approach that relies on a joint DSD diagnostic board with expertise in endocrinology, steroid biochemistry, clinical genetics, and molecular genetics. Reproduced from Alhomaidah *et al.* (1).

CRITERIA FOR A CENTER OF EXPERTISE FOR RARE CONDITION SUCH AS A DSD

These criteria are based on the general criteria recommended by the European Union (EU) Committee of Experts on Rare Diseases (http://www.eucerd.eu/?post_type=document&p=1224).

- Capacity to produce and adhere to good practice guidelines for diagnosis and care
- Quality management in place to assure quality of care and participation in internal and external quality improvement/audit exercises
- High level of expertise evidenced by volume of referrals, second opinions, publications, grants, and teaching and training activities
- Capacity to manage patients with rare conditions
- Contribution to research
- Participation in data collection
- Participation in clinical trials
- Demonstration of multidisciplinary team approach
- Organization of a transitional care pathway to adulthood
- Links and collaborations with other centers of expertise
- Links with patient organizations
- Appropriate pathways for referrals within collaborating centers
- Appropriate arrangements to shorten the time to diagnosis
- E-health solutions, including shared case management systems and tele-health

INTERNATIONAL DSD/CAH REGISTRIES AND THEIR ROLE AS A VIRTUAL NETWORK

The 2005 Chicago Consensus stressed the need for the creation and maintenance of a database. This has also been highlighted as one of the key EU Committee of Experts on Rare Diseases criteria above. Such databases have existed in many centers at local, national, and regional levels and have provided valuable insights into may aspects of DSDs. However, these databases have lacked international interoperability. With the preliminary help of the European Society for Pediatric Endocrinology in 2007 and then the EU in 2008 and the United Kingdom Medical Research Council in 2011, a Web-based registry was developed, which currently exists as the International DSD Registry (www.i-dsd.org). In 2014, this registry developed a sister registry for CAH (www.i-cah.org). The registries consist of >3000 cases of DSDs and CAH entered from >90 centers from all six habitable continents. Not only are these registries fulfilling the function of fruitful research, they are also encouraging the development of a collaborative network and patient-centered service improvement.

WEB SITES

- www.i-dsd.org
- www.i-cah.org
- www.endo-ern.eu
- www.dsdfamilies.org

RECOMMENDED READING

Alhomaidah D, McGowan R, Ahmed SF. The current state of diagnostic genetics for conditions affecting sex development. *Clin Genet.* 2017;**91**(2):157–162.

Cools M, Simmonds M, Elford S, Gorter J, Ahmed SF, D'Alberton F, Springer A, Hiort O; Management Committee of the European Cooperation in Science and Technology Action BM1303. Response to the Council of Europe Human Rights Commissioner's issue paper on human rights and intersex people. *Eur Urol.* 2016;**70**:407–409.

Kyriakou A, Dessens A, Bryce J, Iotova V, Juul A, Krawczynski M, Nordenskjöld A, Rozas M, Sanders C, Hiort O, Ahmed SF. Current models of care for disorders of sex development - results from an international survey of specialist centres. *Orphanet J Rare Dis.* 2016;**11**(1):155.

Lee PA, Nordenström A, Houk CP, Ahmed SF, Auchus R, Baratz A, Baratz Dalke K, Liao LM, Lin-Su K, Looijenga LH III, Mazur T, Meyer-Bahlburg HF, Mouriquand P, Quigley CA, Sandberg DE, Vilain E, Witchel S; Global DSD Update Consortium. Global disorders of sex development update since 2006: Perceptions, approach and care. *Horm Res Paediatr.* 2016;**85**(3):158–180.

Lucas-Herald A, Bertelloni S, Juul A, Bryce J, Jiang J, Rodie M, Sinnott R, Boroujerdi M, Lindhardt Johansen M, Hiort O, Holterhus PM, Cools M, Guaragna-Filho G, Guerra-Junior G, Weintrob N, Hannema S, Drop S, Guran T, Darendeliler F, Nordenstrom A, Hughes IA, Acerini C, Tadokoro-Cuccaro R, Ahmed SF. The long-term outcome of boys with partial androgen insensitivity syndrome and a mutation in the androgen receptor gene. *J Clin Endocrinol Metab.* 2016;**101**(11):3959–3967.

Nixon R, Cerqueira V, Kyriakou A, Lucas-Herald A, McNeilly J, McMillan M, Purvis AI, Tobias ES, McGowan R, Ahmed SF. Prevalence of endocrine and genetic abnormalities in boys evaluated systematically for a disorder of sex development. *Hum Reprod.* 2017;**32**(10):2130–2137.

Rodie ME, Mudaliar MAV, Herzyk P, McMillan M, Boroujerdi M, Chudleigh S, Tobias ES, Ahmed SF. Androgen-responsive non-coding small RNAs extend the potential of HCG stimulation to act as a bioassay of androgen sufficiency. *Eur J Endocrinol.* 2017;**177**(4):339–346.

REPRODUCTIVE ENDOCRINOLOGY

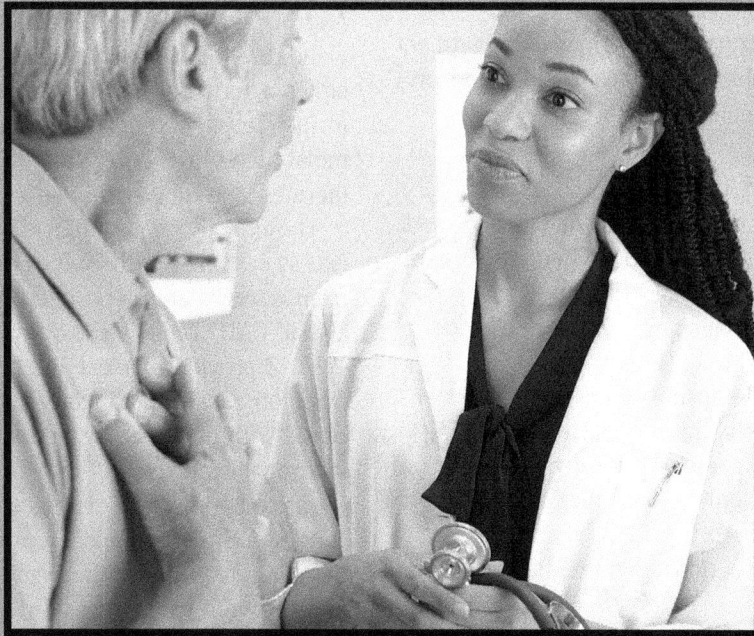

Evaluation and Treatment of Hirsutism

M08
Presented, March 17–20, 2018

David A. Ehrmann, MD. Section of Endocrinology, Diabetes, and Metabolism, The University of Chicago, Chicago, Illinois 60637, E-mail: dehrmann@medicine.bsd.uchicago.edu

SIGNIFICANCE OF THE CLINICAL PROBLEM

- Hirsutism is the term used to describe androgen-dependent excessive male-pattern hair growth in women.
- Hirsutism is among the most common presenting manifestations of androgen excess in women.
- Prevalence of hirsutism varies across populations studied.
- Hirsutism may reflect an important underlying endocrine disorder such as polycystic ovary syndrome (PCOS), nonclassic congenital adrenal hyperplasia (CAH), or rarely an androgen-secreting neoplasm.
- Hirsutism is often refractory to single-modality treatment and may require a combination of medications and/or methods such as photoepilation.

BARRIERS TO OPTIMAL PRACTICE

- Failure to recognize that hirsutism is not merely a cosmetic problem, but may be a manifestation of androgen excess (together with acne and androgenetic alopecia)
- Length of hair growth cycle results in slow/delayed response to treatment
- Failure to distinguish hirsutism from hypertrichosis
- Lack of understanding that race, ethnicity, circulating concentrations of androgens, and sensitivity of the hair follicle to androgens are only some of the determinants of hirsutism
- Suboptimal therapeutic options that are effective for hirsutism

LEARNING OBJECTIVES

As a result of participation in this session, learners should be able to:

- Appreciate the difference between hypertrichosis and hirsutism
- Understand the pathophysiology of hirsutism and generate a differential diagnosis
- Develop diagnostic and therapeutic plans for the evaluation and treatment of hirsutism

SUCCINCT REVIEW

There are three phases in the cycle of hair growth: first, anagen (growth phase); second, catagen (involution phase); and third, telogen (rest phase). Depending on the body site, hormonal regulation may play an important role in the hair growth cycle. Androgen excess in women can lead to increased hair growth in most androgen-sensitive sites except in the scalp region, where hair loss occurs because androgens cause scalp hairs to spend less time in the anagen phase. Hairs grow in non-synchronous cycles, and the growth (anagen) phase, which varies with body area, is about 4 months for facial hair. It is because of the long hair growth cycle that the effects of hormonal therapy require about 6 months for detection and about 9 months to become maximal.

Body hair is categorized as either vellus (fine, soft, and not pigmented) or terminal (long, coarse, and pigmented; Fig. 1). The type of hair produced from a given follicle can vary in response to numerous factors; the correlation between circulating androgen levels and the quantity of hair growth is modest. This is due to the fact that hair growth from the follicle also depends on local growth factors, and there is variability in end-organ pilosebaceous unit (PSU) sensitivity to androgens. Androgens are necessary for terminal hair and sebaceous gland development and mediate differentiation of a PSU into either a terminal hair follicle or a sebaceous gland. In the former case, androgens transform the vellus hair into a terminal hair; in the latter case, the sebaceous component proliferates, and the hair remains vellus.

The etiology is most often idiopathic or a result of androgen excess in women with PCOS. Less often, hirsutism may result from adrenal androgen overproduction, as occurs in non-classic CAH. Table 1 provides a list of causes of hirsutism; Table 2 provides clinical and hormonal features of the most common causes. Cutaneous manifestations commonly associated with hirsutism include acne and male-pattern balding (androgenic alopecia).

Hirsutism must be distinguished from hypertrichosis, the condition of generalized excessive hair growth that may be hereditary or result from certain medications. Hypertrichosis is distributed in a generalized, nonsexual pattern and is not caused by androgen excess (although hyperandrogenemia may aggravate it).

CLINICAL EVALUATION

Obtaining the age at onset and rate of progression of hair growth is important in determining the etiology of hirsutism, as are associated symptoms (*e.g.*, menstrual irregularity) or signs (*e.g.*, acne). Sudden development and rapid progression of hirsutism suggest the possibility of an androgen-secreting neoplasm, in which case virilization (deepening of the voice, clitoromegaly, increased muscle mass) may also be present.

Age at menarche and the timing of menstrual cycles are critical elements in the history; irregular cycles from the time of menarche onward are more likely to result from ovarian

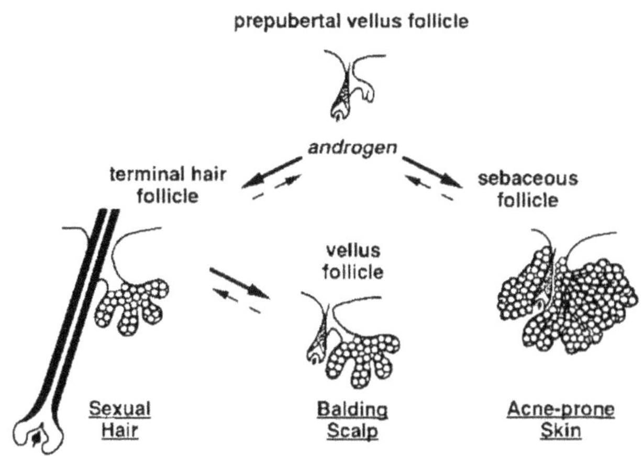

Figure 1. The role of androgen in PSU development. Solid lines indicate the effects of androgens; dotted lines represent the effects of antiandrogens. Hairs are shown in the anagen phase. Modified from Ehrmann and Rosenfield. Clinical review 10: an endocrinologic approach to the patient with hirsutism. *J Clin Endocrinol Metab.* 1990;71(1)1–4.

rather than adrenal androgen excess. The presence of galactorrhea should prompt evaluation for hyperprolactinemia and possibly hypothyroidism. Hypertension, striae, easy bruising, centripetal weight gain, and weakness suggest hypercortisolism. Rarely, patients with acromegaly present with hirsutism. A family history of infertility and/or hirsutism may indicate disorders such as nonclassic CAH, particularly among persons of Eastern European Jewish heritage (Ashkenazi). Use of medications such as phenytoin, minoxidil, and cyclosporine may be associated with androgen-independent excess hair growth (*i.e.*, hypertrichosis; Table 2).

Among women with a body mass index (BMI) >30 kg/m^2, hirsutism may be more common, at least in part because of increased conversion of androgen precursors to testosterone. Elevation in blood pressure may be the result of mineralocorticoid excess from an adrenal source. Cutaneous signs sometimes associated with androgen excess and insulin resistance include acanthosis nigricans and skin tags.

Clinical assessment of hair distribution and quantity is central to the evaluation in any woman presenting with concerns about excessive hair growth. This assessment permits the distinction between hirsutism and hypertrichosis and provides a baseline from which to assess response to treatment. A commonly used method to grade hair growth is the modified scale of Ferriman and Gallwey (Figure 2), in which each of nine androgen-sensitive sites is graded from 0 to 4. Hirsutism in women of reproductive age is indicated by a total score of ≥8 in African American or white women and ≥9 to 10 in Mediterranean, Latino, or Middle Eastern women; the total score varies among Asian women, from ≥2 for Han Chinese women to ≥7 in Southern Chinese women. In those groups that are less likely to manifest hirsutism (*e.g.*, Asian women), additional cutaneous evidence of androgen excess should be sought, including pustular acne and thinning scalp hair. Although widely used, this scoring system has its limitations, which include its subjective nature, the failure to account for a locally high score that does not raise the total score to an abnormal extent, and the lack of consideration of such androgen-sensitive areas as sideburns and the buttocks.

HORMONAL EVALUATION

Androgens are secreted by the ovaries and adrenal glands in response to their respective tropic hormones: luteinizing hormone (LH) and ACTH. Testosterone is the principal circulating steroid involved in the etiology of hirsutism; other steroids that may contribute to the development of hirsutism include androstenedione and dehydroepiandrosterone (DHEA) and its sulfated form (DHEAS). The ovaries and adrenal glands normally contribute approximately equally to testosterone production. Approximately half of the total testosterone originates from direct glandular secretion, and the remainder is derived from the peripheral conversion of androstenedione and DHEA.

Testosterone is converted to the more potent dihydrotestosterone (DHT) by the enzyme 5α-reductase, which is located in the PSU. DHT has a higher affinity for, and slower dissociation from, the androgen receptor. The local production of DHT allows it to serve as the primary mediator of androgen action at the level of the pilosebaceous unit. There are two isoenzymes of 5α-reductase: type 2 is found in the prostate gland and in hair follicles, and type 1 is found primarily in sebaceous glands. This distinction has important implications in considering pharmacologic interventions.

Hyperinsulinemia and/or androgen excess decrease hepatic production of sex hormone–binding globulin (SHBG), resulting in levels of total testosterone within the high to normal range, whereas the unbound hormone is elevated more substantially. Although there is a decline in ovarian testosterone production after menopause, ovarian estrogen production decreases to an even greater extent, and the concentration of SHBG is reduced. Consequently, there is an increase in the relative proportion of unbound testosterone, and it may exacerbate hirsutism after menopause. One approach to testing for the etiology of hirsutism is depicted in Fig. 3. Recent Endocrine Society practice guidelines for the evaluation and treatment of hirsutism in premenopausal women have broadened the suggestion for determining the serum total testosterone concentration to all women with hirsutism and the suggestion for determining the serum free testosterone concentration to hirsute women whose serum total testosterone is normal in the presence of clinical evidence of an endocrine disorder, moderate to severe hirsutism, or progressive sexual hair growth of any degree.

The practice guidelines also recommend testing for elevated androgen levels in the following instances:

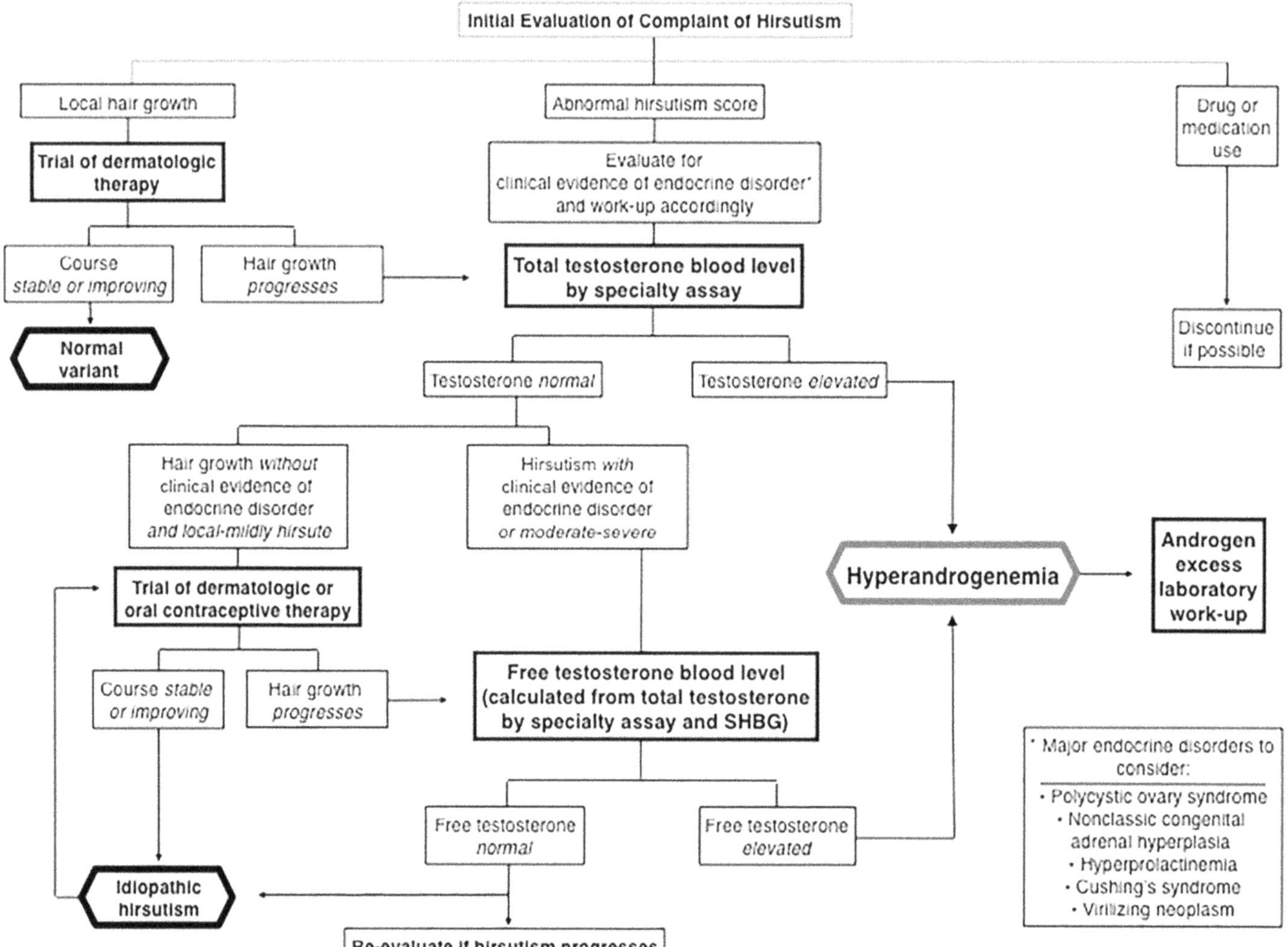

- Hirsutism of any degree associated with any of the following: menstrual irregularity or infertility, central obesity, acanthosis nigricans, clitoromegaly, or sudden onset or rapid progression
- Sexual hair growth of any degree that is progressive with dermatologic therapy or for which hormonal therapy is prescribed
- Serum total testosterone is best assessed by liquid chromatography–tandem mass spectroscopy. With liquid chromatography–tandem mass spectroscopy, the upper limit of normal for serum testosterone in women is in the 45- to 60-ng/dL range (1.6 to 2.1 nmol/L); women with serum testosterone >150 ng/dL require evaluation for the most serious causes of hyperandrogenism (ovarian and adrenal androgen-secreting tumors)

Although DHEAS has been proposed as a marker of predominant adrenal androgen excess, DHEAS is often elevated among women with PCOS. Computed tomography or magnetic resonance imaging should be used to localize an adrenal mass; ultrasound usually suffices to identify an ovarian mass if clinical evaluation and hormonal levels suggest these possibilities.

PCOS is the most common cause of ovarian androgen excess. There are several sets of diagnostic criteria, not to be elaborated upon in this session. Most practitioners use the Rotterdam criteria, as noted below. In all cases, other clinically relevant disorders must be excluded (where clinically indicated, examples include nonclassic CAH and Cushing syndrome) before a diagnosis of PCOS is assigned.

Gonadotropin secretion is altered in PCOS as a consequence of an increase in GnRH pulse frequency relative to the GnRH pulse frequency in women who have normal menstrual cycles. Rapid GnRH favors transcription of the LHβ subunit over the FSHβ subunit, leading the classic increased LH-to-FSH ratio as a criterion for PCOS. Note that progesterone can reduce the frequency of pulses of GnRH.

However, a single measurement of LH and FSH provides little diagnostic sensitivity, because gonadotropin concentrations vary over the menstrual cycle and are released in a pulsatile fashion into the circulation. In routine clinical practice, an elevated level of LH or an elevated ratio of LH to FSH should not be used to diagnose PCOS, and neither is included in any of the currently accepted diagnostic criteria (Table 3).

Table 1. Causes of Hirsutism

Causes
Gonadal hyperandrogenism
Ovarian hyperandrogenism
Polycystic ovary syndrome
Ovarian steroidogenic blocks
Syndromes of extreme insulin resistance (eg, lipodystrophy)
Ovarian neoplasms
Hyperthecosis
Adrenal hyperandrogenism
Premature adrenarche
Functional adrenal hyperandrogenism
Congenital adrenal hyperplasia (nonclassic and classic)
Abnormal cortisol action/metabolism
Adrenal neoplasms
Other endocrine disorders
Cushing syndrome
Hyperprolactinemia
Acromegaly
Peripheral androgen overproduction
Obesity
Idiopathic
Pregnancy-related hyperandrogenism
Hyperreactio luteinalis
Thecoma of pregnancy
Medications
Androgens
Oral contraceptives containing androgenic progestins
Minoxidil
Phenytoin
Diazoxide
Cyclosporine
Valproic acid

The symptoms of PCOS usually begin at about the time of menarche, but onset after puberty may also occur. Chronic anovulation most often manifests as oligomenorrhea or amenorrhea. Anovulatory cycles may lead to dysfunctional uterine bleeding and decreased fertility. A majority of women with PCOS are overweight or obese; in many instances, the BMI is in excess of 40 kg/m^2. Although obesity alone is not thought to be the inciting event in the development of PCOS, excess adiposity can exacerbate associated reproductive and metabolic derangements.

Nonclassic CAH is most often the result of 21-hydroxylase deficiency but can also be caused by autosomal recessive defects in other steroidogenic enzymes necessary for adrenal corticosteroid synthesis. Deficiency of 21-hydroxylase can be excluded by determining a morning 17-hydroxyprogesterone level <6 nmol/L (<2 μg/L; drawn in the follicular phase) or by measuring 17-hydroxyprogesterone 1 hour after the administration of 250 μg of synthetic ACTH (cosyntropin) intravenously.

TREATMENT OF HIRSUTISM

Physical measures to manage hirsutism include methods that remove hair shafts from the skin surface (depilation) and those that extract hairs to above the bulb (epilation). Shaving is a popular depilation method that removes hair down to just below the surface of the skin. Shaving does not affect the rate or duration of the anagen phase or diameter of hair, but it yields a blunt tip (when the growing hair projects beyond the skin surface) rather than the tapered tip of uncut hair, which gives the illusion of thicker hair. Chemical depilatory agents are also commonly used to dissolve the hair. Most depilatories contain sulfur and are malodorous. In addition, irritant dermatitis can occur. Epilation methods, such as plucking or waxing, are relatively safe and inexpensive but cause some discomfort. Scarring, folliculitis, and, particularly in women of color, hyperpigmentation may occur. Although not a method of hair removal, bleaching with products containing hydrogen peroxide and sulfates is a method for masking the presence of undesired hair, particularly facial hair. Adverse effects include irritation, pruritus, and possible skin discoloration.

The goal of pharmacologic therapy is to disrupt one or more of the steps in the pathway of androgen synthesis and action: suppress adrenal and/or ovarian androgen production, increase androgen binding to SHBG, impair the peripheral conversion of androgen precursors to active androgen, and inhibit androgen action at the target-tissue level. Attenuation of hair growth is typically not evident until 4 to 6 months after initiation of medical treatment and in most cases leads to only a modest reduction in hair growth.

Combination estrogen-progestin therapy [oral contraceptive (OCP)] is usually the first-line endocrine treatment of hirsutism and acne, after dermatologic management (depilation, epilation). The estrogenic component of OCPs is either ethinyl estradiol, estradiol valerate, or mestranol. The suppression of LH leads to reduced production of ovarian androgens. The reduced androgen levels also result in a dose-related increase in SHBG, thus lowering the fraction of unbound plasma testosterone. Estrogens also have a direct, dose-dependent suppressive effect on sebaceous cell function.

The choice of a specific OCP should be made on the basis of the progestin component, because progestins vary in their suppressive effect on SHBG levels and in their androgenic potential (Table 4). Ethynodiol diacetate has relatively low androgenic potential, whereas progestins such as norgestrel and levonorgestrel are particularly androgenic, as judged from their attenuation of the estrogen-induced increase in SHBG. Norgestimate exemplifies the generation of progestins that are virtually nonandrogenic. Drospirenone, an analog of spironolactone that has both antimineralocorticoid and

Table 2. Common Conditions in the Differential Diagnosis of Hirsutism/Hyperandrogenism

Condition	Hyperandrogenic	Irregular Menses	Distinguishing Features: Clinical	Distinguishing Features: Hormonal
Nonclassic 21-hydroxylase CAH	Yes	Not typically	Family history of infertility, hirsutism; East Europe Jewish	High basal or ACTH stimulated 17-hydroxyprogesterone
Cushing syndrome	Yes	Yes	HTN, striae, easy bruising	Increase in 24-hour urinary free cortisol
↑ Prolactin	No/mild	Yes	Galactorrhea	Elevated prolactin level
1° Hypothyroidism	No/mild	May be present	Goiter, etc.	Elevated TSH, low T_4/FT_4
Acromegaly	No/mild	Often	Acral enlargement, coarse features, prognathism	Increased IGF1
Primary ovarian insufficiency	No	Yes	Other autoimmune disorder, recurrent miscarriage	Increased FSH, low E2, low AMH
Simple obesity	Often	Variable	Diagnosis of exclusion	None
Virilizing neoplasms	Yes, extreme	Yes	Clitoromegaly, extreme hirsutism, pattern alopecia	Extreme elevation of androgen levels
Medications	Variable	Variable	History	Variable

ACTH, adrenocorticotropic hormone; AMH, anti-Müllerian hormone; FSH, follicle-stimulating hormone; IGF1, insulin-like growth factor 1; TSH, thyroid-stimulating hormone.

antiandrogenic activities, has been approved for use as a progestational agent in combination with ethinyl estradiol.

OCPs are contraindicated in women with a history of thromboembolic disease and women with increased risk of breast or other estrogen-dependent cancers. There is a relative contraindication to the use of OCPs in smokers and those with hypertension or a history of migraine headaches. In most trials, estrogen-progestin therapy alone improves the extent of acne by a maximum of 50% to 70%. The effect on hair growth may not be evident for 6 months, and the maximum effect may require 9 to 12 months because of the length of the hair growth cycle. Improvements in hirsutism are typically in the range of 20%, but there may be an arrest of further progression of hair growth.

Because OCPs are efficacious and have fewer adverse effects, they are recommended over glucocorticoids as first-line treatment for hirsutism in CAH. If the response to OCPs is inadequate, glucocorticoids may be used. The lowest effective dose of glucocorticoid should be used (*e.g.*, dexamethasone 0.2 to 0.5 mg or prednisone 5 to 10 mg), taken at bedtime to achieve maximal suppression by inhibiting the nocturnal surge of ACTH.

Cyproterone acetate is among the most often used antiandrogens in Canada, Mexico, and Europe; it is not available for use in the United States. It acts mainly by competitive inhibition of the binding of testosterone and DHT to the androgen receptor. In addition, it may enhance the metabolic clearance of testosterone by inducing hepatic enzymes. Cyproterone (50 to 100 mg) is administered on days 1 to 15 and ethinyl estradiol (50 μg) is administered on days 5 to 26 of the menstrual cycle. Adverse effects include irregular uterine bleeding, nausea, headache, fatigue, weight gain, and decreased libido.

Spironolactone, which usually is used as a mineralocorticoid antagonist, is also a weak antiandrogen. It is almost as effective as cyproterone acetate when used at high enough doses (100 to 200 mg daily). Patients should be monitored

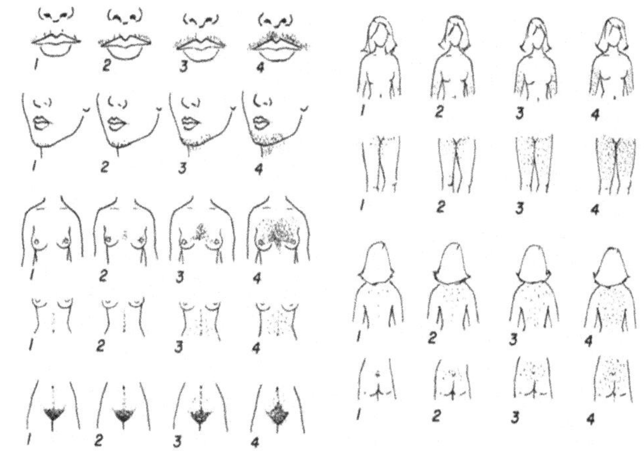

Figure 2. Ferriman-Gallwey hirsutism scoring system (modified). Each of the nine areas most sensitive to the effects of androgen is scored from 0 (no hair growth) to 4 (virilization). The scores are then summed: minimum 0, maximum 36. See text for population-specific norms. Reproduced from Ehrmann and Rosenfield. Clinical review 10: an endocrinologic approach to the patient with hirsutism. *J Clin Endocrinol Metab.* 1990;71(1)1–4.

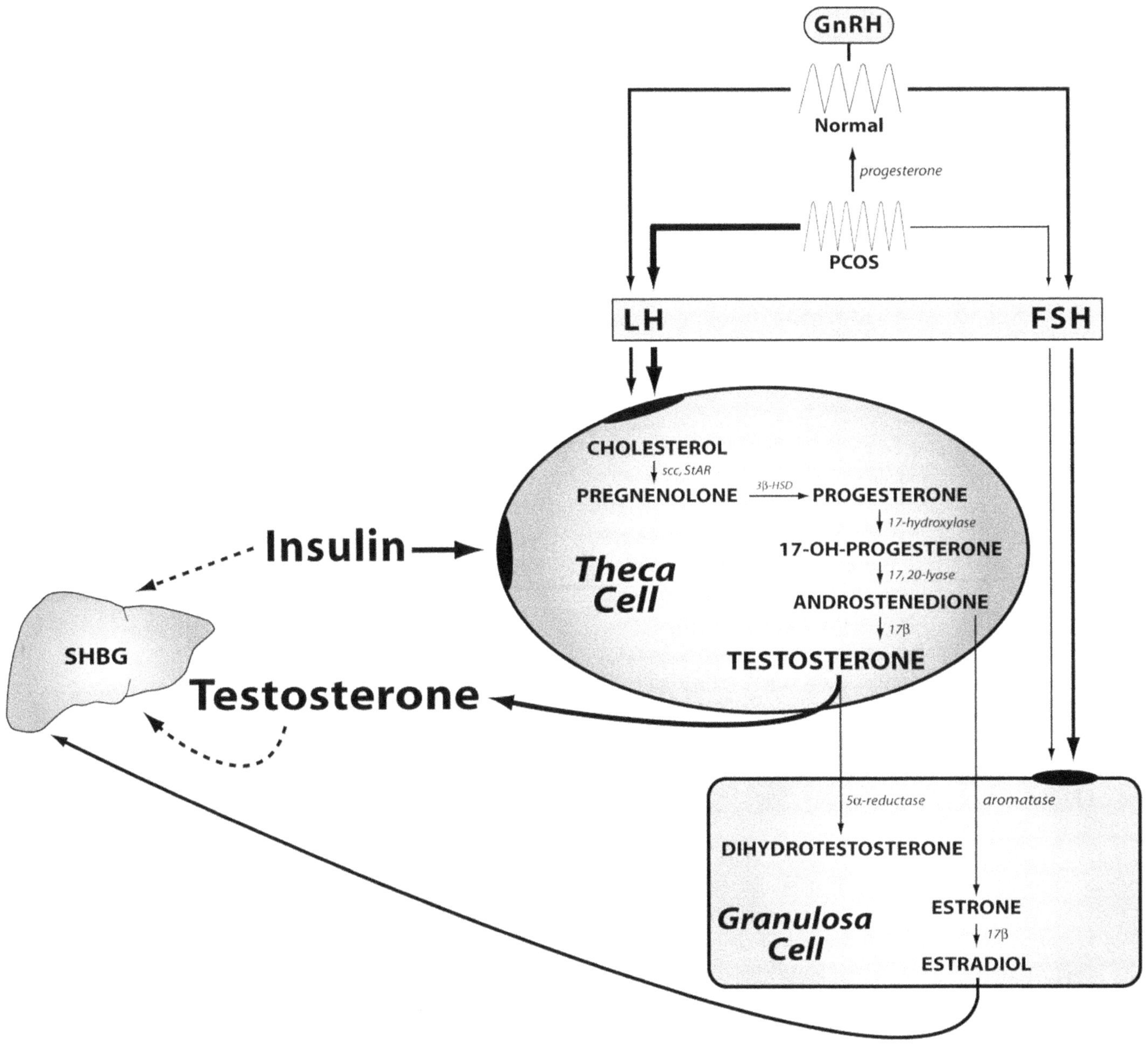

Figure 3. A simplified model of the pathogenesis of PCOS.

intermittently for hyperkalemia or hypotension, although these adverse effects are uncommon. Pregnancy should be avoided because of the risk of feminization of a male fetus. Spironolactone can also cause menstrual irregularity. It often is used in combination with an OCP, which suppresses ovarian androgen production and helps prevent pregnancy.

Table 3. Diagnostic Criteria for PCOS

NIH Consensus Criteria (all required)	Rotterdam Criteria (two of three required)	Androgen Excess PCOS Society Criteria (all required)
Oligo- or anovulation (<6-8 menses/yr)	Oligo- or anovulation (<6-8 menses/yr)	Clinical and/or biochemical signs of hyperandrogenism
Clinical and/or biochemical signs of hyperandrogenism	Clinical and/or biochemical signs of hyperandrogenism	Ovarian dysfunction: oligo- or anovulation (<6-8 menses/yr) and/or polycystic ovaries on ultrasound
Exclusion of other disorders: nonclassic CAH, androgen-secreting tumors, etc.	Polycystic ovaries (by ultrasound)	Exclusion of other androgen excess or ovulatory disorders

Table 4. Relative Androgenic Activity of Progestins in OCPs

Highest Androgenic Activity	Moderate Androgenic Activity	Lowest Androgenic Acitivity
Levonorgesterel	Desogesterel	Ethynodiol diacetate
Norgesterel	Norithindrone acetate	Dienogest
	Norgestimate	Drosperinine

Flutamide is a potent nonsteroidal antiandrogen that is effective in treating hirsutism, but concerns about the induction of hepatocellular dysfunction, even fulminant hepatic failure, have limited its use in the United Sates. Flutamide is often used in Europe. Finasteride is a competitive inhibitor of 5α-reductase type 2. Beneficial effects on hirsutism have been reported, but the predominance of 5α-reductase type 1 in the PSU seems to account for its limited efficacy. Finasteride would also be expected to impair sexual differentiation in a male fetus, and it should not be used in women who may become pregnant.

Dutasteride is an inhibitor of 5α-reductase types 1 and 2. There is some evidence of efficacy for its use in the treatment of hirsutism and alopecia.

Eflornithine cream has been approved as a novel treatment of unwanted facial hair in women, but long-term efficacy remains to be established. It can cause skin irritation under exaggerated conditions of use.

Ultimately, the choice of any specific agent(s) must be tailored to the unique needs of the patient being treated. As noted previously, pharmacologic treatments for hirsutism should be used in conjunction with nonpharmacologic approaches. It is also helpful to review the pattern of female hair distribution in the normal population to dispel unrealistic expectations.

EVALUATION AND TREATMENT OF HIRSUTISM: CASE STUDIES

Case 1

You are asked to see an 18-year-old woman who is concerned about increased hair growth on her face and lower abdomen. Menarche was at age 11 years. For the first year postmenarche, she had approximately four menstrual periods. Between ages 11 and 14 years, her cycles remained unpredictable; she estimates that she had approximately six to seven menses per year. At age 16 years, she began to notice acne on her face and upper back. She consulted a dermatologist who recommended topical clindamycin; after 1 year without a significant improvement, isotretinoin was recommended but the patient decided to seek another opinion and went to see her physician. She was then 17 years old.

She is white and does not smoke, drink alcohol, or use illicit drugs. She graduated high school and will be going to an out-of-state college in September. She lives with her parents and older sister. Her father has type 2 diabetes but is otherwise well. Her mother had thrombophlebitis and a deep vein thrombosis with a pulmonary embolism and is now taking coumadin.

She had never used any form of contraception, but because she was now thinking about becoming sexually active, she inquired about the possibility of using an OCP. Her physical examination at the gynecologist's office was unremarkable with the exception of moderate pustular acne on the chin and upper back. A transvaginal ultrasound showed a 2-cm cyst in the right ovary but no clear evidence of multiple follicles. The ovaries were of normal size and morphology.

On physical examination, she is 5 feet 5 inches (1.65 m) in height; her weight is 211 lbs (95.9 kg); BMI is 35.3 kg/m^2. Blood pressure is 138/94 mm Hg. HR is 104 bpm. She has centripetal obesity but does not have signs of Cushing syndrome. There is no evidence to suggest lipodystrophy. She has acanthosis nigricans on her neck. Her Ferriman-Gallwey score is 7. There is pustular acne on her face and back with evidence of scarring. There is some thinning of her scalp hair but no alopecia.

Questions

1. Does this patient have PCOS?
   a. Yes
   b. No
   c. Not sure, but does it matter?
2. Are additional blood tests required before recommending treatment?
   a. Yes
   b. No
   c. Optional
3. In addition to lifestyle intervention, what treatment(s) would you recommend for her hirsutism and oligomenorrhea?
   a. An OCP
   b. Metformin
   c. A progestin (levonorgesterel)–containing intrauterine device (IUD)
   d. Spironolactone alone
   e. An OCP together with spironolactone
   f. Finasteride
   g. Photoepilation
4. How will you monitor response to treatment?
   a. Measure serum testosterone level in 3 months
   b. Measure serum dihydrotestosterone level in 3 months
   c. Measure LH and FSH
   d. Use a patient-provided self-assessment

Case 2

A 32-year-old woman with a known history of PCOS was referred to you for management. Menarche was at age 10 years.

Her PCOS diagnosis was made when she was 19 years of age on the basis of her history of 9 years of oligomenorrhea together with a serum testosterone that was 2.5× the upper limit of normal in the assay used. She took an OCP intermittently but developed migraine headaches. The OCP was stopped. A progestin-releasing IUD was placed. She has persistent headaches, at times associated with vision disturbances. She is G0P0.

She did have photoepilation of her facial hair growth but is not satisfied with the result. She describes persistent fatigue and a recent weight gain of 12 lbs (5.5 kg) over the last 6 to 8 months.

Her BMI is 37.3 kg/m^2 and blood pressure 162/94 mm Hg. Fasting laboratories include HbA1c of 6.2%, total cholesterol 258 mg/dL, high-density lipoprotein cholesterol 33 mg/dL, triglycerides 194 mg/dL, and low-density lipoprotein cholesterol (calculated) 187 mg/dL. The patient is taking atorvastatin 10 mg/d and amlodipine 10 mg/d.

On examination, she has centripetal obesity with a Ferriman-Gallwey score of 16.

Questions

1. Which, if any, of the following tests are appropriate at this time?
   a. Polysomnography to exclude obstructive sleep apnea
   b. Factor V Leiden assay
   c. Prolactin level
   d. Magnetic resonance imaging of the brain
   e. a, b, c, and d
   f. None of the above
2. What is your treatment recommendation now?
   a. Removal of her IUD
   b. Start metformin with the aim of reaching 2000 mg/d
   c. Start an OCP with close monitoring.
   d. Start spironolactone 100 mg twice per day
   e. Start dutasteride 0.5 mg/d
   f. a and d only
   g. a, b, c, and d

RECOMMENDED READING

Azzouni F, Zeitouni N, Mohler J. Role of 5α-reductase inhibitors in androgen-stimulated skin disorders. *J Drugs Dermatol.* 2013;**12**(2): e30–e35.

Brown DL, Henrichsen TL, Clayton AC, Hudson SB, Coddington CC III, Vella A. Ovarian stromal hyperthecosis: sonographic features and histologic associations. *J Ultrasound Med.* 2009;**28**(5):587–593.

Haak CS, Nymann P, Pedersen AT, Clausen HV, Feldt Rasmussen U, Rasmussen AK, Main K, Haedersdal M. Hair removal in hirsute women with normal testosterone levels: a randomized controlled trial of long-pulsed diode laser vs. intense pulsed light. *Br J Dermatol.* 2010;**163**(5): 1007–1013.

Jung JY, Yeon JH, Choi JW, Kwon SH, Kim BJ, Youn SW, Park KC, Huh CH. Effect of dutasteride 0.5 mg/d in men with androgenetic alopecia recalcitrant to finasteride. *Int J Dermatol.* 2014;**53**(11): 1351–1357.

Martin KA, Anderson RR, Chang RJ, Ehrmann DA, Lobo RA, Murad MH, Pugeat MM, Rosenfield RL. *Evaluation and Treatment of Hirsutism in Premenopausal Women: An Endocrine Society Clinical Practice Guideline.* In Press.

Martin KA, Chang RJ, Ehrmann DA, Ibanez L, Lobo RA, Rosenfield RL, Shapiro J, Montori VM, Swiglo BA. Evaluation and treatment of hirsutism in premenopausal women: an endocrine society clinical practice guideline. *J Clin Endocrinol Metab.* 2008;**93**(4):1105–1120.

McCartney ChR, Marshall JC. Polycystic ovary syndrome. *N Engl J Med.* 2016;**375**(14):1398–1399.

Rosenfield RL, Ehrmann DA. The pathogenesis of polycystic ovary syndrome (PCOS): the hypothesis of PCOS as functional ovarian hyperandrogenism revisited. *Endocr Rev.* 2016;**37**(5):467–520.

Somani N, Turvy D. Hirsutism: an evidence-based treatment update. *Am J Clin Dermatol.* 2014;**15**(3):247–266.

van Zuuren EJ, Fedorowicz Z, Carter B, Pandis N. Interventions for hirsutism (excluding laser and photoepilation therapy alone). *Cochrane Database Syst Rev.* 2015;**4**:CD010334.

Zimmerman Y, Eijkemans MJC, Coelingh Bennink HJT, Blankenstein MA, Fauser BCJM. The effect of combined oral contraception on testosterone levels in healthy women: a systematic review and meta-analysis. *Hum Reprod Update.* 2014;**20**(1):76–105.

Managing Menopause (Including Breast Cancer Survivors)

M18
Presented, March 17–20, 2018

Kathryn A. Martin, MD. Massachusetts General Hospital, Boston, Massachusetts 02114, E-mail: kamartin@mgh.harvard.edu

SIGNIFICANCE OF THE CLINICAL PROBLEM

Menopausal hormone therapy (MHT) has an important role in the management of menopausal symptoms. MHT is highly effective for the management of hot flashes and in many cases, the symptoms of depression that women may experience during the menopausal transition. Low-dose vaginal estrogen, which has minimal systemic absorption, is effective for vulvovaginal atrophy symptoms.

The Endocrine Society's 2015 Clinical Practice Guidelines on treatment of menopausal symptoms agree that MHT is indicated for the management of menopausal symptoms but not for the prevention of cardiovascular disease, osteoporosis, or dementia (1). The benefits of MHT seem to outweigh its risks for most symptomatic women who are either under age 60 years old or <10 years from menopause (and do not have contraindications, such as breast cancer, heart disease, prior stroke, or venous thromboembolism) (1–6).

Although the Women's Health Initiative (WHI) showed adverse cardiovascular effects of hormone therapy in a population of postmenopausal women whose mean age was 63 years old (7–9), this is not the age group that experiences menopausal symptoms or seeks advice on hormone therapy. Almost all women who seek medical therapy for menopausal symptoms do so in their late 40s or 50s.

A number of lines of evidence now suggest that early use of hormone therapy is not associated with an excess risk of coronary heart disease in healthy women ages 50 to 59 years old (or <10 years after menopause). Data include a subgroup analysis from the WHI, a Cochrane review and meta-analysis, and a trial in a subgroup of women in the WHI showing that women in their 50s receiving unopposed estrogen had lower coronary calcium scores than women receiving placebo (8, 9). In addition, data from one trial in younger postmenopausal women (the Kronos Early Estrogen Prevention Study) suggest that intima medial carotid thickness and coronary calcium, markers of subclinical atherosclerosis, are similar in women taking combined estrogen–progestin therapy or placebo (10). In a second trial testing the "timing hypothesis," the progression of intima medial carotid thickness was decreased by estrogen in younger but not older postmenopausal women (<6 or >10 years after menopause, respectively) (2). The WHI recently reported 18-year follow-up data from both trials, and there was no excess mortality (of any type) in either hormone therapy trial. In women ages 50 to 59 years old, there was a decrease in all-cause mortality during the intervention phase (hazard ratio, 0.61) (8).

When counseling women, the clinician should provide estimates for the absolute risks and benefits of hormone therapy for younger postmenopausal women receiving up to 5 years of treatment. Women should be reassured that the absolute risk of complications for healthy, young postmenopausal women (in their 50s or <10 years postmenopausal) is very low (1, 3–6, 11).

After the initial publication of the WHI results in 2002, use of MHT decreased significantly. In a report from the National Health and Nutrition Examination Survey, use of oral MHT in the United States in women over age 40 years old decreased from 22% in 1999 to 2002 to 12% in 2003 to 2004, reaching a low of 4.7% in 2009 to 2010 (12). Unfortunately, this continued decline occurred in spite of reassuring data that the benefits of MHT outweigh the risks for most young menopausal women (within 10 years of menopause or under age 60 years old).

The result of the decline in MHT prescriptions is that many women with significant menopausal symptoms now struggle to find a clinician who is both willing to prescribe and experienced in menopausal care. Current trainees now have little or no experience in menopausal care (13).

BARRIERS TO OPTIMAL PRACTICE

- Lack of awareness of follow-up data from the WHI and meta-analyses of clinical trials showing that women ages 50 to 59 years old (or those <10 years after menopause) who start hormone therapy do not seem to be at increased risk for coronary heart disease
- Many clinicians are unaware that menopausal symptoms, in particular, hot flashes, typically begin during the menopausal transition. In addition, hot flashes persist beyond the age of 70 years old in up to 10% of women; this makes stopping hormone therapy challenging in this subset of women (14)
- Lack of awareness of the increased risk of new-onset depression during the menopausal transition

LEARNING OBJECTIVES

At the end of this presentation, the participant is expected to:

- Identify the absolute risks and benefits for 5 years of hormone therapy use in younger postmenopausal women (in their 50s)
- Identify the most common symptoms of the menopausal transition
- Choose the most appropriate hormone therapy to manage an individual's menopausal symptoms
- Use nonhormonal alternative strategies and medications to treat menopausal symptoms

STRATEGIES FOR DIAGNOSIS, THERAPY, AND/OR MANAGEMENT

The menopausal transition, or perimenopause, begins, on average, 3 to 4 years before the final menstrual period and includes a number of symptoms and physiologic changes that may affect a woman's quality of life. It is characterized by irregular menstrual cycles, hormonal fluctuations, and symptoms that may include hot flashes, mood lability, sleep disturbances, and vaginal dryness. Essentially all women experience irregular menses and hormonal fluctuations before clinical menopause, and up 80% develop hot flashes. However, only 20% to 30% seek medical attention for treatment.

Hot flashes are often associated with arousal from sleep. However, women may experience sleep disturbances even in the absence of hot flashes; it has been estimated that up to 40% of women experience sleep disturbances during the menopausal transition. Primary sleep disorders are common in this population.

Perimenopausal women are also at increased risk for new-onset depression (15–17). The mood symptoms are responsive to estrogen therapy as well as antidepressants.

Estrogen deficiency leads to a decrease in blood flow to the vagina and vulva. This decrease is a major cause of decreased vaginal lubrication and sexual dysfunction in menopausal women. Symptoms of vaginal atrophy (vaginal dryness and dyspareunia) are typically progressive unless vaginal estrogen is given.

The management of common symptoms is described in the cases below.

CASE 1

A 50-year-old woman on hormone therapy for hot flashes and new-onset depression presents for additional management. Her hot flashes have improved, but in spite of multiple adjustments in her estrogen dose, her depression symptoms have not improved. How would you manage this patient?

The patient described in the case may need both hormone therapy and an antidepressant. The next step would be to add a selective serotonin reuptake inhibitor (SSRI). When women present with vasomotor symptoms as well as mood symptoms, one approach is to start by treating the predominant symptom (*e.g.*, if she has severe hot flashes, start with hormone therapy and then add an SSRI if necessary). However, if hot flashes are mild and mood symptoms are severe, one would start with an SSRI and then add estrogen if needed.

CASE 2

A 51-year-old woman whose last period was 4 months ago seeks advice for management of hot flashes. She is awakened at least six to seven times a night and has frequent episodes during the day as well that are interfering with her ability to function at work. She has no history of venous thromboembolism, stroke, or coronary heart disease. She has no family history of breast cancer.

What would you suggest to her?

She is a good candidate for hormone therapy. Although the best approach is to start with low-dose estrogen (*e.g.*, transdermal 17-B estradiol 0.025 mg or oral 17-B estradiol 0.5 mg) and then titrate up as needed for relief of symptoms, higher doses are reasonable for women with severe symptoms. One can then taper the dose later and see if her symptoms can be controlled with a lower dose.

She is started on transdermal 17-B estradiol 0.05 mg with oral micronized progesterone 200 mg days 1 to 12 of the calendar month. She has dramatic improvement of her hot flashes, but she experiences mood symptoms the days that she takes the progesterone. You try a lower dose (100 mg) of progesterone administered daily, but she has trouble tolerating this as well. Subsequent trials of intravaginal progesterone and low doses of medroxyprogesterone acetate also cause mood symptoms. What are her options now?

Progestins are routinely added to estrogen therapy to prevent endometrial hyperplasia in postmenopausal women with an intact uterus. However, many women have trouble tolerating progestins, particularly those with perimenopausal mood symptoms. Progestins can worsen depression or negate the positive effects of estradiol on depression in up to 30% of women. This patient has been unable to tolerate a number of systemic progestin regimens. A reasonable option at this point would be a progestin intrauterine device (IUD) that releases levonorgestrel (18). There are two available doses: a 52-mg device and a 13.5-mg device. They are approved by the Food and Drug Administration for contraception and not for MHT, but for women who cannot tolerate systemic progestins, they are a reasonable off-label use of the IUD. The low-dose IUD has been available in Europe and other countries but is now available in the United States. It is smaller and easier to insert than the higher-dose IUD.

Another option for women who cannot tolerate progestins is the combined conjugated estrogen-bazedoxifine regimen, because this combination of estrogen and a selective estrogen receptor modulator relieves hot flashes, is endometrial protective, and is not associated with breast pain (19). Both oral estrogen and bazedoxifine are associated with an excess of venous thromboembolism. To date, no additive effect on thromboembolism has been observed with conjugated estrogen-bazedoxifine, but longer studies are needed to fully address this risk.

CASE 3

A 63-year-old woman who is posthysterectomy is referred by her primary care physician to discuss management of hot flashes She started on hormone therapy at age 50 years old for severe hot flashes (she most recently was taking 17-B estradiol 0.5 mg orally), but this was discontinued 18 months ago because of a new diagnosis of breast cancer. She is now on tamoxifen and having frequent and severe hot flashes since stopping MHT; they are interfering with sleep and her ability to function at work. She is currently taking black cohosh, isoflavone supplements, and red clover with minimal benefit. A recent thyroid stimulating hormone was normal.

What are her treatment options?

It is not surprising that she had recurrent symptoms after stopping treatment; this is common in women with a prior history of vasomotor symptoms. In addition, she is on tamoxifen, and hot flashes tend to be particularly severe. Given her recent breast cancer, she is no longer a candidate for MHT (20).

There are a number of nonhormonal alternatives for these women (21). Black cohosh, isoflavones, and red clover have not been shown to more effective than placebo (22, 23). If her symptoms were primarily at night, gabapentin would be a good choice (a single bedtime dose starting with 300 mg and titrating up to 900 mg), but if her symptoms occurred throughout the day and if she had any symptoms suggestive of depression, an SSRI/serotonin-norepinephrine reuptake inhibitors would be the first choice (24). Of note, the nonhormonal alternatives, while more effective than placebo, are not as effective as estrogen.

In addition, for women taking tamoxifen, certain SSRIs are contraindicated (paroxetine and fluoxetine), because they are potent inhibitors of Cytochrome P450 2D6 (CYP2D6), the enzyme that converts tamoxifen to its most active metabolite, endoxifen. Although the impact of this effect on breast cancer recurrence or survival is unknown, we suggest not using strong inhibitors of CYP2D6 in women receiving tamoxifen. Less potent inhibitors (citalopram, escitalopram, and venlafaxine) should be used instead.

For her symptoms of vaginal atrophy, water-based lubricants are first-choice therapy (1, 11). Low-dose vaginal estrogen is sometimes an option in breast cancer patients but only after consultation with the patient's oncologist and never in someone on an aromatase inhibitor. Options include 17-B estradiol vaginal tablets or a 17-B estradiol vaginal ring. Estrogen creams are available, but it is difficult to deliver a low-enough dose.

REFERENCES

1. Stuenkel CA, Davis SR, Gompel A, Lumsden MA, Murad MH, Pinkerton JV, Santen RJ. Treatment of symptoms of the menopause: an endocrine society clinical practice guideline. *J Clin Endocrinol Metab.* 2015;**100**(11):3975–4011.
2. Hodis HN, Mack WJ, Henderson VW, Shoupe D, Budoff MJ, Hwang-Levine J, Li Y, Feng M, Dustin L, Kono N, Stanczyk FZ, Selzer RH, Azen SP; ELITE Research Group. Vascular effects of early versus late postmenopausal treatment with estradiol. *N Engl J Med.* 2016; **374**(13):1221–1231.
3. Manson JE; The NAMS 2017 Hormone Therapy Position Statement Advisory Panel. The 2017 hormone therapy position statement of The North American Menopause Society. *Menopause.* 2017;**24**(7): 728–753.
4. Santen RJ, Allred DC, Ardoin SP, Archer DF, Boyd N, Braunstein GD, Burger HG, Colditz GA, Davis SR, Gambacciani M, Gower BA, Henderson VW, Jarjour WN, Karas RH, Kleerekoper M, Lobo RA, Manson JE, Marsden J, Martin KA, Martin L, Pinkerton JV, Rubinow DR, Teede H, Thiboutot DM, Utian WH; Endocrine Society. Postmenopausal hormone therapy: an Endocrine Society scientific statement. *J Clin Endocrinol Metab.* 2010;**95**(7Suppl 1):s1–s66.
5. Martin KA, Manson JE. Approach to the patient with menopausal symptoms. *J Clin Endocrinol Metab.* 2008;**93**(12):4567–4575.
6. Taylor HS, Manson JE. Update in hormone therapy use in menopause. *J Clin Endocrinol Metab.* 2011;**96**(2):255–264.
7. Marjoribanks J, Farquhar C, Roberts H, Lethaby A, Lee J. Long-term hormone therapy for perimenopausal and postmenopausal women. *Cochrane Database Syst Rev.* 2017;**1**:CD004143.
8. Manson JE, Aragaki AK, Rossouw JE, Anderson GL, Prentice RL, LaCroix AZ, Chlebowski RT, Howard BV, Thomson CA, Margolis KL, Lewis CE, Stefanick ML, Jackson RD, Johnson KC, Martin LW, Shumaker SA, Espeland MA, Wactawski-Wende J; WHI Investigators. Menopausal hormone therapy and long-term all-cause and cause-specific mortality: The Women's Health Initiative Randomized Trials. *JAMA.* 2017;**318**(10):927–938.
9. Rossouw JE, Manson JE, Kaunitz AM, Anderson GL. Lessons learned from the Women's Health Initiative trials of menopausal hormone therapy. *Obstet Gynecol.* 2013;**121**(1):172–176.
10. Harman SM, Black DM, Naftolin F, Brinton EA, Budoff MJ, Cedars MI, Hopkins PN, Lobo RA, Manson JE, Merriam GR, Miller VM, Neal-Perry G, Santoro N, Taylor HS, Vittinghoff E, Yan M, Hodis HN. Arterial imaging outcomes and cardiovascular risk factors in recently menopausal women: a randomized trial. *Ann Intern Med.* 2014;**161**(4): 249–260.
11. ACOG. ACOG practice bulletin no. 141: management of menopausal symptoms. *Obstet Gynecol.* 2014;**123**(1):202–216.
12. Sprague BL, Trentham-Dietz A, Cronin KA. A sustained decline in postmenopausal hormone use: results from the National Health and Nutrition Examination Survey, 1999-2010. *Obstet Gynecol.* 2012; **120**(3):595–603.
13. Santen RJ, Stuenkel CA, Burger HG, Manson JE. Competency in menopause management: whither goest the internist? *J Womens Health (Larchmt).* 2014;**23**(4):281–285.
14. Politi MC, Schleinitz MD, Col NF. Revisiting the duration of vasomotor symptoms of menopause: a meta-analysis. *J Gen Intern Med.* 2008; **23**(9):1507–1513.
15. Freeman EW, Sammel MD, Lin H, Nelson DB. Associations of hormones and menopausal status with depressed mood in women with no history of depression. *Arch Gen Psychiatry.* 2006;**63**(4): 375–382.
16. Worsley R, Davis SR, Gavrilidis E, Gibbs Z, Lee S, Burger H, Kulkarni J. Hormonal therapies for new onset and relapsed depression during perimenopause. *Maturitas.* 2012;**73**(2):127–133.
17. Cohen LS, Soares CN, Vitonis AF, Otto MW, Harlow BL. Risk for new onset of depression during the menopausal transition: the Harvard study of moods and cycles. *Arch Gen Psychiatry.* 2006;**63**(4):385–390.
18. Sitruk-Ware R. The levonorgestrel intrauterine system for use in peri- and postmenopausal women. *Contraception.* 2007;**75**(6Suppl): S155–S160.
19. Pinkerton JV, Harvey JA, Pan K, Thompson JR, Ryan KA, Chines AA, Mirkin S. Breast effects of bazedoxifene-conjugated estrogens: a randomized controlled trial. *Obstet Gynecol.* 2013;**121**(5):959–968.
20. Santen RJ, Stuenkel CA, Davis SR, Pinkerton JV, Gompel A, Lumsden MA. Managing menopausal symptoms and associated clinical issues in breast cancer survivors. *J Clin Endocrinol Metab.* 2017;**102**(10):3647–3661.
21. Nelson HD, Vesco KK, Haney E, Fu R, Nedrow A, Miller J, Nicolaidis C, Walker M, Humphrey L. Nonhormonal therapies for menopausal hot flashes: systematic review and meta-analysis. *JAMA.* 2006;**295**(17): 2057–2071.
22. Newton KM, Reed SD, LaCroix AZ, Grothaus LC, Ehrlich K, Guiltinan J. Treatment of vasomotor symptoms of menopause with black cohosh, multibotanicals, soy, hormone therapy, or placebo: a randomized trial. *Ann Intern Med.* 2006;**145**(12):869–879.
23. Nedrow A, Miller J, Walker M, Nygren P, Huffman LH, Nelson HD. Complementary and alternative therapies for the management of menopause-related symptoms: a systematic evidence review. *Arch Intern Med.* 2006;**166**(14):1453–1465.
24. Loprinzi CL, Sloan J, Stearns V, Slack R, Iyengar M, Diekmann B, Kimmick G, Lovato J, Gordon P, Pandya K, Guttuso T Jr, Barton D, Novotny P. Newer antidepressants and gabapentin for hot flashes: an individual patient pooled analysis. *J Clin Oncol.* 2009;**27**(17):2831–2837.

Fertility Induction in Pubertal Boys and Men

M28
Presented, March 17-20, 2018

Richard Quinton, MD, FRCP. Institute of Genetic Medicine, Newcastle University and Department of Endocrinology, Newcastle-upon-Tyne Hospitals, Newcastle-upon-Tyne NE1 4LP, United Kingdom, E-mail: richard.quinton@ncl.ac.uk

SIGNIFICANCE OF THE CLINICAL PROBLEM

Hypogonadotropic hypogonadism (HH) is the only cause of male infertility that can be successfully treated with endocrine [gonadotropin or less commonly, gonadotropin-releasing hormone (GnRH) pump] replacement therapy. Although congenital HH (CHH) and hypopituitarism (combined pituitary hormone deficiency [CPHD]) are rare diseases, affecting approximately one in 4000 and one in 10,000 males, respectively, a significantly larger number of individuals have acquired HH, typically as a result of treatment received for intra- and parasellar tumors. Principles of treatment are similar for males with acquired HH, and fertility outcomes are significantly better. Gonadotropin therapy also has the potential to normalize testicular volume, something that is typically of greater immediate importance than fertility for teenagers and young adults with CHH, and potentially major psychosocial and self-esteem–related benefits arise thereof.

BARRIERS TO OPTIMAL PRACTICE

- Lack of patient and physician awareness of a directly treatable cause of infertility
- Expertise in gonadotropin spermatogenesis induction not usually within the core knowledge and skills for either endocrinology- or obstetrics-and-gynecology–qualified physicians
- Widely used treatment protocols (*e.g.*, American Association of Clinical Endocrinologists guidance) lacking a sound theoretical underpinning and derived in practice from historical clinical trial protocols directed at achieving regulatory approval
- Patchy state- or insurer-based funding for male gonadotropin therapy in most countries

LEARNING OBJECTIVES

As a result of participating in this session, learners should be able to:

- Counsel individual couples on the likelihood of achieving a pregnancy either spontaneously or through assisted reproductive technology (ART) according to recognized prognostic factors related to the male partner with CHH
- Counsel individual couples on the likelihood of a child inheriting CHH
- Prescribe and monitor appropriate and logical gonadotropin treatment regimens
- Decide when to persist with attempts at natural impregnation and when to refer for ART

SCIENTIFIC BACKGROUND UNDERPINNING THERAPY AND MANAGEMENT

Role of Gonadotropins in Human Spermatogenesis

Human spermatogenesis requires the coordinated action of follicle-stimulating hormone (FSH) and endogenous testosterone on the testes. The onset of puberty is marked by sleep-entrained, GnRH-induced pulsatile luteinizing hormone (LH) secretion, with low-frequency nocturnal pulses initially favoring FSH secretion over LH and resulting increases in serum LH, FSH, and testosterone levels progressively extending to the waking hours, culminating in reproductive maturity.

LH and FSH exert differential effects on the compartments of the testes, with LH stimulating maturation of the interstitial Leydig cells that secrete testosterone, and intratesticular testosterone, in concert with FSH, acting on the seminiferous tubules to induce and maintain spermatogenesis. FSH is essential for the development of the tubular compartment where spermatogenesis occurs and stimulates the proliferation of immature Sertoli cells that secrete inhibin B and antimullerian hormone (AMH). The FSH-induced proliferation of immature Sertoli cells has far-reaching effects on fertility potential, with Sertoli cells supporting a species-specific number of germ cells and determining final seminiferous tubule length. Because seminiferous tubules account for ~90% of testicular volume (TV) the size of the testes is a critical indicator of fertility potential.

Minipuberty and Puberty

Inhibin B secreted by mature Sertoli cells is important for negative feedback on FSH in adults. AMH is secreted by immature Sertoli cells; is downregulated by testosterone; and, thus, is highest in early puberty and decreases with rising serum testosterone levels. Of note, Sertoli cells do not express the androgen receptor until age 5 years, so despite the high intratesticular testosterone levels during male minipuberty, the testes do not mature, and spermatogenesis is not initiated. The early neonatal period is thus a key proliferative window for germ cells and immature Sertoli cells.

With the onset of puberty, increasing intragonadal testosterone secretion by Leydig cells ends the proliferative phase. Sertoli cells mature, sex cords develop a lumen in the transition to tubules, and spermatogenesis is initiated. Intratesticular testosterone levels (at the site of production) are ~30 times higher than serum concentration, and these high levels are a requisite for spermatogenesis. This was elegantly demonstrated in a study that showed FSH combined with human chorionic gonadotropin (hCG) induced testosterone production and spermatogenesis in men with CHH, although those who received FSH combined with exogenous testosterone remained azoospermic. Therefore, FSH and LH-induced testosterone are needed to achieve quantitatively and qualitatively normal spermatogenesis.

Hypogonadotropic (Central or Second-Degree) Hypogonadism: LH and FSH Deficiency

HH is treatable with exogenous gonadotropin therapy, but extended treatment periods (≥2 years) may be required, particularly for men with CHH. Although human females already achieve their lifetime supply of oocytes *in utero*, males need to undergo three distinct phases of testicular maturation to develop and sustain spermatogenesis. This complex process is affected by placental hCG, pituitary gonadotropins during the third trimester and perinatal minipuberty, and the onset of puberty in adolescence.

Although men with HH are typically azoospermic, they fall broadly into three prognostic categories with respect to predicted response to spermatogenesis induction therapy. These categories represent a spectrum of GnRH deficiency (*i.e.*, with or without minipuberty) and the degree of spontaneous pubertal development. At the mildest end of the spectrum are men with adult-onset HH (*e.g.*, secondary to structural pituitary disease), and at the most severe end (least favorable) are men with severe CHH or congenital CPHD with a history of bilateral cryptorchidism. Approximately one third of men with CHH exhibit some spontaneous partial puberty at presentation in terms of biochemistry (detectable serum gonadotropins) and TV ≥ 4 mL by Prader orchidometer, constituting an intermediate fertility prognosis group (Table 1).

Positive predictors of outcome for fertility-inducing treatment include no history of cryptorchidism, some spontaneous pubertal development (TV ≥ 4 mL), and higher baseline serum inhibin B levels (>60 pg/mL). Approaches to stimulate gonadal development and fertility include pulsatile GnRH therapy or subcutaneous injections of exogenous gonadotropins. Both approaches are equally effective in inducing spermatogenesis in most men with CHH, but gonadotropins are more readily available because of their obligate use in female superovulation protocols for ART and, unlike GnRH, are effective in men with primary pituitary disease (Table 1).

Table 1: Predicting the Success of Spermatogenesis Induction in Male HH

Positive Predictor	Negative Predictor
HH acquired postpuberty (intact minipuberty)	CHH (absent minipuberty)
TV > 4 mL, consistent with milder deficiency	TV ≤ 4mL, consistent with absent puberty
No history of testicular maldescent	History of bilateral cryptorchidism Thermal and/or surgical trauma effects More sever neuroendocrine deficiency
Higher baseline serum inhibin B level	Baseline serum inhibin B < 60 pg/mL
Good spermatogenetic response in prior cycles	KAL1 mutation (X-linked Kallmann syndrome)
FSH dose titrated to achieve serum levels 4 to 8 IU/L?	hCG therapy preceding FSH?

Pulsatile GnRH Therapy

For patients with CHH who exhibit isolated GnRH deficiency, a logical approach is to replace GnRH. However, this is complicated by the episodic nature of physiological GnRH secretion, with continuous administration resulting in pituitary desensitization and suppression of gonadotropin secretion. Thus, either intravenous or subcutaneous GnRH must be administered in a pulsatile fashion through a programmable mini-infusion pump. Protocols are based on delivering a physiologic regimen of one pulse (discrete bolus) every 2 hours, with dose adjustments aimed at rapidly achieving gonadotropin-stimulated serum testosterone levels within the adult male range.

Pulsatile GnRH induces puberty and fertility, with ~80% of men achieving spermatogenesis on long-term treatment. Men with CHH with TV > 4 mL typically have better outcomes and develop sperm more rapidly (in 6 to 12 months) than those with prepubertal testes, who can require 18 to 24 months of treatment. Despite comparable outcomes to combined gonadotropin therapy, GnRH use is limited by cost, availability of drug, a suitable infusion device, and a diminishing pool of clinicians experienced with this treatment modality. Moreover, GnRH is ineffective for patients with primary pituitary disease.

hCG Monotherapy

hCG is even cheaper than newer testosterone replacement products and, when given by subcutaneous self-injection two to three times per week, achieves stable serum testosterone levels. Monotherapy with hCG is first-line therapy for spermatogenesis induction in men with acquired HH (*e.g.*, post-pituitary surgery, irradiation), typically inducing testicular development, spermatogenesis, and fertility within 3 to 9 months. If spermatogenesis is not achieved or remains suboptimal or if conception has not occurred in this time frame, FSH can be added to the regimen.

However, in CHH, hCG monotherapy is only a viable treatment option for men at the very mildest end of the spectrum (*i.e.*, partial to near-full testicular development) and is much less successful in men with prepubertal testes (TV ≤ 4 mL), of whom only one half develop sperm in the ejaculate even with prolonged treatment; normalization of semen quality [World Health Organization (WHO) criteria] is almost never achieved.

Combined Gonadotropin Therapy With hCG Plus Highly Purified Urinary Gonadotropins/Recombinant FSH

Combined gonadotropin therapy (hCG plus FSH) is the typical regimen for inducing fertility in men with CHH. hCG serves as a long-acting substitute for LH and is combined with FSH in the form of either highly purified urinary gonadotropins (hMGs) or recombinant FSH (rFSH). Like hCG, FSH preparations are given by subcutaneous self- injection. They generally contain 75 IU FSH; although hMG also contains the equivalent of 75 IU LH, this has negligible Leydig cell–stimulating effect. The emergence of long-acting FSH analogs could simplify treatment regimens.

The effectiveness of combined gonadotropin therapy for inducing fertility in HH has been known since the mid-1980s, although drugs, subjects, and dosing schedules were highly variable. Time to develop sperm in the ejaculate ranged from 3 to 19 months, with median times in the 9- to 12-month range. Of note, <40% of men with CHH and TV ≤ 4 mL developed sperm compared with >70% of those with TV > 4 mL. Men with TV ≤ 4 mL were much more likely to have had cryptorchidism (39% *vs* 8%), which is in line with reports that maldescended testes restrict fertility outcomes and that such patients typically require longer treatment to achieve spermatogenesis.

Larger studies performed this century have added more detail that can be summarized as follows: Eighty percent of men with noncryptorchid CHH achieve sperm (mean sperm concentration, 6×10^6/mL); 70% achieve $\geq 1.5 \times 10^6$/mL sperm, which is compatible with spontaneous impregnation in men with CHH, albeit well below WHO criteria of normality; 50% of treatment cycles result in pregnancy, of which just >10% also require ART; a median time of 7 months is needed to achieve sperm in the ejaculate and 28 months to achieve conception; and for those men who had undergone multiple treatment cycles, spermatogenesis is achieved two- to threefold faster in later cycles compared with the initial one.

Implications of Historical Fixed-Dose hCG-First Gonadotropin Therapy Regimes

Approximately three quarters of men with CHH are able to develop sperm with classical historical combined gonadotropin regimes; the majority achieve maximum TV and sperm in the ejaculate within 12 to 18 months of treatment initiation. Despite excluding those with a history of cryptorchidism, at least 20% of men with CHH do not develop sperm in the ejaculate. A number of possible explanations for this treatment failure rate exist. First, absent minipuberty and the irrevocable loss of a critical hormonal stimulus during this window might be an insurmountable obstacle to fertility for some men with CHH. Second, one cannot exclude the possibility that some men might eventually develop sperm with an even longer treatment duration of >3 years. Third, all studies used a fixed-dose FSH regimen (*i.e.*, 225 to 525 IU/wk administered every other day or three times a week) rather than targeting a physiological serum FSH (*e.g.*, target range of 4 to 8 IU/L). Finally, although prior treatment with exogenous testosterone treatment does not affect spermatogenic capacity, the classical approach of starting hCG and then adding FSH could be related to treatment failure.

hCG monotherapy works for men with partial to near-full testicular development, and outcomes are improved by using combined gonadotropin regimens. Until relatively recently, it was reasonable to justify an initial phase of hCG monotherapy in men with CHH who want fertility on the basis of longstanding custom and practice. Indeed, hCG-first protocols were used in all licensing studies for rFSH and FSH analog molecules. To satisfy regulatory authorities' concerns that spermatogenesis was indeed being induced by the investigational FSH product, men with HH who developed sperm during 3 to 6 months of hCG monotherapy were excluded from entry into the combined treatment phase. Moreover, men who did not have normalized serum testosterone levels were excluded to remove patients with a potential underlying primary testicular defect that might confound evaluation of drug effectiveness.

Investigators involved in these studies recalled how hard it was to achieve consistently normal serum testosterone levels during the initial hCG monotherapy phase and how much easier this became once FSH was added. Nearly 20 years ago, the late Mark Vandeweghe presciently noted the uncertain logic and unnecessary complexity of deferring FSH therapy until several months of hCG monotherapy had elapsed; he therefore advocated starting hCG and FSH simultaneously. More recently, one of the very few randomized trials in this area highlighted the possibility that the final spermatogenetic outcome of subsequent combined hCG and FSH (or pulsatile GnRH) treatment might be unwittingly compromised by an initial phase of hCG monotherapy in men with severe CHH.

A Sequential Approach to Spermatogenesis Induction in CHH

Prepubertal TV (≤4 mL) is a strong negative outcome predictor and is compounded by a history of bilateral cryptorchidism, which is common in severe GnRH deficiency. Given that 90% of TV is determined by the seminiferous tubules, factors promoting tubule development (*i.e.*, proliferation of immature Sertoli and germ cells) are critical for optimizing spermatogenic capacity. Therefore, a plausible approach for improving fertility in the most severely affected men with CHH is to provide unopposed FSH treatment with the aim of proliferating immature Sertoli cells before androgen-induced maturation. This also recapitulates the hormonal dynamics of normal puberty, wherein low-frequency GnRH pulses initially favor FSH secretion before stimulating LH-induced testosterone secretion.

In 2013, an open-label randomized study compared 24 months of pulsatile GnRH in gonadotropin-naïve men with noncryptorchid CHH and TV of 4 mL with or without 4 months of rFSH pretreatment. During the 4-month rFSH pretreatment phase, serum inhibin B levels normalized, and TV (ascertained by ultrasound) doubled, whereas histological studies revealed proliferation of Sertoli cells and spermatogonia as well as key cytoskeletal rearrangements. Of note, all men who received rFSH pretreatment ultimately developed sperm in their ejaculate compared with 70% in the GnRH-only group, with the pretreated group also trending toward higher maximal sperm counts.

Given the difficulty of recruiting severely affected patients with CHH without cryptorchidism or prior gonadotropin treatment, this study was insufficiently powered to reach statistical significance, which would have required an estimated 28 participants in each treatment arm. Regardless, these initial studies demonstrated that a sequential treatment approach that uses pretreatment with FSH is successful in inducing testicular growth and fertility in men with CHH and prepubertal testes. However, to definitively demonstrate superiority of this approach, a larger prospective multicenter study would be required. Given the promising benefits for using this approach in the most severely affected men with CHH, a similar protocol could also be applied to those with a history of cryptorchidism who are among the least responsive to gonadotropin therapy.

Patient Monitoring During Spermatogenesis Induction

Fertility-inducing treatment warrants careful clinical and biochemical monitoring, and obtaining expert opinion from clinicians experienced in these specific protocols is highly advisable. Regular assessment of TV through Prader orchidometry is important to evaluate growth, although clinicians tend to slightly overestimate TV by using this technique, whereas sonography in three planes to calculate TV is a reliable and objective metric. Patients should be informed of potential adverse effects of gonadotropin therapy. Gynecomastia is the most common side effect of hCG therapy and is seen in up to one third of patients as a result of excess hCG-induced estradiol (E_2) secretion. It can be avoided by adjusting the hCG dose to avoid inducing supraphysiological E_2 levels; it may be necessary to accept slightly low-normal serum testosterone levels to avoid an excessive rise in serum E_2. Of note, hCG dosing should be based on serum hormone levels, not on subjective reports of energy level and/or libido.

The half-life of hCG is ~36 hours, so trough levels obtained before the subsequent injection are most informative, facilitating closer dose titration and helping to avoid excessive serum testosterone levels that could also result in a raised hematocrit. Therapeutic adherence should be assessed at each visit; patients should be given proper instruction and be able to demonstrate an aseptic self-injection technique. Spermatogenesis can occur even in the setting of modest TV; thus, when TV reaches 5 to 8 mL, regular seminal fluid analysis should be performed after 2 to 3 days of abstinence and repeated every 2 to 3 months thereafter.

hCG Dose Titration

A typical hCG starting dose is ~3000 to 4000 IU/wk, depending on locally available formulations. To ensure stable serum testosterone levels, injections should be spaced (at least twice weekly). The dose may need to be adjusted up or down to find the correct balance between maintaining normal serum testosterone, hemoglobin, hematocrit, and E_2 to minimize risks of testosterone-induced erythrocytosis and E_2-induced gynecomastia. Serum levels should be checked every 4 to 6 weeks, with necessary dose adjustments until steady state has been achieved. As the testes grow, it is often possible to slowly titrate the hCG dose down to minimize potential side effects while maintaining eugonadal serum testosterone levels. Steady-state weekly doses range from 1000 to 10,000 IU/wk. Failure to achieve a serum testosterone response to hCG treatment may result from poor adherence or, rarely, development of antibodies. Measurement of serum hCG levels (except potentially when nonadherence is suspected) is unnecessary, but from our clinical experience, hCG concentrations in the 50 to 150 kU/L range are typical of successful therapy.

FSH (hMG/rFSH) Dose Titration

A typical starting dose of FSH (hMG or rFSH) is 75 IU given on alternate days (or three times a week) by subcutaneous self-injection with the intent of achieving serum FSH levels in the range of 4 to 8 IU/L. It is helpful to monitor serum inhibin B to gauge the response of the Sertoli cells to exogenous FSH. A low baseline serum inhibin B level (<60 pg/mL), which reflects absent testicular development, has been demonstrated to be a negative predictor of outcome. Given that men with CHH have a limited Sertoli cell population (and low testosterone levels), it is expected that baseline serum inhibin B levels are low and AMH levels high.

In men with CHH and severe GnRH deficiency, serial monitoring of serum IB has indicated that levels reach a plateau after 2 months of rFSH treatment (75 IU daily), suggesting that 2 months should be a sufficient pretreatment period with rFSH alone, although a longer period might be beneficial with history of cryptorchidism. Rising serum inhibin B is a positive sign of clinical response. The sharing of improving laboratory measures with patients can be useful for encouraging adherence early in treatment because subtle changes in TV may not yet be evident to the patient.

Although no clear protocol has been established for men with a history of cryptorchidism, it seems reasonable that in such cases the addition of hCG could be deferred until serum inhibin B levels have plateaued on FSH pretreatment. However, a caveat to such an approach that uses prolonged FSH-only therapy is that patients will be hypogonadal for extended periods. Thus, exogenous testosterone, which would not raise intratesticular testosterone levels, could be given to prevent symptoms of hypogonadism during pretreatment to obtain a maximal proliferative benefit, at which time hCG could be introduced, and exogenous testosterone should be stopped.

Relationship Between TV and Spermatogenesis in CHH

Seminal fluid analysis is the key outcome measure and should be repeated every 2 to 3 months within a few months of starting treatment. Assessment of TV is a simple and key clinical indicator of response to fertility treatment. Typically, a TV of 8 to 10 mL indicates spermatogenesis, but men receiving fertility-inducing treatment who attain only limited testicular growth can sometimes have sperm in their ejaculate. The majority of men with CHH will not achieve normal sperm counts as defined by the WHO (*i.e.*, >20 million/mL), yet low sperm counts do not preclude fertility. However, men with smaller testes or a history of cryptorchidism can take 12 to 24 months or even longer with a history of bilateral cryptorchidism. Thus, when discussing fertility planning with patients, couples should be well informed about the potential treatment period necessary to develop fertility (up to 24 months or longer) so that initiation of treatment can be planned accordingly.

Securing the Benefits of Successful Spermatogenesis Induction

Fertility-maintaining treatment typically is continued after conception and into the second trimester because of the possibility of miscarriage early in the pregnancy. If the couple desires to conceive again quickly, hCG alone can be continued to maintain spermatogenesis, although sperm counts and TV tend to diminish over time. Prior gonadotropin treatment results in a two- to threefold shorter time to the appearance of first sperm on subsequent gonadotropin treatment cycles, although success on subsequent cycles cannot be guaranteed. In addition, in some countries like the United Kingdom, entitlement to state-funded fertility treatments ceases with the birth of the first child. Therefore, we recommend that men be encouraged to store sperm (*i.e.*, cryopreservation) before reverting to testosterone replacement. Similarly, for adolescents who receive pubertal induction through gonadotropin therapy, sperm cryopreservation before transitioning to testosterone replacement could be encouraged as an insurance policy of sorts for future fertility.

Role of ART in Men With HH

ART has rapidly advanced, and it is now possible to achieve conception for men with severely impaired sperm counts and/or quality. ART approaches range from relatively less-invasive intrauterine insemination to *in vitro* fertilization and intracytoplasmic sperm injection (ICSI). ICSI was first used in CHH as an approach to shorten treatment duration, and its use should be considered at an early stage where there is suspected dual-factor infertility or because of the age of the female partner or other circumstances.

However, in most cases, the rational approach is to delay ART until maximal testicular development has been achieved. The success rates of ICSI are high in HH, with fertilization rates of 50% to 60% and pregnancy rates of ~30% per cycle. If sperm are consistently absent from the ejaculate, then microtesticular sperm extraction may be effective. Reassuringly, detailed assessment of sperm quality in men undergoing combined gonadotropin treatment revealed that CHH *per se* did not seem to impair DNA integrity or increase the risk of chromosomal aberrations.

ILLUSTRATIVE CLINICAL CASES

Case 1

A 19-year-old male presents with absent puberty and undescended right testis (left-side TV 1 mL). He was anosmic with HH (LH, <0.5 IU/L; FSH, 1.1 IU/L; testosterone, <1.0 nmol/L), confirming Kallmann syndrome. Pubertal induction was initiated with intramuscular testosterone undecanoate, and he was scheduled for right-sided orchidopexy. However, the patient's urologist believed that the procedure would be technically easier and less likely to result in loss of the testis if its volume could be increased.

The patient therefore commenced subcutaneous FSH 150 IU three times a week, and after 2 months, testosterone therapy was replaced with subcutaneous hCG 1500 IU twice a week, achieving normal-range serum levels of hemoglobin, testosterone, E_2, and FSH. After 4 months of combined gonadotropin therapy, his right-side testicle descended spontaneously into the scrotum (right-side TV, 6 mL; left-side TV, 8 mL), so the planned orchidopexy was cancelled. The patient was offered the opportunity to continue therapy and bank sperm for the future, but he did not yet feel emotionally ready for this opportunity.

Question

Is there evidence for gonadotropin therapy in achieving testicular descent?

Answer

The literature relates almost entirely to all-comers with miscellaneous causes of cryptorchidism, which explains why surgery remains the mainstay of treatment. However, for males with CHH (or CPHD) whose cryptorchidism is a direct result of absent minipuberty, combined gonadotropin treatment has a logical basis, and there are increasing numbers of positive case reports. Moreover, even if unsuccessful in achieving testicular descent, the resulting increase in TV undoubtedly will facilitate successful surgery.

Case 2

A 30-year-old man with Kallmann syndrome diagnosed and treated since his late teens was married (young wife, regular menses) and wanted fertility. There was no history of cryptorchidism, TV was 3 mL, and he was azoospermic. He was started on FSH 75 IU daily, and after 2 months, hCG 1500 IU three times a week was added, achieving normal-range serum levels of hemoglobin, testosterone, E_2, and FSH. After 18 months, the testes grew to 20 mL, but he remained azoospermic and so was referred to an andrologist who documented bilateral *vas deferens* agenesis.

The patient's wife received superovulation-ICSI, and at the time of egg collection, the patient underwent a simple testicular aspiration procedure (not microtesticular sperm extraction) that yielded enough high-quality viable sperm to fertilize all available eggs, resulting in a viable singleton pregnancy and a healthy baby boy.

The couple had already received genetic counseling before fertility treatment (although it was difficult to give a definitive opinion because the patient had already screened negative for notable sequence variants in a 20-gene panel). However, the couple wanted to know whether their son inherited the condition. A pediatric opinion was sought, and the child was tested for biochemical minipuberty at 5 weeks of age. Serum levels of LH (2.1 IU/L), FSH (3.2 IU/L), and testosterone (8.1 nmol/L) confirmed eugonadism during the postnatal minipuberty window.

Question
Why was the patient not treated first with hCG monotherapy as per American Association of Clinical Endocrinology guidance?

Answer
TV ≤ 4mL is a signpost of severe gonadotropin deficiency with depleted Sertoli and germ cell population. hCG monotherapy is largely ineffective in this scenario; thus, combined therapy is required. Moreover, it is logical to induce proliferation of these cells with FSH before exposing them to the very high intratesticular testosterone levels induced by hCG and will result in germ and Sertoli cell differentiation.

Question
How common is transmission of CHH with spermatogenesis induction?

Answer
Although well documented, no more than 5% of offspring seem to inherit CHH in this way, which likely reflects the multiallelic genetic basis of most cases of CHH. For male children in particular, confirmation/exclusion of CHH can be confidently achieved by simple biochemical testing during the postnatal minipuberty window.

Case 3
A 30-year-old man who had undergone transphenoidal decompression for pituitary apoplexy 3 years previously was maintained on levothyroxine and testosterone gel treatment of thyrotropin and gonadotropin deficiencies. He had two children with his former wife but was now with a different partner (nulliparous, mid-20s, regular cycles) and wanting fertility. Baseline investigations (off testosterone gel) were LH, 1.2 IU/L; FSH, 2.2 IU/L; and testosterone, 1.2 nmol/L, with azoospermia.

The patient was started on hCG 1500 IU twice a week, achieving normal-range serum levels of hemoglobin, testosterone, E_2, and FSH. Testes grew from 12 to 14 mL, and he achieved sperm counts of 5×10^6/mL at 7 months, 30×10^6/mL at 11 months, and 51.5×10^6/mL at 14 months, at which point his wife was already 14 weeks pregnant. She subsequently delivered a healthy baby girl at term.

Question
Why was hCG monotherapy so successful in this case?

Answer
The patient's testes had previously undergone complete biological development during minipuberty and then puberty as evidenced by a much greater volume than in CHH. Men with acquired HH usually can achieve satisfactory spermatogenesis with hCG monotherapy, and occasionally, they can remain fertile just on testosterone. In many countries, hCG is cheaper than testosterone gels or long-acting intramuscular depot.

LEARNING SUMMARY
Men with CHH have a treatable form of infertility that is amenable to hormonal treatment. Existing data show that ~75% to 80% of these men are able to develop sperm in the ejaculate with appropriate combined gonadotropin treatment or GnRH pump. Evidence suggests that in addition to fertility outcomes, the effects of gonadotropin therapy (*e.g.*, testicular growth) may help to ameliorate some of the psychosocial aspects of CHH and improve some health-related quality-of-life domains in men with CHH.

CHH covers a spectrum of GnRH deficiency, and key factors that affect fertility outcomes include pretreatment TV and whether there is a history of cryptorchidism. Men with some degree of spontaneous pubertal development and larger TV are at the milder end of the disease spectrum. These men are good responders and typically develop sperm within 6 months of starting treatment. In contrast, the most severe cases (*i.e.*, TV ≤ 4 mL and/or a history of bilateral cryptorchidism) have the poorest outcomes, yet results of sequential treatment protocols with FSH pretreatment offer hope for these men. However, a large multicenter study would be required to definitively confirm the superiority of this novel approach.

RECOMMENDED READING

Boehm U, Bouloux P-MG, Dattani MT, de Roux N, Dodé C, Dunkel L, Dwyer AA, Giacobini P, Hardelin JP, Juul A, Maghnie M, Pitteloud N, Prevot V, Raivio T, Tena-Sempere M, Quinton R, Young J. Expert consensus document: European Consensus Statement on congenital hypogonadotropic hypogonadism–pathogenesis, diagnosis and treatment. *Nat Rev Endocrinol.* 2015;**11**(9):547–564.

Dwyer AA, Jayasena CN, Quinton R. Congenital hypogonadotropic hypogonadism: implications of absent mini-puberty. *Minerva Endocrinol.* 2016;**41**(2):188–195.

Dwyer AA, Raivio T, Pitteloud N. Gonadotrophin replacement for induction of fertility in hypogonadal men. *Best Pract Res Clin Endocrinol Metab.* 2015;**29**(1):91–103.

Amenorrhea

M36
Presented, March 17-20, 2018

Magaret E. Wierman, MD. Department of Medicine, Division of Endocrinology, Metabolism, and Diabetes, University of Colorado Anschutz Medical Campus, Aurora, Colorado 80045, E-mail: margaret.wierman@ucdenver.edu

SIGNIFICANCE OF THE CLINICAL PROBLEM

Amenorrhea is the absence of menstrual periods. Oligoamenorrhea is defined as irregular menses, often lighter and less frequent than monthly. Primary amenorrhea refers to the failure to have a first menstrual period, and secondary amenorrhea is defined as cessation of menses after cyclic menses were established. Menstrual disturbances are common, with frequencies of 6% to 10% of women aged 15 to 50 years.

What is normal sexual maturation? Puberty in girls usually begins with breast development at about age 8 years, with onset of menses in the United States at around 12 years. Recent National Health and Nutrition Examination Survey (NHANES) data suggest that the average age of menarche may be decreasing, associated with childhood obesity. African American girls have an earlier onset of breast development than Caucasian girls (8.9 compared with 10.0 years).

The underlying mechanism of pubertal development to trigger normal menstrual cyclicity has been an area of active investigation. Kisspeptin neurons in the hypothalamus send signals to gonadotropin-releasing hormone (GnRH) neurons to secrete increased amounts of the decapeptide in an intermittent fashion to trigger release of the gonadotropins, luteinizing hormone (LH), and follicle-stimulating hormone (FSH) from the pituitary gland. The precise pattern of gonadotropin pulsatility stimulates both gametogenesis and steroidogenesis in the ovary, triggering specific progression of follicular development and secretion of estradiol and later progesterone. The gonadal steroids feed back at both hypothalamic and pituitary targets to modulate further gonadotropin secretion.

The initial cycles in postmenarchal girls are anovulatory and often irregularity persists for up to 12 to 18 months. A final step in the pubertal maturation is the development of a positive feedback effect of higher estrogen levels on the kisspeptin neurons to trigger a GnRH-induced LH surge for monthly ovulation and proper luteal phase function. As the hypothalamic-pituitary-ovarian axis matures, the ovulatory cycles are more frequent and normal adult women usually have ovulatory cycles 10 of 12 months each year.

BARRIERS TO OPTIMAL PRACTICE

The differential diagnosis of the underlying disorder in women who present with amenorrhea or oligoamenorrhea is broad, thus making the initial history, examination, and laboratory collection critical to coming to the appropriate diagnosis and treatment strategy.

LEARNING OBJECTIVES

- Review the normal physiology of the female reproductive axis to understand the approach to the history, exam, and timing of laboratory tests for women presenting with amenorrhea
- List the differential diagnosis of primary compared with secondary amenorrhea and how to confirm or refute each disorder
- Discuss the different treatment strategies for menstrual cycle disorders depending on desire for fertility or not

STRATEGIES FOR DIAGNOSIS, THERAPY, AND/OR MANAGEMENT

It is useful to consider the differential diagnosis of amenorrhea depending on whether it is primary or secondary amenorrhea and then consider the locus of the defect, *i.e.*, hypothalamus, pituitary, gonad, or uterus.

CONCLUSIONS

The approach to the patient who presents with amenorrhea requires careful history with exam and laboratory testing to confirm or refute the diagnosis and then allow appropriate treatment.

CASES

Case 1

A 26-year-old woman presents with a 6-month history of amenorrhea. Her menarche was at age 12 years, and she has had regular menses until recently. She has a history of autoimmune thyroid disease, and a recent thyrotropin measurement was 2.0 mIU/L. The patient reports experiencing dyspareunia, vaginal dryness, and night sweats. Both her mother and maternal aunt had early menopause at age 39 and 40 years, respectively. The patient also has a 19-year-old brother with autism.

On physical examination, her vital signs are normal. She has a small pebbly goiter (about twice normal size). The rest of her examination findings are normal other than an atrophic vaginal lining on pelvic examination.

Laboratory test results were as follows: FSH = 90 mIU/mL (90 IU/L) [reference range, 2.0 to 12.0 mIU/mL (2.0 to 12.0 IU/L)], estradiol = <20 pg/mL (<73.4 pmol/L) [reference range, 22 to 56 pg/mL (80.8 to 206.6 pmol/L)], prolactin = 7 ng/mL (0.30 nmol/L), and karyotype 46,XX.

Which of the following is the most appropriate next test?

A. Qualitative β-human chorionic gonadotropin (β-hCG)
B. Measurement of ovarian antibodies
C. Measurement of thyroperoxidase antibodies
D. Fragile X (*FMR1*) testing
E. Pituitary magnetic resonance imaging

Case 2

A 23-year-old woman presents with irregular menses and then amenorrhea. Her menarche was at age 14 years; her periods were irregular for 18 months and then regular every 28 days. About 2 years ago, her cycle length shortened to 25 days and then to 22 days. She has not had a period in 4 months. She is stressed in her new job. She runs 2 miles three times a week. Her body mass index is 20 kg/m^2. A pregnancy test is negative.

Of the following, which are the best next laboratory tests to obtain?

A. FSH, LH, testosterone, and dehydroepiandrosterone sulfate (DHEA-S)
B. FSH, estradiol, and prolactin
C. FSH, estradiol, and 17-hydroxyprogesterone (17-OHP)
D. FSH, estradiol, and progesterone
E. FSH, adrenocorticotropic hormone, and cortisol

Case 3

A 20-year-old woman presents with oligoamenorrhea. She had early menarche at age 11 years, had hirsutism and acne since age 13 years, and always had irregular menses. She had weight gain from 120 lb (54.5 kg) to 170 lb (77.3 kg) since adolescence. She has a family history of hypertension and type 2 diabetes mellitus.

What is not in the differential diagnosis for this patient?

A. Polycystic ovary syndrome (PCOS)
B. Premature ovarian insufficiency
C. Congenital adrenal hyperplasia
D. Obesity-induced hyperandrogenic anovulation
E. Ovarian tumor

DISCUSSION OF CASES AND ANSWERS

Case 1. Take Home Point: Understand the Extended Diagnostic Differential in Women Presenting With Premature Ovarian Insufficiency

Answer: D (fragile X [*FMR1*] testing). This case presents with premature ovarian insufficiency. It is useful to review the differential diagnosis (1–4). In this case, the history and laboratories direct you to a diagnosis of a potential genetic disorder, and fragile X premutation screening should be performed, especially in those who have a family history of male relatives with learning disorders, autism, or mental retardation or family members with ataxia and/or dementia (suggestive of fragile X–related ataxia) (5). The screening is accomplished by *FMR1* genetic testing (answer D). In fragile X carriers, CGG repeats are in the premutation range.

Pregnancy would not elevate FSH, so qualitative β-hCG (answer A) is not necessary. Ovarian antibodies (answer B) have not been identified as a cause of this type of premature ovarian insufficiency. As currently developed, their measurement is not clinically useful and has no predictive value. Thyroid antibodies (answer C) are very useful in predicting thyroid disease but are not relevant to this clinical scenario. There is no indication for pituitary magnetic resonance imaging (answer E) given the patient's presentation, because an FSH-secreting pituitary tumor mimicking premature ovarian insufficiency is rare. Gonadotrope-secreting pituitary tumors are more common in men than in women. In premenopausal women, they may present with ovarian hyperstimulation due to biologically active FSH and persistently elevated estradiol levels (6). In postmenopausal women, they present with mass effects, headaches, vision changes, and often pituitary dysfunction because of tumor size. Usually, the tumors in postmenopausal women blunt the rise in gonadotropins (*i.e.*, postmenopausal FSH and LH levels are instead in the premenopausal range).

Antimüllerian hormone (AMH) is a marker of ovarian reserve and follicular number. Infertility specialists have used it extensively in clinical practice to evaluate older women with borderline elevated FSH levels to predict response to *in vitro* fertilization and to diagnose premature ovarian insufficiency. A woman with PCOS would have a high AMH level and a lower FSH level. AMH levels are lower in women with impending premature ovarian insufficiency (with higher FSH levels). Importantly, women with hypothalamic amenorrhea also have a low AMH level but a low-normal FSH level. These caveats should be remembered in checking an AMH level.

Case 2. Take Home Point: Hypothalamic Amenorrhea Is a Diagnosis of Exclusion. History Is Most Important With Exam and Laboratories Helping You to Exclude Other Diagnoses

Answer: B (FSH, estradiol, and prolactin). Hypothalamic amenorrhea is a diagnosis of exclusion (7, 8). Excessive stress, exercise, herbal therapy, supplements, and drugs may alter the GnRH pulse generator, thereby altering the necessary switch of pulse frequency and amplitude across the menstrual cycle to induce ovulation and ensure regular periods. Hyperprolactinemia due to mild thyroid dysfunction, medications, or tumors can turn off the GnRH pulse generator and present as hypothalamic amenorrhea. Estrogen is low in the settings of hypothalamic amenorrhea and hyperprolactinemia, but it would be high if the patient were pregnant. The best laboratory tests to order next are measurements of FSH, estradiol, and prolactin (answer B).

Androgens would be measured in a patient who has acne and hirsutism (thus, answer A is incorrect). A stimulated 17-OHP measurement is the best test to assess for congenital adrenal hyperplasia, but there is no reason to suspect that in this vignette because the patient did not describe hyperandrogenic symptoms or early pubic hair (thus, answer C is incorrect). Progesterone is measured to assess ovulation and luteal-phase function in women attempting fertility (thus, answer D is incorrect). Cushing syndrome may result in amenorrhea due to inhibition of gonadotropin secretion by excess cortisol, and its measurement is not indicated in this case (thus, answer E is incorrect).

If the patient had presented as primary amenorrhea with low estradiol and low gonadotropins, genetic causes of hypothalamic amenorrhea would be considered. In the last 10 years, our understanding of the genetic causes of GnRH deficiency, including both anosmic idiopathic hypogonadotropic hypogonadism and normosmic idiopathic hypogonadotropic hypogonadism, has greatly expanded (9–14). In this patient with absent sexual maturation and no sense of smell, the associated abnormalities point to a defect in the gene encoding fibroblast growth factor 8 (*FGF8*) or its receptor, the fibroblast growth factor receptor 1 (*FGFR1*). Autosomal dominant disorders are of the *FGF* pathway. Mutations in the *FGF* pathway are more common than mutations in *KAL1*, which also presents with anosmia. Because *KAL1* is located on the X chromosome, women with *KAL1* mutations are not usually symptomatic. The *FGF* system cross-talks with anosmin (product of *KAL1*) during GnRH neuron migration to ensure targeting of the GnRH neurons to the hypothalamus. Patients with *KAL1* or *FGF* pathway mutations often have midline defects, such as cleft palate. *KISS1R* (previously known as *GPR54*) is a G-protein–coupled receptor now called the kisspeptin receptor. Together with its ligand, kisspeptin, this pathway has been identified as an upstream activator of GnRH secretion at the time of puberty. Very few cases of *KISS1R* mutations have been identified. However, a constitutively active *KISSR1* mutation was identified as a putative cause of precocity in a young girl, which is further evidence of the importance of this ligand/G-protein–coupled receptor signaling to activate pubertal development. Mutations in the gene encoding the makorin ring finger protein 3 (*MKRN3*) result in familial precocious puberty. This novel imprinted gene is thought to function as a ubiquitin ligase and act as an epigenetic regulator of pubertal development (15). Its exact role in GnRH neuron biology is under active investigation. Mutations in the gene encoding leptin (*LEP*) or its receptor (*LEPR*) result in morbid obesity and failure to undergo puberty. Although leptin signals fat stores to the brain, it is necessary but not sufficient for pubertal development.

Despite an explosion of new research in the genetics of pubertal development, fewer than 40% of all patients with idiopathic hypogonadotropic hypogonadism have a known genetic mutation. New approaches such as exome sequencing of families and large cohorts of probands will increase our discovery of new players in the control of the reproductive axis.

Case 3. Take Home Point: Most Women With Hyperandrogenism Present With Oligoamenorrhea. Again the History and Laboratory Will Help Narrow the Diagnosis and Point to the Appropriate Treatment

Answer: B (Premature ovarian insufficiency would not present in this fashion and thus is the correct diagnosis. These patients have normal menarche and cycles until their cycles shorten and stop. They have signs and symptoms of estrogen deficiency.) PCOS (answer A) is a common disorder that occurs in 6% to 8% of women. Affected patients usually present with hirsutism, acne, and irregular menses (16–18). Sixty percent of affected women become obese. Occasionally, girls with PCOS can exercise and implement lifestyle interventions to mask the symptoms of the disorder and actually induce a picture of hypothalamic amenorrhea. Their PCOS phenotype then manifests when their diet, lifestyle, or exercise regimen is modified or they stop therapy with oral contraceptives.

Several definitions have been used to define PCOS. The National Institutes of Health criteria includes oligoovulation and clinical and/or biochemical hyperandrogenism after excluding congenital adrenal hyperplasia, hyperprolactinemia, Cushing syndrome, and other disorders. The revised Rotterdam criteria added the criterion of ultrasonography with at least 12 to 15 small cysts around the periphery of the ovary or an increased ovarian volume. This patient has not had ultrasonography, but she fits the criteria with hirsutism and anovulation.

Women with PCOS are at risk for impaired glucose tolerance and type 2 diabetes mellitus, with a risk 5 to 10 times that of age-matched control women. In women with PCOS, the prevalence of impaired glucose tolerance is 30% to 35% and the prevalence of type 2 diabetes mellitus is 3% to 10%. The risk of prediabetes and diabetes is higher in those women who are obese. For example, in normal-weight women with PCOS, the risk is 10% to 15% for impaired glucose tolerance and 1% to 2% for diabetes. But, taken together, all women with PCOS have increased risk compared with that of age-matched and weight-matched control women. Metabolic complications are more common when there is a family history of type 2 diabetes mellitus. The recent Endocrine Society guidelines recommend use of a 75-g oral glucose tolerance test to screen for impaired glucose intolerance in women with PCOS because of increased sensitivity but state that hemoglobin A_{1c} measurement may be more practical and cost effective.

Studies have suggested that women with PCOS are at risk for endometrial hyperplasia and endometrial cancer at an earlier age. In addition, women with PCOS have a higher risk of nonalcoholic fatty liver disease, but it is unclear whether treatment strategies alter this risk. Recently, investigators have emphasized the increased risk of obstructive sleep apnea in women with PCOS. The risk is worse with concomitant obesity, but it is also increased when compared with body mass index–matched control women. If a patient undergoes ovulation induction with antiestrogens (clomiphene) or the preferred aromatase inhibitor (letrozole) or gonadotropins, she will have increased risk of multiple gestations. Pregnancy complications in women with PCOS include gestational diabetes mellitus, preterm delivery, and preeclampsia. Despite an increase in metabolic syndrome and cardiac risk factors, studies have not yet shown an increased risk of cardiovascular disease in women with PCOS.

Patients with nonclassical congenital adrenal insufficiency (answer C) can present with signs and symptoms similar to PCOS, *i.e.*, hirsutism, acne, and irregular menses. Few studies have followed women with congenital adrenal hyperplasia prospectively to ask the incidence of insulin resistance, weight gain, and metabolic complications long-term. A 17-OHP >200 ng/dL would suggest this diagnosis and trigger additional testing. Obesity-induced hyperandrogenism (answer D) is not well studied in the literature but is seen clinically in women with regular menses to gain weight to a critical threshold and then develop hirsutism, acne, irregular menses, and/or amenorrhea. This scenario is the opposite end of the spectrum from anorexia-induced amenorrhea. The androgens are thought to result from the 5α-reductase activity in the excess fat tissue. This case does not have this history. We treat these women with interventions that help with weight loss and insulin sensitization, and often if they lose weight, their menses will return. An ovarian tumor (answer E) producing androgens (only 10% of tumors make hormones) would present with a more rapid onset of hirsutism, acne, and virilization (male pattern balding, alopecia, and clitoromegaly). A vaginal ultrasound would help identify the tumor, which can be small. Adrenal tumors usually make high levels of DHEA-S, whereas ovarian tumors usually make male levels of testosterone. Premature ovarian insufficiency (answer B) would not present in this fashion.

REFERENCES

1. Silva CA, Yamakami LY, Aikawa NE, Araujo DB, Carvalho JF, Bonfá E. Autoimmune primary ovarian insufficiency. *Autoimmun Rev.* 2014; **13**(4-5):427–430.
2. Welt CK. Primary ovarian insufficiency: a more accurate term for premature ovarian failure. *Clin Endocrinol (Oxf).* 2008;**68**(4): 499–509.
3. Del Mastro L, Ceppi M, Poggio F, Bighin C, Peccatori F, Demeestere I, Levaggi A, Giraudi S, Lambertini M, D'Alonzo A, Canavese G, Pronzato P, Bruzzi P. Gonadotropin-releasing hormone analogues for the prevention of chemotherapy-induced premature ovarian failure in cancer women: systematic review and meta-analysis of randomized trials. *Cancer Treat Rev.* 2014;**40**(5):675–683.
4. Webber L, Davies M, Anderson R, Bartlett J, Braat D, Cartwright B, Cifkova R, de Muinck Keizer-Schrama S, Hogervorst E, Janse F, Liao L, Vlaisavljevic V, Zillikens C, Vermeulen N; European Society for Human Reproduction and Embryology (ESHRE) Guideline Group on POI. ESHRE Guideline: management of women with premature ovarian insufficiency. *Hum Reprod.* 2016;**31**(5):926–937.
5. Wang T, Bray SM, Warren ST. New perspectives on the biology of fragile X syndrome. *Curr Opin Genet Dev.* 2012;**22**(3):256–263.
6. Macchia E, Simoncini T, Raffaelli V, Lombardi M, Iannelli A, Martino E. A functioning FSH-secreting pituitary macroadenoma causing an ovarian hyperstimulation syndrome with multiple cysts resected and relapsed after leuprolide in a reproductive-aged woman. *Gynecol Endocrinol.* 2012;**28**(1):56–59.
7. Gordon CM. Clinical practice. Functional hypothalamic amenorrhea. *N Engl J Med.* 2010;**363**(4):365–371.
8. Santoro N. Update in hyper- and hypogonadotropic amenorrhea. *J Clin Endocrinol Metab.* 2011;**96**(11):3281–3288.
9. Caronia LM, Martin C, Welt CK, Sykiotis GP, Quinton R, Thambundit A, Avbelj M, Dhruvakumar S, Plummer L, Hughes VA, Seminara SB, Boepple PA, Sidis Y, Crowley WF, Jr, Martin KA, Hall JE, Pitteloud N. A genetic basis for functional hypothalamic amenorrhea. *N Engl J Med.* 2011;**364**(3):215–225.
10. Melmed S, Casanueva FF, Hoffman AR, Kleinberg DL, Montori VM, Schlechte JA, Wass JA; Endocrine Society. Diagnosis and treatment of hyperprolactinemia: an Endocrine Society clinical practice guideline. *J Clin Endocrinol Metab.* 2011;**96**(2):273–288.
11. Wierman ME, Kiseljak-Vassiliades K, Tobet S. Gonadotropin-releasing hormone (GnRH) neuron migration: initiation, maintenance and cessation as critical steps to ensure normal reproductive function. *Front Neuroendocrinol.* 2011;**32**(1):43–52.
12. Warren MP. Endocrine manifestations of eating disorders. *J Clin Endocrinol Metab.* 2011;**96**(2):333–343.
13. Sykiotis GP, Pitteloud N, Seminara SB, Kaiser UB, Crowley WF, Jr. Deciphering genetic disease in the genomic era: the model of GnRH deficiency. *Sci Transl Med.* 2010;**2**(32):32rv2.
14. Bianco SD, Kaiser UB. The genetic and molecular basis of idiopathic hypogonadotropic hypogonadism. *Nat Rev Endocrinol.* 2009;**5**(10): 569–576.
15. Abreu AP, Dauber A, Macedo DB, Noel SD, Brito VN, Gill JC, Cukier P, Thompson IR, Navarro VM, Gagliardi PC, Rodrigues T, Kochi C, Longui CA, Beckers D, de Zegher F, Montenegro LR, Mendonca BB, Carroll RS, Hirschhorn JN, Latronico AC, Kaiser UB. Central precocious puberty caused by mutations in the imprinted gene MKRN3. *N Engl J Med.* 2013;**368**(26):2467–2475.
16. Legro RS, Arslanian SA, Ehrmann DA, Hoeger KM, Murad MH, Pasquali R, Welt CK; Endocrine Society. Diagnosis and treatment of polycystic ovary syndrome: an Endocrine Society clinical practice guideline. *J Clin Endocrinol Metab.* 2013;**98**(12):4565–4592.
17. Tasali E, Chapotot F, Leproult R, Whitmore H, Ehrmann DA. Treatment of obstructive sleep apnea improves cardiometabolic function in young obese women with polycystic ovary syndrome. *J Clin Endocrinol Metab.* 2011;**96**(2):365–374.
18. Ramezani-Binabaj M, Motalebi M, Karimi-Sari H, Rezaee-Zavareh MS, Alavian SM. Are women with polycystic ovarian syndrome at a high risk of non-alcoholic fatty liver disease; a meta-analysis. *Hepat Mon.* 2014;**14**(11):e23235.

Diagnosis and Management of Male Hypogonadism

M37
Presented, March 17-20, 2018

Bradley D. Anawalt, MD. University of Washington School of Medicine, Seattle, Washington 98195, E-mail: banawalt@medicine.washington.edu

SIGNIFICANCE OF THE CLINICAL PROBLEM

The male gonad has two primary functions: spermatogenesis and sex hormone steroidogenesis. Defects in spermatogenesis occur in ~10% of men, and men with abnormal spermatogenesis can be described as having male hypogonadism (1). However, for this Meet the Professor, I will use the term "male hypogonadism" to describe men with testosterone deficiency. Male hypogonadism may be caused by decreased sensitivity to testosterone, but it is much more commonly due to decreased production and secretion of testosterone, resulting in a low serum testosterone concentration. A low serum testosterone concentration is not sufficient to make the diagnosis of hypogonadism; the diagnosis requires symptoms or signs of testosterone deficiency and a low circulating testosterone concentration in an early morning blood sample on at least two occasions.

The prevalence of male hypogonadism has not been determined, but it is common. The prevalence of low serum testosterone concentrations is very high and increases with age (2, 3), but the prevalence of symptoms of hypogonadism plus low serum testosterone is much lower (4, 5). In middle-aged and older men, the prevalence of male hypogonadism is probably 2% to 5% (5). In young men, the prevalence is lower, but there are few data on the true prevalence in men <50 years old.

Although the diagnosis of male hypogonadism is generally straightforward in men with known hypothalamic, pituitary, or testicular disease, it is difficult to make the diagnosis in men without a known cause for testicular deficiency. The development of new formulations of testosterone replacement therapy has made the management of male hypogonadism more convenient. However, successful marketing of testosterone therapy as a potential cure for many common symptoms such as fatigue, decreased sense of well-being, and age-related declines in sexual, physical, and mental function has increased the requests for and prescription of testosterone replacement therapy in the United States and, to a lesser degree, in other parts of the world. Clinicians are often in the quandary of whether to assess gonadal function in men with symptoms that are not specific for hypogonadism and how to manage low serum testosterone concentrations in these men who do not clearly meet the criteria for the diagnosis of male hypogonadism.

BARRIERS TO OPTIMAL PRACTICE

- Lack of access to an accurate and precise testosterone assay with a validated and universal normal range
- Public misconceptions about the positive and negative effects of testosterone replacement therapy *vs.* pharmacological use of androgens
- Lack of well-designed, long-term studies of the beneficial and adverse effects of testosterone therapy on young and older men with hypogonadism
- Disparity of access for all men to all formulations of testosterone therapy

LEARNING OBJECTIVES

- To describe an approach on how to make an accurate diagnosis of male hypogonadism in individual patients
- To distinguish the temporal effects of testosterone replacement therapy on sexual function, erythropoiesis, muscle, and bone density
- To understand when and how to prescribe exogenous testosterone therapy for hypogonadal men with a history of cardiovascular disease, prostate disease, or higher risk of thromboembolic disease

STRATEGIES FOR DIAGNOSIS, THERAPY, AND/OR MANAGEMENT

When male hypogonadism is suspected based on symptoms or signs, the clinician should request measurement of total testosterone on a blood sample obtained in the early morning. The blood sample should be obtained when the patient is at baseline health and not acutely ill. Because of substantial variability in day-to-day blood testosterone concentrations and variability in the measurement, low serum testosterone concentrations must be confirmed with at least one more early morning blood sample in the fasting state. The assessment of serum free testosterone concentrations should be made using an accurate method (*e.g.,* calculated free testosterone or direct measurement after equilibrium dialysis). There are several methods of calculating free testosterone concentrations (based on total testosterone and circulating testosterone-binding proteins), but it is not known which method is the best method for clinical use (6–8). In general, the three commonly advocated methods (including the Vermuelen method) correlate well with values obtained by equilibrium dialysis. All three methods of calculating free testosterone concentrations rely upon an accurate assay for total testosterone.

The clinician should know the quality of their local laboratory's total and free testosterone assays. Specifically, it is important that the clinician use a US Centers for Disease Control and Prevention (CDC)–validated testosterone assay (or an assay that has been verified by a similar external quality control program) (9). Total testosterone is most accurately measured by liquid chromatography tandem mass spectroscopy, but many fluoroimmunoassays are accurate within the ranges of total testosterone commonly seen in clinical practice. The fluoroimmunoassays are less accurate when testosterone concentrations are very low or very high. Platform assays that measure free testosterone concentrations directly are notoriously inaccurate and often underestimate the true free testosterone concentration.

After confirmation that the early morning serum testosterone concentration is reproducibly and unequivocally low, a careful assessment for the cause of hypogonadism must be performed. Primary hypogonadism is characterized by elevated gonadotropins [serum follicle-stimulating hormone (FSH) > serum luteinizing hormone (LH)]. For some men with primary hypogonadism, karyotyping (to detect an extra X chromosome) may be useful. Secondary hypogonadism is characterized by low serum testosterone and low or inappropriately normal serum gonadotropins. Common causes of secondary hypogonadism include sellar tumors, hyperprolactinemia, iron overload syndromes, and Cushing syndrome.

Before initiation of testosterone therapy, men should be counseled on the potential side effects. Acne and erythrocytosis are known side effects. All forms of androgen therapy are associated with suppression of serum HDL cholesterol, but the clinical significance of this effect is unknown. The major areas of controversy regarding the potential adverse effects of testosterone therapy are the effects on the risk of cardiovascular events, prostate disease, and thromboembolic disease.

Although two recent epidemiological studies demonstrated an association between testosterone therapy and increased risk of cardiovascular events in higher-risk men, two other recent large epidemiological studies showed no increased risk (10–13). The recently completed US Testosterone Trial demonstrated no substantial difference in cardiovascular events in the group of older men treated with testosterone *vs.* those treated with placebo after 1 year of therapy (14). The Testosterone Trial also demonstrated a significantly greater increase in coronary artery noncalcified plaque volume in the testosterone-treated group compared with placebo (15). However, there was >50% baseline difference in noncalcified plaque volume between the two groups, a difference that suggests a clinically important baseline difference between the two groups.

Exogenous testosterone therapy increases serum prostate-specific antigen concentrations by 0.3 to 0.5 ng/mL (9). Testosterone rarely significantly worsens symptoms of bladder outlet obstruction due to benign prostatic hyperplasia, and there is weak evidence suggesting a benefit for such symptoms (16). There is little evidence that exogenous testosterone therapy increases the risk of developing prostate cancer, but testosterone therapy is contraindicated in men with untreated aggressive (Gleason 8 to 10) prostate cancer or extracapsular prostate cancer 1 (17). There is controversy about testosterone therapy in hypogonadal men who have been treated effectively for less aggressive prostate cancer or prostate cancer confined to the prostate.

Although the US Food and Drug Administration requires a label warning about the potential increased risk of venothrombotic events with testosterone therapy, two large database studies published in 2016 demonstrated no association between idiopathic venothrombotic events and any form of testosterone therapy (18, 19).

MAIN CONCLUSIONS

For symptomatic hypogonadal men, the known benefits of testosterone therapy generally exceed the potential adverse effects. For men with mild hypogonadism, the benefits of testosterone therapy are less impressive. For eugonadal men, the long-term benefit and safety of testosterone therapy are unknown.

STRATEGIES FOR DIAGNOSIS, THERAPY, AND/OR MANAGEMENT

Case 1

The Patient Who Is Already Taking Androgen Therapy

You are consulted for a second opinion about whether a 38-year-old man should continue testosterone therapy. One year ago, he reported increased fatigue, depressed mood, and decreased sexual desire. His serum total testosterone concentration on an early morning blood sample was 310 ng/dL (10.8 nmol/L; normal, 335 to 975 ng/dL, 11.8 to 33.8 nmol/L). The repeat measurement (with the same assay) was 295 ng/dL (10.2 nmol/L). Calculated free testosterone was low. Serum gonadotropin concentrations were normal. His primary care clinician recommended testosterone therapy. Eight months ago, the man started testosterone gel therapy, but he did not feel better and did not like applying the gel daily. He switched to testosterone enanthate, 150 mg intramuscularly, every 14 days about 3 months ago. He continues to report fatigue, depressed mood, and decreased sexual desire.

Physical Examination

The patient's height is 72 inches (183 cm) and body mass index (BMI) is 28 kg/m^2. He has a beard. There is no gynecomastia or nipple discharge. He has a normal penis and his testes are 12 mL bilaterally.

Laboratories

The patient's hematocrit is 40% (normal 38% to 46%).

What is the best course of management?

A. Continue testosterone therapy at current dosage with no further evaluation

B. Continue testosterone therapy at current dosage but order sella magnetic resonance imaging

C. Increase testosterone enanthate to 200 mg every 14 days

D. Discontinue testosterone therapy and reassess gonadal axis with a different testosterone assay in 1 month

Discussion

Answer: D. This man is likely to be eugonadal, and he is not clearly benefiting from testosterone therapy. The assay that was used to diagnose hypogonadism in this man has an unusual normal range, and this unusual range suggests either an inaccurate assay or an inappropriate control group for the normal range. Clinicians should be aware that the CDC has a standardization program for testosterone assays. Assays that have been validated by this program have a normal range of 264 to 916 ng/dL (9.2 to 31.8 nmol/L) for the 2.5th and 97.5th percentile and 303 to 852 ng/dL (10.5 to 29.5 nmol/L) for the 5th and 95th percentile (20). Clinicians should use an assay that has been validated by the CDC (or a similar accuracy-based external validation quality control program).

Healthy, young eugonadal men who are treated with exogenous testosterone will recover their gonadal axis function after discontinuation of testosterone therapy. The recovery occurs within 1 month after cessation of intramuscular testosterone enanthate or cypionate (unpublished data from several male hormonal contraceptive trials). The time of recovery is shorter with testosterone formulations with shorter half-lives (transdermal formulations) and longer in formulations with longer half-lives (testosterone undecanoate).

Answers A, B, and C are not correct because the man is likely eugonadal and is not benefitting from testosterone therapy after an adequate trial for his symptoms; a longer trial or higher dosage of testosterone is not going to result in improved energy, mood, or sexual function.

Case 2

The Older Man With Decreased Libido and Low Serum Testosterone Concentrations

A 67-year-old man reports a progressive decline in libido and sexual satisfaction over the past 2 years. He is able to attain and maintain erections enough to have sexual activity, but he would like "harder erections". He reports a satisfying relationship with his longtime sexual partner/spouse.

He has no history of coronary artery disease, prostate cancer, or fracture. He has no additional risk factors for osteoporosis.

Physical Examination

The patient's height is 72 inches (183 cm) and BMI is 28 kg/m^2. Blood pressure is 132/72 and heart rate is 68. He has a normal cardiac and pulmonary examination. There is no gynecomastia or nipple discharge. He has a normal penis and his testes are 20 mL bilaterally.

Laboratories (From an Early Morning Blood Sample)

The patient's serum total testosterone is 255 ng/dL (8.8 nmol/L) (CDC-validated testosterone assay); 5th and 95th percentile = 264 to 916 ng/dL (9.2 to 31.8 nmol/L). Calculated free testosterone is low. Serum T4, thyrotropin, FSH, and LH are normal. Hematocrit is 35% (normal 38% to 46%). He has a normal serum ferritin iron saturation, B12, and folate and a slightly low reticulocyte count. Repeat early morning testosterone is 265 ng/dL (9.2 nmol/L).

Imaging

Bone densitometry (dual-energy X-ray absorptiometry) reveals a T-score of −1.7 in the left hip and −2.0 in the lumbar spine.

In this man, what is the best course of management?

A. Initiation of testosterone at one-half the usual replacement dosage for 3-month trial
B. Initiation of testosterone at full replacement dosage for 3-month trial
C. Initiation of testosterone at one-half the usual replacement dosage for 12-month trial
D. Initiation of testosterone at usual replacement dosage for 12-month trial
E. Initiation of alendronate weekly and sildenafil as needed

Discussion

Answer: B. This man's primary complaint is low libido, and he has a low-normal serum testosterone concentration that has been confirmed on two early morning blood samples. He also has anemia and osteopenia. In the Testosterone Trial, testosterone replacement therapy improved erectile function and overall sexual satisfaction compared with placebo. The effect on erectile function was considered modest (with an improvement on the International Index of Erectile Function score of about half that seen with sildenafil) (14). In addition, the Testosterone Trial demonstrated that testosterone replacement therapy significantly increased hematocrit in men with unexplained anemia. The effects on sexual function and hematocrit are seen within ~3 months (14, 21). Finally, the Testosterone Trial demonstrated that testosterone increased bone mineral density after 1 year of therapy (22). For this man, a 3-month trial will suffice to determine if there is a positive effect on sexual function and erythropoiesis. If there is no improvement in either of these two outcomes, then testosterone therapy could be discontinued.

Answers A and C are incorrect because full dosage replacement therapy is warranted in this man who appears to be hypogonadal, and it is unlikely that low-dosage testosterone therapy would increase his testosterone concentrations enough to confer benefit. (It should be noted that some men have substantial increases in serum testosterone with low dosages of testosterone therapy.) Answer D is incorrect because there is no need to commit a 12-month trial of testosterone for this patient. His primary problem is sexual dysfunction; he has osteopenia that does not necessarily require pharmacotherapy (23). It is true that the full effects of testosterone therapy on bone mineral density take 1 to

2 years. Therefore, a trial of at least 12 months would be required if the primary desired outcome was increased bone mineral density. The sexual benefits of testosterone therapy tend to wane at 12 months (14). If this man has improved sexual function at 3 months that disappears at 12 months, then continuation of testosterone therapy might be based on the positive effects on bone (22, 23). Answer E is incorrect because it requires two drugs (and greater expense) and because pharmacotherapy for osteopenia might not be warranted for this man.

Case 3

The Hypogonadal Man With a History of Possible Contraindications to Testosterone Therapy

A 64-year-old man is diagnosed with hypogonadism based on typical symptoms and signs, including a marked decrease in libido and muscle strength. His laboratory tests are consistent with severe primary hypogonadism: very low serum testosterone concentration and elevated (FSH > LH) gonadotropins.

His past medical history is remarkable for localized prostate cancer (Gleason 7) that was treated with radical prostatectomy 6 years ago. Surgical margins were clear, and follow-up imaging and serum prostate-specific antigen (PSA) measurements have shown no sign of recurrence. He has history of lower extremity deep venous thrombosis after an ankle fracture ipsilateral to the thrombosis.

Physical Examination

The patient's height is 69 inches (175 cm) and BMI is 31 kg/m^2. Blood pressure is 130/82 and heart rate is 76. He has normal secondary sexual characteristics. He has a normal cardiac and pulmonary exam. There is no gynecomastia or nipple discharge. He has a normal penis and his testes are 20 mL bilaterally.

Laboratories

Serum PSA is undetectable. Bone densitometry (dual-energy X-ray absorptiometry) reveals a T-score of −1.5 in the left hip and −2.2 in the lumbar spine.

What is the best management of this man's hypogonadism?

A. Initiate low-dosage testosterone replacement therapy
B. Initiate full-dosage testosterone replacement therapy
C. Initiate clomiphene
D. Initiate generic alendronate

Discussion

Answer: B. This patient has severe primary hypogonadism, and testosterone therapy should be considered. According to the 2018 Endocrine Society Guidelines, testosterone therapy should not be administered to men with prostate cancer, but the authors acknowledge that there is controversy about androgen replacement therapy in men with a history of localized prostate cancer that has been treated with radical prostatectomy and evidence of recurrent disease (undetectable PSA and negative imaging) (9). In this man with severe primary hypogonadism, there are clear benefits of androgen replacement therapy on bone, muscle, and sexual function. He can be followed for evidence of recurrent prostate cancer with serum PSA measurements. If after (written) informed consent, he wishes to proceed with androgen replacement therapy, I would prescribe testosterone and measure a serum PSA within 3 months of initiation of testosterone replacement therapy and at least annually thereafter.

Although the best evidence (17, 18) suggests that testosterone therapy does not increase the risk of deep venous thrombosis, it is possible that testosterone therapy increases the risk of thromboembolic events in men with underlying thrombophilia. This man has a history of a deep venous thrombosis associated with lower extremity trauma and surgery, and he is very unlikely to have underlying thrombophilia. Testosterone therapy will not increase his risk of recurrent venous thrombosis. In women, selective estrogen receptor modulators such as raloxifene and clomiphene increase the risk of venous thrombosis. It is not known whether clomiphene increases the risk of venous thrombosis in men.

Low-dosage testosterone replacement therapy (answer A) will not confer the full benefits of testosterone on bone and muscle, and there is no evidence that low-dosage testosterone is safer than full-dosage testosterone replacement therapy. Clomiphene (answer C) is ineffective in primary hypogonadism and is not approved or proven to be safe and effective for secondary hypogonadism in large, well-designed, randomized, placebo-controlled trials. Alendronate (answer D) would be effective for decreasing the risk of fractures in this man with severe hypogonadism and osteopenia if testosterone therapy is not initiated (23). Answer D is not incorrect *per se*, but it will not treat this man's sexual dysfunction or weakness due to hypogonadism.

REFERENCES

1. Anawalt BD. Approach to male infertility and induction of spermatogenesis. *J Clin Endocrinol Metab.* 2013;**98**(9):3532–3542.
2. Araujo AB, O'Donnell AB, Brambilla DJ, Simpson WB, Longcope C, Matsumoto AM, McKinlay JB. Prevalence and incidence of androgen deficiency in middle-aged and older men: estimates from the Massachusetts Male Aging Study. *J Clin Endocrinol Metab.* 2004;**89**(12):5920–5926.
3. Harman SM, Metter EJ, Tobin JD, Pearson J, Blackman MR; Baltimore Longitudinal Study of Aging. Longitudinal effects of aging on serum total and free testosterone levels in healthy men. *J Clin Endocrinol Metab.* 2001;**86**(2):724–731.
4. Araujo AB, Esche GR, Kupelian V, O'Donnell AB, Travison TG, Williams RE, Clark RV, McKinlay JB. Prevalence of symptomatic androgen deficiency in men. *J Clin Endocrinol Metab.* 2007;**92**(11):4241–4247.
5. Wu FC, Tajar A, Beynon JM, Pye SR, Silman AJ, Finn JD, O'Neill TW, Bartfai G, Casanueva FF, Forti G, Giwercman A, Han TS, Kula K, Lean ME, Pendleton N, Punab M, Boonen S, Vanderschueren D, Labrie F, Huhtaniemi IT; EMAS Group. Identification of late-onset hypogonadism in middle-aged and elderly men. *N Engl J Med.* 2010;**363**(2):123–135.

6. Zakharov MN, Bhasin S, Travison TG, Xue R, Ulloor J, Vasan RS, Carter E, Wu F, Jasuja R. A multi-step, dynamic allosteric model of testosterone's binding to sex hormone binding globulin [published correction appears in *Mol Cell Endocrinol.* 2017;454:167]. *Mol Cell Endocrinol.* 2015;**399**:190–200.
7. Vermeulen A, Verdonck L, Kaufman JM. A critical evaluation of simple methods for the estimation of free testosterone in serum. *J Clin Endocrinol Metab.* 1999;**84**(10):3666–3672.
8. Sartorius G, Ly LP, Sikaris K, McLachlan R, Handelsman DJ. Predictive accuracy and sources of variability in calculated free testosterone estimates. *Ann Clin Biochem.* 2009;**46**(Pt. 2):137–143.
9. Bhasin S, Brito JP, Cunningham GR, Hayes FJ, Hodis HN, Matsumoto AM, Snyder PJ, Swerdloff RS, Vesper HW, Wu FC, Yialamas MA. Testosterone therapy in men with androgen deficiency syndromes: an Endocrine Society clinical practice guideline. *J Clin Endocrinol Metab.* 2018. In press.
10. Vigen R, O'Donnell CI, Barón AE, Grunwald GK, Maddox TM, Bradley SM, Barqawi A, Woning G, Wierman ME, Plomondon ME, Rumsfeld JS, Ho PM. Association of testosterone therapy with mortality, myocardial infarction, and stroke in men with low testosterone levels. *JAMA.* 2013;**310**(17):1829–1836.
11. Finkle WD, Greenland S, Ridgeway GK, Adams JL, Frasco MA, Cook MB, Fraumeni JF Jr, Hoover RN. Increased risk of non-fatal myocardial infarction following testosterone therapy prescription in men. PLoS One. 2014;9(1):e85805.
12. Shores MM, Smith NL, Forsberg CW, Anawalt BD, Matsumoto AM. Testosterone treatment and mortality in men with low testosterone levels. *J Clin Endocrinol Metab.* 2012;**97**(6):2050–2058.
13. Baillargeon J, Urban RJ, Kuo YF, Ottenbacher KJ, Raji MA, Du F, Lin YL, Goodwin JS. Risk of myocardial Infarction in older men receiving testosterone therapy. *Ann Pharmacother.* 2014;**48**(9):1138–1144.
14. Snyder PJ, Bhasin S, Cunningham GR, Matsumoto AM, Stephens-Shields AJ, Cauley JA, Gill TM, Barrett-Connor E, Swerdloff RS, Wang C, Ensrud KE, Lewis CE, Farrar JT, Cella D, Rosen RC, Pahor M, Crandall JP, Molitch ME, Cifelli D, Dougar D, Fluharty L, Resnick SM, Storer TW, Anton S, Basaria S, Diem SJ, Hou X, Mohler ER III, Parsons JK, Wenger NK, Zeldow B, Landis JR, Ellenberg SS; Testosterone Trials Investigators. Effects of testosterone treatment in older men. *N Engl J Med.* 2016;**374**(7):611–624.
15. Budoff MJ, Ellenberg SS, Lewis CE, Mohler ER III, Wenger NK, Bhasin S, Barrett-Connor E, Swerdloff RS, Stephens-Shields A, Cauley JA, Crandall JP, Cunningham GR, Ensrud KE, Gill TM, Matsumoto AM, Molitch ME, Nakanishi R, Nezarat N, Matsumoto S, Hou X, Basaria S, Diem SJ, Wang C, Cifelli D, Snyder PJ. Testosterone treatment and coronary artery plaque volume in older men with low testosterone. *JAMA.* 2017;**317**(7):708–716.
16. Jarvis TR, Chughtai B, Kaplan SA. Testosterone and benign prostatic hyperplasia. *Asian J Androl.* 2015;**17**(2):212–216.
17. Parker C, Gillessen S, Heidenreich A. Horwich A; ESMO Guidelines Committee. Cancer of the prostate: ESMO Clinical Practice Guidelines for diagnosis, treatment and follow-up. *Ann Oncol.* 2015;**26**(Suppl. 5): v69–v77.
18. Li H, Benoit K, Wang W, Motsko S. Association between use of exogenous testosterone therapy and risk of venous thrombotic events among exogenous testosterone treated and untreated men with hypogonadism. *J Urol.* 2016;**195**(4 Pt. 1):1065–1072.
19. Martinez C, Suissa S, Rietbrock S, Katholing A, Freedman B, Cohen AT, Handelsman DJ. Testosterone treatment and risk of venous thromboembolism: population based case-control study. *BMJ.* 2016;**355**: i5968.
20. Travison TG, Vesper HW, Orwoll E, Wu F, Kaufman JM, Wang Y, Lapauw B, Fiers T, Matsumoto AM, Bhasin S. Harmonized reference ranges for circulating testosterone levels in men of four cohort studies in the United States and Europe. *J Clin Endocrinol Metab.* 2017; **102**(4):1161–1173.
21. Roy CN, Snyder PJ, Stephens-Shields AJ, Artz AS, Bhasin S, Cohen HJ, Farrar JT, Gill TM, Zeldow B, Cella D, Barrett-Connor E, Cauley JA, Crandall JP, Cunningham GR, Ensrud KE, Lewis CE, Matsumoto AM, Molitch ME, Pahor M, Swerdloff RS, Cifelli D, Hou X, Resnick SM, Walston JD, Anton S, Basaria S, Diem SJ, Wang C, Schrier SL, Ellenberg SS. Association of testosterone levels with anemia in older men: a controlled clinical trial. *JAMA Intern Med.* 2017;**177**(4): 480–490.
22. Snyder PJ, Kopperdahl DL, Stephens-Shields AJ, Ellenberg SS, Cauley JA, Ensrud KE, Lewis CE, Barrett-Connor E, Schwartz AV, Lee DC, Bhasin S, Cunningham GR, Gill TM, Matsumoto AM, Swerdloff RS, Basaria S, Diem SJ, Wang C, Hou X, Cifelli D, Dougar D, Zeldow B, Bauer DC, Keaveny TM. Effect of testosterone treatment on volumetric bone density and strength in older men with low testosterone: a controlled clinical trial. *JAMA Intern Med.* 2017;**177**(4):471–479.
23. Watts NB, Adler RA, Bilezikian JP, Drake MT, Eastell R, Orwoll ES, Finkelstein JS; Endocrine Society. Osteoporosis in men: an Endocrine Society clinical practice guideline. *J Clin Endocrinol Metab.* 2012; **97**(6):1802–1822.

Opiate-Induced Endocrinopathies

M42
Presented, March 17–20, 2018

Niki Karavitaki, FRCP. Institute of Metabolism and Systems Research, College of Medical and Dental Sciences University of Birmingham, Birmingham B15 2TT, United Kingdom, and Centre for Endocrinology, Diabetes and Metabolism, Birmingham Health Partners, Birmingham B15 2TH, United Kingdom, E-mail: n.karavitaki@bham.ac.uk

SIGNIFICANCE OF THE CLINICAL PROBLEM

The availability and use of opiates, particularly for the management of noncancer pain, has increased substantially over the last decades (1). The prescribing of opiate analgesics for pain management has increased more than fourfold in the United States since the mid-1990s (2), and review of the opiate prescription patterns in a US industrial cohort between 2003 and 2013 showed that opiate prescribing nearly doubled during this period (3). Possible contributing factors include changes in medication formulations, marketing of the pharmaceutical industry, and the aging population (4). It is of note that prescribers involve a wide range of health professionals, including pain physicians, family physicians, orthopedic surgeons, anesthesiologists, psychiatrists, physical medicine, and rehabilitation specialists (1). It has been shown that long-acting opiates prescribed for chronic noncancer pain are linked to increased mortality from not only unintentional overdose but also from cardiovascular causes (5). Furthermore, the 2014 National Survey on Drug Use and Health (NSDUH) revealed that 27 million Americans were current users of illicit drugs [including marijuana/hashish, cocaine (including crack), heroin, hallucinogens, inhalants, or prescription-type psychotherapeutics (pain relievers, tranquilizers, stimulants, and sedatives)] (6). The endocrine consequences of opiates are numerous, requiring alertness among the specialists to avoid harmful long-term consequences.

BARRIERS/CHALLENGES TO OPTIMAL CLINICAL PRACTICE

- Lack of robust data on the prevalence of opiate-induced endocrinopathies and on predictive factors for the development of them
- Lack of evidence-based protocols on the diagnosis and management of endocrinopathies in patients on opiates

LEARNING OBJECTIVES

As a result of participating in this session, learners should be able to recognize the risk of hypogonadism and adrenal insufficiency in patients on opiates and diagnose and manage it effectively.

STRATEGIES FOR DIAGNOSIS, THERAPY, AND/OR MANAGEMENT

Opiates have a plethora of actions on the human endocrine system leading to stimulatory or inhibitory effects on hormone release. Acute administration of opiates in humans results in increased secretion of growth hormone (4). On the other hand, chronic administration has different effects. In a study of patients with severe chronic pain treated with intrathecal opiates, severe growth hormone deficiency was diagnosed with 15% of them (7). The impacts of dose and route of opiates and of the extent of pain on the growth hormone dynamics have not been clarified, and the clinical significance of the detected deficit remains to be elucidated.

Acute administration of opiates increases prolactin, and a similar effect may occasionally be seen in chronic use (7).

Chronic opiate administration reduces luteinizing hormone and follicle-stimulating hormone mainly by inhibiting hypothalamic gonadotropin-releasing hormone secretion. Direct inhibition of the gonadotropin release at the pituitary level has also been proposed. Furthermore, sex steroid hormones have major modulating effects on the sensitivity of the hypothalamo-pituitary-gonadal axis to opiates, explaining why the effects of these drugs vary not only within the menstrual cycle but also with puberty and menopause (4). The reported prevalence of hypogonadism ranges between 21% and 86%, regardless of the route of administration (oral, intrathecal, or transdermal) (8–13). Higher prevalence in men than women has been described (11). Based on a small number of studies, testosterone treatment has been shown to provide benefits in males. Aloisi *et al.* (14) demonstrated that 1 year of testosterone replacement therapy in nine male patients suffering from a severe form of chronic noncancer pain requiring epidural morphine and diagnosed with morphine-induced hypogonadism resulted in substantial improvement of total, free, and bioavailable testosterone levels, as well as of several other parameters of pain and andrological and psychological outcomes. In the first double-blind, randomized, placebo-controlled trial of testosterone replacement in men with opiate-induced androgen deficiency, 14 weeks of testosterone administration was associated with improved pain sensitivity to multiple modalities of experimentally induced noxious stimuli, including pressure algometry and repetitive noxious punctate stimuli. In addition, males in the testosterone group showed substantial improvement in sexual desire, as well as a reduction in fat mass and an improvement in lean body mass compared with those in the placebo group (15). Published series on the management of opiate-induced hypogonadism and relevant outcomes in females are not available.

Exogenous opiates also have a negative impact on bone health. This could be partly explained by the opiate-induced hypogonadism, as well as by the inhibition of the osteoblast function via opiate receptors. Notably, a recent small observational study demonstrated that 50% of patients who received intrathecal opiate therapy had osteopenia and 21.4% of them had osteoporosis (16).

In humans, exogenous opiates have a predominantly inhibitory role in the regulation of the hypothalamo-pituitary-adrenal axis, in both acute and chronic settings. Single administration of various opiates (morphine, heroin, buprenorphine, and remifentanil) results in suppression of adrenocorticotropic hormone (ACTH) and glucocorticoid secretion, blunted pituitary-adrenal response to corticotropin-releasing hormone, and diminished cortisol response to psychosocial or surgical stress in normal subjects. Chronic use of different types or formulations of opiates in chronic pain patients leads to decreased ACTH and cortisol levels and to cortisol insufficiency (defined as basal morning plasma cortisol level <100 nmol/L or a cortisol response to synthetic ACTH stimulation <430 nmol/L) in 8.3% of them (17,18). Intrathecal administration of morphine or hydromorphine in patients with nonmalignant pain resulted in basal cortisol levels <5 μg/dL and peak cortisol <18 μg/dL during an insulin tolerance test in 9.2% and 14.8% of them, respectively (7). In addition, 33.3% of chronic pain patients receiving spinal morphine and 50% of those on oral morphine demonstrated hypoadrenalism (stimulated cortisol levels during insulin tolerance test <18 μg/dL) (19). Furthermore, several case reports documenting secondary adrenal insufficiency after oral or transdermal opiate administration have been published. Factors predicting the development of abnormal adrenal stress response are not as yet known. The altered hypothalamo-pituitary-adrenal axis function of opiate users returns to normal after discontinuation of the drug. It has also been suggested that methadone maintenance treatment may restore the axis among heroin-dependent patients (20).

MAIN CONCLUSIONS

Opiates can affect the endocrine system in multiple ways. The most clinically substantial consequences of exogenous opiates are hypogonadism and hypoadrenalism, which need to be diagnosed and managed early, particularly in cases of chronic use. Factors predicting the development of hormone deficits have not been as yet established.

CASES

Case 1

A 52-year-old man has a history of chronic back pain attributed to disc prolapse for which he has been on various analgesics in the last 3 years. In the last 9 months, his general practitioner has put him on fentanyl patches 50 μg/72 h. In the last 6 months, he has noticed erectile dysfunction. How would you approach this problem?

A. Referral to psychologist
B. Stop fentanyl
C. Arrange pituitary magnetic resonance imaging
D. Offer sildenafil
E. Arrange measurement of 9:00 AM serum testosterone, follicle-stimulating hormone, luteinizing hormone, and prolactin

The correct answer is E. Fentanyl patches, like many opiates, are associated with secondary hypogonadism, and, on the first instance, biochemical confirmation of this diagnosis is required. Once this is confirmed, further investigations should be arranged (including imaging of the hypothalamo-pituitary area), aiming to establish the etiology of the gonadotropin deficiency. If fentanyl patches are finally responsible for the patient's erectile dysfunction, testosterone replacement could be a management option. Discussion of the necessity of treatment with opiates and alternative therapeutic approaches should be also done with the relevant specialists.

Case 2

A 45-year-old man has been offered morphine for back pain after a road traffic accident 5 months ago. He is currently on 30 mg daily, and in the last 3 months, he suffers from tiredness and low energy levels. His blood pressure shows postural drop from 110/80 mm Hg to 90/65 mm Hg. Before the road traffic accident, his blood pressure measurements were 130/85 mm Hg. What are your next steps?

A. Review the patient in 4 weeks to check if his symptoms persist
B. Change to another opiate
C. Offer fludrocortisone
D. Arrange assessment of the hypothalamo-pituitary-adrenal axis as soon as possible
E. Stop the morphine immediately

The correct answer is D. Exogenous opiates can inhibit the hypothalamo-pituitary-adrenal axis and can lead to cortisol deficiency. Prompt diagnosis of this condition is required, aiming to avoid the devastating consequences of untreated adrenal insufficiency. Changing to another opiate may have similar effects, and abrupt cessation of morphine can be dangerous. The management of the secondary hypoadrenalism requires glucocorticoid replacement.

REFERENCES

1. Manchikanti L, Kaye AM, Knezevic NN, McAnally H, Slavin K, Trescot AM, Blank S, Pampati V, Abdi S, Grider JS, Kaye AD, Manchikanti KN, Cordner H, Gharibo CG, Harned ME, Albers SL, Atluri S, Aydin SM, Bakshi S, Barkin RL, Benyamin RM, Boswell MV, Buenaventura RM, Calodney AK, Cedeno DL, Datta S, Deer TR, Fellows B, Galan V, Grami V, Hansen H, Helm Ii S, Justiz R, Koyyalagunta D, Malla Y, Navani A, Nouri KH, Pasupuleti R, Sehgal N, Silverman SM, Simopoulos TT, Singh V, Solanki DR, Staats PS, Vallejo R, Wargo BW, Watanabe A, Hirsch JA. Responsible, safe, and effective prescription of opioids for chronic

non-cancer pain: American Society of Interventional Pain Physicians (ASIPP) Guidelines. *Pain Physician.* 2017;**20**(2S):S3–S92.

2. Volkow N, Benveniste H, McLellan AT. Use and misuse of opioids in chronic pain [published online ahead of print October 13, 2017]. *Annu Rev Med.* doi:10.1146/annurev-med-011817-044739.
3. Pensa MA, Galusha DH, Cantley LF. Patterns of opioid prescribing and predictors of chronic opioid use in an industrial cohort, 2003 to 2013 [published online ahead of print November 13, 2017]. *J Occup Environ Med.* doi:10.1097/JOM.0000000000001231.
4. Vuong C, Van Uum SH, O'Dell LE, Lutfy K, Friedman TC. The effects of opioids and opioid analogs on animal and human endocrine systems. *Endocr Rev.* 2010;**31**(1):98–132.
5. Ray WA, Chung CP, Murray KT, Hall K, Stein CM. Prescription of long-acting opioids and mortality in patients with chronic noncancer pain. *JAMA.* 2016;**315**(22):2415–2423.
6. Center for Behavioral Health Statistics and Quality. Behavioral Health Trends in the United States: Results from the 2014 National Survey on Drug Use and Health. Washington, DC: US Department of Health and Human Services; 2015. HHS publication no. SMA 15-4927, NSDUH series H-50.
7. Abs R, Verhelst J, Maeyaert J, Van Buyten JP, Opsomer F, Adriaensen H, Verlooy J, Van Havenbergh T, Smet M, Van Acker K. Endocrine consequences of long-term intrathecal administration of opioids. *J Clin Endocrinol Metab.* 2000;**85**(6):2215–2222.
8. Daniell HW. Opioid-induced androgen deficiency. *Curr Opin Endocrinol Diabetes.* 2006;**13**(3):262–266.
9. Finch PM, Roberts LJ, Price L, Hadlow NC, Pullan PT. Hypogonadism in patients treated with intrathecal morphine. *Clin J Pain.* 2000;**16**(3): 251–254.
10. Daniell HW, Lentz R, Mazer NA. Open-label pilot study of testosterone patch therapy in men with opioid-induced androgen deficiency. *J Pain.* 2006;**7**(3):200–210.
11. Fraser LA, Morrison D, Morley-Forster P, Paul TL, Tokmakejian S, Larry Nicholson R, Bureau Y, Friedman TC, Van Uum SH. Oral opioids for chronic non-cancer pain: higher prevalence of hypogonadism in men than in women. *Exp Clin Endocrinol Diabetes.* 2009;**117**(1):38–43.
12. Duarte RV, Raphael JH, Labib M, Southall JL, Ashford RL. Prevalence and influence of diagnostic criteria in the assessment of hypogonadism in intrathecal opioid therapy patients. *Pain Physician.* 2013;**16**(1): 9–14.
13. Daniell HW. Opioid endocrinopathy in women consuming prescribed sustained-action opioids for control of nonmalignant pain. *J Pain.* 2008;**9**(1):28–36.
14. Aloisi AM, Ceccarelli I, Carlucci M, Suman A, Sindaco G, Mameli S, Paci V, Ravaioli L, Passavanti G, Bachiocco V, Pari G. Hormone replacement therapy in morphine-induced hypogonadic male chronic pain patients. *Reprod Biol Endocrinol.* 2011;**9**(1):26.
15. Basaria S, Travison TG, Alford D, Knapp PE, Teeter K, Cahalan C, Eder R, Lakshman K, Bachman E, Mensing G, Martel MO, Le D, Stroh H, Bhasin S, Wasan AD, Edwards RR. Effects of testosterone replacement in men with opioid-induced androgen deficiency: a randomized controlled trial. *Pain.* 2015;**156**(2):280–288.
16. Duarte RV, Raphael JH, Southall JL, Labib MH, Whallett AJ, Ashford RL. Hypogonadism and low bone mineral density in patients on long-term intrathecal opioid delivery therapy. *BMJ Open.* 2013;**3**(6): e002856.
17. Gibb FW, Stewart A, Walker BR, Strachan MW. Adrenal insufficiency in patients on long-term opioid analgesia. *Clin Endocrinol (Oxf).* 2016; **85**(6):831–835.
18. Aloisi AM, Buonocore M, Merlo L, Galandra C, Sotgiu A, Bacchella L, Ungaretti M, Demartini L, Bonezzi C. Chronic pain therapy and hypothalamic-pituitary-adrenal axis impairment. *Psychoneuroendocrinology.* 2011;**36**(7):1032–1039.
19. Valverde-Filho J, da Cunha Neto MB, Fonoff ET, Meirelles ES, Teixeira MJ. Chronic spinal and oral morphine-induced neuroendocrine and metabolic changes in noncancer pain patients. *Pain Med.* 2015;**16**(4): 715–725.
20. Yang J, Li J, Xu G, Zhang J, Chen Z, Lu Z, Deng H. Elevated hair cortisol levels among heroin addicts on current methadone maintenance compared to controls. *PLoS One.* 2016;**24:11**(3):e0150729.

Oncofertility

M53
Presented, March 17–20, 2018

Teresa K. Woodruff, PhD. Department of Obstetrics and Gynecology, Northwestern University, Chicago, Illinois 60611, E-mail: tkw@northwestern.edu

SIGNIFICANCE OF THE CLINICAL PROBLEM

Facing a cancer diagnosis at any age is devastating. However, young cancer patients have the added burden that life-preserving cancer treatments, including surgery, chemotherapy, and radiotherapy, may compromise their future fertility (1–4). The possibility of reproductive dysfunction as a consequence of cancer treatment has a negative impact on the quality of life of cancer survivors. The field of oncofertility, which merges the clinical specialties of oncology and reproductive endocrinology, was developed to explore and expand fertility preservation options and better manage the reproductive status of cancer patients. Fertility preservation for females has proved to be a particular challenge, because mature female gametes are rare and difficult to acquire (5–7). The purpose of this presentation is to provide a comprehensive overview of how cancer treatments affect the female reproductive axis, delineate the diverse fertility preservation options that are currently available or being developed for young women, and describe current measures of ovarian reserve that can be used pre- and postcancer treatment.

BARRIERS TO OPTIMAL PRACTICE

Barriers to care include a lack of common provider knowledge and resources as well as the potential of financial toxicity in fertility preservation care. The successful perpetuation of oncofertility practice requires the increased availability of clinical and scientific training in oncofertility as well as strengthened networks between fields.

It is the purpose of my work and the work of the Oncofertility Consortium to reduce these barriers and create educational opportunities for physicians and researchers who are looking to provide fertility preservation care to cancer patients as well as patients with nonmalignant conditions facing infertility.

LEARNING OBJECTIVES

As a result of participating in this session, learners should be able to do the following.

- Provide a comprehensive overview of how cancer treatments affect the female reproductive axis
- Delineate the diverse fertility preservation options that are currently available or being developed for young women
- Describe current measures of ovarian reserve that can be used pre- and postcancer treatment

BENCH TO BEDSIDE CONSIDERATIONS

As a basic scientist, I do not directly manage patients, and therefore, the discussion in this article will be about research models that are prismatic to future clinical care.

RESEARCH CASE 1: METHOD TO MATURE FIRST HUMAN EGG COMPLETELY *IN VITRO*

All advanced reproductive technologies, like *in vitro* fertilization, require *in vivo* maturation of an oocyte. For the first time, we have created an *in vitro* follicle growth paradigm that allowed a dynamic human follicle growth environment *in vitro*. Follicles developed from the preantral to antral stage and for the first time, produced meiotically competent metaphase II oocytes after *in vitro* maturation (8). Similar methods in mouse, caprine, bovine, feline, and nonhuman primate are similarly advancing our fundamental understanding of follicle maturation paradigms.

RESEARCH CASE 2: METHOD TO MONITOR 28-DAY OVARIAN CYCLE IN A MICROFLUIDIC DISH

The endocrine system dynamically controls tissue differentiation and homeostasis but has not been studied using dynamic tissue culture paradigms. Here, we show that a microfluidic system supports murine ovarian follicles to produce the human 28-day menstrual cycle hormone profile, which controls human female reproductive tract and peripheral tissue dynamics in single, dual, and multiple unit microfluidic platforms (MFPs; solo MFP, duet MFP, and quintet MFP, respectively) (9). These systems simulate the *in vivo* female reproductive tract and the endocrine loops between organ modules for the ovary, fallopian tube, uterus, cervix, and liver, with a sustained circulating flow between all tissues. The reproductive tract tissues and peripheral organs integrated into an MFP, termed EVATAR, represent a powerful new *in vitro* tool that allows organ-organ integration of hormonal signaling as a phenocopy of menstrual cycle and pregnancy-like endocrine loops and has great potential to be used in drug discovery and toxicology studies.

RESEARCH CASE 3: DISCOVERY OF ZINC SPARK AT TIME OF FERTILIZATION MARKS DEVELOPMENTAL CAPACITY

Egg activation refers to events required for transition of a gamete into an embryo, including establishment of the polyspermy block, completion of meiosis, entry into mitosis, selective recruitment and degradation of maternal messenger RNA, and pronuclear development. Here, we show that zinc fluxes accompany human egg activation. We monitored calcium and zinc dynamics in individual human eggs using selective fluorophores after activation with calcium-ionomycin, ionomycin, or phosopholipase C isoform ζ complementary RNA microinjection. These egg activation methods, as expected, induced rises in intracellular calcium levels and also triggered the coordinated release of zinc into the extracellular space in a prominent "zinc spark" (10). The ability of the gamete to mount a zinc spark response was meiotic-stage dependent. Moreover, chelation of intracellular zinc alone was sufficient to induce cell cycle resumption and transition of a meiotic cell into a mitotic one. Together, these results show critical functions for zinc dynamics and establish the zinc spark as an extracellular marker of early human development.

RESEARCH CASE 4: DEVELOPMENT OF A BIOPROSTHETIC OVARY

Emerging additive manufacturing techniques enable investigation of the effects of pore geometry on cell behavior and function. Here, we three-dimensionally print microporous hydrogel scaffolds to test how varying pore geometry, accomplished by manipulating the advancing angle between printed layers, affects the survival of ovarian follicles (11); 30° and 60° scaffolds provide corners that surround follicles on multiple sides, whereas 90° scaffolds have an open porosity that limits follicle-scaffold interaction. As the amount of scaffold interaction increases, follicle spreading is limited, and survival increases. Follicle-seeded scaffolds become highly vascularized, and ovarian function is fully restored when implanted in surgically sterilized mice. Moreover, pups are born through natural mating and thrive through maternal lactation. These findings present an *in vivo* functional ovarian implant designed with three-dimensional printing and indicate that scaffold pore architecture is a critical variable in additively manufactured scaffold design for functional tissue engineering.

Taken together, these basic science breakthroughs are setting the stage for clinical care.

REFERENCES

1. De Vos M, Smitz J, Woodruff TK. Fertility preservation in women with cancer. *Lancet.* 2014;**384**(9950):1302–1310.
2. Jeruss JS, Woodruff TK. Preservation of fertility in patients with cancer. *N Engl J Med.* 2009;**360**(9):902–911.
3. Salama M, Woodruff TK. Anticancer treatments and female fertility: clinical concerns and role of oncologists in oncofertility practice. *Expert Rev Anticancer Ther.* 2017;**17**(8):687–692.
4. Woodruff TK. Fertility lost-fertility found: narratives from the leading edge of oncofertility. *Narrat Inq Bioeth.* 2017;**7**(2):147–150.
5. Duncan FE, Pavone ME, Gunn AH, Badawy S, Gracia C, Ginsberg JP, Lockart B, Gosiengfiao Y, Woodruff TK. Pediatric and teen ovarian tissue removed for cryopreservation contains follicles irrespective of age, disease diagnosis, treatment history, and specimen processing methods. *J Adolesc Young Adult Oncol.* 2015;**4**(4):174–183.
6. Duncan FE, Zelinski M, Gunn AH, Pahnke JE, O'Neill CL, Songsasen N, Woodruff RI, Woodruff TK. Ovarian tissue transport to expand access to fertility preservation: from animals to clinical practice. *Reproduction.* 2016;**152**(6):R201–R210.
7. Johnson EK, Finlayson C, Rowell EE, Gosiengfiao Y, Pavone ME, Lockart B, Orwig KE, Brannigan RE, Woodruff TK. Fertility preservation for pediatric patients: current state and future possibilities. *J Urol.* 2017; **198**(1):186–194.
8. Xiao S, Zhang J, Romero MM, Smith KN, Shea LD, Woodruff TK. In vitro follicle growth supports human oocyte meiotic maturation. *Sci Rep.* 2015;**5**(1):17323.
9. Xiao S, Coppeta JR, Rogers HB, Isenberg BC, Zhu J, Olalekan SA, McKinnon KE, Dokic D, Rashedi AS, Haisenleder DJ, Malpani SS, Arnold-Murray CA, Chen K, Jiang M, Bai L, Nguyen CT, Zhang J, Laronda MM, Hope TJ, Maniar KP, Pavone ME, Avram MJ, Sefton EC, Getsios S, Burdette JE, Kim JJ, Borenstein JT, Woodruff TK. A microfluidic culture model of the human reproductive tract and 28-day menstrual cycle. *Nat Commun.* 2017;**8**:14584.
10. Duncan FE, Que EL, Zhang N, Feinberg EC, O'Halloran TV, Woodruff TK. The zinc spark is an inorganic signature of human egg activation. *Sci Rep.* 2016;**6**(1):24737.
11. Laronda MM, Rutz AL, Xiao S, Whelan KA, Duncan FE, Roth EW, Woodruff TK, Shah RN. A bioprosthetic ovary created using 3D printed microporous scaffolds restores ovarian function in sterilized mice. *Nat Commun.* 2017;**8**:15261.

Endocrine Assessment and Management of Adult Patients With DSD and CAH

M56
Presented, March 17–20, 2018

Richard J. M. Ross, MBBS, MD, FRCP. University of Sheffield, Sheffield S10 2RX, United Kingdom, E-mail: r.j.ross@sheffield.ac.uk

SIGNIFICANCE OF THE CLINICAL PROBLEM

The title for this MTP arose in the context of the increasing number of adult endocrinologists providing cross-sex hormone therapy for transgender individuals who may also see patients with disorder of sex development (DSD). The Meet the Professor session considers the appropriate evaluation of adults presenting for hormone treatment with DSD or gender dysphoria. Thus, this session is not about the management of adults with gender identity disorder; rather, it is a session that considers the management of DSDs in the light of referrals from the general community that may include adults with gender identity disorder.

There has been much debate and controversy regarding the terms used to describe gender identity, that is, a person's fundamental sense of being a man, a woman, or of indeterminate sex. Here are some of the terms generally used in the medical literature.

Infants with a congenital discrepancy between external genitalia, gonadal, and chromosomal sex are classified as having DSD. Although the term DSD has been accepted by the medical community, patients and support groups question its usefulness and appropriateness based on three criticisms: first, that DSD is an overly broad term that applies to conditions in which no sexual or gender disruption is expected [*e.g.*, Turner syndrome, trisomy X, many females with congenital adrenal hyperplasia (CAH), and others]; second, that the use of the word disorder is seen as pejorative by some; and third, that an umbrella term like DSD lacks sufficient specificity to be helpful diagnostically and is therefore unnecessary. Many of these groups do not accept the DSD designation and feel that it should be abandoned by the medical community. Until a consensus is reached on this issue, the term DSD is used in the medical literature. DSDs with genital abnormalities sufficient to prompt evaluation occur in approximately one in 1000 to 4500 live births. Manifestations may include bilateral cryptorchidism, scrotal or perineal hypospadias, clitoromegaly, posterior labial fusion, phenotypic female appearance with a palpable gonad (with or without inguinal hernia), or hypospadias with a unilateral nonpalpable gonad. Infants with discordant genitalia and sex chromosomes are also considered to have DSDs.

The terms transgender and gender incongruence describe a situation where an individual's gender identity differs from external sexual anatomy at birth. The prevalence of transgender depends upon the definition used to classify a person as transgender. In studies that included only individuals who had undergone hormone therapy or gender-affirming surgery or had diagnostic codes documenting transgender, the reported prevalence of transgender was seven to nine per 100,000 people. However, studies that included transgender status based upon self-report indicate a prevalence of transgender of approximately 871 per 100,000 people. Gender identity disorder is a Diagnostic and Statistical Manual of Mental Disorders, Fourth Edition, Text Revision, diagnosis. This psychiatric diagnosis is made when a strong and persistent cross-gender identification, combined with a persistent discomfort with one's sex or sense of inappropriateness in the gender role of that sex, causes clinically significant distress. Transsexual people identify as, or desire to live and be accepted as, a member of the gender opposite to that assigned at birth; the term male-to-female transsexual person refers to a biological male who identifies as, or desires to be, a member of the female gender; a female-to-male transsexual person refers to a biological female who identifies as, or desires to be, a member of the male gender.

BARRIERS TO OPTIMAL PRACTICE

- DSDs with genital abnormalities sufficient to prompt evaluation at birth occur in approximately one in 1000 to 4500 live births, but most are rare, and the most common cause, CAH, occurs in one in 12,000 to 15,000 live births. Diagnosis, management, and treatment are undertaken in infancy and childhood, and there are therefore few centers that have experience in assessing and treating adults with DSD and CAH.
- There is considerable debate and controversy about terminology and treatment within both the medical community and general population and in many cases little is known about the cause and there is a limited evidence base for treatment.

LEARNING OBJECTIVES

As a result of participating in this session, learners should be able to:

- Explain the complexity of managing DSD, CAH, and gender dysphoria, that is, the distress and unease experienced if gender identity and sex are not completely congruent

STRATEGIES FOR MANAGEMENT

The optimal care for adults with DSD requires an experienced multidisciplinary team (MDT). The team may exist as a clinical network with links between more than one specialist center. As a minimum standard, the clinical team should include specialists in endocrinology, gynecology and/or urology, clinical psychology/psychiatry, and nursing. Support groups can provide ongoing support to affected individuals, including opportunities to gather and explore information, promote autonomy, and build knowledge and self-confidence regarding the diagnosis of DSD. Support groups can provide a range of such information via Web sites and newsletters as well as through telephone helplines and group meetings for both families and professionals. They can also work in collaboration with the MDT to help families as well as affected people in seeking appropriate medical care and improve patients' understanding of their condition as well as the reasons for medical therapy. Alongside the formal psychological support provided by the specialist clinical psychologist, support groups can also offer invaluable peer support to families and individuals affected by DSD. By being in touch with others with a similar condition and belonging to a support group, people can gain a sense of empowerment, and the whole experience may also normalize a condition that may have previously been perceived as a source of stigma. Health care professionals rely on support groups for providing guidance on the development of health care strategy as well as for providing the opportunity to interact with affected people at national support group meetings and conferences. Contact details of national support groups and Web resources such as the AIS (androgen insensitivity syndrome) Support Group, the CAH Support Group, and dsdfamilies should be supplied routinely as part of any written information. Some patients may not wish to access support groups or meet other families, and the members of the MDT should also be aware of and, over time, review these wishes.

AIS results from androgen receptor dysfunction and is a common cause of DSD. The AIS phenotype largely depends on the degree of residual androgen receptor activity. Hormone replacement therapy is needed after gonadectomy. Patients who choose to retain the gonads are at risk for developing germ cell tumors. Complete AIS (CAIS) commonly presents as primary amenorrhea in a female adolescent. It may present earlier when testes are found in a female infant having an inguinal hernia repair. The issues are wide ranging and include establishing a diagnosis, providing information about the condition in an appropriate manner, monitoring puberty, considering the need for and timing of gonadectomy, and aiming to support the affected adult to achieve adequate sexual function and optimal quality of life. Sex of rearing is universally female in CAIS. It is well established that there is a higher risk of developing germ cell tumors in the category of DSD when Y-chromosomal material is present in the karyotype. In CAIS, the tumor risk is considered to be low, at least until adolescence, but it increases thereafter with age. Puberty occurs spontaneously in CAIS with retained gonads due to excess testosterone being aromatized to estrogen from lutenizing hormone–induced steroidogenesis. For this reason, it is currently generally recommended that gonads be removed once puberty is completed if CAIS presents early in childhood. If the gonads are removed before puberty, hormone induction of puberty is similar to that used for girls with Turner syndrome. Because women with CAIS do not have a uterus, treatment can be used with continuous, unopposed estrogen. The vagina is generally hypoplastic in CAIS. Consequently, self-dilatation therapy may be needed to enable sexual intercourse. This is the first-line treatment option and is effective in a majority of patients. Some women with CAIS prefer to take supplemental testosterone after gonadectomy because they report an improvement in well-being. Serum testosterone and luteinizing hormone levels in women with CAIS and intact gonads are within or above the normal ranges for adult males, whereas follicle-stimulating hormone levels are not elevated. Serum estradiol and sex hormone binding globulin are within the usual adult male and adult female reference ranges, respectively. Serum gonadotropin levels increase further after gonadectomy but are only partially suppressed with estrogen substitution. This observation suggests resistance to the negative-feedback effect of androgens on hypothalamic-pituitary control of gonadotropin secretion in CAIS, but maintenance of a partial negative feedback by estrogens.

CAH is the most common genetic endocrine disorder, and mutations in the *CYP21A2* gene encoding the enzyme 21-hydroxylase account for 95% of patient cases. In 21-hydroxylase deficiency, failure in cortisol synthesis results in reduced cortisol feedback and consequently increased pituitary adrenocorticotropic hormone release, which in turn promotes overproduction of 17-hydroxyprogesterone, progesterone, and adrenal androgens. Thus, patients with CAH have two major problems: cortisol deficiency and androgen excess, and many patients also have mineralocorticoid deficiency, because 21-hydroxylase mediates a key step in aldosterone synthesis. Glucocorticoid replacement in CAH aims to both replace cortisol and prevent the adrenocorticotropic hormone–driven androgen excess. This is challenging, because therapy aimed at normalizing androgen levels frequently results in excess glucocorticoid exposure, with associated complications including short stature, obesity, hypertension, osteoporosis, and an adverse metabolic profile. The conundrum facing the physician is striking a balance between too much and too little glucocorticoid treatment to avoid complications of glucocorticoid excess and life-threatening adrenal crisis. CAH is a lifelong chronic disorder.

Subfertility occurs frequently in women with CAH, which is explained by a range of factors including poorly controlled disease and abnormalities of the genital tract structures. Insufficient glucocorticoid replacement can lead to anovulation resulting from hyperandrogenemia, and polycystic ovaries in women with CAH are common. Sexual activity in many women has been shown to be reduced and associated with poor surgical reconstruction of genital malformations. In men who receive no or inadequate treatment, subfertility may arise from overproduction of adrenal androgens, which inhibits gonadotrophin secretion and consequent spermatogenesis. Perhaps as many men experience subfertility as women, but this may not be recognized. Testicular adrenal rest tissue is another factor that may lead to male subfertility by blocking the seminiferous tubules resulting in azoospermia and Leydig cell failure.

MAIN CONCLUSIONS

- Optimal care for adults with DSD requires an experienced MDT.
- Sex of rearing is female in CAIS, and timing of gonadectomy and hormone replacement therapy is important.
- Glucocorticoid replacement in CAH is challenging, because therapy aimed at normalizing androgen levels frequently results in excess glucocorticoid exposure, and insufficient glucocorticoid replacement can lead to infertility in men and women.

DISCUSSION OF CASES AND ANSWERS

Case 1

A 25-year-old bearded man who is a recent refugee from Iran is referred with ambiguous genitalia, having had no previous endocrine investigations. Discussion will include:

- Which investigations should be undertaken: chromosomes, gonadal steroids and gonadotrophins, and imaging of the pelvis
- Interpretation of investigations: causes of ambiguous genitalia
- Differentiating gender identity disorder from DSD: does the patient have gender incongruence
- Importance of psychological counseling in diagnosis and management

Case 2

A 50-year-old woman presents with female pattern hair loss and primary amenorrhea. Discussion will include:

- Which investigations should be undertaken, including: chromosomes, gonadal steroids and gonadotropins, and imaging of the pelvis
- Interpretation of investigations: cause of androgen insensitivity
- How to advise patients with androgen insensitivity who do not wish to undergo orchidectomy
- The causes of female pattern hair loss

Case 3

A 30-year-old woman with salt-wasting classic CAH who presented at birth with ambiguous genitalia now requests fertility support. Discussion will include:

- A history of any surgery should be taken and the patient examined by an experienced gynecologist to exclude any physical barriers to pregnancy.
- Both the patient and male partner should have genetic testing for CAH and be counseled about the risks of having a baby with CAH.
- To maximize fertility, the patient should have optimal control of adrenal androgens and progesterone, which may require treatment with increased doses of hydrocortisone and or prednisolone with monitoring of androgens and progesterone.
- If the male partner is a CAH carrier, the couple should be counseled about preimplantation diagnosis and dexamethasone treatment during pregnancy.
- During pregnancy, the patient should continue her regular glucocorticoid replacement; there is no need to monitor androgens. Patient may need an increased dose of glucocorticoid during the final trimester and should observe the sick-day rules. During labor, the patient should receive intramuscular hydrocortisone.

RECOMMENDED READING

Ahmed SF, Achermann JC, Arlt W, Balen A, Conway G, Edwards Z, Elford S, Hughes IA, Izatt L, Krone N, Miles H, O'Toole S, Perry L, Sanders C, Simmonds M, Watt A, Willis D. Society for Endocrinology UK guidance on the initial evaluation of an infant or an adolescent with a suspected disorder of sex development (revised 2015). *Clin Endocrinol (Oxf).* 2016;**84**(5):771–788.

Cools M, Looijenga L. Update on the pathophysiology and risk factors for the development of malignant testicular germ cell tumors in complete androgen insensitivity syndrome. *Sex Dev.* 2017;**11**(4):175–181.

Cousen P, Messenger A. Female pattern hair loss in complete androgen insensitivity syndrome. *Br J Dermatol.* 2010;**162**(5):1135–1137.

Han TS, Walker BR, Arlt W, Ross RJ. Treatment and health outcomes in adults with congenital adrenal hyperplasia. *Nat Rev Endocrinol.* 2014;**10**(2):115–124.

Hembree WC, Cohen-Kettenis P, Delemarre-van de Waal HA, Gooren LJ, Meyer WJ III, Spack NP, Tangpricha V, Montori VM; Endocrine Society. Endocrine treatment of transsexual persons: an Endocrine Society clinical practice guideline. *J Clin Endocrinol Metab.* 2009;**94**(9):3132–3154.

Mongan NP, Tadokoro-Cuccaro R, Bunch T, Hughes IA. Androgen insensitivity syndrome. *Best Pract Res Clin Endocrinol Metab.* 2015;**29**(4):569–580.

UpToDate. Available at: https://www.uptodate.com/contents/search.

THYROID

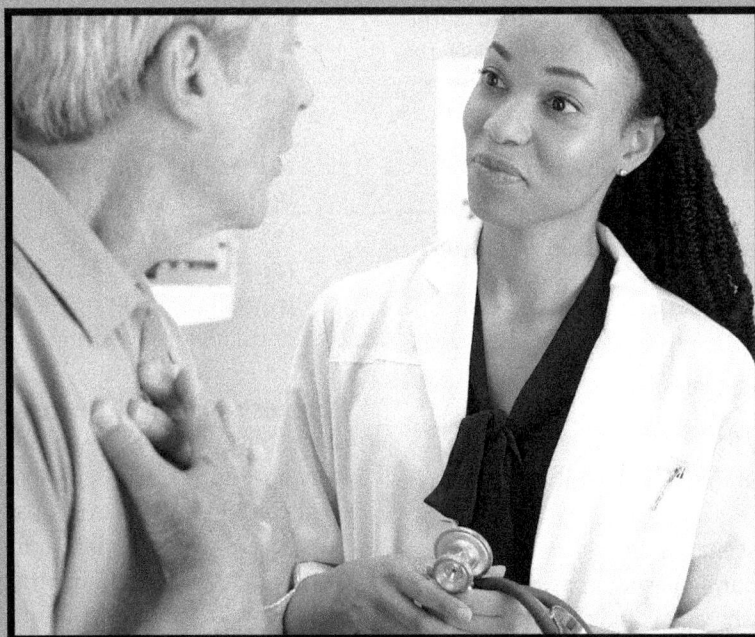

Graves Disease and Pregnancy

M02
Presented, March 17–20, 2018

Susan J. Mandel, MD, MPH. Perelman School of Medicine, University of Pennsylvania, Philadelphia, Pennsylvania 19104, E-mail: susan.mandel@uphs.upenn.edu

SIGNIFICANCE OF THE PROBLEM

Graves disease affects 1 in 500 to 1000 gestations, and the optimal treatment is challenging. Both maternal antithyroid drugs (ATDs) and thyrotropin (TSH) receptor antibodies (TRAbs) cross the placenta and affect fetal thyroid function, with variable effects depending gestational age, maternal disease activity, and ATD dosage. In addition, reports have detailed the potential hepatotoxicity of propylthiouracil (PTU) as well as the teratogenic effects of methimazole (MMI)/carbimazole and PTU. Therefore, an important clinical issue is how and when to treat hyperthyroid pregnant mothers. Although untreated moderate to severe hyperthyroidism adversely affects the pregnancy, new recommendations support that untreated mild hyperthyroidism may be safe for both the mother and the fetus.

BARRIERS TO OPTIMAL PRACTICE

1. The interpretation of maternal thyroid function tests (TFTs) to both diagnose hyperthyroidism and titrate ATD dosage is challenging, because gestational physiology differs from the nonpregnant state.
2. Concerns exist regarding ATD safety during gestation with respect to fetal outcomes.

LEARNING OBJECTIVES

As a result of participating in this session, learners should be able to:

1. Differentiate clinical scenarios in which ATD therapy may be discontinued during gestation from those in which continued ATD therapy is indicated
2. Describe the optimal ATD regimen and dose titration for pregnant hyperthyroid women when therapy is required
3. Understand fetal risks from ATD therapy and placental transfer of maternal TRAbs
4. Recognize how to monitor for fetal and neonatal thyrotoxicosis

STRATEGIES FOR DIAGNOSIS, THERAPY, AND MANAGEMENT

Normal Gravid Physiology

A background of increased renal iodine clearance (increase in glomerular filtration rate) and transplacental iodine passage exists.

Thyroxine-binding globulin increases ~2.5-fold, with peak levels at 15 to 20 weeks of gestation because of estrogen-induced glycosylation, decreasing hepatic clearance.

Total thyroxine (T_4) and total triiodothyronine (T_3) increase through midgestation and are associated with thyroxine-binding globulin rise. Normal range in pregnancy is 1.5× the nonpregnant reference range (1).

A transient increase in free T_4 (FT_4) may occur late in the first trimester when FT_4 levels are positively correlated with human chorionic gonadotropin (hCG) levels. However, using the automated FT_4 assays, serum FT_4 levels progressively decrease throughout gestation. In addition, there is significant interassay variation in measurement. By the third trimester, up to 70% of women may have FT_4 levels below the nonpregnant reference range (1). Commercial assays should provide trimester-specific ranges.

Reciprocal changes are seen in TSH and hCG as a function of gestational age, with peak hCG and nadir TSH levels at the end of the first trimester. TSH is suppressed below normal levels (<0.4 mIU/L) in 9% of normal pregnancies (2). hCG shares an α subunit and is a thyroid stimulator. If trimester-specific ranges not available for the commercial assay, at the end of the first trimester, upper and lower normal limits should be decreased by 0.5 mIU/L and 0.4 mIU/L, respectively, so that the normal gestational range is 0.1 to 0.4 mIU/L (3). In the second and third trimesters, TSH gradually returns to nonpregnant normative reference ranges.

Diagnosis of Graves Disease

Graves disease may present for the first time in the first trimester or it may relapse in the first trimester after a woman has been in remission, or a patient with pre-existing Graves disease may conceive. Similar to other autoimmune disorders, Graves disease usually improves throughout gestation and may remit in the third trimester, which is a time of immune tolerance in up to 35% of women. Clinical diagnosis of Graves disease may be confounded by the hyperadrenergic state of pregnancy. A serum TSH of <0.1 mIU/L can occur in up to 5% of normal pregnancies (4). Any subnormal TSH must be evaluated with full thyroid hormone testing with comparison to the pregnancy reference range and measurement of TRAbs, which, together with the usually distinct clinical presentation, will help to differentiate from gestational thyrotoxicosis.

Risks

Uncontrolled hyperthyroidism is associated with pregnancy loss, pregnancy-induced hypertension, preterm labor, intrauterine growth restriction, placental abruption, stillbirth, and maternal congestive heart failure (1, 3, 5). With appropriate maternal therapy, these risks can be substantially reduced (6). Importantly, maternal subclinical hyperthyroidism has not been reported to be associated with adverse gestation outcomes (7). Fetal/neonatal hypo- and hyperthyroidism are discussed later.

Treatment

ATDs are the mainstay of treatment of maternal Graves therapy. ^{131}I is contraindicated in pregnancy, and surgery is an option only for those patients who remain significantly thyrotoxic on ATD therapy, are nonadherent, or present allergic reactions or severe ATD-related side effects. Beta-blockers may be used in low doses to control hyperadrenergic symptoms until euthyroidism is achieved.

The initial ATD dose depends on the degree of hyperthyroidism, and the equivalent potency of MMI to PTU is about 1:20 (10 mg/d MMI = 200 mg/d PTU). The ATD side effects in pregnant women do not differ from those in nonpregnant patients. However, in 2010, the US Food and Drug Administration issued an advisory about hepatotoxicity in patients taking PTU and recommended limiting the use of PTU to (1) the first trimester of pregnancy (because of the MMI-associated embryopathy; see below); (2) those patients with MMI allergy; or (3) those in thyroid storm (8).

The larger concern with MMI use in pregnancy is its associated embryopathy (aplasia cutis, choanal atresia, tracheoesophageal fistulae, and abdominal wall defects). Recent studies from Denmark using national population registries reported that MMI therapy in the first trimester is associated with 2 to 4 excess birth defects per 100 live births, more frequent than previously thought. PTU was also found to be associated with birth defects in 2% to 3% of children, but these were generally milder (face and neck cysts) (9). The fetus is at highest risk for embryopathy when maternal drug exposure occurs between 6 and 10 weeks' gestation.

Therefore, American Thyroid Association guidelines (3, 10) recommend that women of childbearing age with Graves disease on ATD therapy have preconception counseling with their endocrinologist regarding the complexities of disease management during gestation, as well as the ATD association with embryopathy. Options of ^{131}I therapy, surgery, and medical management should be reviewed. When a woman chooses to remain on ATDs, the option of switching from MMI to PTU preconception should be discussed. For those on ATDs, pregnancy should be confirmed by testing as soon as possible, and the pregnant women should contact their treating care provider.

For women who require ATD therapy for Graves disease during pregnancy, the recent 2017 American Thyroid Association pregnancy guidelines provide the following recommendations (3):

PTU is recommended for the treatment of maternal hyperthyroidism through 16 weeks of pregnancy. *Strong recommendation, Moderate-quality evidence.*

Pregnant women receiving MMI who require ATD therapy should be changed to PTU as early as possible. *Weak recommendation, Low-quality evidence.*

When shifting from MMI to PTU, a dose ratio of ~1:20 should be used (*e.g.*, MMI 10 mg/d = PTU 100 mg twice a day). *Strong recommendation, Moderate-quality evidence.*

If ATD therapy is required after 16 weeks' gestation, it remains unclear whether PTU should be continued or therapy changed to MMI; because both medications are associated with potential adverse effects and shifting potentially may lead to a period of less-tight control, no recommendation regarding switching ATD drug medication can be made at this time. *No Recommendation, Insufficient evidence.*

It is important to remember that remission occurs in up to 60% of patients with Graves disease who have been on ATD therapy for over 12 months. Although some may experience relapse, the measurement of TRAbs has been demonstrated to be helpful in predicting duration of remission. In a Norwegian study, only 5% of TRAb-negative patients relapsed in the first 8 weeks after stopping ATD therapy (11). Therefore, in pregnancy, in which a goal is to try to limit ATD exposure during organogenesis, cessation of ATD therapy should be considered in those TRAb-negative women who have been on ATD for longer than 6 months and are biochemically euthyroid on low doses of MMI (5 to 10 mg/d) or PTU (<100 to 200 mg/d) (10). If relapse occurs, ATD therapy can be reinitiated, but this would generally be beyond the window of risk for fetal anomalies. Frequent administration of maternal TFTs, every 1 to 2 weeks initially, allows the detection of those few who relapse, and ATD with PTU can be started if prior to 16 weeks' gestation.

Even if ATD therapy is required in the first and second trimesters, it is critical to remember that during the third trimester, a time of immune tolerance, up to 35% of patients may go into remission and the ATD dosage can be lowered or discontinued (1).

Subtotal thyroidectomy is usually only considered during pregnancy as therapy for maternal Graves disease when consistently high levels of ATD are required to control maternal hyperthyroidism, when a patient is nonadherent or allergic to ATD therapy, or when severe ATD-related side effects such as agranulocytosis have occurred. Thyroidectomy is usually performed in the second trimester, and preparation with a low dose of potassium iodide (50 to 100 mg/d) can be used (3, 12).

ATD Dosage Titration

ATD therapy for maternal hyperthyroidism using either PTU or MMI has implications for the fetus because of transplacental passage and subsequent inhibition of fetal thyroid function. Studies have not demonstrated a maternal ATD dose–fetal thyroid response effect in this scenario, which should not be surprising. The fetal thyroid is subject to the same two influences as the maternal thyroid: the inhibitory effect of the ATD and the stimulatory effect of the TRAbs. Furthermore, the relative contribution of each factor may vary as the pregnancy progresses with changes in TRAb levels. Therefore, the mother's thyroid serves as the biosensor to judge the relative contribution of ATD inhibition and antibody stimulation. To best illustrate this concept, the study by Momotani *et al.* correlated maternal and cord FT_4 levels. All babies born to mothers who had increased FT_4 at delivery had fetal FT_4 levels in the normal range, and of those babies born to mothers with FT_4 in the upper third of normal range, 90% had normal FT_4 levels. Over 50% of babies born to mothers with normal FT_4 had either a low FT_4 or an elevated TSH (13).

Therefore, ATD should be adjusted to the lowest possible dose to maintain maternal TFTs so that the total T_4 and T_3 level is at or slightly above the pregnancy reference range (1.5× the nonpregnant range) or the FT_4 is at or above the trimester-specific reference range. If serum TSH becomes detectable, it should be below the lower limit of the pregnant reference cutoff (1, 3, 10).

Fetal Goiter and TRAb Testing

Fetal goiter may represent either fetal hypo- or hyperthyroidism and, again, reflects the relative balance between maternal TRAb stimulation and maternal ATD inhibition. Fetal Graves disease is reported to complicate 1% of all pregnancies in women with either active Graves disease or in those who have previously undergone radioiodine ablation or surgery. The mechanism is the transplacental transfer of maternal TRAbs at the end of the second or the early third trimester, and levels threefold elevated are most predictive of this condition (14).

Measurement of TRAbs should be performed in women with (1) active Graves disease in pregnancy (either untreated or taking ATD); (2) a prior history of Graves disease treated with either surgery or ^{131}I; and (3) prior delivery of an infant with hyperthyroidism (15). TRAbs should initially be checked in the first trimester (a time of Graves disease stimulation) and, if negative, no further testing during pregnancy is required if a woman is not receiving ATD. For both those requiring continued ATD therapy and those with a history of previously ablated Graves disease, a recheck of TRAbs at 20 to 23 weeks will identify pregnancies at risk for fetal hyperthyroidism; if positive at that time, subsequent testing at 30 to 34 weeks assesses for neonatal hyperthyroidism risk (3).

A fetal ultrasound to assess heart rate (HR), growth, amniotic fluid, and the presence of fetal goiter should be performed in the second half of pregnancy when either maternal hyperthyroidism is uncontrolled or the maternal TRAb level is >3× the upper limit of normal. When a fetal goiter is present, fetal thyrotoxicosis is suggested by diffuse goiter vascularity in conjunction with fetal tachycardia and advanced bone age, whereas fetal hypothyroidism is associated with peripheral blood flow in the goiter and delayed bone age, but fetal bradycardia is not generally present (16). The clinical scenario generally indicates the likely diagnosis:

- Mom with active Graves disease overtreated with ATD with inappropriately "normal" or low TFTs → **Fetal HYPOthyroidism**
- Mom with active Graves disease untreated or not controlled on ATD → **Fetal HYPERthyroidism**
- Hypothyroid Mom with history of Graves disease after surgery or ^{131}I ablation → **Fetal HYPERthyroidism**

Cordocentesis by maternal fetal medicine specialists can be performed in rare situations if required, to differentiate fetal hypo- from hyperthyroidism in the setting of maternal ATD therapy.

The maternal transfer of TRAbs to the fetus that continues until term may result in neonatal hyperthyroidism, which persists for the duration of maternal immunoglobulin G, until about 3 months of life. However, if the mother is receiving ATD at delivery, neonatal TFTs will likely be normal until the maternal ATD dissipates from the newborn, and then the TRAb effect is unopposed; therefore, neonatal thyrotoxicosis often does not become clinically evident until 1 to 2 weeks of life. A recent study from France measured cord TRAb levels in 33 infants born to TRAb-positive mothers taking ATD at term. Thirty percent were TRAb negative and had normal neonatal thyroid function. Of the 24 infants with detectable cord TRAb levels, only 7 (21%) developed neonatal hyperthyroidism at a mean age of 5 days of life, and all had TRAb levels >2× the upper normal limit (14).

MAIN CONCLUSIONS

1. Consider stopping ATD therapy in the first trimester for TRAb-negative women with Graves disease who have been on ATDs for longer than 6 months and are biochemically euthyroid on low doses of MMI (5 to 10 mg/d) or PTU (<100 to 200 mg/d).
2. If ATD is required during pregnancy, because of its association with embryopathy, MMI should not be used in the first trimester, and PTU should be substituted. Because maternal ATDs also can inhibit fetal thyroid hormone synthesis via transplacental passage, ATDs should be titrated to the lowest dose to maintain maternal TFTs so that the total T_4 and T_3 levels are at or slightly above the pregnancy reference range (1.5× the nonpregnant range) or the FT_4 is at or above the trimester-specific reference range. If serum TSH becomes detectable, it should be below the lower limit of the pregnant reference cutoff.
3. Placental passage of maternal TRAbs may cause fetal and neonatal thyrotoxicosis, and this may occur when maternal levels are >3× the upper limit of normal.
4. Fetal ultrasound to assess HR, growth, amniotic fluid, and the presence of fetal goiter should be performed in

the second half of pregnancy when either maternal hyperthyroidism is uncontrolled or the maternal TRAb level is >3× the upper limit of normal; sonographic evaluation with help differentiate when a fetal goiter is associated with hyper- vs hypothyroidism. Maternal fetal medicine should be consulted in these challenging clinical cases.

CASE

A 32-year-old female was diagnosed with hyperthyroidism due to Graves disease 8 months ago.

- Her initial examination was notable for a HR of 96 bpm, no orbitopathy, a diffuse goiter of ~60 g with bruit, hyperreflexia, and proximal muscle weakness.
- Her initial FT_4 was 4.7 ng/dL (normal range, 0.8 to 1.8 ng/dL); T_3 was 432 ng/dL (normal range, 80 to 200 ng/dL); TSH was <0.01 mIU/L; thyroid-stimulating immunoglobulin was 350% (normal level, <149%); and she had a TRAb level of 4.2 (normal level, <0.9).
- She was started on propranolol 20 mg twice a day and MMI 20 mg once a day, and her most recent TFTs from 2 months ago showed an FT_4 of 1.9 ng/dL, a T_3 of 195 ng/dL, and a TSH of <0.01 mIU/L.
- She telephones you to tell you that she just found out that she is pregnant and is at about 6 weeks' gestation.

You see her in the office and evaluate her.

Scenario 1

She has a HR of 92 bpm, a persistent but smaller goiter (40 g without a bruit), a TSH of <0.02 mIU/L, an FT_4 of 2.3 ng/dL, and a total T_3 of 320 ng/dL on MMI 20 mg/d.

How should she be treated?

A. Continue MMI 20 mg daily
B. Discontinue MMI and start PTU 100 mg three times a day (tid)
C. Discontinue MMI and start PTU 50 mg tid
D. Discontinue MMI and start potassium iodide 1 drop tid

Scenario 2

She has a HR of 76 bpm and her thyroid is now normal size. She tells you she stopped propranolol 3 months ago. She has a TSH of 0.21 mIU/L, an FT_4 of 1.53 ng/dL, and a total T_3 of 200 ng/dL on MMI 20 mg/d.

What is the next best step?

A. Decrease MMI to 10 mg/d
B. Change to PTU 50 mg tid
C. Check TRAb or thyroid-stimulating immunoglobulin level
D. Change to potassium iodide 1 drop tid

Discussion

For Both Scenarios

Because she was of childbearing age at diagnosis, an initial discussion about conception planning, with a review of the complexities of Graves disease management during gestation and the potential risks of therapy, should have occurred. A review of therapeutic options, including ^{131}I and potential surgery, should be included in the discussion.

Scenario 1

In early pregnancy, she is persistently thyrotoxic on MMI 20 mg/d, with a goiter and with detectable TRAbs. This constellation of findings is consistent with the need for continued ATD therapy during gestation, albeit with careful monitoring so that maternal overtreatment does not occur. She is currently taking MMI, which is associated with the described embryopathy. Therefore, B is the best answer: her ATD therapy should be changed to PTU (the ratio of MMI to PTU is ~1:20); PTU 100 mg tid is the best option because the other PTU dose would be too low. Potassium iodide has been shown to be an option in a small Japanese study (17), and may be a possibility if she has an adverse effect from PTU. She will require TRAb measurement again at 20 to 24 weeks to assess for fetal thyrotoxicosis and, if present, a fetal ultrasound is indicated.

Scenario 2

In early pregnancy, she is clinically and biochemically euthyroid after 8 months of ATDs. Therefore, this raises the possibility that she may not require ATD therapy, at least for the next 2 months, during the time of organogenesis. The best answer here is C: check the TRAb level to confirm that her disease is not very active. If the TRAb result is negative, even though her MMI dosage is moderate (20 mg/d), the options would be to either stop the MMI and recheck TFTs in 1 week or lower the MMI to 10 mg/d and recheck TFTs in 1 week.

REFERENCES

1. Chan GW, Mandel SJ. Therapy insight: management of Graves' disease during pregnancy. *Nat Clin Pract Endocrinol Metab.* 2007;**3**(6):470–478.
2. Glinoer D, de Nayer P, Bourdoux P, Lemone M, Robyn C, van Steirteghem A, Kinthaert J, Lejeune B. Regulation of maternal thyroid during pregnancy. *J Clin Endocrinol Metab.* 1990;**71**(2):276–287.
3. Alexander EK, Pearce EN, Brent GA, Brown RS, Chen H, Dosiou C, Grobman WA, Laurberg P, Lazarus JH, Mandel SJ, Peeters RP, Sullivan S. 2017 Guidelines of the American Thyroid Association for the Diagnosis and Management of Thyroid Disease During Pregnancy and the Postpartum. *Thyroid.* 2017;**27**(3):315–389.
4. Lambert-Messerlian G, McClain M, Haddow JE, Palomaki GE, Canick JA, Cleary-Goldman J, Malone FD, Porter TF, Nyberg DA, Bernstein P, D'Alton ME; FaSTER Research Consortium. First- and second-trimester thyroid hormone reference data in pregnant women: a FaSTER (First- and Second-Trimester Evaluation of Risk for aneuploidy) Research Consortium study. Am J Obstet Gynecol. 2008;199(1):62.e1–6.
5. Millar LK, Wing DA, Leung AS, Koonings PP, Montoro MN, Mestman JH. Low birth weight and preeclampsia in pregnancies complicated by hyperthyroidism. *Obstet Gynecol.* 1994;**84**(6):946–949.
6. Aggarawal N, Suri V, Singla R, Chopra S, Sikka P, Shah VN, Bhansali A. Pregnancy outcome in hyperthyroidism: a case control study. *Gynecol Obstet Invest.* 2014;**77**(2):94–99.
7. Casey BM, Dashe JS, Wells CE, McIntire DD, Leveno KJ, Cunningham FG. Subclinical hyperthyroidism and pregnancy outcomes. *Obstet Gynecol.* 2006;**107**(2, Pt 1):337–341.

8. Bahn RS, Burch HS, Cooper DS, Garber JR, Greenlee CM, Klein IL, Laurberg P, McDougall IR, Rivkees SA, Ross D, Sosa JA, Stan MN. The role of propylthiouracil in the management of Graves' disease in adults: report of a meeting jointly sponsored by the American Thyroid Association and the Food and Drug Administration. *Thyroid.* 2009; **19**(7):673–674.
9. Laurberg P, Andersen SL. Therapy of endocrine disease: antithyroid drug use in early pregnancy and birth defects: time windows of relative safety and high risk? *Eur J Endocrinol.* 2014;**171**(1): R13–R20.
10. Ross DS, Burch HB, Cooper DS, Greenlee MC, Laurberg P, Maia AL, Rivkees SA, Samuels M, Sosa JA, Stan MN, Walter MA. 2016 American Thyroid Association Guidelines for Diagnosis and Management of Hyperthyroidism and Other Causes of Thyrotoxicosis. *Thyroid.* 2016; **26**(10):1343–1421.
11. Nedrebo BG, Holm PI, Uhlving S, Sorheim JI, Skeie S, Eide GE, Husebye ES, Lien EA, Aanderud S. Predictors of outcome and comparison of different drug regimens for the prevention of relapse in patients with Graves' disease. *Eur J Endocrinol.* 2002;**147**(5):583–589.
12. Momotani N, Hisaoka T, Noh J, Ishikawa N, Ito K. Effects of iodine on thyroid status of fetus versus mother in treatment of Graves' disease complicated by pregnancy. *J Clin Endocrinol Metab.* 1992;**75**(3): 738–744.
13. Momotani N, Noh J, Oyanagi H, Ishikawa N, Ito K. Antithyroid drug therapy for Graves' disease during pregnancy. Optimal regimen for fetal thyroid status. *N Engl J Med.* 1986;**315**(1):24–28.
14. Besançon A, Beltrand J, Le Gac I, Luton D, Polak M. Management of neonates born to women with Graves' disease: a cohort study. *Eur J Endocrinol.* 2014;**170**(6):855–862.
15. Laurberg P, Nygaard B, Glinoer D, Grussendorf M, Orgiazzi J. Guidelines for TSH-receptor antibody measurements in pregnancy: results of an evidence-based symposium organized by the European Thyroid Association. *Eur J Endocrinol.* 1998;**139**(6):584–586.
16. Huel C, Guibourdenche J, Vuillard E, Ouahba J, Piketty M, Oury JF, Luton D. Use of ultrasound to distinguish between fetal hyperthyroidism and hypothyroidism on discovery of a goiter. *Ultrasound Obstet Gynecol.* 2009;**33**(4):412–420.
17. Yoshihara A, Noh JY, Watanabe N, Mukasa K, Ohye H, Suzuki M, Matsumoto M, Kunii Y, Suzuki N, Kameda T, Iwaku K, Kobayashi S, Sugino K, Ito K. Substituting potassium iodide for methimazole as the treatment for Graves' disease during the first trimester may reduce the incidence of congenital anomalies: a retrospective study at a single medical institution in Japan. *Thyroid.* 2015;**25**(10):1155–1161.

Challenges in Interpretation of Thyroid Function Tests

M15
Presented, March 17-20, 2018

Gregory A. Brent, MD. David Geffen School of Medicine at UCLA, VA Greater Los Angeles Healthcare System, Los Angeles, California 90095, E-mail: gbrent@mednet.ucla.edu

SIGNIFICANCE OF THE CLINICAL PROBLEM

Thyroid function tests are the most frequently ordered endocrine tests. In the majority of patients, the results provide a clear and consistent message of the underlying diagnosis or response to treatment (1). In some patients, however, the results are discordant with the clinical impression, inconsistent over time, or difficult to interpret. The underlying factor can be related to the specific hormone assay used; the presence of an interfering substance; unexpected changes in the course of the underlying thyroid disease; a genetic defect in the thyroid signaling pathway; or, in some cases, a combination of multiple factors.

BARRIERS TO OPTIMAL PRACTICE

- The expanding number of drugs targeting pathways that secondarily influence thyroid function both directly and as a consequence of activation of thyroid autoimmunity and promotion of thyroid disease
- The spectrum of thyroid autoantibodies with stimulating and blocking properties in the patient, including those that can be transferred vertically during pregnancy to a developing fetus and produce neonatal thyroid disease
- The challenge of evaluating patients with erratic thyroid studies associated with suspected impairment of levothyroxine absorption
- Interpretation of serum thyrotropin (TSH) results in conditions associated with differences between TSH bioactivity and measured TSH immunoreactivity, such as central hypothyroidism
- Recognition of genetic defects in thyroid signaling pathways that can lead to a disparity between clinical thyroid status and thyroid function tests

LEARNING OBJECTIVES

As a result of participating in this session, learners should be able to:

- Describe a systematic approach to evaluating thyroid function when the test results are discordant with each other or are inconsistent with the clinical impression
- Understand the factors that can interfere with measurements of thyroxine (T4) and TSH
- Describe the range of thyroid autoantibodies associated with thyroid disease and their functional consequences
- Describe an approach to evaluating a patient with hypothyroidism with erratic serum TSH and suspected levothyroxine malabsorption
- Identify the clinical and laboratory test profile of a patient with defects in thyroid hormone receptor (THR) signaling

STRATEGIES FOR DIAGNOSIS, THERAPY, AND/OR MANAGEMENT

Challenges in interpretation of thyroid function tests occur in a variety of settings. Thyroid function test results can be inconsistent with the clinical impression or symptoms of the patient being evaluated. Symptoms of thyroid disease are not specific and are found in patients without thyroid disease, and patients with authentic thyroid disease may not have typical symptoms, especially elderly patients (2). When thyroid tests are discordant with the clinical presentation, thyroid studies are repeated, or a test that is more specific for a thyroid disease process, such as thyroid autoantibodies, is added. Functional measurements of thyroid activity, such as radioiodine uptake or ultrasound to assess blood flow, can favor a diagnosis of primary thyroid disease. Repeating thyroid studies after an interval of time, especially mildly abnormal TSH results, often produces a normal reference-range follow-up. Thyroid tests can be discordant with each other, such as a normal or an elevated serum TSH concentration and an elevated serum T4 level or a normal or suppressed TSH concentration and a low serum T4 level. The option in such a situation is repeat testing, sometimes by using a different laboratory or an assay that recognizes the possibility of an antibody or substance that interferes with the assay. The same test can be performed with a different assay system or by a different laboratory, or a specific investigation for the interfering factor can be initiated. More-precise laboratory measurements, such as free T4 (FT4) or free triiodothyronine (FT3) by dialysis, can be performed, although these are typically more expensive and may require sending the specimen to a reference laboratory. Interference of biotin ingestion with thyroid testing has been well documented (3). The impact of drugs and exogenous substances that interfere with thyroid testing and T4 absorption as well as that trigger primary thyroid disease is well recognized (4). Among drugs, the much wider use of immune checkpoint inhibitors in cancer treatment has led to a high fraction of associated thyroid disease (5, 6). Interpretation of thyroid function tests may be further complicated by genetic disorders, which can disrupt essentially every component of thyroid signaling pathways (7). Although in most cases of challenging thyroid function tests a single factor can be identified, multiple diseases or other factors can be present. Patients have been reported with resistance to thyroid hormone (RTH) and an additional disease, including Hashimoto disease, Graves disease, and TSH-secreting pituitary adenoma (8).

CASES

Case 1: A Pregnant Woman With Hashimoto Disease and a Fetus With Tachycardia

A 31-year-old female was diagnosed with Hashimoto disease at age 18 years and has been on continuous T4 replacement since (9). She is pregnant and takes levothyroxine 0.125 mg/d. She is in excellent health and has no history of other medical conditions, medication use, tobacco, and alcohol or substance abuse. Thyroid function tests showed a reduced serum TSH concentration of 0.09 mU/L (reference range, 0.10 to 2.50 mU/L, trimester-specific range) and normal-range FT4 and FT3 levels. Antithyroperoxidase antibody was 600 U/mL (normal, ≤20 U/mL) and antithyroglobulin antibody, 788 U/mL (normal, <2.5 U/mL), which is consistent with autoimmune thyroiditis. Evaluation of the fetus showed thyroid gland enlargement and persistent tachycardia that ultimately required treatment of the mother with combined levothyroxine and methimazole (MMI) until delivery. The fetus was delivered by caesarean section at 36 weeks as a result of profound fetal distress. Umbilical cord blood tests showed pronounced neonatal thyrotoxicosis [TSH, 0.01 mU/mL (reference range, 5.12 to 14.6 mU/mL); FT4, 5.30 ng/dL (reference range, 0.66 to 2.17 ng/dL); FT3, 13.44 pg/mL (reference range, 1.97 to 7.87 pg/mL)].

Which of the following is the most likely etiology of hyperthyroidism in this infant?

A. Excessive dose of levothyroxine given to the mother
B. Transplacental passage of maternal TSH receptor–stimulating antibody (TRAb)
C. Germline TSH receptor gene–activating mutation in the fetus
D. Excessive maternal doses of MMI

Case 1: Discussion

The answer is B, "Transplacental passage of maternal TSH receptor–stimulating antibody (TRAb)." This patient has a history of hypothyroidism and a thyroid autoantibody pattern consistent with Hashimoto thyroiditis (9). Vertical transmission of TRAb is well described in mothers with hypothyroidism treated with levothyroxine when they have ablative treatment of Graves disease and persistent TRAb (10). The recent American Thyroid Association guidelines on thyroid disease in pregnancy recommend measurement of TRAb at initial thyroid testing in euthyroid women with a history of Graves disease and then again, if elevated, between weeks 18 and 22 of gestation, and if elevated, regular fetal evaluation and monitoring is performed (10). It is very unlikely that maternal levothyroxine supplementation at this low level, especially with administration of MMI, would produce this degree of neonatal thyrotoxicosis (answer A). Germline TSH receptor gene–activating mutations are rare but have been reported. The clinical presentation of thyroid disease, however, is later in life and would not fit this clinical profile (answer C). Excessive doses of MMI would produce neonatal hypothyroidism, the opposite of the pattern seen in this infant (answer D). This patient does not have a history of Graves disease, yet the pattern of thyroid disease and the fetus is most consistent with transplacental passage of TRAb (answer B). The spectrum of thyroid autoantibodies in autoimmune thyroid disease is such that substantial overlap has been reported. Patients with Graves disease often have antithyroperoxidase and antithryoglobulin antibodies, and a small subset patients with Hashimoto disease have TSH receptor–blocking antibodies (11). The presence of TRAb in a patient with Hashimoto disease, as in this case, is rare but has been previously reported (12). Why did this patient not have clinical Graves disease with hyperthyroidism? The most likely explanation is that the predominant pattern of thyroid destruction with longstanding Hashimoto disease did not leave sufficient tissue for the TRAb to stimulate.

Case 2: Erratic TSH in a Patient With Levothyroxine-Treated Hypothyroidism: Poor Adherence or Reduced Absorption?

A 68-year-old man is followed for hypothyroidism after radioiodine treatment of Graves disease and is taking levothyroxine. Titration to a consistent levothyroxine dose has been difficult, and for the last 3 years, the patient has been taking levothyroxine doses of 0.300 to 0.375 mg/d, with TSH values ranging from 0.3 to 53 mU/L (reference range, 0.4 to 4.3 mU/L). Despite the patient's claims of continued compliance, his TSH values over the past several months were 12 to 53 mU/L, with a serum FT4 in the lower normal reference range. He has underlying depression and a history of alcohol abuse and is taking a variety of medications, including lithium.

Which of the following would you recommend as the next step to manage this patient's chronically abnormal thyroid function tests?

A. Increase levothyroxine dose until TSH normalizes
B. Separate all other medications at least 1 hour before or after levothyroxine ingestion
C. Perform a levothyroxine absorption test
D. Supervise levothyroxine administration
E. Provide intravenous or intramuscular levothyroxine

Case 2: Discussion

The answer is C, "Perform a levothyroxine absorption test." The patient with hypothyroidism treated with levothyroxine replacement with erratic or difficult-to-normalize TSH, despite reported good compliance, is a common clinical challenge. Such patients also may have a discordance between TSH and FT4, depending on the timing of testing and dose of levothyroxine. A first step in such patients is to ensure that the patient has overt hypothyroidism and that endogenous thyroid hormone is not being produced. This patient may need a higher dose of levothyroxine, but he is already on a high dose, and if the underlying problem is not identified and changes, the dose could become excessive (answer A). Identification of factors that can interfere with absorption is reasonable, and separating levothyroxine from ingestion of food is a good step to take (answer B), but this patient has been having erratic TSH levels for 3 years, and this solution is unlikely. Supervised levothyroxine administration, often given as a weekly single dose (answer D), also is a reasonable option and should address whether adherence is the primary problem. Intravenous or intramuscular levothyroxine (answer E) can be used short term in the hospital if enteral administration is not possible, but it is quite expensive and not a practical long-term solution. Given the duration of time and failure of previous interventions, a levothyroxine absorption test is recommended (answer C). There are a number of different approaches, including a single large dose with timed blood tests for T4 (13) or combining an absorption test with weekly administration (14). In this patient, an abnormal absorption test was documented, and he was switched to liquid capsule Tirosint (Akrimax Pharmaceuticals, Cranford, NJ), which in select patients is better absorbed and results in consistent normalization of his serum TSH (15).

Case 3: Patient With Subclinical Hypothyroidism Where TSH Normalizes With Treatment, but FT4 Does Not Improve

A 72-year-old male with hyperlipidemia and hypertension is seen for routine health maintenance. His cholesterol and blood pressure have been in good control. On review of systems, he complains of some reduced energy and sleeping more than usual. His vital signs are normal, and he has no thyroid enlargement. Laboratory evaluation, including electrolytes, complete blood cell counts, lipids, and liver function tests, is normal. The patient's thyroid function tests results are TSH, 5.49 mIU/L (normal range, 0.35 to 4.50 mIU/L); FT4, 0.56 ng/dL (normal range, 0.89 to 1.76 ng/dL), and thyroperoxidase (TPO) antibodies, 5 IU/mL (normal, <20 IU/mL). Levothyroxine 0.025 mg/d is begun for subclinical hypothyroidism. He has no change in symptoms, and repeat laboratory results 2 months later show a TSH of 3.25 mIU/L and FT4 of 0.54 ng/dL.

Which of the following is the next step to further evaluate or adjust therapy in this patient?

A. Increase levothyroxine dose by 0.025 mg and follow up TSH and FT4 measurements in 6 to 8 weeks
B. Evaluate anterior pituitary function
C. Reinforce the importance of compliance with patient and taking levothyroxine on an empty stomach and then repeat follow-up TSH and FT4 measurement in 6 to 8 weeks
D. Switch to a different brand of levothyroxine or Tirosint capsules

Case 3: Discussion

The answer is B, "Evaluate anterior pituitary function." On initial review of the thyroid studies and clinical profile, the patient could be viewed as having fairly typical subclinical hypothyroidism, which is frequently seen in elderly men. The increase in the upper reference TSH range seen with age likely makes this TSH of 5.9 mIU/L a normal reference range adjusted for older age (14). The FT4 level, however, is reduced and actually much lower than one would expect in subclinical hypothyroidism. The TPO antibodies are also negative, which can be seen in a small fraction of patients with Hashimoto disease but further raises concerns about an underlying process not related to primary thyroid disease. Furthermore, the normal TSH seen in follow-up may be independent of the very small dose of levothyroxine. In a recent study of subclinical hypothyroidism in older adults, among subjects with an initial abnormally elevated TSH, 62% had a normal TSH after several months of repeat testing (16). An increase in the levothyroxine dose (answer A), reinforcing the optimal circumstances for taking levothyroxine (answer C), or even switching preparations (answer D), is potentially reasonable in the presence of a low serum T4 concentration. These approaches, however, do not account for the inappropriately normal serum TSH, despite subnormal serum T4, suggesting central hypothyroidism (17). This patient had a nonfunctioning pituitary macroadenoma and had central hypothyroidism along with central hypogonadism and central hypoadrenalism. The TSH in central hypothyroidism can have altered glycosylation and reduced bioactivity, measurable in the reference range or slightly elevated, but is not fully bioactive (17, 18).

Case 4: Teenager With Pubertal Delay and Suspected Hypothyroidism but Normal TSH

A 16-year-old male is referred for suspected hypothyroidism but has a normal TSH (19). He was evaluated by his pediatrician for possible delayed puberty. He has cranial hyperostosis, delayed dentition, height at the 50th percentile, bone age 2.7 standard deviations below normal, constipation, and anemia. His thyroid function tests are TSH, 3.20 mIU/L (reference range, 0.27 to 4.20 mIU/L); FT4, 9.0 pmol/L (reference range, 12 to 22 pmol/L); and FT3, 8.0 pmol/L (reference range, 3.9 to 6.7 pmol/L).

Which of the following is the most likely cause of the patient's clinical findings and thyroid function test pattern?

A. Hypothalamic or pituitary process producing central hypothyroidism
B. RTH-THRβ
C. RTH-THRα
D. Substance interfering with the assay, artificially lowering the measured TSH

Case 4: Discussion

The answer is C, "RTH-THRα." The patient has clinical features of early-onset hypothyroidism with developmental delay, abnormalities of bone growth, and mildly delayed growth and puberty (19). Thyroid function tests showed a normal-range TSH, reduced FT4, and elevated FT3. The reduced FT4 should be a stimulus for increased TSH secretion, but this was not seen in the patient. On the basis of the normal TSH and low FT4, the possibility of blunted TSH secretion secondary to a pituitary or hypothalamic lesion (answer A) should be considered and could fit with clinical hypothyroidism. The elevated FT3, though, would not be expected. When serum T4 falls, there is an increase in T4-to-T3 conversion as a result of increased activity of 5′-deiodinase type 2, but there should not be an excess of T3, as seen in this patient. RTH-THRβ (answer B) may have some bony deformities different from those in the current patient and growth delays, but the serum FT4 is elevated in this condition, which is not seen in this patient. Interference with the TSH assay is possible (answer D). Biotin, for example, has been shown to lower TSH and raise serum T4 and T3 concentrations, but that does not fit the normal-range TSH in this patient (3). This also would not explain the elevated serum T3. The clinical profile suggests reduced thyroid hormone action during bone growth and cognitive development, despite normal or elevated serum T3 and normal serum TSH, and is consistent with a genetic defect of thyroid hormone signaling. Thyroid transport defects, such as MCT8 mutations, have low serum T4 and high serum T3 but profound developmental neurologic deficits (7). Although rare, several families have THRα gene mutations (20). Because the THRβ signaling is not affected, feedback to TSH is normal, and the axis does not "reset" to a higher level of serum T4, as is seen with THRβ gene mutations (21). In patients with developmental manifestations of thyroid hormone deficiency and thyroid studies with a normal TSH, reduced serum FT4, and elevated FT3, RTH-THRα should be considered (answer C). The clinical manifestations vary by the specific THRα mutation but include bony deformities, reduced cognitive function, constipation, and anemia.

REFERENCES

1. Brent GA, ed. *Thyroid Function Testing.* New York, NY: Springer; 2010.
2. Carlé A, Pedersen IB, Knudsen N, Perrild H, Ovesen L, Andersen S, Laurberg P. Hypothyroid symptoms fail to predict thyroid insufficiency in old people: a population-based case-control study. *Am J Med.* 2016;**129**(10):1082–1092.
3. Kummer S, Hermsen D, Distelmaier F. Biotin treatment mimicking Graves' disease. *N Engl J Med.* 2016;**375**(7):704–706.
4. Barbesino G. Drugs affecting thyroid function. *Thyroid.* 2010;**20**(7): 763–770.
5. Torino F, Barnabei A, Paragliola R, Baldelli R, Appetecchia M, Corsello SM. Thyroid dysfunction as an unintended side effect of anticancer drugs. *Thyroid.* 2013;**23**(11):1345–1366.
6. González-Rodríguez E, Rodríguez-Abreu D; Spanish Group for Cancer Immuno-Biotherapy (GETICA). Immune Checkpoint inhibitors: review and management of endocrine adverse events. *Oncologist.* 2016; **21**(7):804–816.
7. Visser WE, van Mullem AA, Visser TJ, Peeters RP. Different causes of reduced sensitivity to thyroid hormone: diagnosis and clinical management. *Clin Endocrinol (Oxf).* 2013;**79**(5):595–605.
8. Teng X, Jin T, Brent GA, Wu A, Teng W, Shan Z. A patient with a thyrotropin-secreting microadenoma and resistance to thyroid hormone (P453T). *J Clin Endocrinol Metab.* 2015;**100**(7):2511–2514.
9. Kiefer FW, Klebermass-Schrehof K, Steiner M, Worda C, Kasprian G, Diana T, Kahaly GJ, Gessl A. Fetal/neonatal thyrotoxicosis in a newborn from a hypothyroid woman with Hashimoto thyroiditis. *J Clin Endocrinol Metab.* 2017;**102**(1):6–9.
10. Alexander EK, Pearce EN, Brent GA, Brown RS, Chen H, Dosiou C, Grobman WA, Laurberg P, Lazarus JH, Mandel SJ, Peeters RP, Sullivan S. 2017 Guidelines of the American Thyroid Association for the diagnosis and management of thyroid disease during pregnancy and the postpartum. *Thyroid.* 2017;**27**(3):315–389.
11. Diana T, Krause J, Olivo PD, König J, Kanitz M, Decallonne B, Kahaly GJ. Prevalence and clinical relevance of thyroid stimulating hormone receptor-blocking antibodies in autoimmune thyroid disease. *Clin Exp Immunol.* 2017;**189**(3):304–309.
12. McKenzie JM, Zakarija M. Fetal and neonatal hyperthyroidism and hypothyroidism due to maternal TSH receptor antibodies. *Thyroid.* 1992;**2**(2):155–159.
13. Sherman SI, Malecha SE. Absorption and malabsorption of levothyroxine sodium. *Am J Ther.* 1995;**2**(10):814–818.
14. Chaker L, Bianco AC, Jonklaas J, Peeters RP. Hypothyroidism. *Lancet.* 2017;**390**(10101):1550–1562.
15. Colucci P, D'Angelo P, Mautone G, Scarsi C, Ducharme MP. Pharmacokinetic equivalence of a levothyroxine sodium soft capsule manufactured using the new Food and Drug Administration potency guidelines in healthy volunteers under fasting conditions. *Ther Drug Monit.* 2011;**33**(3):355–361.
16. Stott DJ, Rodondi N, Kearney PM, Ford I, Westendorp RGJ, Mooijaart SP, Sattar N, Aubert CE, Aujesky D, Bauer DC, Baumgartner C, Blum MR, Browne JP, Byrne S, Collet TH, Dekkers OM, den Elzen WPJ, Du Puy RS, Ellis G, Feller M, Floriani C, Hendry K, Hurley C, Jukema JW, Kean S, Kelly M, Krebs D, Langhorne P, McCarthy G, McCarthy V, McConnachie A, McDade M, Messow M, O'Flynn A, O'Riordan D, Poortvliet RKE, Quinn TJ, Russell A, Sinnott C, Smit JWA, Van Dorland HA, Walsh KA, Walsh EK, Watt T, Wilson R, Gussekloo J; TRUST Study Group. Thyroid hormone therapy for older adults with subclinical hypothyroidism. *N Engl J Med.* 2017;**376**(26):2534–2544.
17. Beck-Peccoz P, Rodari G, Giavoli C, Lania A. Central hypothyroidism: a neglected thyroid disorder. *Nat Rev Endocrinol.* 2017;**13**(10): 588–598.
18. Estrada JM, Soldin D, Buckey TM, Burman KD, Soldin OP. Thyrotropin isoforms: implications for thyrotropin analysis and clinical practice. *Thyroid.* 2014;**24**(3):411–423.
19. Moran C, Agostini M, McGowan A, Schoenmakers E, Fairall L, Lyons G, Rajanayagam O, Watson L, Offiah A, Barton J, Price S, Schwabe J, Chatterjee K. Contrasting phenotypes in resistance to thyroid hormone alpha correlate with divergent properties of thyroid hormone receptor α1 mutant proteins. *Thyroid.* 2017;**27**(7):973–982.
20. Moran C, Agostini M, Visser WE, Schoenmakers E, Schoenmakers N, Offiah AC, Poole K, Rajanayagam O, Lyons G, Halsall D, Gurnell M, Chrysis D, Efthymiadou A, Buchanan C, Aylwin S, Chatterjee KK. Resistance to thyroid hormone caused by a mutation in thyroid hormone receptor (TR)α1 and TRα2: clinical, biochemical, and genetic analyses of three related patients. *Lancet Diabetes Endocrinol.* 2014; **2**(8):619–626.
21. Brent GA. Mechanisms of thyroid hormone action. *J Clin Invest.* 2012; **122**(9):3035–3043.

Medullary Thyroid Cancer

M31
Presented, March 17-20, 2018

Jaydira Del Rivero, MD. Rare Tumor Initiative, National Cancer Institute, National Institutes of Health, Bethesda, Maryland 20892, E-mail: jaydira.delrivero@nih.gov

INTRODUCTION

Medullary thyroid cancer (MTC) is a neuroendocrine tumor of the parafollicular or C cells of the thyroid gland. MTC accounts for approximately 4% of thyroid carcinomas. Its estimated incidence in the United States for 2010 is about 1300 to 2200 patients. Sporadic MTC accounts for about 75% of all cases of the disease. The typical age of presentation is in the fifth or sixth decade, and there may be a slight female preponderance. Hereditary MTC is divided into three distinct clinical subtypes. Multiple endocrine neoplasia (MEN) type 2A, or Sipple syndrome, is the most common subtype, accounting for approximately 70% to 80% of patients with hereditary MTC. MEN2A is characterized by MTC in 100% of affected individuals, by pheochromocytoma in 50%, and by primary hyperparathyroidism in 20%. MTC is usually the first manifestation of the syndrome. Patients typically present with a thyroid nodule or neck mass by age 15 to 20 years, but MTC can appear as early as age 5 years. MEN2B is less common than MEN2A, accounting for approximately 5% of MTC cases. It is characterized by (1) a clinically more aggressive form of MTC that is manifest at a younger age (second decade) and that occurs in 100% of affected individuals; (2) by pheochromocytoma in 50%; and (3) by characteristic dysmorphic features including distinctive mucosal neuromas on the tongue, lips, and subconjunctival areas, diffuse ganglioneuromas of the gastrointestinal tract, and marfanoid habitus. Hyperparathyroidism is not associated with MEN2B. Familial MTC is the third clinical subtype of inherited MTC. It accounts for 10% to 20% of hereditary MTC cases and is defined by the presence of MTC in kindreds, with 4 to 10 or more affected members and with objective evidence of the absence of adrenal and parathyroid gland involvement. This form of hereditary MTC is less aggressive and has an older age at onset, usually between 20 and 40 years, compared with MEN2A and MEN2B. MTC most often produces both immunoreactive calcitonin (CTN) and carcinoembryonic antigen (CEA), and these can be used as tumor markers.

SIGNIFICANCE OF THE CLINICAL PROBLEM

Total thyroidectomy with central lymph node dissection is the appropriate surgery. Surgery and/or external beam radiotherapy can be used for residual or recurrent disease treatment; however, the survival benefit for either modality is unclear. Unlike differentiated thyroid cancer, MTC does not uptake iodine, and I-131 radioactive iodine is ineffective. Patients with metastatic disease are candidates for approved agents that include either vandetanib or cabozantinib, but toxicity (with substantial morbidity) limits their use and eventually generates resistance. It is important to establish specific criteria to determine which patients may benefit from systemic therapies.

BARRIES TO OPTIMAL PRACTICE

- MTC is uncommon compared with differentiated thyroid cancer, making it more difficult for general practitioners to develop expertise in their care.
- Managing metastatic MTC requires the participation of a multidisciplinary group of specialties available in referral centers.
- Reconciling available therapies associated with MTC.
- With the new approval of targeted therapies for metastatic or recurrent MTC, endocrinologists and oncologists are working on defining the effect of these therapies on the patient's disease course and the impact on quality of life and survival benefit.

LEARNING OBJECTIVES

As a result in participating in this session, learners should be able to:

- Recognize the three distinct clinical subtypes of hereditary MTC
- Define the role of localized therapies in the management of MTC
- Recognize the importance of a multidisciplinary approach to the management of advanced MTC
- Define the indications, toxicities, and role of novel molecular targeted therapies in the management of metastatic MTC

STRATEGIES FOR DIAGNOSIS, THERAPY, AND/OR MANAGAMENT

MTC is a CTN-producing tumor derived from thyroid parafollicular or C cells, which derive from the neural crest. MTC presents worldwide as part of an autosomal dominant inherited disorder in about 20% to 25% of cases and as sporadic tumor in about 75% of cases. Sporadic tumors tend to be solitary, whereas familial tumors tend to be bilateral and multifocal. Activating mutations of the rearranged during transfection (RET) proto-oncogene are characteristic, with germline-activating RET mutations (as seen in familial MTC and MEN2) being a predisposing factor (the somatic RET codon M918T mutation in sporadic MTC appears to portend an aggressive clinical course and a poor prognosis). MTC most often produces both immunoreactive CTN and CEA, and these can be used as tumor markers.

Patients with MTC typically present with an asymptomatic thyroid mass. Some may also have local symptoms such as dysphagia, dyspnea, or hoarseness. Approximately 10% will present with systemic symptoms usually consisting of bone pain, flushing, and/or diarrhea. Approximately 50% of patients present with regional lymphadenopathy. Distant metastases typically occur in late-stage disease and usually involve lung, liver, bones, and adrenal glands. If fine-needle aspiration findings are suggestive of MTC, further evaluation should consist of CTN and CEA measurement and genetic testing for germline *RET* mutations. Surgery is the only curative treatment of MTC and consists of total thyroidectomy with bilateral central lymphadenectomy, but only when it is performed at a time when the tumor is confined to the thyroid gland. There is no treatment (apart from complete surgical removal) that has been shown to be effective for recurrent or persistent MTC. Long-term outcomes in patients undergoing repeat neck operations have been fairly good, with excellent prevention of recurrence in the central neck. External beam radiation can be used for residual or recurrent disease; however, the survival benefit is still unclear.

The growth rate of MTC is estimated by using Response Evaluation Criteria in Solid Tumors; however, we can also determine the growth rate by measuring serum levels of CTN and CEA over multiple time points to determine the CTN doubling time, which plays an important role in the follow-up and management of MTC. CTN doubling times of >2 years seem to be associated with a better long-term prognosis than those of <6 months. The CTN doubling time is a better predictor of survival than the CEA doubling time (the American Thyroid Association provides a calculator to determine doubling times of serial serum CTN and CEA measurements). In patients with detectable serum levels of CTN and CEA after thyroidectomy, the levels of the markers should be measured at least every 6 months to determine their doubling times. Furthermore, systemic therapy should not be administered to patients who have increasing serum CTN and CEA levels but no documented evidence of metastatic disease. Moreover, systemic therapy given to patients with stable low-volume metastatic disease as determined by anatomical imaging studies and serum CTN and CEA doubling times >2 years is not recommended.

Metastatic MTC is the most common cause of death in patients with MEN2A, MEN2B, or familial MTC, and the tumor is relatively unresponsive to conventional doses of radiation therapy and to standard or novel chemotherapeutic regimens. Until recently, doxorubicin was the only US Food and Drug Administration (FDA)-approved treatment of patients with advanced thyroid cancer. Doxorubicin has resulted in transient tumor response rates in up to 20% of patients with MTC and is associated with substantial toxicity. There is no treatment (apart from complete surgical removal) that has been shown to be effective for recurrent or persistent MTC. External beam radiation can be used for residual or recurrent disease; however, the survival benefit is still unclear. Furthermore, several tyrosine kinase inhibitors (TKIs) such as axitinib, cabozantinib, gefitinib, imatinib, motesanib, sorafenib, sunitinib, and vandetanib have been evaluated in phase 1, 2, and 3 clinical trials of patients with advanced MTC.

Vandetanib, an oral inhibitor of vascular endothelial growth factor receptor (VEGFR), RET, and epidermal growth factor receptor, was approved in April 2011 by the FDA for the treatment of advanced (metastatic or unresectable locally advanced) MTC based on an international randomized phase 3 trial. In a preliminary report of results (median follow-up of 24 months), the median progression-free survival (PFS) was improved in patients randomly assigned to vandetanib vs placebo [hazard ratio, 0.45; 95% confidence interval (CI), 0.30 to 0.69]. The overall response rate was 45%. Objective responses were durable on the basis of the median duration of response not being reached at 24 months of follow-up. Its toxicity profile is extensive, including diarrhea, rash, nausea, hypertension, headache, fatigue, and decreased appetite; the grade 3 toxicities reported are diarrhea, hypertension, and fatigue. Therefore, toxicity can limit its use in patients with small-volume, asymptomatic, or indolent disease.

Cabozantinib, a TKI of hepatocyte growth factor receptor, VEGFR 2, and RET, demonstrated clinical activity in patients with MTC. A double-blind, phase 3 trial comparing cabozantinib to placebo in 330 patients with documented radiographic progression of metastatic MTC was performed. The estimated median PFS was 11.2 months for cabozantinib vs 4.0 months for placebo (hazard ratio, 0.28; 95% CI, 0.19 to 0.40; $P < 0.001$). Prolonged PFS with cabozantinib was observed across all subgroups, including by age, prior TKI treatment, and RET mutation status (hereditary or sporadic). The response rate was 28% for cabozantinib and 0% for placebo; responses were seen regardless of RET mutation status. Kaplan-Meier estimations of patients alive and progression-free at 1 year were 47.3% for cabozantinib and 7.2% for placebo. Common cabozantinib-associated adverse events included diarrhea, palmar-plantar erythrodysesthesia, decreased weight and appetite, nausea, and fatigue and resulted in dose reductions in 79% and dosing delays in 65% of patients. Adverse events led to treatment discontinuation in 16% of cabozantinib-treated patients. Both vandetanib and cabozantinib have recently been approved by the FDA for the treatment of advanced MTC based on improvement in PFS in phase 3 trials. No improvement in overall survival has been demonstrated; therefore, patients with indolent disease should consider observation until their disease becomes necessary to treat.

MAIN CONCLUSIONS

- Hereditary MTC is divided into three distinct clinical subtypes—MEN2A, MEN2B, and familial MTC—and genetic screening and disease-specific screening are imperative.
- A multidisciplinary approach is needed for the optimal management of localized and advanced MTC.
- Novel targeted therapies can provide an effective alternative for properly selected patients with rapidly progressive MTC; however, for approved agents that include either vandetanib or cabozantinib, toxicity limits their use.

CASES WITH QUESTIONS

Case 1

A 23-year-old man with a history of MEN2A and MTC presents for follow-up. He was originally diagnosed 5 years ago when a thyroid mass was noted incidentally after a car accident. He subsequently underwent a total thyroidectomy with central and right neck dissections. Today, his review of systems is negative. On physical examination, his neck is notable for well-healed surgical scars and no palpable nodules or lymph nodes. The rest of the examination is unremarkable. Laboratory studies reveal normal serum chemistries, complete blood count, and thyrotropin (TSH). His CTN measurement from today is 93 pg/mL (normal, ≤14.3 pg/mL), and this level has been stable since his thyroidectomy. Which of the following is the most appropriate next step in his management?

A. Radioactive iodine whole-body scan and treatment with radioactive iodine if the scan is positive for disease.
B. Contrast-enhanced computed tomography or magnetic resonance imaging of the neck, chest, and abdomen with liver protocol for initial staging, followed by treatment with vandetanib 300 mg daily. Repeat CTN measurement in 2 to 3 months.
C. Contrast-enhanced computed tomography or magnetic resonance imaging of the neck, chest, and abdomen with liver protocol for staging. If imaging results are negative, repeat serum CTN measurement in 6 months.
D. Treat his neck with external beam radiotherapy.
E. Increase his levothyroxine dose to suppress TSH to <0.1 μIU/mL (normal, 0.27 to 4.20 μIU/mL). Remeasure his CTN and TSH levels in 6 weeks.

Case 2

A 50-year-old woman with a history of metastatic medullary carcinoma of the thyroid presented for routine follow-up. She was originally diagnosed with MTC about 10 years ago and was treated initially with total thyroidectomy. Soon after diagnosis, she was found to have asymptomatic nodules that remained relatively stable, so she was followed with active surveillance. Recently, she received external beam radiation therapy to palliate pain related to a new bone lesion and was found at that time to have enlargement of bilateral pulmonary nodules. Tumor marker levels, including CTN and CEA, have also doubled in the last 6 months. Which of the following is the most appropriate treatment option for this patient?

A. Lenvatenib
B. Radioactive iodine
C. Doxorubicin and cisplatin
D. Vandetanib

DISCUSSION WITH CASES AND ANSWERS

Case 1

The purpose of this question is to recognize the appropriate time to initiate therapy with a kinase inhibitor in advanced MTC. Vandetanib and cabozantinib are TKIs that are approved for the treatment of symptomatic or progressive MTC in patients with unresectable locally advanced or metastatic disease. Both were approved based on improvement in PFS compared with placebo but demonstrated no improvement in overall survival. Therefore, given the treatment-related risks, their use in patients with indolent, asymptomatic, or slowly progressing disease is typically not recommended. Answer B is incorrect because we do not know the results of his imaging. Asymptomatic patients with elevated CTN and negative imaging results should not receive vandetanib. If disease is present, there are several options to be considered depending on the disease burden and location. They include surgical resection if feasible, localized therapy such as radiofrequency ablation or chemoembolization, and vandetanib or cabozantinib therapy. Answers A and E are incorrect because MTC is derived from parafollicular or C cells. This cell type does not incorporate iodine or have TSH receptors. Therefore, TSH suppression and radioactive iodine are not effective therapies. Answer D is incorrect because although external beam radiation is sometimes used, it is not done empirically without imaging to assess for resectable disease. Further, MTC is not particularly radiosensitive. Answer C is the best answer. If his imaging results are negative, measurement of his CTN should be repeated in 3 to 6 months. If it is stable, no further imaging is indicated. If it continues to rise, it rapidly increases, or he develops new symptoms, further imaging should be done.

Case 2

Vandetanib is the treatment of choice for metastatic MTC. It was approved in April 2011 by the FDA for the treatment of advanced (metastatic or unresectable locally advanced) MTC based on the international randomized phase 3 trial. Lenvatenib is FDA approved for the treatment of iodine refractory metastatic papillary thyroid cancer but not for metastatic MTC. Doxorubicin is an FDA- approved cytotoxic agent approved for the treatment of metastatic differentiated thyroid cancer and does not have a role in the management of MTC. Although cytotoxic therapy should be discouraged in patients with metastatic MTC, it may be considered in selected patients with rapidly progressive disease not amenable for clinical trials. Clinical trials with cytotoxic agents have shown limited efficacy with best responses of partial remission generally in the range of 10% to 20%, and these responses are short lived. Radioactive iodine therapy does not have a role in the management of MTC.

RECOMMENDED READING

Brandi ML, Gagel RF, Angeli A, Bilezikian JP, Beck-Peccoz P, Bordi C, Conte-Devolx B, Falchetti A, Gheri RG, Libroia A, Lips CJ, Lombardi G, Mannelli M, Pacini F, Ponder BA, Raue F, Skogseid B, Tamburrano G, Thakker RV, Thompson NW, Tomassetti P, Tonelli F, Wells SA Jr, Marx SJ. Guidelines for diagnosis and therapy of MEN type 1 and type 2. *J Clin Endocrinol Metab.* 2001;**86**(12):5658–5671.

Eng C, Mulligan LM, Healey CS, Houghton C, Frilling A, Raue F, Thomas GA, Ponder BA. Heterogeneous mutation of the RET proto-oncogene in subpopulations of medullary thyroid carcinoma. *Cancer Res.* 1996; **56**(9):2167–2170.

Kouvaraki MA, Shapiro SE, Perrier ND, Cote GJ, Gagel RF, Hoff AO, Sherman SI, Lee JE, Evans DB. RET proto-oncogene: a review and update of genotype-phenotype correlations in hereditary medullary thyroid cancer and associated endocrine tumors. *Thyroid.* 2005;**15**(6): 531–544.

Kurzrock R, Sherman SI, Ball DW, Forastiere AA, Cohen RB, Mehra R, Pfister DG, Cohen EE, Janisch L, Nauling F, Hong DS, Ng CS, Ye L, Gagel RF, Frye J, Müller T, Ratain MJ, Salgia R. Activity of XL184 (cabozantinib), an oral tyrosine kinase inhibitor, in patients with medullary thyroid cancer. *J Clin Oncol.* 2011;**29**(19):2660–2666.

Lodish MB, Stratakis CA. Rare and unusual endocrine cancer syndromes with mutated genes. *Semin Oncol.* 2010;**37**(6):680–690.

Saad MF, Fritsche HA Jr, Samaan NA. Diagnostic and prognostic values of carcinoembryonic antigen in medullary carcinoma of the thyroid. *J Clin Endocrinol Metab.* 1984;**58**(5):889–894.

Saad MF, Ordonez NG, Rashid RK, Guido JJ, Hill CS Jr, Hickey RC, Samaan NA. Medullary carcinoma of the thyroid: a study of the clinical features and prognostic factors in 161 patients. *Medicine (Baltimore).* 1984; **63**(6):319–342.

Wells SA Jr, Asa SL, Dralle H, Elisei R, Evans DB, Gagel RF, Lee N, Machens A, Moley JF, Pacini F, Raue F, Frank-Raue K, Robinson B, Rosenthal MS, Santoro M, Schlumberger M, Shah M, Waguespack SG. Revised American Thyroid Association guidelines for the management of medullary thyroid carcinoma: the American Thyroid Association Guidelines Task Force on Medullary Thyroid Carcinoma. *Thyroid.* 2015;**25**(6):567–610.

Wells SA Jr, Robinson BG, Gagel RF, Dralle H, Fagin JA, Santoro M, Baudin E, Elisei R, Jarzab B, Vasselli JR, Read J, Langmuir P, Ryan AJ, Schlumberger MJ. Vandetanib in patients with locally advanced or metastatic medullary thyroid cancer: a randomized, double-blind phase III trial. *J Clin Oncol.* 2012;**30**(2):134–141.

Thyroid Hormone Resistance

M61
Presented, March 17–20, 2018

W. Edward Visser, MD, PhD. Department of Endocrinology, Academic Centre of Thyroid Diseases, Erasmus Medical Centre, 3015 CN Rotterdam, The Netherlands, E-mail: w.e.visser@erasmusmc.nl

INTRODUCTION

Thyroid hormone is crucial for metabolism and development. Cellular thyroid hormone homeostasis requires adequate function of (1) thyroid hormone transporter proteins, (2) deiodinating enzymes, and (3) nuclear receptors. Defects in any of these processes give rise to distinct syndromes, collectively called resistance to thyroid hormone (RTH) syndromes.

Currently, four RTH syndromes have been recognized: (1) RTH-β ("classical" RTH), due to mutations in thyroid hormone receptor β (TRβ); (2) RTH-α, due to mutations in thyroid hormone receptor α (TRα); (3) MCT8 deficiency; and (4) SBP2 deficiency. These disorders are characterized by tissue-specific changes in thyroid state accompanied by abnormal thyroid function tests (TFTs). Diagnosis and management is challenging in many cases. Basic, translational, and clinical studies have advanced the understanding of RTH syndromes and contributed to optimizing therapeutic strategies.

The clinical and biochemical phenotypes, imaging modalities, underlying mechanisms, and treatment options are discussed for the different RTH syndromes (Table 1).

SIGNIFICANCE OF THE CLINICAL PROBLEM

The clinical features of RTH syndromes are the composite of hypothyroid, euthyroid, and hyperthyroid tissues, which are accompanied by abnormal TFTs in the blood. Given the essential role of thyroid hormone in development, early detection is paramount in order to initiate therapy for alleviating or preventing disease-specific outcomes.

BARRIERS TO OPTIMAL PRACTICE

Proper diagnosis of RTH syndromes can be challenging. Recognizing RTH syndromes from other disorders [*e.g.*, central hypothyroidism and thyrotropin (TSH)-producing pituitary tumors] is crucial for optimal management and treatment possibilities (1). Because RTH syndromes often present to endocrinologists with abnormal TFTs, it is crucial to distinguish RTH syndromes from assay interference (*e.g.*, drugs and antibodies).

Clinical management can be difficult because an optimal balance between thyroid hormone deficiency and excess has to be achieved.

LEARNING OBJECTIVES

As a result of participating in this session, learners should be able to:

- Recognize the clinical and biochemical features associated with the distinct RTH syndromes
- Apply the general management principles in RTH syndromes

STRATEGIES FOR DIAGNOSIS, THERAPY, AND/OR MANAGEMENT

RTH-β

Diagnosis

RTH-β is caused by mutations in *THRB* (2, 3). Patients with RTH-β display a variable phenotype, including goiter, tachycardia, raised energy expenditure, hyperactive behavior, delayed bone age, and learning disabilities. Symptoms are due to a combination of thyroid hormone action in predominantly TRβ-expressing tissues (*e.g.*, pituitary and liver) and thyroid hormone overexposure in TRα-expressing tissues (*e.g.*, heart, brain, gut, and bone). Patients who receive treatment (*e.g.*, antithyroid drugs or radioactive iodine) to normalize triiodothyronine (T_3) and thyroxine (T_4) concentrations often develop typical symptoms of hypothyroidism.

RTH-β is characterized by elevated serum T_3 and T_4 concentrations with nonsuppressed TSH concentrations. The distinction between RTH-β and a TSH-producing pituitary adenoma (TSHoma) can be challenging because, in both conditions, the free T_4 (FT_4) and free T_3 (FT_3) will be elevated independent of the method used. Dynamic testing [*e.g.*, thyrotropin-releasing hormone (TRH)-test] is useful to differentiate between both disorders. Genetic testing confirms the diagnosis of RTH-β, although in 10% to 15% of patients with classical RTH, no mutation in *THRB* can be detected.

Management

In many patients, treatment is not necessary because the resistance seems to be adequately compensated by the elevated levels of T_4 and T_3. Given the large variability in symptoms, therapy should be individually tailored to alleviate symptoms. Tachycardia and tremor as symptoms of hyperthyroidism can be adequately treated using beta-adrenergic blockers. Standard preventive medicine can be considered for dyslipidemia and reduced bone mineral density. In some cases, treatment with the T_3 analog 3,5,3′-triiodothyroacetic acid, or Triac, which has a higher affinity for TRβ than for TRα, can be used to lower serum TSH and thyroid hormone levels, thereby reducing the clinical symptoms of hyperthyroidism (4).

RTH-α

Diagnosis

Mutations in *THRA* result in RTH-α, which is characterized by reduced sensitivity in TRα-expressing tissues (5). Prominent

Table 1. Overview of biochemical and key clinical features in the different resistance to thyroid hormone disorders

	RTH-β	RTH-α	MCT8-def	SBP2-def
TSH	↑/=	=	= (↑)	=
FT4	↑	↓ (=)	↓(=)	↑
T3	↑/=	↑/=	↑	↓
rT3	↑	↓ (=)	↓	↑
Other	Goitre, tachycardia, anxiety/AHDS	Delayed growth, mild anemia, skin tags	Intellectual disability, dystonia, central hypotonia, low body weight	Delayed milestones, delayed growth, photosensitivity, neuropathy
Treatment	Beta-blockers Triac	T_4	Supportive (T3 analogues)	Vitamin E

features include dysmorphic facies, abnormal bone development (*e.g.*, growth retardation and macrocephaly), constipation, and variable neurocognitive symptoms (*e.g.*, dyspraxia, ataxia, and intellectual disability).

Abnormal TFTs include low/low-normal (F)T_4, high/high-normal T_3, low reverse T_3 (rT_3), but normal TSH levels. A substantial proportion of RTH-α cases have very subtle abnormalities. Mild anemia and elevated creatine kinase levels are frequently observed.

Therapy

T_4 therapy can improve constipation, energy expenditure, and general well-being in adults. Initiation of T_4 treatment during childhood has the potential to improve growth velocity, bone development, and neurocognitive outcomes.

SBP2 Deficiency

Diagnosis

Selenoproteins form a distinct group of 25 proteins, including the three deiodinases and different proteins involved in antioxidant function. Selenoproteins recode the UGA codon into a selenocystein residue, for which normal SBP2 function is indispensable. Deficiency in SBP2 gives rise to a multisystem disorder that includes delayed growth, myopathy, and sensorineural hearing loss. Central obesity, primary infertility, delayed developmental milestones, and enhanced skin photosensitivity have variably been reported (6).

SBP2-deficient patients display a typical biochemical fingerprint due to diminished deiodinase function. Serum (F)T_4 and rT_3 levels are elevated, whereas (F)T_3 levels are low or low-normal, causing a frankly elevated T_4:T_3 ratio. TSH concentrations are either in the upper-normal range or slightly elevated. Serum selenium concentrations are reduced.

Management

There is no standard treatment of patients with SBP2 deficiency. Neither standard T_3 administration nor selenium supplementation in SBP2-deficient patients is recommended. Vitamin E treatment can be considered in order to reduce elevated peroxidation products.

MCT8 Deficiency

Diagnosis

MCT8 deficiency (also called Allan-Herndon-Dudley syndrome) is an X-linked disease that results from absent/impaired thyroid hormone transport by defective MCT8 (7). The phenotype of this disorder has a central or neurocognitive part and a peripheral or endocrine part. The delayed neurocognitive development results in severe intellectual and motor disability, axial hypotonia, and dystonia. The peripheral component is characterized by a progressive decline in body weight, muscle wasting, and tachycardia.

The combination of increased (F)T_3 and decreased (F)T_4 and rT_3 serum concentrations is characteristic for MCT8 deficiency.

Management and Therapy

The current treatment modalities consist mainly of supportive care including physical, occupational, and speech therapies; dietary supplementation; and medical treatment of dystonia and seizures. Frequent orthopedic follow-up is required to monitor the development and progression of scoliosis.

The ideal treatment should restore thyroid hormone signaling in hypothyroid tissues that rely on MCT8 (MCT8-dependent tissues) for their cellular thyroid hormone uptake while alleviating the T_3 thyrotoxicity in MCT8-independent tissues (4, 8). T_4 monotherapy should be discouraged. T_4 administration in combination with propylthiouracil (PTU) may have beneficial effects on T_3 concentration and body weight but will not change neurocognitive outcomes. PTU reduces the type 1 deiodinase, thereby inhibiting T_4-to-T_3 conversion. Long-term administration of PTU accumulates the risk of severe side effects. T_3 analogs that bypass MCT8 but mimic T_3 action hold potential. The effects of Triac in MCT8-deficient patients are currently being investigated in a clinical trial (NTC02060474).

MAIN CONCLUSIONS

1. RTH syndromes have clinical features that arise from tissue-specific reduced thyroid hormone sensitivity or from thyroid hormone excess.
2. Apart from general supportive measures, disease-specific therapies include T_4 therapy (RTH-α), T_3 analog therapy

(RTH-β and MCT8 deficiency), and vitamin E supplementation (SBP2 deficiency).

DISCUSSION OF CASES AND ANSWERS

Case 1

A 39-year-old woman is referred because of abnormal TFTs. She has no overt clinical symptoms, except a mild tachycardia and palpitations during exercise. Physical examination reveals a small goiter. Her TFTs reveal a TSH concentration of 4.3 mU/L (normal, 0.4 to 4.5 mU/L) and an FT_4 concentration of 39 pmol/L (normal, 11 to 25 pmol/L). Previous samples 6 and 12 months ago had similar results.

Question

Which drugs could explain the above-mentioned tests? (1) amiodarone, (2) furosemide, (3) prednisone, (4) low-molecular-weight heparin

A. 1 and 2
B. 3 and 4
C. 1, 2, and 4
D. None of the drugs
Answer C

Glucocorticoids decrease TSH concentrations. Amiodarone inhibits T_4-to-T_3 conversion, typically resulting in elevated FT_4 concentrations and low or low-normal (F)T_3 concentrations. TSH concentrations can be normal or high-normal. Furosemide displaces T_4 from binding proteins, thereby increasing the free fraction. The furosemide-induced increase in the FT_4 fraction is progressively lost with sample dilution. Heparin and low-molecular-weight heparin induce lipoprotein lipase from endothelium *in vivo*, which leads to increased nonesterified fatty acids *in vitro*, which subsequently displace T_4 from thyroxine-binding globulin.

Question

Assume that no drugs are responsible for this combination of TFTs. All of the following conditions explain these TFTs, except:

A. Resistance to thyroid hormone
B. Nonthyroidal illness
C. Familial dysalbuminemic hyperthyroxinemia
D. TSHoma
Answer B

Nonthyroidal illness typically presents with low (F)T_3 and (F)T_4 concentrations accompanied by low or low-normal TSH concentrations.

Question

What is the most adequate test to distinguish between RTH-β and a TSHoma?

A. T_3:rT_3 ratio
B. TSH response in a TRH-test
C. Sex hormone–binding globulin concentrations
D. Pituitary hormones
Answer B

Upon TRH intravenous administration, the TSH response evaluation can help to differentiate TSHoma from RTH-β. A <1.5-fold increase is concordant with a TSHoma, whereas a larger-than-fivefold increase is associated with RTH-β.

Question

A genetic test reveals a mutation in *THRB*. Which additional tests have value for the management of RTH-β? (1) 24-hour electrocardiographic analysis, (2) dual-energy X-ray absorptiometry scan (bone mineral density assessment), (3) magnetic resonance imaging of the brain, (4) blood lipid concentrations, (5) liver ultrasound

A. 1, 2, and 3
B. 2, 4, and 5
C. 1, 2, and 4
D. 3, 4, and 5
Answer C

Although RTH-β can be associated with anxiety or attention deficit hyperactivity disorder, magnetic resonance imaging of the brain will not reveal gross abnormalities that dictate treatment. Although the liver has important TRβ expression, and dyslipidemia is associated with RTH-β, a liver ultrasound has no additional value. Tachycardia or atrial fibrillation can be documented with an electrocardiogram, whereas thyrotoxic effects on bone mineral density can be assessed by dual-energy X-ray absorptiometry scan; heart and bone are TRα-expressing tissues.

Question

What medical treatment option can be considered if this patient does have RTH-β?

A. Radioactive iodine therapy
B. Methimazole
C. Metoprolol
D. No medical treatment
Answer C

Supportive therapy is the mainstay in the treatment of RTH-β. Palpitations or tachycardia can be relieved with symptomatic treatment. Aiming at FT_4 levels within the reference range by means of radioactive iodine therapy or antithyroid drugs will result in hypothyroid symptoms.

Case 2

The consultant neurologist has referred a male to your clinic. He has a syndrome comprising a severe neurocognitive delay and extrapyramidal signs. In the diagnostic workup, the neurologist has tested TSH and FT_4. The TSH concentration is 3.5 mU/L (normal, 0.4 to 4.5 mU/L) and the FT_4 concentration is 7 pmol/L (normal, 11 to 25 pmol/L). The specific request is whether T_4 therapy should be started.

Question

What initial explanation(s) come across your mind?

A. Central hypothyroidism
B. MCT8 deficiency
C. Mutations in TRα
D. All the above-mentioned diagnoses
Answer D

Question

What additional tests will you order?

A. Vitamin E
B. Total T_4
C. Total T_3
D. No additional test
Answer C

There are two RTH disorders that have normal TSH and low/low-normal FT_4 levels with neurodevelopmental delay. Because total T_3 and FT_3 levels can be elevated in both RTH-α and MCT8 deficiency, these are useful additional tests when either of these diagnoses is suspected. Central hypothyroidism is a possibility, although it generally is not associated with intellectual disability.

REFERENCES

1. Koulouri O, Moran C, Halsall D, Chatterjee K, Gurnell M. Pitfalls in the measurement and interpretation of thyroid function tests. *Best Pract Res Clin Endocrinol Metab.* 2013;**27**(6):745–762.
2. Dumitrescu AM, Refetoff S. The syndromes of reduced sensitivity to thyroid hormone. *Biochim Biophys Acta.* 2013;**1830**(7):3987–4003.
3. Refetoff S, Weiss RE, Usala SJ. The syndromes of resistance to thyroid hormone. *Endocr Rev.* 1993;**14**(3):348–399.
4. Groeneweg S, Peeters RP, Visser TJ, Visser WE. Therapeutic applications of thyroid hormone analogues in resistance to thyroid hormone (RTH) syndromes. *Mol Cell Endocrinol.* 2017;**458**:82–90.
5. Moran C, Chatterjee K. Resistance to thyroid hormone due to defective thyroid receptor alpha. *Best Pract Res Clin Endocrinol Metab.* 2015; **29**(4):647–657.
6. Schoenmakers E, Agostini M, Mitchell C, Schoenmakers N, Papp L, Rajanayagam O, Padidela R, Ceron-Gutierrez L, Doffinger R, Prevosto C, Luan J, Montano S, Lu J, Castanet M, Clemons N, Groeneveld M, Castets P, Karbaschi M, Aitken S, Dixon A, Williams J, Campi I, Blount M, Burton H, Muntoni F, O'Donovan D, Dean A, Warren A, Brierley C, Baguley D, Guicheney P, Fitzgerald R, Coles A, Gaston H, Todd P, Holmgren A, Khanna KK, Cooke M, Semple R, Halsall D, Wareham N, Schwabe J, Grasso L, Beck-Peccoz P, Ogunko A, Dattani M, Gurnell M, Chatterjee K. Mutations in the selenocysteine insertion sequence-binding protein 2 gene lead to a multisystem selenoprotein deficiency disorder in humans. *J Clin Invest.* 2010;**120**(12): 4220–4235.
7. Visser WE, Friesema EC, Visser TJ. Minireview: thyroid hormone transporters: the knowns and the unknowns. *Mol Endocrinol.* 2011; **25**(1):1–14.
8. Visser WE, van Mullem AA, Visser TJ, Peeters RP. Different causes of reduced sensitivity to thyroid hormone: diagnosis and clinical management. *Clin Endocrinol (Oxf).* 2013;**79**(5):595–605.

MISCELLANEOUS

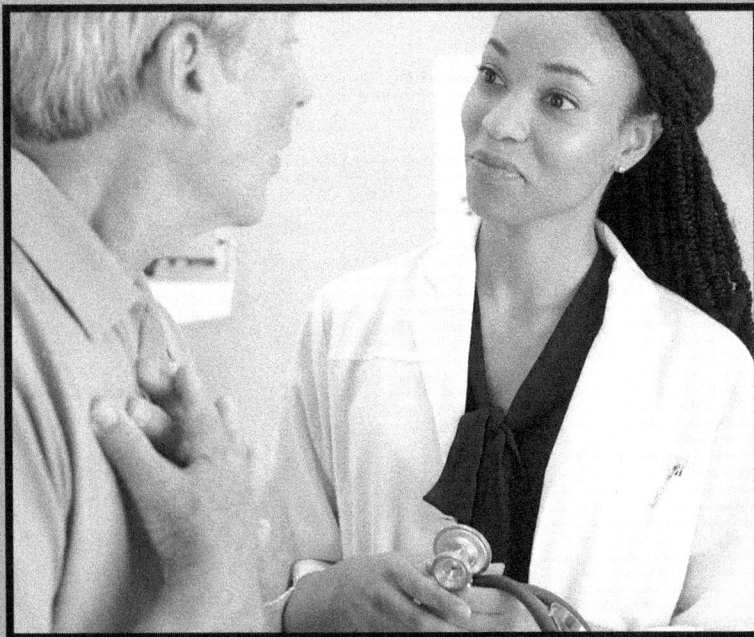

Debunking Internet Myths: What Is the Best Approach?

M24
Presented, March 17–20, 2018

Jonathan D. Leffert, MD. North Texas Endocrine Center, Dallas, Texas 75231, E-mail: jleffert@leffertmail.com

SIGNIFICANCE OF THE CLINICAL PROBLEM

In our current health care system, 60% of the public uses the Internet for health information, and 35% are engaged in online diagnosis (1, 2). Fifty-three percent of online diagnosers talk with a clinician about their diagnosis, and 41% have their diagnosis confirmed. Nonspecific diagnosis that includes fatigue, weight gain, and other vague symptoms often will lead self-diagnosers to an endocrine diagnosis such as hypothyroidism, adrenal abnormalities, and testosterone deficiency (3, 4). Patients with these symptoms present to endocrinologists, armed with information they find on the Internet, for an evaluation for an endocrine cause for their symptoms. These patients require a considerable amount of a physician's time to adequately evaluate their symptoms and physical findings and to obtain appropriate laboratory tests.

BARRIERS TO OPTIMAL PRACTICE

- Information from the Internet on endocrine disease that is inaccurate and unfiltered
- Patients with a diagnosis other than endocrine disorder who have been either unable or unwilling to obtain a diagnosis and are frustrated by not feeling well
- Patients with symptoms that are nonspecific on the basis of laboratory findings for some diagnoses that have broad ranges with diurnal and assay variability

LEARNING OBJECTIVES

As a result of participating in this session, learners should be able to:

- Discuss the background and status of the Internet's effect on health care information seeking
- Recognize the frustrated patient who is searching for answers to symptoms and obtain an appropriate endocrine workup with the goal of addressing the patient's unmet medical needs

STRATEGIES FOR DIAGNOSIS, THERAPY, AND/OR MANAGEMENT

The Internet has been both a blessing and a curse for endocrinologists over the last 20 years. Since starting in practice in 1991, I have experienced a marked increase in the number of patients who present with vague symptoms and laboratory tests that were not specific but may indicate an endocrine disorder. Patients with symptoms of fatigue and weight gain have looked for a simple solution in the form of a thyroid pill to alleviate their symptoms. Now, as a result of readily accessible information, patients self-diagnose and insist on obtaining the laboratory tests required to confirm their "diagnosis" of thyroid disease.

The confluence of often inaccurate Internet information, easy-to-use testosterone medications, wide-ranging testosterone assays with biological variability, and society's high value placed on youth has resulted in an explosion of patients with testosterone deficiency. This group of patients with high expectations for treatment benefit is challenging to treat. In my clinical experience, this group has a difficult-to-define disease biochemically, and if treated with testosterone replacement, most often do not experience treatment benefit.

Patients with symptoms and lack of biochemical specificity for diagnosis are those with self-diagnosed adrenal fatigue or Cushing syndrome. Most of the time in this group, few signs, symptoms, or biochemical findings are consistent with adrenal insufficiency. In patients with self-diagnosed Cushing syndrome, I am wary of pursuing this diagnosis because of false-positive biochemical test results. If I pursue this diagnosis, I use the most-specific screening test for the clinical setting to try to avoid the false-positive finding.

Management of self-diagnosed patients is challenging, and we must evaluate the patient with the same rigor we apply to all patients. I take a history, including reviewing previous records and laboratory results, perform the physical examination, and discuss my findings with the patient. I discuss the laboratory evaluation for each condition listed above, using a minimalist approach to try to avoid false positives findings. This is particularly true in patients who, in my evaluation, are unlikely to have an endocrine disorder.

Finally, and most importantly, I explain at length and nonjudgmentally my methodology of evaluation for their condition. I tell patients about my approach to clinical medicine, which is based on the scientific method and associated clinical guidelines. At this point, I ask the patient whether I met his or her expectations and whether he or she has additional questions for me. During our consultation, I attempt to address the issues the patient brought from the Internet, and when I am finished, most of the time the patient is less frustrated.

Case Presentation and Discussion

Case 1

A 21-year-old woman with history of fatigue and weight gain presented to her naturopath. She had no previous medical or surgical history. On physical examination, her BMI was 19 kg/m^2, her thyroid gland was not enlarged, and the rest of the examination was unremarkable. Her thyroid test showed a free thyroxine level of 1.2 ng/dL, thyrotropin level of 1.4 mIU/L, and an elevated reverse triiodothyronine (T3) level. The patient then consulted the Internet about the reverse T3 elevation. From this source, her naturopath recommended additional evaluation and consideration of thyroid hormone treatment.

Discussion

In this case, the patient focused on the reverse T3 as a marker of thyroid hormone deficiency, which she had researched and found to be an important factor in thyroid function. I discussed in detail with the patient the physiology of thyroid metabolism and the lack of significance of an elevated reverse T3 as a biochemical marker for thyroid dysfunction. Finally, I gave her alternative diagnostic possibilities for her symptoms and suggestions for referral.

Case 2

A 30-year-old man presents for evaluation of low testosterone. He was seen by a low testosterone center initially for fatigue without any symptoms of sexual dysfunction. His initial testosterone level was 280 ng/dL on one sample drawn in the afternoon. He was started on testosterone cypionate 75 mg every week initially and increased to 100 mg/wk because of lack of improvement in symptoms. On physical examination, the patient appears plethoric and has decreased testicular size. In addition to weekly testosterone injections, he takes an aromatase inhibitor to decrease his potential risk of gynecomastia. He presents to discuss the cause of his low testosterone and the duration of treatment.

Discussion

Discussion of low testosterone in healthy young men taking high-dose testosterone replacement is a challenge. These men often are eugonadal and looking for symptom relief for other underlying psychological or body dysmorphic issues. I emphasize the importance of evaluation of the underlying cause of hypogonadism as the initial step in a diagnostic evaluation. To accomplish this goal, I discontinue the testosterone replacement therapy and ask the patient to return in 3 months for repeat evaluation of his pituitary gonadal axis. I emphasize that if in fact, he is hypogonadal that he will require lifelong treatment with testosterone with its known and potential consequences. Most patients at this point opt to discontinue the testosterone and return for future testing.

Case 3

A 45-year-old woman presents for discussion of exhaustion, mood changes, and muscle aches after seeing a chiropractor. The chiropractor ordered a panel of laboratory tests, including salivary cortisol obtained over a period of several hours. The salivary cortisol values were consistent with adrenal fatigue. Her medical history and physical examination are unremarkable. The patient is interested in treatment for adrenal fatigue.

Discussion

It is difficult to deal with a disease entity that patients presume to be endocrinological as promoted by individuals outside the specialty. This situation requires time and patience to explain the underlying physiology of the pituitary-adrenal axis at the patient's educational level. From this explanation, the patient understands that outside the disease entity of adrenal insufficiency, adrenal fatigue does not exist as a diagnosis. I explain the underlying paradigm of all medical illness that without a diagnosis, I do not have an endocrine treatment. Finally, I suggest diagnostic possibilities and make referrals.

REFERENCES

1. Sbaffi L, Rowley J. Trust and credibility in Web-based health information: a review and agenda for future research. *J Med Internet Res.* 2017;**19**(6):e218.
2. Fox S, Duggan M; Pew Research Center. One in three American adults have gone online to figure out a medical condition. Available: http://www.pewinternet.org/2013/01/15/health-online-2013. Accessed 3 June, 2017.
3. Mueller J, Jay C, Harper S, Davies A, Vega J, Todd C. Web use for symptom appraisal of physical health conditions: a systematic review. *J Med Internet Res.* 2017;**19**(6):e202.
4. Tan SS, Goonawardene N. Internet health information seeking and the patient-physician relationship: a systematic review. *J Med Internet Res.* 2017;**19**(1):e9.

Endocrine Manifestations of HIV Disease

M29
Presented, March 17–20, 2018

Steven K. Grinspoon, MD. Harvard Medical School and Massachusetts General Hospital, Boston, Massachusetts 02114, E-mail: sgrinspoon@partners.org

SIGNIFICANCE OF THE CLINICAL PROBLEM

HIV disease affects up to 37 million patients worldwide and over 1.4 million in the United States. Endocrine and metabolic abnormalities have been commonly reported in HIV. HIV itself, related infectious organisms, immune activation, cytokines, and antiretroviral medications may all affect endocrine function. Endocrine disorders in HIV disease, for example hypogonadism, adrenal insufficiency, diabetes mellitus (DM), and bone loss, may cause substantial morbidity and are thus important to diagnose (1). Interactions between antiretroviral therapy (ART) and specific medication may also contribute to endocrine disturbances. Endocrine strategies may improve quality of life and long-term mortality through effects on critical metabolic and body composition parameters, and fat redistribution with loss of peripheral and abdominal subcutaneous fat and relative or absolute gains in central (visceral) adiposity among some patients. However, diagnosis and treatment may be difficult due to varying nutritional conditions and effects of the varied medications used to treat HIV disease. As HIV patients live longer due to the success of antiretroviral medications, adverse effects resulting from these very medications and HIV-related immune dysfunction have resulted in increased cardiovascular risk and metabolic changes that require intervention and long-term management by the endocrine specialist. This MTP session will focus on key topics of interest to endocrine practitioners who care for HIV-infected patients.

BARRIERS TO OPTIMAL PRACTICE

- Endocrine abnormalities are often difficult to recognize in HIV patients who may be on numerous medications unfamiliar to the endocrine practitioner.
- Treatment of endocrine disorders in HIV patients may involve coordinated care with HIV practitioners, especially if this care involves changing antiretroviral medications or interactions between ART and endocrine therapies.

LEARNING OBJECTIVES

As a result of participating in this session, learners should be able to:

- Understand the spectrum of adrenal, gonadal, and thyroid disorders among HIV-infected patients and recognize the specific effects of antiretroviral medications on these conditions
- Recognize that insulin resistance, DM, and dyslipidemia are common among HIV-infected patients, may present with unique laboratory abnormalities, may require unique therapeutic strategies, and may contribute to increased cardiovascular disease (CVD) in HIV

STRATEGIES FOR DIAGNOSIS, THERAPY, AND MANAGEMENT

Adrenal Function

Adrenal dysfunction may be suspected in the patient with advanced HIV disease because of fatigue, hyponatremia, and other features of adrenal insufficiency. Biochemical evidence of adrenal insufficiency is relatively common among hospitalized AIDS patients, with 17% of 74 hospitalized AIDS patients screened by cosyntropin test demonstrating inadequate adrenal stimulation (1-hour cortisol <18 μg/dL) in an early study. In contrast, fewer patients demonstrate clinical symptoms of adrenal insufficiency (2). Among patients with clinical symptoms, a higher percentage, up to 30%, may demonstrate inadequate testing using cosyntropin (3). Adrenal insufficiency occurring in the context of advanced HIV disease is most often caused by tissue destruction of the adrenal glands from opportunistic infections. Cytomegalovirus (CMV) adrenalitis is the most common etiology, seen in ~40% to 90% of patients with CMV infections at autopsy. However, adrenocortical destruction caused by CMV is usually $<50\%$ and therefore unlikely to cause adrenal insufficiency (4), and CMV disease is rare with well-preserved immune function in patients on newer potent ARTs. Other organisms and processes that have been associated with adrenal destruction in HIV disease include *Mycobacterium tuberculosis*, *Mycobacterium avium intracellulare*, *Cryptococcus*, and hemorrhage. Additionally, pituitary/hypothalamic destruction resulting in secondary adrenal insufficiency may be caused in rare instances by opportunistic infection (*e.g.*, toxoplasmosis, *Cryptococcus*, and CMV).

Medications may contribute to adrenal insufficiency in HIV patients. Ketoconazole, an antifungal agent, inhibits side-chain cleavage enzyme and 11-β-hydroxylase. These effects are not generally seen with fluconazole, itraconazole, and more recently introduced imidazole derivatives. Phenytoin, opiates, and rifampin, among other drugs, affect cortisol metabolism. For example, adrenal insufficiency may be precipitated by the use of rifampin for treatment of tuberculosis in patients with reduced adrenal reserve. Megestrol acetate, a potent synthetic progestational derivative used as an appetite stimulant, has glucocorticoid properties and decreases adrenocorticotropic hormone (ACTH). Abrupt withdrawal of megestrol acetate may precipitate adrenal insufficiency, and such patients should be tested for adrenal insufficiency and receive physiologic glucocorticoid administration as needed after megestrol withdrawal. In addition, megestrol acetate can decrease gonadal function, which should also be monitored during and after therapy. Cases of Cushing syndrome have been described with the concomitant use of fluticasone and ritonavir, via inhibition of CYP3A4 by ritonavir and resultant reduction in metabolism of fluticasone. This combination of medications can result in symptoms of severe cortisol excess and potential severe adrenal insufficiency with discontinuation of fluticasone (5). Such patients demonstrate very low measured cortisol and ACTH levels, despite symptoms of hypercortisolemia, due to suppression of the endogenous hypothalamic-pituitary-adrenal axis by increased concentrations of circulating fluticasone. After discontinuation of the fluticasone, long-term physiologic steroid replacement is necessary until the hypothalamic-pituitary-adrenal axis recovers. In addition, adrenal insufficiency has been reported in ~5% of patients receiving intra-articular steroids while on protease inhibitors (PIs), particularly ritonavir, with increasing risk seen among those with more than two injections within the prior 6 months (6).

HIV-infected patients with symptoms of adrenal insufficiency and particularly those with hyponatremia and risk factors for adrenal insufficiency, *e.g.*, known disseminated CMV or recent use of megestrol acetate, should be evaluated. Evaluation of the cortisol axis should proceed as in other patients with suspected adrenal dysfunction. Cosyntropin testing is usually an adequate first step, except in those patients in whom hypothalamic or pituitary insufficiency of recent onset is suspected. In such patients, use of morning cortisol levels, metyrapone, or insulin tolerance testing may be necessary, if there are no contraindications. After adrenal insufficiency is documented, ACTH testing and appropriate imaging are used to localize the defect. In patients with symptoms of adrenal excess and low cortisol and ACTH levels, exogenous steroid use or interactions with ART should be suspected.

Gonadal Function

Gonadal dysfunction is common among HIV-infected men with weight loss and advanced illness. Initial studies indicated biochemical hypogonadism in ~50% of men with AIDS, in association with increased disease severity. Among HIV-infected men with low weight, hypogonadism was seen in 20% (7). More recent studies suggest a lower prevalence of hypogonadism of ~9% to 16% (8–10). The mechanisms of hypogonadism in HIV-infected patients may relate to severe illness and/or effects of undernutrition on gonadotropin secretion, medication effects, or, more rarely, tissue destruction from opportunistic infections. Most often, hypogonadism is secondary, with low or inappropriately normal gonadotropin levels, as seen in 91% of patients with reduced free testosterone levels during initiation of highly active ART (11). Primary hypogonadism is seen less often. Among young men, median age 45 years, using a morning total testosterone as a cutoff to define hypogonadism, Rochira *et al.* (9) demonstrated that gonadotropins were elevated in 16% of patients. In addition, opportunistic infections of the testes have rarely been reported, and up to 25% of HIV-infected patients with AIDS will demonstrate testicular involvement of widespread opportunistic infection or systemic neoplasms, including CMV, toxoplasmosis, Kaposi sarcoma, and testicular lymphoma; although there is little data to suggest that primary hypogonadism develops in all such cases (12). Among women, amenorrhea and anovulation are common.

In addition, a number of medications may affect the hypothalamic-pituitary-gonadal axis. Ketoconazole inhibits side-chain cleavage enzyme and other critical enzymes in testicular steroidogenesis. Megestrol acetate is used to increase appetite, but as a synthetic progestational agent, it suppresses gonadotropin secretion and results in hypogonadism. Opiate therapy affects gonadotropin-releasing hormone secretion and may result in hypogonadotropic hypogonadism. PIs may increase prolactin levels and result in galactorrhea.

Sex hormone–binding globulin (SHBG) levels are increased in 30% to 55% of HIV-infected patients. Therefore, the use of bioavailable or free testosterone is recommended to diagnose hypogonadism, because use of total testosterone assays may underestimate the prevalence of true hypogonadism in this population. In patients in whom acute and chronic illness may contribute to hypogonadism, retesting of gonadal function by measuring an early morning bioavailable testosterone level is recommended upon resolution of the illness, as endogenous function may return with improved health. In patients who remain hypogonadal, administration of physiologic testosterone replacement after appropriate workup is appropriate.

Thyroid Function

Altered thyroid function tests are common in HIV-infected patients. Thyroid-binding globulin (TBG) levels are increased in HIV-infected patients and correlate inversely with CD4 counts (13). Abnormal thyroid function test results may be caused by the stress of illness in patients with advanced disease or concomitant morbidities, as found in other patients with "euthyroid sick syndrome". However, among adults, some studies have shown that reverse T3 levels do not rise in association with decreasing T3 levels, as one would expect in nonthyroidal illness (3). Patients with progressive HIV disease therefore exhibit decreased T3 levels, increased TBG, and decreased reverse T3 levels with increasing illness. In addition to the euthyroid sick syndrome, large screening studies have demonstrated an increased prevalence of primary hypothyroidism in HIV-infected patients. Recent studies have investigated the prevalence of thyroid dysfunction in the current era of highly active ART. In one study of 1565 HIV-infected patients, the prevalence of overt hypothyroidism was 2.5% and of overt hyperthyroidism 1%. A higher percentage of patients demonstrated subclinical hypothyroidism (4%) and nonthyroidal illness (17%) (14). Recently, thyroid dysfunction has been described with an immune reconstitution syndrome, in which autoimmune thyroid disease occurs in association with use of potent ART and improved immune function, typically, 12 to 36 months after ART is initiated (15). Graves disease is most often reported in this context. The estimated prevalence for immune reconstitution thyroid disease with initiation of highly active antiretroviral therapy (HAART) was 3% for women and 0.2% for men (16). In addition, thyroid disease related to anatomic replacement and infection of the thyroid has been reported in HIV-infected patients. *Pneumocystis* thyroiditis has been reported to cause a painful thyroiditis-like picture. Medications may affect thyroid function. Rifampin influences hepatic clearance of thyroxine, and interferon is associated with an increased incidence of autoimmune hypothyroidism.

Metabolic Changes in HIV-Infected Patients

Lipid abnormalities are highly prevalent among HIV-infected patients, particularly those with changes in fat distribution and increased visceral fat and upper trunk fat. Hypertriglyceridemia has long been associated with HIV infection and was observed prior to the introduction of potent ART and is related in part to increased very-low-density lipoprotein secretion and decreased clearance (17). The etiology of these changes is not known but may relate to the effects of viral infection itself, microbial translocation via lipopolysaccharide (18), altered cytokines, including IFN-α (19), or increased apolipoprotein E (20). In longitudinal studies, reductions in high-density lipoprotein (HDL), total, and low-density lipoprotein (LDL) cholesterol are observed with seroconversion. With antiretroviral treatment, cholesterol and LDL rise to preinfection levels, but low HDL levels persist (21). Among patients with changes in fat distribution, 57% demonstrated hypertriglyceridemia and 46% low HDL in comparison with an age- and body mass index (BMI)–matched cohort from the Framingham Offspring Study (22). Recent studies also suggest more atherogenic small dense LDL among HIV-infected patients with lipodystrophy (23). Severe dyslipidemia among HIV-infected patients may result from the effects of antiretroviral drugs, including specific PIs, such as ritonavir, which have been shown to increase triglyceride (TG) levels.

Insulin resistance and DM are relatively common among HIV-infected patients. In an early longitudinal study, DM was 3.1 times more likely to develop in HIV-infected patients receiving combination ART than in control subjects (24). More recent studies confirm increased risk of DM prior to 2000 but equivalent rates among HIV-infected and non–HIV-infected individuals in the era of modern ART with agents less likely to contribute to glucose abnormalities (25). Hyperinsulinemia in such patients is consistent with insulin resistance as the primary mechanism for impaired glucose tolerance and DM. In addition, increased BMI, lipodystrophy, low CD4 counts, and exposure to specific, older ART medications, including stavudine and indinavir, are also predictive of DM in the HIV population (25). Hemoglobin A_{1c} has been shown to underestimate glucose in HIV-infected patients. In one study, use of a hemoglobin A_{1c} cutoff of 5.8% optimized the area under the curve for the diagnosis of DM and increased sensitivity from 40.9% to 88.8% while decreasing specificity from 97.5% to 77.5% compared with the use of a cutoff of 6.5% (26).

The mechanisms of insulin resistance among HIV-infected patients may be caused by the abnormal fat distribution itself (*e.g.*, increased central adiposity), loss of peripheral subcutaneous fat, altered cytokines (*e.g.*, low adiponectin), or other factors, including mitochondrial dysfunction, increased lipolysis (27), and accumulation of fat in the muscle and liver. Increased inflammation after initiation of ART is associated with development of DM among HIV-infected patients (28), and metabolic changes may result from microbial translocation and increased LPS, despite viral suppression (29). In addition, substantial evidence suggests direct effects of specific antiretroviral therapy to reduce insulin sensitivity. PIs have now been shown to decrease glucose uptake by inhibiting the transport function of GLUT-4 (30). Nucleoside reverse transcriptase inhibitors (NRTIs) are associated with insulin resistance, which may relate to mitochondrial toxicity (31) or through effects on subcutaneous fat (32).

MAIN CONCLUSIONS

- There is a wide spectrum of adrenal, thyroid, and gonadal disorders among HIV-infected patients, which may result from specific medication effects, subacute/acute infections, immune reconstitution, or severe illness.
- Insulin resistance, DM, and dyslipidemia are common among HIV-infected patients and may contribute to increased CVD in this population.

DISCUSSION OF CASES AND ANSWERS

Case 1

A 56-year-old male with HIV/AIDS (CD_4 = 521 cells/mm^3) and viral load suppressed on ART presents for follow-up. He notes improved pain in right shoulder after steroid injection for avascular necrosis (1 month prior) but also notes new appetite over the past month, and he is increasingly concerned regarding his increased supraclavicular fat pads. His medications include ritonavir-boosted darunavir, tenofovir and FTC, and raltegravir. On physical exam, soft, full supraclavicular spaces were noted bilaterally, more pronounced than on prior exams.

Question 1 for Case 1

What is the most likely diagnosis?

1. Ongoing lipodystrophic changes due to ART

2. Madelung disease occurring in the context of HIV, due to NRTI therapy
3. Endogenous Cushing developing in an HIV patient
4. Iatrogenic Cushing due to exogenous therapy and interaction with ART ←

Explanation of the Best Answer

This patient most likely has an interaction between a steroid injected into his right shoulder and ritonavir. Ritonavir can prolong the metabolism of exogenous steroids in HIV patients, resulting in a Cushingoid syndrome. Specifically, PIs downregulate CYP3A4 activity and can increase concentrations of exogenously administered glucocorticoid. Iatrogenic Cushing has been most often described with simultaneous administration of triamcinolone and ritonavir, but can be seen in the context of administration of ritonavir and other steroids. The rapid worsening of already present fat pads suggests a new insult on top of existing lipodystrophy. A rapid worsening of lipodystrophy without a change in HIV medications would be unusual. Madelung disease does present with supraclavicular fullness but is not associated with NRTI therapy *per se* and is not a common feature of HIV patients. Endogenous Cushing could be occurring in this HIV patient, but this is less likely than an interaction between his HIV medications and exogenous steroid administered.

Question 2 for Case 1

What initial diagnostic tests would be most useful to confirm the diagnosis?

1. Midnight salivary cortisol
2. Dexamethasone/corticotropin-releasing hormone testing
3. Triamcinolone level
4. Morning cortisol and ACTH ←

Explanation of the Best Answer

The best option would be a morning cortisol and ACTH, both of which would be expected to be suppressed in the case of Cushing due to an exogenous steroid, in this case triamcinolone, potentiated by an interaction with an HIV medicine. The exogenous steroid would be expected to decrease endogenous steroid and ACTH levels, which is diagnostic in the setting of increased Cushingoid symptoms. A cortrosyn stimulation test might be useful, if enough time has passed that the adrenal axis is fully suppressed from the exogenous insult, but a morning cortisol and ACTH are the best initial tests. Testing a midnight cortisol, which is already at nadir, would not yield useful information. Dexamethasone/corticotropin-releasing hormone testing is inappropriate in this context and is best used to distinguish true Cushing syndrome from pseudo-Cushing. A triamcinolone level may be useful as a confirmatory test and to determine blood levels of the offending agent, after the diagnosis of Cushing due to exogenous steroids has been made, with a morning cortisol and ACTH level. Other causes of a low ACTH and cortisol would be due to infiltrative or infectious processes in the pituitary but would be associated with true adrenal insufficiency, in contrast with this patient who had symptoms of adrenal excess. Primary adrenal insufficiency would be associated with a low cortisol and increased ACTH, and similarly not be associated with signs of adrenal excess.

In terms of follow-up, this patient was placed on physiological steroid replacement for his adrenal insufficiency, his HIV medications were changed in consultation with his infectious disease physician, and his Cushingoid features slowly resolved over 6 months.

Case 2

A 58-year-old man (health care system executive) presented for care; his HIV disease was diagnosed in 1985 due to a transfusion. He had known cured hepatitis C (treated with sofosbuvir/ribavirin in 2014), hypothyroidism after interferon treatment, hypertension, and hypertriglyceridemia. His current medications included dolutegravir/rilpivirine/emtricitabine, synthroid, atenolol, amlodipine, lisinopril, hydrochlorothiazide, omega-3 fatty acids, and famotidine. His diet was generally healthy, and he exercised by cycling. On physical exam, his blood pressure was 130/87 mm Hg and BMI 29.9 kg/m^2. He was a well-appearing man with moderate features of lipodystrophy, including mild fat loss in cheeks and bitemporal regions, with abdominal fat accumulation and lipoatrophy of extremities. His waist circumference was 110 cm. Laboratory data demonstrated a CD4 of 385 cells/mm^3, an HIV viral load <20 copies/mL, and a creatinine of 1.2 mg/dL. His lipids included a total cholesterol of 238 mg/dL, HDL of 37 mg/dL, LDL of 156 mg/dL, and TG of 224 mg/dL. Previously his glucose was 125 mg/dL, with a 2-hour oral glucose tolerance test glucose of 195 mg/dL. He now has occasional random glucoses above 200s, with fasting glucoses in 120s. His hemoglobin A_{1c} was recently 6.9%.

Question 1 for Case 2

Which statement is true?

1. DM is seen in HIV at the same prevalence as in non-HIV
2. Diagnosis with hemoglobin A_{1c} can underestimate glucose in HIV ←
3. Metformin can be used as in non-HIV, without regard to ART regimen

Explanation of the Best Answer

DM is seen at increased frequency among patients with HIV, with a prevalence ratio of 4.6 among HIV patients on HAART compared with non-HIV in the Multicenter AIDS Cohort Study (MACS). Potential mechanisms include fat redistribution and altered adipokines, PI effects to reduce glucose transporter (GLUT-4), impaired mitochondrial function from NRTIs, increased inflammation and inflammatory cytokines, and coinfections with hepatitis C. Metformin is generally very well tolerated in HIV but can interact with dolutegravir, which can increase metformin levels. Lower doses of metformin should be administered to HIV patients on dolutegravir.

Case 3

A 45-year-old man with HIV infection diagnosed 14 years ago presented for care. He had no other major medical problems and no history of CVD. His current medications include boosted atazanavir, emtricitabine, and tenofovir. His prior medications included indinavir, lamivudine, and zidovudine. His mother had myocardial infarction (MI) at age 61 years. He smokes one pack per day and does not exercise routinely. On physical exam, his blood pressure was 110/70 mm Hg, pulse was 70 beats/min, and BMI 21.2 kg/m^2, and he exhibited mild abdominal fat accumulation. His laboratory data included a CD4 of 455 cells/mm^3 and a viral load of 467 copies/mL. His lipids included a total cholesterol of 178 mg/dL, HDL 35 mg/dL, LDL 102 mg/dL, and TG 203 mg/dL. The fasting glucose was 101 mg/dL. The calculated Framingham 10-year risk of MI was 8%. Using the 2013 American College of Cardiology (ACC) risk calculator, the 10-year risk was 6.3%.

Question 1 for Case 3

Does this patient have substantial CVD risk?

1. Yes
2. No
3. Not by traditional risk calculators, but he may have unique HIV-specific risk factors ←

Explanation of the Best Answer

By traditional risk scores, including the Framingham and ACC risk calculators, the risk is not significantly increased. However, neither of these equations takes into account unique factors that may increase CVD risk in HIV, including inflammation and immune activation. Therefore, the best answer is the one that recognizes this potential increased risk not included in current risk calculators. Numerous epidemiological studies suggest that CVD risk is increased in HIV 50% to 100% compared with non-HIV, in relationship to nontraditional risks, including inflammation. Imaging studies have suggested increased arterial inflammation using fluorodeoxyglucose positron emission tomography and noncalcified vulnerable plaque on computed tomography angiography.

The patient in question underwent cardiac computed tomography as part of a research study, which revealed plaque in the left anterior descending artery, left circumflex artery, and right coronary artery, with severe stenosis of the proximal left anterior descending artery and left circumflex artery as well as akinesis of the inferolateral wall consistent with prior MI. He was evaluated by cardiology, and findings were confirmed by cardiac catheterization. The patient underwent successful coronary artery bypass surgery and he was placed on a statin, beta-blocker, and aspirin.

Question 2 for Case 3

Should statins be used for primary CVD prevention in HIV without increased LDL?

1. Yes
2. No
3. Not enough data ←

Explanation of the Best Answer

Statins have not yet been tested for primary CVD prevention in HIV. Statins may have potential benefit in HIV as they reduce monocyte chemoattraction and inflammation, beyond effects on LDL. In HIV, statins have been shown to reduce noncalcified plaque as well as markers of arterial inflammation. Statins have been shown to effectively reduce LDL in HIV, but no studies have as yet determined potential effects to prevent CVD events. To address this question, the National Institutes of Health recently funded a large, multicenter, randomized, placebo-controlled primary CVD prevention trial of statins in HIV. When considering use of statins in HIV, it should be recognized that PIs downregulate CYP3A4 activity and increase concentrations of CYP3A4-metabolized drugs, including certain statins. Pitavastatin and pravastatin, which are not metabolized through CYP3A4, may be ideal choices in HIV. Atorvastatin and rosuvastatin may be used in those on a PI but initiated at low doses and titrated carefully. Efavirenz can induce statin metabolism, resulting in lower statin levels.

This work is adopted from *Williams Textbook of Endocrinology*, 13th Edition, Chapter 41, The Endocrinology of HIV/AIDS, Grinspoon, Steven K.

REFERENCES

1. Grinspoon S. The endocrinology of HIV/AIDS. In: Melmed S, Polonsky KS, Larsen PR, Kronenberg HM, eds. *Williams Textbook of Endocrinology.* 13th ed. Philadelphia, PA: Elsevier; 2016:1776–1798.
2. Membreno L, Irony I, Dere W, Klein R, Biglieri EG, Cobb E. Adrenocortical function in acquired immunodeficiency syndrome. *J Clin Endocrinol Metab.* 1987;**65**(3):482–487.
3. Grinspoon SK, Bilezikian JP. HIV disease and the endocrine system. *N Engl J Med.* 1992;**327**(19):1360–1365.
4. Glasgow BJ, Steinsapir KD, Anders K, Layfield LJ. Adrenal pathology in the acquired immune deficiency syndrome. *Am J Clin Pathol.* 1985; **84**(5):594–597.
5. Foisy MM, Yakiwchuk EM, Chiu I, Singh AE. Adrenal suppression and Cushing's syndrome secondary to an interaction between ritonavir and fluticasone: a review of the literature. *HIV Med.* 2008;**9**(6):389–396.
6. Hyle EP, Wood BR, Backman ES, Noubary F, Hwang J, Lu Z, Losina E, Walensky RP, Gandhi RT. High frequency of hypothalamic-pituitary-adrenal axis dysfunction after local corticosteroid injection in HIV-infected patients on protease inhibitor therapy. *J Acquir Immune Defic Syndr.* 2013;**63**(5):602–608.
7. Rietschel P, Corcoran C, Stanley T, Basgoz N, Klibanski A, Grinspoon S. Prevalence of hypogonadism among men with weight loss related to human immunodeficiency virus infection who were receiving highly active antiretroviral therapy. *Clin Infect Dis.* 2000;**31**(5):1240–1244.
8. Monroe AK, Dobs AS, Palella FJ, Kingsley LA, Witt MD, Brown TT. Morning free and total testosterone in HIV-infected men: implications for the assessment of hypogonadism. *AIDS Res Ther.* 2014;**11**(1):6.
9. Rochira V, Zirilli L, Orlando G, Santi D, Brigante G, Diazzi C, Carli F, Carani C, Guaraldi G. Premature decline of serum total testosterone in HIV-infected men in the HAART-era. *PLoS One.* 2011;**6**(12):e28512.

10. Moreno-Pérez O, Escoín C, Serna-Candel C, Portilla J, Boix V, Alfayate R, González-Sánchez V, Mauri M, Sánchez-Payá J, Picó A. The determination of total testosterone and free testosterone (RIA) are not applicable to the evaluation of gonadal function in HIV-infected males. *J Sex Med.* 2010;**7**(8):2873–2883.
11. Wunder DM, Bersinger NA, Fux CA, Mueller NJ, Hirschel B, Cavassini M, Elzi L, Schmid P, Bernasconi E, Mueller B, Furrer H; Swiss HIV Cohort Study. Hypogonadism in HIV-1-infected men is common and does not resolve during antiretroviral therapy. *Antivir Ther.* 2007; **12**(2):261–265.
12. Hutchinson J, Murphy M, Harries R, Skinner CJ. Galactorrhoea and hyperprolactinaemia associated with protease-inhibitors. *Lancet.* 2000;**356**(9234):1003–1004.
13. Bourdoux PP, De Wit SA, Servais GM, Clumeck N, Bonnyns MA. Biochemical thyroid profile in patients infected with the human immunodeficiency virus. *Thyroid.* 1991;**1**(2):147–149.
14. Madge S, Smith CJ, Lampe FC, Thomas M, Johnson MA, Youle M, Vanderpump M. No association between HIV disease and its treatment and thyroid function. *HIV Med.* 2007;**8**(1):22–27.
15. Hoffmann CJ, Brown TT. Thyroid function abnormalities in HIV-infected patients. *Clin Infect Dis.* 2007;**45**(4):488–494.
16. Chen F, Day SL, Metcalfe RA, Sethi G, Kapembwa MS, Brook MG, Churchill D, de Ruiter A, Robinson S, Lacey CJ, Weetman AP. Characteristics of autoimmune thyroid disease occurring as a late complication of immune reconstitution in patients with advanced human immunodeficiency virus (HIV) disease. *Medicine (Baltimore).* 2005;**84**(2):98–106.
17. Hellerstein MK, Grunfeld C, Wu K, Christiansen M, Kaempfer S, Kletke C, Shackleton CH. Increased de novo hepatic lipogenesis in human immunodeficiency virus infection. *J Clin Endocrinol Metab.* 1993; **76**(3):559–565.
18. Timmons T, Shen C, Aldrovandi G, Rollie A, Gupta SK, Stein JH, Dubé MP. Microbial translocation and metabolic and body composition measures in treated and untreated HIV infection. *AIDS Res Hum Retroviruses.* 2014;**30**(3):272–277.
19. Grunfeld C, Pang M, Doerrler W, Shigenaga JK, Jensen P, Feingold KR. Lipids, lipoproteins, triglyceride clearance, and cytokines in human immunodeficiency virus infection and the acquired immunodeficiency syndrome. *J Clin Endocrinol Metab.* 1992;**74**(5):1045–1052.
20. Grunfeld C, Doerrler W, Pang M, Jensen P, Weisgraber KH, Feingold KR. Abnormalities of apolipoprotein E in the acquired immunodeficiency syndrome. *J Clin Endocrinol Metab.* 1997;**82**(11):3734–3740.
21. Riddler SA, Smit E, Cole SR, Li R, Chmiel JS, Dobs A, Palella F, Visscher B, Evans R, Kingsley LA. Impact of HIV infection and HAART on serum lipids in men. *JAMA.* 2003;**289**(22):2978–2982.
22. Hadigan C, Meigs JB, Corcoran C, Rietschel P, Piecuch S, Basgoz N, Davis B, Sax P, Stanley T, Wilson PW, D'Agostino RB, Grinspoon S. Metabolic abnormalities and cardiovascular disease risk factors in adults with human immunodeficiency virus infection and lipodystrophy. *Clin Infect Dis.* 2001;**32**(1):130–139.
23. Srisawasdi P, Suwalak T, Sukasem C, Chittamma A, Pocathikorn A, Vanavanan S, Puangpetch A, Santon S, Chantratita W, Kiertiburanakul S, Kroll MH. Small-dense LDL cholesterol/large-buoyant LDL cholesterol ratio as an excellent marker for indicating lipodystrophy in HIV-infected patients. *Am J Clin Pathol.* 2013;**140**(4):506–515.
24. Brown TT, Cole SR, Li X, Kingsley LA, Palella FJ, Riddler SA, Visscher BR, Margolick JB, Dobs AS. Antiretroviral therapy and the prevalence and incidence of diabetes mellitus in the multicenter AIDS cohort study. *Arch Intern Med.* 2005;**165**(10):1179–1184.
25. Rasmussen LD, Mathiesen ER, Kronborg G, Pedersen C, Gerstoft J, Obel N. Risk of diabetes mellitus in persons with and without HIV: a Danish nationwide population-based cohort study. *PLoS One.* 2012; **7**(9):e44575.
26. Eckhardt BJ, Holzman RS, Kwan CK, Baghdadi J, Aberg JA. Glycated hemoglobin A(1c) as screening for diabetes mellitus in HIV-infected individuals. *AIDS Patient Care STDS.* 2012;**26**(4):197–201.
27. Carper MJ, Cade WT, Cam M, Zhang S, Shalev A, Yarasheski KE, Ramanadham S. HIV-protease inhibitors induce expression of suppressor of cytokine signaling-1 in insulin-sensitive tissues and promote insulin resistance and type 2 diabetes mellitus. *Am J Physiol Endocrinol Metab.* 2008;**294**(3):E558–E567.
28. Brown TT, Tassiopoulos K, Bosch RJ, Shikuma C, McComsey GA. Association between systemic inflammation and incident diabetes in HIV-infected patients after initiation of antiretroviral therapy. *Diabetes Care.* 2010;**33**(10):2244–2249.
29. Pedersen KK, Pedersen M, Trøseid M, Gaardbo JC, Lund TT, Thomsen C, Gerstoft J, Kvale D, Nielsen SD. Microbial translocation in HIV infection is associated with dyslipidemia, insulin resistance, and risk of myocardial infarction. *J Acquir Immune Defic Syndr.* 2013;**64**(5): 425–433.
30. Noor MA, Seneviratne T, Aweeka FT, Lo JC, Schwarz JM, Mulligan K, Schambelan M, Grunfeld C. Indinavir acutely inhibits insulin-stimulated glucose disposal in humans: a randomized, placebo-controlled study. *AIDS.* 2002;**16**(5):F1–F8.
31. Fleischman A, Johnsen S, Systrom DM, Hrovat M, Farrar CT, Frontera W, Fitch K, Thomas BJ, Torriani M, Côté HC, Grinspoon SK. Effects of a nucleoside reverse transcriptase inhibitor, stavudine, on glucose disposal and mitochondrial function in muscle of healthy adults. *Am J Physiol Endocrinol Metab.* 2007;**292**(6):E1666–E1673.
32. Mallon PW, Unemori P, Sedwell R, Morey A, Rafferty M, Williams K, Chisholm D, Samaras K, Emery S, Kelleher A, Cooper DA, Carr A; SAMA Investigators. In vivo, nucleoside reverse-transcriptase inhibitors alter expression of both mitochondrial and lipid metabolism genes in the absence of depletion of mitochondrial DNA. *J Infect Dis.* 2005; **191**(10):1686–1696.

Weaning Off Unnecessary Hormones

M34
Presented, March 17–20, 2018

Simon Aylwin, MA, MB, BChir, PhD, FRCP. Department of Endocrinology, King's College Hospital, London SE5 9RS, United Kingdom, E-mail: simonaylwin@nhs.net

John Miell, MD, DM, FRCPE, FRCP. Department of Endocrinology, Lewisham and Greenwich NHS Trust, London SE13 6LH, United Kingdom, E-mail: johnmiell@yahoo.co.uk

SIGNIFICANCE OF THE PROBLEM

Natural and bioidentical hormones and synthetic hormone agonists are widely used for both physiological replacement and for pharmacological therapy. For each endocrine axis, there are circumstances in which the requirement for a specific agent needs to be revised and the consideration of treatment withdrawal arises. This article examines the scenarios in which the safe and timely withdrawal of hormone therapy is appropriate, the pitfalls and hazards associated with cessation of treatment, and a clinical approach for the practicing clinician.

For each hormone axis, we discuss the clinical approach and evaluate the evidence when salient, specifically addressing the following questions:

- Was the indication for therapy valid?
- Is the indication for therapy still present?
- Has the age or status of the patient altered such that hormone therapy is no longer appropriate?
- Was treatment being given as physiological replacement or for a pharmacological purpose?
- Has prolonged treatment led to the suppression of the endogenous axis?
- Is weaning preferred to abrupt cessation and what is the appropriate weaning schedule?
- What investigations should be performed before and/or after therapy cessation?

These generic concepts are discussed with specific reference to common clinical scenarios.

Scenario 1

Arabella, a 29-year-old woman, has been on long-term thyroxine since her teenage years but remains fatigued. She has been advised by a naturopath that she should try alternative treatment. Can she suspend her levothyroxine treatment? Practice point: Short-term withdrawal of levothyroxine for 3 to 4 weeks has a modest impact on quality of life and is sufficient to allow thyrotropin to rise in athyreotic subjects (1).

Scenario 2

Belinda, a 32-year-old woman, stopped taking an oral contraceptive 5 months ago and remains amenorrheic. She is concerned about fertility. Her partner has a 4-year-old child from a previous relationship. What investigations should be undertaken and when? Practice point: Most women will have restored menstrual function 6 months after discontinuation of oral contraceptive pills and are not disadvantaged in terms of future fecundity (2).

Scenario 3

Chuck is a 28-year-old man who practices mixed martial arts. He admits to long-term anabolic steroid hormone use but now wishes to start a family. What are his chances and how can we help manage the withdrawal of exogenous androgens (3)? Practice point: Withdrawal of androgens can be associated with substantial morbidity and the suppression of spermatogenesis (4). A number of approaches have been described to stimulate recovery, although the evidence base remains poor.

Scenario 4

Donald, a 60-year-old man, has been on treatment with prednisolone for polymyalgia and is now on 6 mg daily. How should he come off therapy? Practice point: Withdrawal of glucocorticoids should be undertaken in parallel with the use of biochemical assessment to gauge the extent of recovery of the hypothalamic-pituitary-adrenal axis (5).

Scenario 5

Enrico, age 35 years, had been on antiretroviral therapy for 10 years. He has developed clinical steroid excess and adrenal suppression due to concurrent steroid inhalers (6). How should his iatrogenic Cushing syndrome be managed with withdrawal of therapy? Practice point: Augmentation of the effect of exogenous glucocorticoid due to retroviral therapy can lead to Cushing syndrome, and reduction should be handled with caution.

Scenario 6

Fabrice is an 18-year-old man who has been treated for growth hormone (GH) deficiency since the age of 9 years. He is unsure of the original indication for GH therapy. His parents want him to continue but he wants to know if he can stop (7); please advise. Practice point: In adolescents with GH deficiency, quality of life does not appear to be affected and the principle issues relate to lean body mass composition after discontinuation (8).

Scenario 7

Germaine is a 54-year-old woman who has been on hormone replacement therapy (estrogen patch and sequential oral progestogen) for 6 years but is now concerned about the health risks because her daughter has had breast cancer (9). How should she best withdraw treatment? Practice point: Women should be warned that withdrawal of hormone replacement therapy may lead to rebound of psychological symptoms, although the effects may not be sustained (10).

Scenario 8

Hilary has "normo-thyroxinemic hypothyroidism," T_4/T_3 deiodinase deficiency, "adrenal fatigue," postural orthostatic tachycardia syndrome, and chronic fatigue. She is taking T_4/T_3 combination, hydrocortisone, fludrocortisone, and dehydroepiandrosterone. Where do you start?

REFERENCES

1. Davids T, Witterick IJ, Eski S, Walfish PG, Freeman JL. Three-week thyroxine withdrawal: a thyroid-specific quality of life study. *Laryngoscope.* 2006;**116**(2):250–253.
2. Cronin M, Schellschmidt I, Dinger J. Rate of pregnancy after using drospirenone and other progestin-containing oral contraceptives. *Obstet Gynecol.* 2009;**114**(3):616–622.
3. Wenker EP, Dupree JM, Langille GM, Kovac J, Ramasamy R, Lamb D, Mills JN, Lipshultz LI. The use of hCG-based combination therapy for recovery of spermatogenesis after testosterone use. *J Sex Med.* 2015; **12**(6):1334–1337.
4. Kanayama G, Hudson JI, DeLuca J, Isaacs S, Baggish A, Weiner R, Bhasin S, Pope HG Jr. Prolonged hypogonadism in males following withdrawal from anabolic-androgenic steroids: an under-recognized problem. *Addiction.* 2015;**110**(5):823–831.
5. Walsh JP, Dayan CM. Role of biochemical assessment in management of corticosteroid withdrawal. *Ann Clin Biochem.* 2000;**37**(3): 279–288.
6. Valin N, De Castro N, Garrait V, Bergeron A, Bouche C, Molina JM. Iatrogenic Cushing's syndrome in HIV-infected patients receiving ritonavir and inhaled fluticasone: description of 4 new cases and review of the literature. *J Int Assoc Provid AIDS Care (JIAPAC).* 2009; **8**(2):113–121.
7. Elbirt D, Mahlev-Guri K, Gradstein S, Zung A, Asher I, Werner B, Radain-Sade S, Burke M, Sthoeger ZM. Adrenal suppression and Cushing's syndrome due to the interaction between ritonavir and inhaled fluticasone. *J Allergy Clin Immunol.* 2010;**125**(2 Suppl 1): AB79.
8. Savage MO, Drake WM, Carroll PV, Monson JP. Transitional care of GH deficiency: when to stop GH therapy. *Eur J Endocrinol.* 2004; **151**(Suppl 1):S61–65.
9. Perrone G, Capri O, Galoppi P, Patacchioli FR, Bevilacqua E, de Stefano MG, Brunelli R. Menopausal symptoms after the discontinuation of long-term hormone replacement therapy in women under 60: a 3-year follow-up. *Gynecol Obstet Invest.* 2013;**76**(1): 38–43.
10. Schmidt PJ, Ben Dor R, Martinez PE, Guerrieri GM, Harsh VL, Thompson K, Koziol DE, Nieman LK, Rubinow DR. Effects of estradiol withdrawal on mood in women with past perimenopausal depression: a randomized clinical trial. *JAMA Psychiatry.* 2015;**72**(7): 714–726.

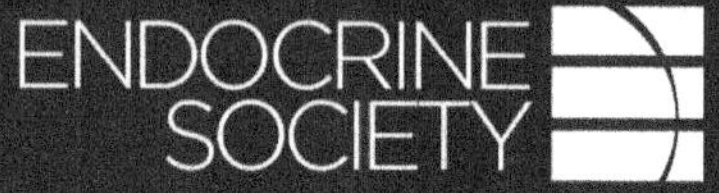
ENDOCRINE
SOCIETY

www.ingramcontent.com/pod-product-compliance
Lightning Source LLC
Chambersburg PA
CBHW080928220326
41598CB00034B/5718